Clinical Practice Guidelines for Midwifery & Women's Health
Third Edition

Nell L. Tharpe, MS, CNM, CRNFA, FASCCP

Cindy L. Farley, PhD, CNM, FACNM

Midwifery Institute

Philadelphia University

Philadelphia, Pennsylvania

JONES AND BARTLETT PUBLISHERS

Sudbury, Massachusetts

BOSTON   TORONTO   LONDON   SINGAPORE

World Headquarters
Jones and Bartlett Publishers
40 Tall Pine Drive
Sudbury, MA 01776
978-443-5000
info@jbpub.com
www.jbpub.com

Jones and Bartlett Publishers
Canada
6339 Ormindale Way
Mississauga, Ontario L5V 1J2
Canada

Jones and Bartlett Publishers
International
Barb House, Barb Mews
London W6 7PA
United Kingdom

Jones and Bartlett's books and products are available through most bookstores and online booksellers. To contact Jones and Bartlett Publishers directly, call 800-832-0034, fax 978-443-8000, or visit our website, www.jbpub.com.

Substantial discounts on bulk quantities of Jones and Bartlett's publications are available to corporations, professional associations, and other qualified organizations. For details and specific discount information, contact the special sales department at Jones and Bartlett via the above contact information or send an email to specialsales@jbpub.com.

Copyright © 2009 by Jones and Bartlett Publishers, LLC

All rights reserved. No part of the material protected by this copyright may be reproduced or utilized in any form, electronic or mechanical, including photocopying, recording, or by any information storage and retrieval system, without written permission from the copyright owner.

The authors, editor, and publisher have made every effort to provide accurate information. However, they are not responsible for errors, omissions, or for any outcomes related to the use of the contents of this book and take no responsibility for the use of the products and procedures described. Treatments and side effects described in this book may not be applicable to all people; likewise, some people may require a dose or experience a side effect that is not described herein. Drugs and medical devices are discussed that may have limited availability controlled by the Food and Drug Administration (FDA) for use only in a research study or clinical trial. Research, clinical practice, and government regulations often change the accepted standard in this field. When consideration is being given to use of any drug in the clinical setting, the health care provider or reader is responsible for determining FDA status of the drug, reading the package insert, and reviewing prescribing information for the most up-to-date recommendations on dose, precautions, and contraindications, and determining the appropriate usage for the product. This is especially important in the case of drugs that are new or seldom used.

Library of Congress Cataloging-in-Publication Data
Tharpe, Nell, 1956-
  Clinical practice guidelines for midwifery & women's health / Nell L. Tharpe and Cindy L. Farley. — 3rd ed.
     p. ; cm.
  Clinical practice guidelines for midwifery and women's health
  Includes bibliographical references and index.
  ISBN-13: 978-0-7637-5013-8 (alk. paper)
  ISBN-10: 0-7637-5013-1 (alk. paper)
  1. Midwifery—Standards. 2. Maternity nursing—Standards. 3. Gynecologic nursing—Standards. I. Farley, Cindy L. II. Title. III. Title: Clinical practice guidelines for midwifery and women's health.
  [DNLM: 1. Midwifery—Practice Guideline. 2. Genital Diseases, Female—Practice Guideline. 3. Pregnancy Complications—Practice Guideline. 4. Women's Health—Practice Guideline. WQ 165 T3675c 2008]
  RG950.T476 2008
  618.2—dc22
                                    2008000611

6048

Production Credits
Publisher: Kevin Sullivan
Acquisitions Editor: Emily Ekle
Acquisitions Editor: Amy Sibley
Editorial Assistant: Patricia Donnelly
Editorial Assistant: Rachel Shuster
Associate Production Editor: Amanda Clerkin
Associate Marketing Manager: Rebecca Wasley

Manufacturing and Inventory Control Supervisor: Amy Bacus
Composition: Arlene Apone
Cover Design: Anne Spencer
Cover Image Credit: © Photos.com
Printing and Binding: Courier Stoughton
Cover Printing: Courier Stoughton

Printed in the United States of America
12 11 10 09 08   10 9 8 7 6 5 4 3 2 1

This edition is dedicated to my granddaughter, *Charlie Kathleen McLellan*. From your mother's womb to my waiting hands, you opened my eyes anew to the ever-present need for midwives to accompany women on their journeys and hear their stories. Never has the need for woman-centered midwifery care been so apparent; not simply serving the generations of women who have gone before, but safeguarding the processes and practices of midwifery for generations of women yet to come.

Deep appreciation goes to my colleague and friend Cindy Farley for joining me on this journey. What an adventure we've had!

Nell L. Tharpe, MS, CNM, CRNFA, FASCCP

This edition is dedicated to courage.

To Nell's courage in providing steadfast service to midwives and in inviting others to help shape her work;

To the courage of midwives in facing the daily triumphs and challenges of bringing a special human connection to health care;

To the courage of women in persevering through trying times and circumstances to nourish themselves and their families.

"What makes the muskrat guard his musk?
Courage!"

The Cowardly Lion, *The Wizard of Oz*

I am grateful for the support of my colleagues and my students; my children, Kyle and Katy McEvoy; my sister, Becky Doherty; and my mother, Carol Farley. In special memory of my dear father, Lloyd M. Farley.

Cindy L. Farley, PhD, CNM, FACNM

Contents

Preface

DISCLAIMER

The third edition of *Clinical Practice Guidelines for Midwifery & Women's Health* provided here represents a broad range of practices that include evidence-based, traditional, and empiric care from a wide variety of sources. The *Clinical Practice Guidelines for Midwifery & Women's Health* reflects current practice and provides support and guidance for day-to-day clinical practice with diverse populations. Regional differences in practice styles occur; therefore the guidelines are broadly based and designed to reflect current practice and literature as much as possible.

Both the American College of Nurse–Midwives (ACNM) and the Midwives Alliance of North America (MANA) recommend that midwives utilize written policies and/or practice guidelines. The *Clinical Practice Guidelines for Midwifery & Women's Health* has grown out of a need for a concise reference guide to meet that recommendation. However, no text on midwifery and women's health is all-inclusive; therefore there may be additional safe and reasonable practices that are not included in *Clinical Practice Guidelines for Midwifery & Women's Health*.

The *Clinical Practice Guidelines for Midwifery & Women's Health* is used voluntarily, and the authors expect each women's health professional to temper her or his use with sound clinical judgment, knowledge of patient or client preferences, national and local practice standards, and application of sound risk management principles. By accepting the *Clinical Practice Guidelines for Midwifery & Women's Health*, midwives and other women's health professionals are not restricted to their exclusive use.

This book is written for all the midwives, wherever they practice, and the women, children, and families they serve.

Acknowledgments

The authors gratefully acknowledge the following contributors to the third edition of *Clinical Practice Guidelines for Midwifery & Women's Health:*

Mamie Guidera, CNM, MSN
Midwife, Hospital of University of Pennsylvania
Faculty, University of Pennsylvania

Joan Slager, CNM, MSN, CPC, FACNM
Director, Nurse–Midwifery
Bronson Women's Service

Donna Walls, RN, BSN, IBCLC
Master Herbalist, Aromatherapist
Lactation Consultant

Many thanks to the hard-working and enthusiastic class 10 students in the Master's of Science with a concentration in midwifery degree completion program of the Midwifery Institute of Philadelphia University, under the supervision of their faculty, Cindy L. Farley, PhD, CNM, FACNM:

Lisa Arrington, CNM, BSN
Kathryn Austin, RN, BSN
Jamie Donenfield, CNM, BSN
Deirdre East, RN, BA, DipEd, DipClinNsg
    (Midwifery) (Australia)
Jacqueline Gayle-Nicholson, CNM, BSN
Trina Haywood, RN, BSN
Tina Ingram, RN, BSN
Cyndia Johnson, CNM, BSN
Cheryl Kohrs, RN, BSN, ADM
    (South Africa)
Mary Milkey, CNM, BBA, BSN

Lakesha Moore, CNM, BSN
Carol-Ann Rademeyer, RN,
    BSN, RM (South Africa)
Brigitte Rhody, RN, BSEd
Ebony Roebuck, RN, BSN
Frances Sahrphillips, RN, BSN
Kaye Sanford, RN, BSN
Barbara Smith-Foy, CNM, BA
Susan Studebaker, RNC, CHES, MS
Sivan Veksler, RN, BSN
Paula Wiens, RN, CPM, BA

A Short History of the Clinical Practice Guidelines for Midwifery & Women's Health

The *Clinical Practice Guidelines for Midwifery & Women's Health* grew out of an idea that germinated in the mind of Nell Tharpe and blossomed in the fertile soil of isolated midwifery practice in rural Maine.

As a new midwife practicing in a small coastal community in the days before widespread computer access and remote from healthcare resources or colleagues, Nell relied on a handful of dog-eared texts and well-marked copies of the *Journal of Nurse–Midwifery* for her clinical information. She longed for a quick-reference text that would guide her through the clinical challenges that women presented in her diverse full-scope practice, and provide a means to keep current with the state of midwifery and women's health.

Over the years, Nell collected a file of resources and a wealth of experience (at one point, for over three years, she was the sole birth attendant at her local 17-bed community hospital). Sitting down to her computer, with her notes and her experiences Nell wrote the first draft of what would become the *Clinical Practice Guidelines for Midwives* in one very full week. She printed and sold it one copy at a time.

The response was immediate: midwives wanted this type of reference book. Over the next six years Nell wrote two additional editions that were professionally printed and bound before deciding that the business of running a publishing business while maintaining a practice was overwhelming. Jones and Bartlett Publishers were approached, and happily took over book sales and contracted for the next edition of what was now titled the *Clinical Practice Guidelines for Midwifery & Women's Health*.

In the meantime, Nell completed her MS in Midwifery at Philadelphia University, honing her writing and research skills under the superb teaching of midwife Cindy Farley. As the next edition was being written, Nell realized that her time for doing this important work was limited. She immediately thought of Cindy, and invited her to work collaboratively on the following edition.

Cindy became aware of Nell's clinical practice guidelines at an American College of Nurse–Midwives (ACNM) annual meeting, long before Nell was her student. She was delighted to know that a midwife was providing a needed service to support midwives in practice. After all, midwives should be placing their energies into the creative and interpersonal aspects of their care and their practice, not into writing guidelines for standard care for selected, commonly encountered clinical conditions. And who better to understand issues facing midwifery than a midwife peer? In Cindy's humble opinion, this was a brilliant idea!

In 2000, when Cindy had the opportunity to open a new midwifery practice, she purchased Nell's clinical practice guidelines for this practice and has purchased updated versions since that time. She was particularly impressed with the alternative therapies section and the suggestions for further diagnostic testing as being very midwife-friendly. Cindy would sometimes make copies of a particular clinical practice guideline and give it to the woman under her care so the woman would know her options in care as well as standard treatments. Additionally, these guidelines were helpful in meeting local and national ACNM criteria for peer review.

Cindy was thrilled to have Nell in her master's classes and the two formed a bond of mutual respect and friendship. Cindy jumped at the chance to become involved in the revision of a book she has admired for years. Additionally, Cindy is always looking for real world experiences for her Master's in Midwifery students to combine academic course objectives and research critique skills in projects that have relevance to practicing midwives. Updating the evidence base and revising selected clinical practice guidelines was a perfect class research project for her students. Cindy also tapped her former students, Mamie Guidera and Joan Slager, and her colleague, Donna Walls, to contribute their expertise to selected sections of the book.

Nell and Cindy strive to make this on-going work-in-progress as helpful and user-friendly as possible. If you have any suggestions for additions or improvements for the next edition of this book, please email Nell at midwifepub@gwi.net or Cindy at cfarley@woh.rr.com.

Essential Midwifery Practice

1

Exemplary midwifery practice is woman oriented and focuses on excellence in the processes of providing women's health care, improving maternal and child health, and promoting the discipline of midwifery through professionalism for the benefit of women and their families.

Midwives are blessed with a passion for their work. It is this passion, coupled with the patience and perseverance of each individual midwife, that women under their care so appreciate and that has helped the discipline of midwifery grow. It is the authors' hope that this book will make your professional practice simpler and more rewarding, allowing you more time for the expression of your passion and less time on the mundane tasks common to most midwifery practices.

The *Clinical Practice Guidelines for Midwifery & Women's Health* was designed with the busy midwife in mind. It condenses and outlines selected aspects of the art and science of essential midwifery. You may find it convenient to have several copies: one for your exam room(s), one for your birth setting, and another by the phone at home. These Guidelines are a working practice tool designed to provide you with the latest evidence for specific clinical conditions that midwives frequently encounter in an easy-to-follow format. These Guidelines are only one reference of many that should inform your practice as a midwife. Although these Guidelines are updated on a regular basis, it is incumbent upon you to stay current with the latest evidence pertaining to midwifery care practices and to determine how to best incorporate this evidence into your own midwifery practice.

PURPOSE OF CLINICAL PRACTICE GUIDELINES

Clinical practice guidelines are used to define and delineate parameters for care in specific clinical conditions. How these guidelines are applied in practice may be influenced by a number of things, such as the accepted standards of the midwife's or women's health care provider's professional organization(s) and your own practice preferences. State laws, both statutes and regulations, may affect the scope of practice, as may hospital bylaws, birth center rules and regulations, health insurance contracts, and liability insurance policies. Each individual midwife must determine her or his scope of practice within these legal and professional boundaries based on philosophy of midwifery practice, educational preparation, experience, skill level, and the individual practice setting. A midwife's scope of practice may vary from one practice location to another and may change throughout her or his career.

Each client who comes to a midwife for care has the right to information regarding the midwife's scope of practice, usual practice location(s), and provisions for access to medical or obstetric care should this become necessary. Development of working relationships with area health care providers can be a valuable asset in fostering continuity of care for the women you serve.

Evidence-based practice is the catchword of the day. Evidence-based practice is "the explicit, judicious and conscientious use of current best evidence from health care research in decisions about the care of individuals and populations" (Sackett et al., 1997). To apply an evidence-based approach in practice, you need to

- Ask clinically focused questions
- Conduct focused published literature review
- Critically appraise this literature
- Apply the results of this appraisal to clinical practice (Lydon-Rochelle et al., 2003).

There are evidence-based resources available that summarize and synthesize the latest information for busy practitioners, such as the Cochrane Database and the regular feature on evidence-based practice in the *Journal of Midwifery & Women's Health*. However, the analytical practitioner should be cautious and judicious in applying new evidence in practice. Scientific evidence is developed with clearly defined populations of patients in narrow focused areas and is expressed in terms of numerical probabilities; our care is delivered to one woman at a time in the context of her specific life situation and is expressed in terms

of hopeful possibilities. Evidence as well as our philosophy, beliefs, and knowledge should guide and inform us as we go about the daily business of providing midwifery care to women and their families.

All midwives are encouraged to be lifelong learners and reflective practitioners. Reflection in practice involves looking to our experiences, connecting with our feelings, and attending to our theories in use. It entails building new understandings to inform our actions in the situation that is unfolding (Schon, 1983). Clinical expertise is developed over time and with attention to practice. New practitioners or novices are encouraged to maintain heightened awareness of their evolving expertise to set safe boundaries of practice for themselves. Experienced practitioners are encouraged to remain current in their knowledge base and to protect their passion for this work to avoid the complacency or cynicism that sometimes accompanies the ongoing demands of practicing midwifery in challenging settings.

WOMEN FIRST

Midwives and other women's health professionals practice within a health care system that is increasingly complex. Often, women do not have an adequate frame of reference to allow the formulation of clear questions regarding health issues that concern them. Many clients need guidance to obtain access to necessary health care. Women look to their care provider to provide guidance that is consistent with their perceived needs and internal beliefs. Teasing out the health concerns important to each individual woman requires skill in active listening, sensitivity to cultural issues, and knowledge of common health practices, procedures, and preferences. Meeting women's health needs requires consideration of varied options for care or treatment and necessitates cultivation of a broad-based network of professional collaborative relationships.

Midwifery and women's health is first and foremost about caring for women. Every woman deserves to receive care that is safe, satisfying, and fosters her ability to care for herself. Such care, to be effective, must address women's own cultural and developmental needs. As midwives caring for women in our country's diverse communities, the ability to listen and to integrate women's concerns into the care provided is an integral component of essential midwifery practice. The aim is to provide care based on the woman's expressed and identified needs through a plan of care that is mutually developed and supported by both the woman and the midwife.

ENVIRONMENT OF CARE

The environment of care affects health practices and outcomes. The environment includes the physical surroundings, sociocultural milieu, and the caring efforts provided by the attending practitioners. A woman's autonomy and her sense of control are shaped by her environment. Power dynamics between client and provider vary in different environments. A woman's physiologic response may be affected, mediated by her sense of safety and by the release of powerful stress hormones. This can be particularly striking in environments for labor and birth (Lothian, 2004).

Midwives practice in many different environments in America, such as hospitals of various acuity levels, offices, birth centers, clinics, and homes. Additionally, some midwives find themselves practicing abroad in impoverished and low resource settings. Practice principles typically remain the same regardless of environment, but services and procedures offered vary with access to resources, equipment, and qualified personnel. Within an ideal supportive health care system, midwives would have access to the full range of services, environments, and providers necessary for their client's care, including true collaborative practice based on meeting the needs of the client.

No matter where we stand ourselves on the continuum of health care practices and environments of care, it remains imperative that we understand the broad range of services that are available to the women who come to us for care. The women who come to us for care, our clients, do not live in the health care world. Their awareness of what services are available may be influenced by issues of access, impact of advertising, social and cultural beliefs, the experiences of their friends or relatives, and the ever-present popular media. Unless we become knowledgeable of the many options available to our clients, we may be poorly prepared to listen and understand what health care choices women are making, thereby decreasing our effectiveness in addressing their needs.

Midwifery care is traditionally based on providing care that fosters the physiologic process of labor and birth. Modern midwifery and women's health care stems from physiologic noninterventionist care and includes interventions only as necessary and medically indicated. Deciding what interventions are "necessary" and when they are "indicated" defines our individual practice as midwives yet may be a function of the environment of care in which the midwife practices.

Clients whose primary orientation is toward complementary and alternative care may be guided toward mainstream medical care when it is indicated through a trusting relationship with their midwife or health care provider. In a situation of trust, clients whose point of reference is mainstream medical care may be empowered to become more autonomous in their health care decision-making. With ready access to medical care ensured, some women are able to embrace noninterventionist care for normal labor and birth.

HOW TO USE THIS BOOK

Use of a systematic approach is essential to providing optimum women's health care in today's busy health care environment. A consistently applied method of organization is central to providing comprehensive women's health care that is most likely to meet the client's need in a thorough and optimal fashion. The *Clinical Practice Guidelines for Midwifery & Women's Health* uses a

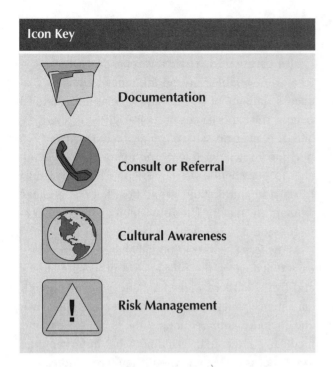

Icon Key

Documentation

Consult or Referral

Cultural Awareness

Risk Management

system of organization consistent with the way most health care providers are taught to gather, interpret, and act on the data obtained in the individual client encounter. By using this format the Guidelines promote a methodical and consistent approach for client assessment, problem identification, and treatment or referral. Clear identification of documentation essentials and practice pitfalls act as reminders to the busy professional. Although the term *midwife* is used frequently throughout this book, the content and recommendations are equally relevant for other women's health care professionals.

When used in lieu of practice-specific practice guidelines, the text may be individualized by including dated and initialed written additions and deletions, highlighting, and so on. A reference copy allows you to refer back to your current practice parameters should you be called to describe your practice at a future date.

Symbols are used throughout the text to indicate key areas that require particular attention. The purpose of the symbols is to heighten awareness, stimulate critical thinking in areas that are potentially

problematic, and encourage comprehensive record keeping and interdisciplinary communication.

 Cultural Awareness

The world is fast becoming a global society. No matter where we practice, it is likely that each of us will provide care to women who come from different countries or cultures from ourselves or from locations other than where we obtained our basic midwifery education and training.

Use of this symbol highlights a need for cultural awareness. Cultural awareness is essential for quality care of women in our multicultural world. We need to consider each woman as an individual who exists not only in our practice settings but also in the context of her own life circumstances and background. Cultural influences may affect birth choices, birth control methods, sexual orientation, self-care preferences, and more. Cultural awareness includes consideration of the client's race, religion, ethnic heritage, age, generation, geographic factors, and cultural mores. Additionally, we need to remember that not everyone from a particular culture embraces the typical beliefs and behavior patterns associated with their culture and that people can be members of several different subculture groups, some with conflicting beliefs. A client's health beliefs and cultural traditions should be explored and verified as a plan of care is being developed.

 Risk Management

Risk management includes the thoughtful consideration of factors that potentially increase risk to the mother or baby, to the well woman, or to the midwife providing care. Identification of risk factors is the first step in reducing their potential impact on outcomes. Risk management as applied to midwifery practice includes careful documentation of care provided. Integral components of the midwifery risk management plan include active listening to each woman as an individual and clearly stated expectations for your role as a midwife and the woman's role when receiving care.

Use of this symbol highlights a need for determining whether a risk is modifiable by particular actions on the part of the client or the midwife. Steps should then be taken to reduce such risk. For risks that are inherent in the client or care practice, careful attention to risk/benefit information and detailed documentation are in order.

 ### Consultation or Referral

Consultations and referrals provide for continuity of care when problems develop or when additional expertise is required. Consultations may range from informal conversations to problem-oriented evaluation of the client by the consultant. When midwives consult with OB/GYN physicians, they need to remember that the physician practices a different specialty and may not have a similar approach to the problem as the midwife.

Use of this symbol highlights a need for considering whether a client is best served by the involvement of other professionals in her care, such as dieticians or social workers; whether her condition requires additional expertise to supplement midwifery care through consultation and collabora-

tion; or whether her needs are best met by referral to specialty care for treatment of a specific condition or for transfer for complete ongoing care.

 ### Documentation in Action

Documentation of care is one of the basic building blocks that supports midwifery practice. Documentation skills allow the midwife or other women's health professional to review the care provided at a later date. If documentation is the key to validating quality care, then documentation skills are essential to midwifery practice. Careful and complete documentation serves as your legal record of events that have occurred. Standardizing the documentation format frees the midwife to concentrate on the content of the client encounter and documentation or note.

Use of this symbol highlights a need for careful documentation practices in accordance with institutional standards and national documentation recommendations. For those midwives or students who seek to improve documentation skills, additional recommendations for documentation are addressed later in this chapter (Table 1-1).

Understand that your client's chart continues long after you finish your entries about the care you provided to this woman, and it will pass

Table 1-1   Clinical Practice Guidelines Format
Client history: Components of the history and chart review
Physical examination: Components of the physical exam to consider
Clinical impression: Differential diagnoses and code groups to consider
Diagnostic testing: Diagnostic tests and procedures to consider
Providing treatment: Therapeutic measures to consider
Providing treatment: Alternative measures to consider
Providing support: Education and support measures to consider
Follow-up care: Follow-up measures to consider
Collaborative practice: Consider consultation or referral

through many hands. Other providers caring for your client at a later date, billing and coding personnel, quality improvement officers, the Joint Commission, and perinatal morbidity and mortality reviewers are just some examples of people who may read the chart to see what care you provided during your encounter with the client.

Comprehensive descriptions of the categories of information that might be obtained during client assessment, evaluation, and development of a midwifery management plan are provided below in the format that you will find throughout the Guidelines.

The "midwifery management plan" reflects the overall plan of care so if the midwife is unable to provide continued care, it is clear to another health care provider what the intended plan is and the client's understanding of that plan. The midwifery management plan is not comprised exclusively of the *treatment* plan but includes all the following components: diagnostic testing, which directs therapeutic measures (treatments) used; client education and support; the plan for continued care or follow-up; and consults or referrals.

Client History: Components of the History and Chart Review

The client history is obtained through chart review and client or family interviews. The client history is commonly divided into various categories based on the nature of the encounter, the environment of care, the scope of the practitioner, and the goal or objective of the client visit. Categories may include the comprehensive health history, the interval history, and the problem-oriented or event-specific history. The comprehensive health history can be further subdivided into the client's past medical and surgical history, social history, and family medical history. These subtypes of the history can be again subdivided to allow for focus on specific areas of concern, such as menstrual history, obstetric history, or genetic history.

The review of systems (ROS) is a review of the major body systems with the client to determine the presence or absence of signs and symptoms of

health conditions, illness, or disease. The comprehensive review of systems includes the following categories: constitutional symptoms (weight loss, fever, malaise, fatigue); eyes, ears, nose, mouth, and throat; skin; respiratory; cardiovascular; gastrointestinal; genitourinary; musculoskeletal; endocrine; lymphatic/hematologic; immunologic/allergic; psychiatric; and neurologic systems (American Medical Association [AMA], 2004).

Identifying which components of the history to further explore with the client is a skill that can assist the midwife in efficiently identifying problems or concerns and in developing a working list of potential differential diagnoses. Components of the history that are included in the client interview should be documented, including, when applicable, the client's stated attitude and the observed affect, or emotional state. The skilled diagnostician is an active listener who can discern which client responses are pertinent and use directed inquiry to elicit further information.

Review of the medical record is an integral part of the client's health history. Many clients provide a limited and necessarily subjective accounting of their health history. The medical record serves to provide an objective overview of the client's health status and may reveal essential details omitted during the client interview. However, the medical record is an imperfect data source that may contain errors and omit or condense a great deal of important information relevant to understanding your client's needs.

Physical Examination: Components of the Physical Exam to Consider

Every body system has both general and specific elements that may be evaluated during the physical examination. Thorough evaluation of the area(s) of concern is an integral part of client or patient evaluation. Components that are included during the physical examination are based on the nature of the presenting problem or health condition and the individual midwife's scope of practice. Although many midwives care primarily for women during the childbearing year, others provide comprehensive women's health care, including evaluation and treatment of gynecologic and/or primary care problems and conditions.

Both performance and documentation of the physical examination is most frequently organized in a head-to-toe fashion. Using a consistent technique allows for systematic client evaluation and comprehensive documentation of results and facilitates review of pertinent information. Standard medical terms are used to describe the presence or absence of findings in an objective manner consistent with the anatomic area under evaluation. "Normal" is not an objective finding, because the range of normal varies widely from client to client.

Standard terminology is used to identify areas of note (i.e., right lower quadrant, periumbilical, substernal). Left and right are clearly identified when applicable. Instruments and tests used during the physical examination are identified when necessary to describe the technique used for evaluation, for example: "A speculum was inserted in the vagina to expose the cervix" or alternatively, "Speculum exam demonstrated . . .".

The language should be clear, descriptive, and indicate clinical findings and any unusual client response to the examination. Notes reflect the midwife's critical thinking process during the examination (italicized in the example that follows): "The left breast was noted to have an irregular fixed mass in the upper outer quadrant, extending into the axillary tail. The mass is approximately 2 × 3 cm, with bluish discoloration over the area, *which may represent increased vascularity*. The mass is firm but not hard; however, it is fixed to the chest wall and accompanied by palpable axillary lymph nodes. *The clinical picture is highly suspicious for breast cancer in spite of a negative mammogram last week*."

Clinical Impression: Differential Diagnoses and Code Groups to Consider

The clinical impression may be more familiar as the assessment or diagnostic impression. The differential diagnosis includes a brief summary of the possible diagnoses that should be considered given the presenting symptoms or condition of the client. Differential diagnoses are often documented in the medical record as a running list from most to least important or likely. You need to consider that more than one diagnosis may be possible due to shared symptomatology, such as the dual diagnosis of bacterial vaginosis and trichomonas in the case of vaginal discharge, pruritus and foul odor.

The clinical impression identifies the midwife's assessment of the client's health status based on the client history, physical examination, and any testing performed on-site. The clinical impression and differential diagnosis then direct further evaluation and testing, plans for continued care, and indications for consultation or referral. The plan should be consistent with the differential diagnoses noted. A firm diagnosis may not yet have been made, making testing part of the overall midwifery plan.

The clinical impression is used for coding purposes. Although useful to document the clinician's thinking, the term "rule out" is not acceptable for coding purposes; however, it may be used as a way of clarifying diagnostic testing recommendations to confirm or eliminate ("rule out") a specific differential diagnosis under consideration. Common International Classification of Diseases diagnosis codes are provided in each guideline. The International Classification of Diseases, Ninth Revision, Clinical Modification (ICD-9-CM) is the official system of assigning codes to diagnoses and procedures associated with hospital utilization in the United States.

ICD-9 codes or code groups are provided after most diagnoses under this section of each guideline throughout the book (Box 1-1). Midwives are responsible for accurately coding the services they provide to their clients (Slager, 2004). Coding decisions are complex and establish the medical necessity for the services provided. The codes provided are intended to provide a starting point for diagnosis code decision-making; other codes may be more appropriate. The midwife must use the code that best describes the

---

Box 1-1 Examples of Differential Diagnoses

1. Preventive health visit, not otherwise specified (NOS) (ICD-9 code V70)
2. Urinary burning, urgency, and frequency (ICD-9 code 788)
3. Pregnancy, 10 weeks gestation by LMP (ICD-9 code V22)
4. Breast mass, L (ICD-9 code 611.72)
5. Pregnancy, at 12 weeks with RLQ pain. (ICD-9 code V22.2 and 789.03) Rule out:
   - Round ligament pain
   - Appendicitis
   - Ectopic pregnancy
   - Ovarian cyst

Source: icd9data.com, 2006

---

unique situation of the patient. Codes are updated each year with *no grace period* so the midwife must obtain the newest version of coding resources each year. Establishing medical necessity is vital to getting paid—if codes do not make sense, are not supported by documentation, or are non-specific, this will result in downgrades or denials. There is a difference between coding and billing. You can always find a code, but billing rules may prohibit its use—such is the case with some diagnoses that are used with or without a pregnancy. Always check a current resource for the most up-to-date ICD-9 codes. Codes can be obtained from http://icd9data.com/.

Diagnostic Testing: Diagnostic Tests and Procedures to Consider

Diagnostic testing includes any tests or procedures performed to elicit additional information to accurately diagnose a problem or to evaluate an ongoing treatment plan. Testing should be documented in a brief and straightforward manner with additional explanations necessary only in unusual situations. Testing is often documented as a numbered list using standard terminology. Each test ordered must be clearly identifiable by other health care professionals. One area in which confusion may occur is when diagnosis or screening *panels* are ordered, the names or components of which may

not be consistent from facility to facility. For example, the panel "PIH labs" (pregnancy-induced hypertension or preeclampsia panel) may include different arrays of tests at different locations. This becomes especially important when a transfer of care is necessary and test results are pending.

Test results should be clearly documented in an easy to find location, especially when they pertain to ongoing care of a problem. Test results come under the heading of "Objective Findings" when you are writing or dictating a note. Anticipatory thinking regarding potential diagnostic test results should be documented in the record to allow continuity of care should another clinician become responsible for providing continued care.

Providing Treatment: Therapeutic Measures to Consider

Therapeutic measures include the administration, ordering, or prescription of medications or accepted medical treatments. Documentation of medications should include the medication name, indication for use, dosage, timing, and route of administration. When off-label medication use is prescribed it should be documented as such and should include documentation of relevant discussions with the client regarding clinician recommendations for off-label medication use and informed consent for such use. Other treatments, such as physical therapy or respiratory therapy treatments, should be documented as ordered, including the indication for the treatment.

Providing Treatment: Alternative Measures to Consider

Alternative treatment measures include complementary and alternative therapies, such as acupuncture, acupressure, homeopathy, herbal remedies, and massage. These treatments are not considered to be prescribed because they are easily available to clients for self-treatment. However, the midwife should be aware of these therapies to point out treatment options and current evidence regarding safety and effectiveness of these treatments and to provide any cautionary advice for their use. When possible, sources should be cited for suggested measures and client instruction and pertinent discussion regarding alternative, traditional, and empiric treatments documented. For more information on the use of herbal treatments, see Appendix A.

Lack of randomized controlled trials may limit use of alternative measures in some practices, whereas in other practices these time-honored methods of caring for women may be used on a regular and frequent basis. Ethical midwifery practice requires discussion of known risks and benefits of therapeutic measures as well as the limits of our knowledge and documentation of the same. Consider the following example:

> Client, G3, P2002, inquired about use of castor oil to stimulate labor at 41½ weeks. The FHR was reactive today, cervix is soft and 1 cm. We discussed her options: expectant care, herbal or homeopathic remedies to stimulate cervical change, and the parameters for use of cervical ripening medications and/or induction of labor. She expressed interest in castor oil and was provided with information and instructions for use of P.O. castor oil for cervical ripening (McFarlin et al., 1999). She was instructed to call with the onset of labor or return to the office in the am if no labor ensues for monitoring of maternal/fetal well-being.

Providing Support: Education and Support Measures to Consider

Client education and support are integral elements of midwifery practice and as such should be clearly documented. Use of standardized client education materials can make documentation of education simpler and less time consuming. A master file should be kept of regularly used client education materials so the midwife may refer back as needed to see what materials were used during a specific time period. Documentation should indicate whether education and support measures were provided verbally, in writing, or both. A teaching checklist is an efficient way to document standard teaching provided. The use of written instructions or recommendations allows the client to refer back to them after the visit and to refresh her memory regarding instructions or information provided at the visit.

Client support may include coordination of recommended care, such as scheduling of diagnostic tests and coordination of referrals. Although review of diagnostic test results and clinical planning based on those results fall under the category of *follow-up*, interaction with the client that includes information about test results, options for care, discussion of alternatives, and a compassionate listening ear occurs within the client support and education framework.

Follow-up Care: Follow-up Measures to Consider

Follow-up includes the actual process of documentation of care that has been provided, anticipatory thinking, and recommendations for future care. It also clearly indicates the timing of the next recommended appointment for further care. This serves to ensure that the midwife, as well as other clinicians, has a clear impression of the client visit, the care provided, and the anticipated next steps in the ongoing care of this individual.

Instructions for the client's next visit are a critical element in documentation of the midwifery plan of care. Clients must know what is expected of them to follow through with recommendations for care. Follow-up may include such things as returning for a scheduled visit (i.e., a routine prenatal visit) or a plan for the midwife to contact the client after receipt of a test result (i.e., a mammogram performed on a client with a suspicious breast mass). Clients should also be reminded to call or present for care if mild symptoms at the time of the examination persist or worsen (i.e., nasal congestion that develops into a productive cough with fever or scant vaginal spotting that turns bright red and heavy), along with instructions on how to reach on-call personnel and where to present for urgent or emergency care.

When a deviation from normal or expected findings occurs, a detailed plan for follow-up is documented. In the example above of a woman with a breast mass, the documentation might include the date that results were received; discussion with the client about her options for care; referral to a breast specialist; the date and time of the specialist appointment; documentation of the consult request, including records transferred to the specialist with written client consent; and a mechanism to follow-up to verify client follow-through.

For midwives who provide comprehensive women's health care, a *follow-up file* may be necessary to track clients and their problems. In this instance, documentation in the client record that the follow-up file has been utilized can help with tracking. A follow-up file may be a calendar, a cross-referenced index card file, or a software program that automatically generates reminders, identifies no-shows, and provides a comprehensive record of problems and follow-up contacts. Tracking of clients with ongoing treatment of unresolved problems is an integral part of any midwifery risk management plan.

Collaborative Practice: Consider Consultation or Referral

Midwifery practice occurs within the context of a health care system. A consultation is any request for collaboration with another health care professional

to provide care for a client. Documentation of a consultation or referral in the client's medical record includes the name and specialty of the provider, how the contact was made (e.g. phone, letter, or directly by the client), the indication for the consultation or referral, and expectations for care.

Consultations or referrals are made for many types of services, such as counseling, smoking cessation, nutritional evaluation, physical therapy, psychiatric care, substance abuse treatment, alternative therapies, and medical or surgical evaluation of reproductive or other health problems.

Written consultation or referral requests typically include a brief history of the problem, essential information about the client, the type of service for which the client is being referred, and expectations regarding care. A copy of the request is maintained in the client medical record. Including information about scheduled consultation or referral appointments is often helpful when following up on problems.

When a consultation is obtained, the consultant's opinion must be documented. If the consultant provides this service via telephone, the midwife is responsible for documenting the content of the consultation, the consultant's recommendations for care, and the relevance or application of those recommendations to the midwifery plan of care. When the consultant evaluates the client in person, the consultant is responsible for documenting his or her opinion and any care rendered.

DOCUMENTATION OF MIDWIFERY AND WOMEN'S HEALTH CARE

Thoughtful documentation can highlight inherent differences between the midwifery and medical models of providing women's health care. This in turn encourages outcomes-based research that demonstrates positive outcomes for clients cared for by midwives, as shown in seminal midwifery care studies described by Farley (2005). The recommendations that follow provide a general guideline for documenting midwifery care (Table 1-2).

Table 1-2   Documentation Standards

STANDARD	PERFORMANCE MEASURES
1. Elements in the client's medical record are organized in a consistent manner.	• Client record is organized in a clear and systematic fashion. • Records are entered in chronologic order.
2. Client medical records are maintained and stored in a manner that protects the safety of the records and the confidentiality of the information.	• All medical records are stored out of reach and out of view of unauthorized persons. (see related standard Maintenance, Disclosure, and Disposal of Confidential Information).
3. Client name or identification number is on each document in the record.	• Client name or identification number is found on each document in the record.
4. Entries are legible.	• Handwritten entries are legible. • Notes use a consistent standardized format and language that allows the reader to review care without the use of separate legend/key.
5. Entries are dated. In addition, entries are timed and dated when time is a critical factor in the plan of care.	• Each entry to the record is dated. • Entries generated by an outside source (e.g., referrals, consults) are also dated when reviewed. • Notes related to client encounters are in the record within 72 hours or 3 business days of occurrence.
6. Entries are initialed or signed by author.	• Entries are initialed or signed by the author. Author identification may be a handwritten signature, unique electronic identifier, or initials. This applies to practitioners and members of the office staff who contribute to the record. • When initials are used, there is a designation of signature and status maintained in the office. • Entries generated by an outside source (e.g., referrals, consults) are also initialed or signed when reviewed.
7. Personal and biographical data are included in the record.	• Includes information necessary to identify client and insurer and to submit claims. • Includes information related to client need for language or cultural interpreter or other communication mechanisms as necessary to ensure appropriate client care. • Information may be maintained in a computerized database, as long as it is retrievable and can be printed as needed to transfer the record to another practitioner or for monitoring purposes. • Name of the client's primary care provider is clearly indicated in the record.

(continues)

Table 1-2   Documentation Standards (continued)

STANDARD	PERFORMANCE MEASURES
8. **A.** Initial history and physical examinations for new patients are recorded within 12 months of a patient first seeking care or within three visits, whichever occurs first.	• **A.** Initial history and physical examination for new clients is recorded within 12 months of the first visit or within three visits, whichever occurs first. If applicable, there is written evidence that the practitioner advised client to return for a physical examination. The record of a complete history and physical, included in the medical chart and done within the past 12 months by another practitioner is acceptable. Well-child exams meet this standard.
B. Past medical history is documented and includes serious accidents, operations, and illnesses.	• **A and B.** History and physical documentation contains pertinent information such as age, height, vital signs, past medical and behavioral health history, preventive health maintenance and risk screening, physical examination, medical impression, and documentation related to the ordering of appropriate diagnostic tests, procedures, and/or medications. Self-administered client questionnaires are an acceptable way to obtain baseline past medical history and personal information. There is written documentation to explain the lack of information contained in the medical record regarding the history and physical (e.g., poor historians, patient's inability or unwillingness to provide information).
C. Family history is documented.	• **C.** Patient record contains immediate family history or documentation that it is noncontributory.
D. Birth history is documented for patients aged 6 years and under.	• **D.** Infant records should include gestational and birth history and should be age and diagnosis appropriate.
9. Allergies and adverse reactions are prominently listed or noted as "none" or "NKA."	• Medication allergies or history of adverse reactions to medications or other substances, such as latex, are displayed in a prominent and consistent location or noted as "none" or "NKA." (Examples of where allergies may be prominently displayed include on coversheet inside the chart, at the top of every visit page, or on a medication record in the chart.) • When applicable and known, there is documentation of the date the allergy was first discovered, related symptoms, previous treatments, and preventive measures required (such as a latex-free environment).
10. Information regarding social history is recorded.	• Practitioner must have documentation in the record regarding social history, such as sexual orientation and behaviors, and use of tobacco, alcohol, or illicit drugs (or lack thereof) in clients 12 years of age and older who have been seen three or more times.

Table 1-2	Documentation Standards (continued)

STANDARD	PERFORMANCE MEASURES
10. Information regarding social history is recorded. *(continued)*	• Cultural and developmental issues are clearly documented when present. • Health care habits and preferences are noted, including use of alternative therapies, herbal remedies, and dietary supplements.
11. An updated problem list is maintained.	• A problem list, which summarizes important client medical information, such as major diagnoses, past medical and/or surgical history, and recurrent complaints, is documented and maintained by all practitioners in the practice. • The problem list is clearly visible and accessible. • Continuity of care between multiple practitioners in the same practice is demonstrated by documentation and review of pertinent medical information.
12. Client's chief complaint or purpose for visit is clearly documented.	• The client's chief complaint or the purpose of the visit is recorded as stated by the client. • Documentation supports that the client's perceived needs and/or expectations were addressed. • Documented history and physical are relevant to the client's reason for visit. • Telephone encounters relevant to medical issues are documented in the medical record and reflect practitioner review, including phone triage handled by office staff.
13. Clinical assessment and/or physical findings are recorded. Working diagnoses are consistent with findings.	• Clinical assessment and physical examination are documented and correspond to the client's chief complaint, purpose for seeking care, and/or ongoing care for chronic illnesses. • Documentation supports working diagnoses or clinical impressions that logically follow from clinical assessment and physical examination findings.
14. Plan of action/treatment plan is consistent with diagnosis(es).	• Proposed treatment plans, therapies, or other regimens are documented and logically follow previously documented diagnoses and clinical impressions. • Rationale for treatment decisions appears appropriate and is substantiated by documentation in the record. • Follow-up diagnostic testing is performed at appropriate intervals for diagnoses.

(continues)

Table 1-2   Documentation Standards (continued)

STANDARD	PERFORMANCE MEASURES
15. Informed consent is obtained for the indicated, proposed diagnostic and therapeutic measures.	• The medical record shows clear justification for diagnostic and therapeutic measures. • Risks related to recommended diagnostic and therapeutic measures, as well as alternative options, including doing nothing, are discussed with the client using accepted parameters for informed consent and clearly documented in the record.
16. Unresolved problems from previous visits are addressed in subsequent visits.	• Continuity of care from one visit to the next is demonstrated when a problem-oriented approach to unresolved problems from previous visits is documented in subsequent visit notes.
17. Follow-up instructions and time frame for follow-up or the next visit are recorded as appropriate.	• Return to office in a specified amount of time is recorded at time of visit or following consultation, laboratory, or other diagnostic reports. • Follow-up is documented for clients who require prenatal/postpartum care, periodic visits for a chronic illness, or reassessment following an episodic illness. • Client participation in the coordination of care is demonstrated through client education, follow-up, and return visits. • Implementation of a follow-up plan is documented for clients with critical values or acute conditions who do not return for care as described in the practice's risk management policy.
18. Current medications are documented in the record, and notes reflect that long-term medications are reviewed at least annually by the practitioner and updated as needed.	• Information regarding current medications is readily apparent from review of the record. • Changes to medication regimen are noted as they occur. When medications appear to remain unchanged, the record includes documentation of at least annual review by the practitioner. • There is documentation of consideration of medication, herbal, or dietary supplement interactions.
19. Health care education is noted in the record and periodically updated as appropriate.	• Education is age, developmental, and culturally appropriate. • Education may correspond directly to the reason for the visit, to specific diagnosis-related issues, to address client concerns, or to clarify and amplify age-appropriate health promotion recommendations. • Education provided to clients, family members, or designated caregivers is documented. • Examples of patient noncompliance are documented.

Table 1-2	Documentation Standards (continued)

STANDARD	PERFORMANCE MEASURES
20. Screening and preventive care practices are in accordance with current recommendations from national standard setting organizations.	• Each record includes documentation that preventive services were ordered and performed or that the practitioner discussed preventive services with the client and the client chose to defer or decline them. • Current immunization and screening status is documented. • Practitioners may document that a patient reported receiving preventive services from another practitioner (e.g., family practitioner) and should request records as indicated.
21. An immunization record is completed for members 18 years and under.	• The record includes documentation of immunizations administered from birth to present for clients 18 years and under. • When prior records are unavailable, practitioners may document that a child's parent or guardian affirmed that immunizations were administered by another practitioner and the approximate age or date the immunizations were given.
22. Requests for consultation are consistent with clinical assessment/physical findings.	• The clinical assessment supports the decision for a referral. • Referrals are provided in a timely manner according to the severity of the patient's condition. • Referral requests and expectations are clearly documented.
23. Laboratory and diagnostic reports reflect practitioner review.	• Results of all laboratory tests and other diagnostics are documented in the medical record. • Records demonstrate that the practitioner reviews laboratory and diagnostic reports and makes treatment decisions based on report findings. • Reports within the review period are initialed and dated by the practitioner, or another system of ensuring practitioner review is in place and clearly delineated in the practice's risk management policy.
24. Client notification of laboratory and diagnostic test results and instruction regarding follow-up, when indicated, are documented.	• Clients are notified of abnormal laboratory and diagnostic results and advised of recommendations regarding follow-up or changes in treatment. • The record documents patient notification of abnormal results. A practitioner may document that the client is to call regarding results; however, the practitioner is responsible for ensuring that the client is advised of any abnormal results and recommendations for continued care.

(continues)

Table 1-2 Documentation Standards (continued)	
STANDARD	**PERFORMANCE MEASURES**
25. There is evidence of continuity and -coordination of care between primary and specialty care practitioners or other providers.	• Consultation reports reflect practitioner review. • Primary care provider records include consultation reports/summaries (within 60–90 days) that correspond to specialist referrals or documentation that there was a clear attempt to obtain reports that were not received. Subsequent visit notes reflect results of the consultation as may be pertinent to ongoing client care. • Specialist records include a consultation report/summary addressed to the referral source. • When a client receives services at or through another provider such as a hospital, emergency care, home care agency, skilled nursing facility, or behavioral health specialist, there is evidence of coordination of care through consultation reports, discharge summaries, status reports, or home health reports. The discharge summary includes the reason for admission, the treatment provided, and the instructions given to the client on discharge.

Adapted from the following sources:

Commission on Office Laboratory Accreditation. Retrieved January 4, 2008 from http://www.cola.org/

CareFirst BlueCross BlueShield. *Medical record documentation standards.* Retrieved January 4, 2008 from http://www.carefirst.com/providers/attachments/BOK5129.pdf

American Cancer Society. *Screening recommendations.* Retrieved January 4, 2008 from http://www.cancer.org/docroot/PED/content/PED_2_3X_ACS_Cancer_Detection_Guidelines_36.asp?sitearea=PED

National Institutes of Health. *National guidelines clearinghouse.* Retrieved January 4, 2008 from http://www.guideline.gov/index.aspx

National Heart, Lung, and Blood Institute. *Clinical practice guidelines.* Retrieved January 4, 2008 from http://www.nhlbi.nih.gov/guidelines/

U.S. Preventive Services Task Force. *Topic index A–Z.* Retrieved January 4, 2008 from http://www.ahrq.gov/clinic/uspstf/uspstopics.htm

The ideal medical record provides the reader with a clear view of the client's presentation, the midwife's evaluation process, and the implementation and results of treatment or recommendations. Meticulous documentation also allows other professionals to follow the course of care provided and to gain insight into the client's response. Client health records are an essential communication tool in a group practice and during consultation or referral. This section explores the process of documentation from several points of view:

• Documentation using current procedural terminology (CPT) evaluation and management (E/M) criteria; a method of documentation developed by the AMA that reflects the complexity and level of care provided to meet current reimbursement criteria

• Documentation as an essential communication tool; a method of recording events and findings for future reference that follows accepted standards

• Documentation as a means of demonstrating application of risk management and collaborative practice processes

• Documentation as a reflection of the midwifery model of care; describing care that reflects the philosophy and standards of the practice of midwifery

Evaluation and Management Criteria

The AMA publishes the CPT handbook, which is used to assist in choosing a code for a service or procedure based on the documentation of the service or procedure during coding and billing. Midwives should become familiar with this book as well as the ICD-9 code books because they are essential for accurate coding practices and for receiving appropriate reimbursement for services.

The CPT system lists codes for services provided by clinicians using specific criteria that must be present in the documentation of care provided. E/M codes are based on the level of service provided. The level of E/M services provided are determined by the amount of history, physical examination, medical decision-making (critical thinking), counseling and coordination of care (client education and support), nature of the presenting problem, and the amount of time required to provide care.

The history and physical examination and the complexity of critical thinking are the key components used to determine the level of E/M service provided. The nature of the presenting problem, along with the provision of client education and support, are considered contributory, whereas time spent is considered separately. Time criteria used in E/M is based on the time spent during the face-to-face client visit. However, the time required for review of diagnostic testing, follow-up, and coordination of care is factored into the time component (AMA, 2004).

The CPT book clearly outlines the required components for the level of care provided. A brief overview is provided here.

The E/M evaluation considers four types of history and physical examination. The *problem-focused visit* is limited to a brief history of the reason for the encounter and an examination that is limited to the affected area. The *expanded problem focused visit* adds a pertinent system review and examination of additional body systems that might be affected by the presenting problem. The *detailed visit* adds pertinent history related to the reason for the encounter and a thorough examination of the affected area and related organ systems. The *comprehensive visit* adds a complete review of systems, comprehensive review of the client history and risk assessment, and either a comprehensive physical examination or thorough examination of a single organ system.

The complexity of medical decision-making required is based on the complexity of reaching a diagnosis and/or of formulating a management plan. The more medical records, tests, or other information to be reviewed, the more complex the evaluation becomes. The greater the number of differential diagnoses and potential plans to be considered, the more complex the management decision-making becomes. The higher the risk of complications, morbidity, mortality, or comorbidity related to health problems or recommended testing, the more complex the management decision-making becomes. Decision-making is evaluated as being straightforward or of low, moderate, or high complexity (AMA, 2004).

Documentation of the Midwifery Model of Care

As professionals, midwives continually work toward the goal of educating clients and colleagues about how midwifery differs from medicine and nursing. Midwifery educators strive to ensure that these differences are reflected in midwifery education programs and the clinical experiences of those learning midwifery (American College of Nurse-Midwives [ACNM], 2007). Midwifery encompasses the belief that birth is essentially normal, that women have the right to be listened to and heard, and that birth and well-woman care are important events in the lives of women. These beliefs translate into subtle and overt behavioral differences in maternity and women's health practice that should be reflected in the client's medical record.

As a profession that performs many of the same practice procedures as obstetrics and gynecology, midwives need to demonstrate and clearly reflect through documentation how midwifery differs from obstetrics and gynecology. Although many of the behaviors that a midwife, a physician, a nurse practitioner, or a physician's assistant demonstrate when providing women's health care may be similar, the origins, attitudes, and client perception of the care may be substantially different. Documentation of midwifery care should reflect the essence of midwifery: woman-oriented care focused on excellence in the processes of providing care with attentiveness to outcomes.

Standards for Documentation

Documentation standards have been developed to allow use of the client's medical record as an effective means of communication between professionals, verification of services provided for billing and reimbursement purposes, and analysis of care provided for quality and appropriateness. To objectively evaluate medical record content, standardized criteria have been developed that are relevant to specific objectives (Johnson, 2001). Each organization that utilizes the medical record has set detailed criteria for evaluation of the content, which is based on their needs.

Documentation as Communication: Skills and Techniques

Thorough documentation provides midwives and other health care professionals with a clear view of each woman's individual presentation, concerns, and preferences for care. The client record also serves as a means of following the midwife's thought processes regarding development of the working diagnosis and ongoing plans for continued client care. Clear concise documentation is the key to validating quality care and is an integral part of the midwife's risk management program.

The goal of each note is to present a record of care provided and other essential information to guide the midwife and other health care professionals in the event of a transfer of care, such as might occur after problem-oriented referral, transfer to physician care for a high-risk condition, or simple cross-coverage arrangements.

In the event of legal action, the ideal medical record provides a clear picture of the client presentation, concerns, participation in care decisions, and response to care or treatment. The medical record identifies the midwife's evaluation process and working diagnoses; it also includes her or his anticipatory thinking and planning for diagnosis, treatment, and continued care. The midwifery plan for follow-up care and evaluation includes relevant parameters for initiation of collaborative practice when indicated or applicable.

Both ACNM and the Midwives Alliance of North America (MANA) offer clinical data sets that can be used as tools to evaluate the adequacy of standardized client record forms used in midwifery practice and that contribute to a national database to document and describe midwifery care. These data sets have been developed to provide standardized and validated tools for collecting data about the care midwives provide. Midwives seeking to improve their documentation skills may also use the clinical data sets as a self-evaluation instrument by performing retrospective chart or medical record audits to determine process or documentation weaknesses and areas for improvement.

Thorough and complete documentation is concise and focused; rarely is it necessary to provide lengthy notes. Although notes may be handwritten, typed, entered into a computer data collection system, or dictated and transcribed, they must be legible to the average reader. They may be written on a form that provides a preset format, such as a labor flow sheet, or written on a blank sheet of paper, such as a progress note. Notes should reflect pertinent findings and the critical thinking that occurs during the care of each client. All notes should have, at a minimum, the following information:

- Client identification: Name, date of birth, and medical record number where applicable
- Date of service: Date and time are necessary for time-sensitive situations such as labor care or during newborn resuscitation

- Reason for encounter: Often described in the client's own words (e.g., "It burns when I pee") or as a simple statement (e.g., "onset of labor")
- Client history: An expansion of the reason for the encounter, commonly known as the "chief complaint" or the "history of present illness"; includes all relevant history and subjective information provided by the client or family, including, as applicable, the review of systems, past history (chart review), family, and social history
- Objective findings: Includes the results of the physical examination, mental status evaluation, and/or laboratory work, ultrasound, or other testing as indicated by the history and physical
- Clinical impression: Also known as the "assessment" or "working diagnosis"; may include several differential diagnoses under consideration pending laboratory or testing results; may be documented as "primary symptoms" or "conditions" with differential diagnoses listed to validate testing and communicate anticipatory thinking
- Midwifery plan of care: May be subdivided into several categories; essentially outlines all diagnostic, therapeutic, and educational measures initiated at the visit, along with further actions anticipated based on potential results and specific needs of the client; should end with a recommendation for the timing of the next visit

Documentation as Risk Management

Exemplary midwifery practice includes understanding and implementing essential components of a risk management program to enhance midwifery care and client outcomes. Thorough documentation using a standardized format allows objective evaluation of the care provided. Each note should be written from the objective outside observer point of view. Thorough but concise documentation is the ideal. Use of fill-in-the-blank forms can be a useful way to quickly record essential information, particularly for routine encounters; a common example of this is the prenatal flow

sheet. These notes are best supplemented with a narrative note whenever there are unusual circumstances or findings.

The *problem list* is a convenient way to highlight ongoing acute or chronic problems. It should be kept in an easily seen location enabling all clinicians caring for the client to identify at a glance potential factors that may influence the care provided. This decreases the potential for a problem to be missed and focuses providers on important current and resolved health issues for this client. The *medication list* is often adjacent to the problem list. Risk may be reduced by reviewing and updating both lists at each visit.

A follow-up file is a useful way to track clients with problems that require future care. Although not part of the client medical record per se, it comprises a significant part of the midwife's risk management plan. When notification of abnormal results is documented in the medical record, a plan must be formulated. The follow-up file system tracks whether clients return for recommended care and generates reminders to document clinician notification of clients who are noncompliant. The midwife's risk management plan should describe the follow-up process and clearly indicate the procedure for utilizing the midwife's follow-up system.

Documenting Culturally Competent Care

Midwives and other health professionals have a legal and moral obligation to provide culturally competent care. An excellent resource for women's health providers is *Caring for Women Cross-Culturally* (Hill et al., 2003). Cultural competence is the ability to professionally step outside of your own culture and obtain the vision and skills necessary to provide care in a context that is appropriate for the women who come to you for care.

The attitudes and behaviors needed to do this include a sincere interest in other cultures, the ability to communicate, and a sense of honor for the customs of others. On a more practical level, the ability to access interpreter services is a key behavior that is both essential and legally mandated. Each midwife is expected to obtain or to have access to information regarding specific health care problems that are racially or ethnically mediated. Each midwife should become familiar with historical events and cultural practices that may also affect health in the populations served. Each of these components should be addressed in the medical record when they are applicable. It can be a simple check box, such as "☑ Interpreter service offered."

Documentation of cultural competence may include a detailed description, such as when the informed consent process is provided through an interpreter before surgery or a procedure. It may be culturally appropriate to excuse the father from the birth room or to ensure a family member is present as a chaperone during intimate examinations. Documentation of the cultural indications for changes or variations from usual care serves to protect the midwife and to reinforce the need for respect and awareness of cultural differences.

The essential characteristic of the culturally competent midwife is an ability to embrace diversity while retaining one's sense of personal cultural identity. To do this, it may be necessary to relinquish control in select client encounters. Feelings of discomfort, failure, fear, frustration, anger, or embarrassment may serve to indicate a need for the midwife to examine her own personal viewpoint to become more culturally sensitive. The midwife might consider thoughtful and deliberate examination of challenging intercultural exchanges as a means to foster personal growth.

Women may come from settings where there is very limited access or availability of health care and accept whatever care is provided. Other women may have a strong need to direct their health care and mandate their active participation in all health-related decisions. Most women fall somewhere between these two extremes.

Awareness and sensitivity to cultural practices and beliefs can enhance client satisfaction and build a trusting professional relationship. Cultural diversity encompasses a wide range of reference points, which may include social and emotional development, age, race, religion, sexual orientation, ethnic heritage, country of origin, geographic location, and cultural beliefs and mores. Becoming culturally competent involves a certain level of interest, inquiry, and awareness of cultural differences. It involves sensitivity to the customs of the social groups the woman belongs to but also an awareness that she may not conform to the common perceptions of those groups' behaviors and beliefs.

Cultural differences may be considered cross-cultural, meaning the midwife and the client come from different ethnic or racial backgrounds, or they may be intercultural, where the midwife and the client come from similar ethnic or social backgrounds but have developed disparate views and beliefs, especially with regard to health care. Examples of this include the home birth midwife whose client reveals she wants access to pharmacological pain relief for labor or a hospital-based midwife whose client calls to request an in-home examination for possible labor.

Cultural competence requires that the midwife remains open-minded, cultivates active listening skills, and evaluates each woman's needs according to the environment of care. Access to culturally competent interpreters to translate language, social customs, and mores related to women's health care is extremely helpful. A minimum standard requires that language interpreters be available. Literal translation, however, may not always provide correct or accurate information. Individualizing care also involves taking into account the woman's chronologic age, her developmental stage, emotional development, sexual orientation and preferences, cultural background, and other social factors.

Developmental Considerations

Attention to developmental changes throughout a woman's life is essential to address the concerns that may be most pressing to her. The needs of adolescent women are very different from those of women of childbearing age, as are those of the woman who is past menopause—even when they each present for the same type of visit. Midwives who frequently care for the medically underserved should remember that the effects of poverty, abuse, low self-esteem, or marginal nutrition may adversely impact a woman's developmental growth.

Adolescents　Young women in their teens may present at various developmental stages based on age, emotional development, ethnicity, and other social and cultural factors. Compliance is frequently an issue as authority is challenged and the young woman seeks to explore the boundaries and limits of her situation. Parental presence and involvement may indicate support and guidance for the teen and her choices or it may be a reflection of dysfunctional parent–teen dynamics.

Older Women　After the childbearing years have passed, women often have a change of focus from reproductive health care to concerns surrounding general health and well-being. Many women celebrate the freedom of mature adulthood. They may explore new attitudes, become more adventurous, and find that their confidence flourishes. Many older women live alone, by choice or by necessity. Women, more than men, are affected as they age by increasing poverty and diminished resources to cope with illness or disability.

The Mentally Challenged　Such women may require coordination of specialized services to be provided appropriate reproductive health care. Intimate examinations may require sedation or anesthesia to avoid emotional trauma, especially in the mentally challenged woman with a history of sexual abuse.

The Physically Challenged　Physically handicapped women may or may not have developmental delays depending on the cause of the physical challenge. Individual assessment is necessary to determine the client's developmental level and provide developmentally appropriate services. Examinations may be made more challenging by physical limitations, and ample time should be scheduled to allow for this.

Immigrant and Refugee Women　These women may have culturally mediated variations in devel-

opment, which may make interpretation of developmental stages more challenging. Accessing resources to learn about cultural variations may aid in appropriate client assessment.

Socioeconomic Challenges　Various socioeconomic challenges may impact the rate and progression of a woman's physical, emotional, and social development. Remaining nonjudgmental offers the optimum opportunity to determine how best to identify each individual's unique needs and provide or direct women to the services that might best meet those needs.

Informed Consent

Informed consent is a specific process designed to ensure that clients receive full information to participate in health care decision-making regarding a recommended treatment or procedure. The midwife is expected to recommend a course of action and share her or his reasoning process with the client. Client understanding of the information provided is as important as the information itself. Discussion should be carried on in lay person's terms, and client understanding should be assessed along the way.

Complete informed consent includes discussion of the following elements (Rozovsky, 2001):

- Indications for the recommended procedure, medication, or treatment
- Accepted or experimental use of the proposed procedure, medication, or treatment
- Potential or anticipated benefits, actions, or effects of the proposed course of action
- Potential risks and adverse effects of the proposed course of action
- Potential risks and adverse effects of declining the proposed course of action
- Any urgency to undergoing the proposed course of action
- Alternatives to the proposed course of action, including potential effectiveness, risk, and benefit

- Client understanding of discussion, best demonstrated by the client paraphrasing information received and documented by direct quote (e.g., "You're going to try to turn my baby so she isn't butt first.")
- Client acceptance of the recommendation

Midwife and client signatures are preferably witnessed by a third party. Many midwives who practice in the out-of-hospital setting opt to use the informed consent process to present information on birth centers or home birth. This provides opportunity for questions, discussion, and documentation of client participation in decisions.

In most cases it is clear whether or not the client is competent to make her own decisions. The midwife should assess the client's ability to understand the nature of the problem, to understand the risks associated with the problem and the recommended course of action, and to communicate her decision based on that understanding.

Competent clients have the right to refuse treatment after the informed consent process. This right may be limited when the client is pregnant and her decision affects her unborn child. Treatment refusal may be an indicator that further discussion is necessary to gain insight into the client's emotional response, beliefs, and understanding about the nature of the problem and recommendations for care (University of Washington School of Medicine, 1999).

Components of Common Medical Notes

When documenting care provided, each category should be addressed, using either appropriate details or the phrase "not applicable." This serves two purposes: It maintains the expected format of the note, and it clearly indicates what clinical components the midwife included while caring for the client.

Office Visit or Progress Note

This format is typically used for problem-oriented and well-woman office visits as well as for progress notes during labor and postpartum. Standardized prenatal care forms typically vary from this format;

however, it becomes useful during evaluation of a problem or complication during pregnancy.

- Subjective: Client interview and record review
- Objective: Physical examination and diagnostic or screening test results
- Assessment: Differential or working diagnosis
- Plan: Evaluation, treatment, education, and follow-up care including coordination of care, consultations, and/or referrals

Procedure Note

The procedure note is used to provide detailed information about a procedure such as endometrial biopsy, intrauterine device insertion, colposcopic examination, external version, or circumcision. This format is appropriate to use to document a procedure regardless of location or environment of care and includes the following:

- Procedure performed
- Indication for procedure: Include diagnosis and any relevant history of present problem
- Informed consent: Include any relevant discussion
- Anesthesia, if used
- Estimated blood loss, in milliliters; minimal is accepted for estimated blood loss less than 10 ml.
- Complications: Describe with treatment and client response to treatment
- Technique: Describe techniques used, including instruments, anesthesia technique and amount used, sequence of events, and rationale for technique choices, when appropriate
- Findings: Describe clinical findings, specimens collected and disposition of same, and client post-procedure status

Medical Consultation or Referral

The purpose of the formal consultation or referral request is to provide the consultant with adequate information about the client in advance to allow the consultant to focus on the problem or condition. Referral requests may be verbal or written (commonly in letter format) and often include the following:

- Client introduction: Name, date of birth, indication for consult or referral
- History of present problem or illness
- Type of consultation requested
- Brief client history: Allergies, medications, illnesses, surgeries, relevant social history
- Expectation for care: Advises the consultant of any client education provided regarding the problem or illness; appropriate to advocate for the client's preferences when stating expectations for care

Admission History and Physical Examination

The admission history and physical is typically used when admitting a client to the hospital with an obstetric, gynecologic, or medical problem. However, it is also appropriate to use when admitting a client to midwifery care in labor in any environment of care.

- Admission diagnosis
- History of present condition or illness
- Past OB/GYN history
- Past medical history
- Past surgical history
- Current medications
- Allergies
- Social history
- Family history
- Review of systems
- Physical findings
- Diagnostic testing
- Plan of care
- Anticipated course of care
- Consults
- Plan for reevaluation

Delivery Note

The delivery note is designed to summarize the pregnancy, labor, and birth in a brief but comprehensive overview of the pregnancy and labor, including detailed information about the birth and immediate postpartum and newborn periods. A typical delivery note includes the following:

- Brief review of prenatal course
- Admission status
- Course of labor
  - Length of each stage
  - ROM: time, color, fetal heart rate
  - Maternal and fetal response during labor
  - Labor events or interventions
  - Complications and treatment
- Delivery information
  - Time, date, location
  - Route and method of birth
  - Maternal and fetal position
  - Techniques or interventions used with indication, such as
    - Anesthesia, type, and dose
    - Episiotomy or laceration
    - Type of suture and technique of repair if done
    - Medications if used
    - Complications and treatment, including client response
  - Evaluation of placenta
  - Estimated blood loss
  - Maternal status postdelivery
- Newborn information
  - Gender
  - Resuscitation, if indicated
  - Apgar
  - Weight
  - Bonding
  - Feeding, voiding, stooling
  - Newborn status postdelivery

Discharge Summary

This is an appropriate format to use after a hospital admission, but it may be used for summarizing a birth center admission or home birth encounter as well.

- Admission diagnosis
- Discharge diagnosis
- History of present condition or illness
- Past medical history

- Past surgical history
- Current medications
- Allergies
- Social history
- Family history
- Review of systems
- Physical findings
- Diagnostic testing
- Treatments and procedures
- Hospital course
- Complications
- Discharge medications
- Discharge instructions
- Condition on discharge
- Plan for continued care

Documentation is an essential skill for midwifery and women's health practice that should be attended to with the same care and attention given to other components of clinical practice. Meticulous documentation accurately reflects the scope and nature of midwifery care and enhances communication among health professionals who care for and about women. The information contained within the client's medical record forms a basis for planning continued care. Continuity of care is enhanced through the interdisciplinary documentation of care and services provided. This includes communication between the health care provider and the client and the health care provider and other health professionals contributing to the client's care. Other uses of the medical record, such as internal hospital audits for quality assurance purposes and for protection of the legal interests of the client and health care professionals who provided care, are addressed in the next section on Risk Management.

RISK MANAGEMENT

Risk management is a dynamic process based on assessing probabilities of untoward outcomes or events and on developing strategies to reduce or manage these events. In health care this phrase is often used to refer to health risks to the client,

health or professional risks to the practitioner, or financial risks to the institution or practice. Application of sound risk management principles to midwifery and women's health practice includes providing and monitoring quality health care to the women we serve while practicing in a manner that protects the midwife from undue risk, whether it be from infectious disease, malpractice litigation or financial insolvency.

This section identifies ways to safeguard your practice while providing quality care in our litigious society. Risk management means identifying and managing the potential risk to each woman we care for, to every unborn and newborn infant, to ourselves as midwives, and to each of the other health professionals that become involved in the care of the women and families we serve (National Association for Healthcare Quality, 1998).

Developing a Collaborative Practice Network

Midwives do not practice in isolation. Every midwife, regardless of practice location, needs a network of contacts to help provide ongoing care and services. The collaborative practice model allows for a wide variety of professional relationships that range from informal to highly structured arrangements.

Development of professional relationships with physicians and other health care providers in your area begins with you. Make arrangements to meet at a convenient time and introduce yourself. Bring practice brochures or business cards so that these providers and their office staff members understand the services you offer and how to reach you. Make good eye contact, shake hands firmly, and present yourself as a competent, skilled, professional colleague. Your goal is to initiate a relationship so that when you have a client who needs care, your credibility has been established. It is not required that you agree on philosophy of care or management styles, but it is important that you establish a good working relationship. It is also good practice to nurture your relationship with the office staff for those times when you may need them to prioritize your requests for assistance during office hours.

Determining in advance what type of consult is indicated affects what information you provide. Present the consultation request in terms that direct the care you are seeking for your client. If you do not provide this direction, the physician will likely manage your client as she or he would her or his usual patients.

The AMA Evaluation and Management Services Guidelines state "A consultation is a type of service provided by a physician whose opinion or advice regarding evaluation and/or management of a specific problem is requested by another physician or other appropriate source" (AMA, 2004). Forms of consultation that the midwife may use include the following types:

- Informational: "Just letting you know that Mrs. B is here in labor. She is a G3, P2002 at term and is at 5 cm after 1 hour of labor. The fetal heart rate is in normal range with good variability, estimated fetal weight is 7½ pounds, and I expect a spontaneous vaginal birth shortly." In this instance you have already established a professional relationship with a defined collaborating individual that includes notification in specific circumstances or as indicated according to your professional judgment. This may also include proactive consultation to provide information when there is potential for an emergency that may require additional support or expertise.
- Request for information or opinion: "Ms. K has atypical glandular cells on her most recent Pap smear. I've never seen this before. What do you recommend for her follow-up?" In this instance you are looking for information from your consultant physician to guide your client's care when you have reached the limits of your experience and knowledge. This is a good time to discuss future management of such patients and to determine your own needs for continuing education.
- Request for evaluation: "I'm sending Mrs. S to you for evaluation of her enlarged uterus. She

is a 47-year-old G2, P2002 who has had severe menorrhagia for the past 5 months. We have discussed potential treatments, and she is interested in exploring endometrial ablation to treat her menorrhagia." In this instance the client has a problem that requires evaluation and treatment that is not within your scope of practice. Clearly stating previous discussions, client preferences, and your expectations for care can influence the care provided to the client. The expectation is that the client will return to you for care once the problem has resolved or been treated. This is a more formal consultation and a consult form, as well as release of supporting clinical documents with patient permission, should be initiated.

- Transfer of care: "Mrs. R has a large lesion consistent with cervical cancer. I am transferring her to you for care of this problem." In this instance the client has a problem that necessitates ongoing physician management. Transfer of care means that the client is released from midwifery care and the consultant is expected to assume responsibility for her ongoing medical care. In an emergency (e.g., "Ms. P has a postpartum hemorrhage. I believe she has retained placental parts. Her EBL is currently at 1000 ml. Please come to L & D immediately."), the nature of the problem requires immediate action on the part of the consultant. Expectations for immediate physician evaluation of a client must be clearly stated. For those midwives who practice in the out-of-hospital setting, calling the OB/GYN or pediatrician on-call may be preferable to simply calling 911 or the emergency room. If you have an established working relationship, a direct admission to the maternity unit may be possible.
- Other collaborative practice relationships: Primary care providers commonly care for midwifery clients in the event of a general medical problem such as hypertension, diabetes, or heart disease. Although some midwives have

expanded their practice to include primary care services, this is often limited to treatment of acute minor conditions, such as back pain and upper respiratory infections. Midwives may initially manage selected chronic conditions, such as mild depression, and refer if no improvement occurs with standard measures, or they may continue management of selected stable chronic conditions, such as mild asthma, and refer if the condition destabilizes.

Every practitioner caring for women, regardless of their scope of practice, should develop a network of care providers that may include physicians, chiropractors, naturopaths, acupuncturists, dieticians, mental health professionals, social service personnel, clergy, support and self-help groups, local emergency services, homeless shelters, and addiction centers. This network provides the mechanism by which midwives may address the varied needs of the women who come to them for care.

A key element to providing woman-oriented care is to connect women with the services they require and may not know how to access. This may include a combination of mainstream medical care, alternative or complementary modalities, and nonmedical services. The role of the midwife is to listen to women, clarify their needs, and facilitate meeting those needs in a caring and nonjudgmental manner. Your individual philosophy of midwifery care should guide the care you provide.

Clear discussion of the parameters of midwifery practice, the practice location(s), practice limitations or boundaries required by collaborative relationships, practice agreements, and clinical options of midwifery care (including privileges) goes a long way toward evaluating whether a particular midwifery practice is appropriate for the individual client.

Collaborative practice connects midwives to additional health professionals who provide ongoing or specialty care that is not within the midwife's scope of practice. Additionally, these other specialists become aware of the services you offer to women and can be a source of referrals to your practice as well. Women's health care forms a continuum that extends from home birth and alternative care, through general medical and community-based medicine and midwifery, to high-tech tertiary care and specialty services.

Collaborative practice means that a working relationship is formed between the attending midwife and the physician or other health care provider. Midwives function as an integral part of the health care system. Not all services are appropriate for all women. Midwives have a responsibility to provide access to services as indicated by the individual woman's health, preferences, and the midwife's scope of practice. The primary goal of the collaborative relationship is accessing the best care for each client as needed.

The ACNM joint statement with the American College of Obstetricians and Gynecologists clearly states the following: "When obstetrician-gynecologists and certified nurse-midwives/certified midwives collaborate, they should concur on a clear mechanism for consultation, collaboration, and referral based on the individual needs of the patient" (ACNM, 2002).

The process of providing care can be broken into several discrete components that occur after a client or situational assessment and that are relevant to risk management (American Academy of Family Physicians, 2004):

- Identification of conditions that may increase client risk or potential risk (working diagnosis)
- Potential for significant adverse effects directly related to the actual or potential risk (assessment of risk related to diagnosis)
- Potential impact of the adverse effects on the client and the provider (client- and midwife-specific hazard analysis)
- Management of risk (midwifery plan of care and provider risk management strategy)

Risk to the Client

Quantification of risk for an individual is a difficult task and requires careful counseling that avoids absolutes. When a client is "at risk," it is important to specify what condition or complication she is at risk for and to then give a probability of both its occurrence and its nonoccurrence. For example, if a woman undergoing amniocentesis has a 1% chance of rupture of membranes during the procedure, then she has a 99% chance of no rupture during the procedure. However, even with reliable odds to share with a woman regarding her choices and their potential sequelae, the experience she will have is 100%—she will either 100% rupture or 100% not rupture her membranes.

New data are continually being compiled about risks associated with race, ethnicity, genetics, lifestyle, behaviors, and other factors. By keeping abreast of new data and incorporating it into your knowledge base, you are then able to provide clients with information relevant to health care decisions and options that are appropriate for them. Frank discussions about the relative risk of options for care should include the potential for unexpected outcomes, the unpredictability of individual response, and the impact and importance of self-determination.

Risk to the Unborn and Newborn

Calculating risk to the unborn, and by extension to the newborn, is also difficult and fraught with emotions as parents try to make the best decisions possible on behalf of their child. Pregnant women and their families look to their midwives as skilled professionals with the ability to identify potential problems, discuss the various options open to them, involve them in decision-making, and take corrective action to safeguard their babies in the womb.

How information is presented during pregnancy and women's health care visits may influence the client's attitude about her body, the safety of birth, the ability of the health care system to meet her and her baby's needs, and her ability to parent. Risk should be addressed in a realistic fashion that is supportive of women and birth and does not undermine traditional, alternative, or mainstream medical providers. You can foster the concept that women's bodies and birth work while still addressing the fact that there are no guarantees of perfect outcomes, and that access to basic and advanced medical services is available.

Risk to the Midwife

Each midwife needs to determine what is included in her own individual scope of practice. Not every midwife provides every service. A scope of practice is a dynamic entity, one that changes with experience, practice location, fatigue, staffing, distance to specialty care, and so on. Each midwife must manage individual professional risk by constantly assessing the scope of her or his midwifery practice and whether it meets the midwife's needs as well as those of the community of women served.

Identification of a woman with risk factors may impact midwifery management of risk in a number of respects: It may result in a transfer of care, a consultation, or continued independent management of the woman's care. It depends on the midwife's expertise and self-determined scope of practice, state laws regarding midwifery practice, and the midwife's comfort in caring for the particular risk factor in this individual, health care setting, community, and legal climate.

Standards of practice define the expected knowledge and behaviors of the midwife according to her education, certification, and licensure status. Midwives are held accountable to national, state, and local standards. Each midwife should maintain familiarity with the professional standards, state laws, and rules that govern her midwifery practice. Professional standards are defined by the ACNM, MANA, and the International Confederation of Midwives. Each of them requires knowledge of the following:

- Midwifery practice standards and recommendations
- Pathophysiology and treatment of commonly encountered conditions
- Indications for and access to medical consultation

Risk Management Plan

The term *risk management* has acquired a negative connotation in recent years, because many liability insurance companies use this term to identify risk factors that may indicate an increased likelihood for a poor outcome and litigation. A comprehensive and realistic midwifery practice risk management plan demonstrates to the liability insurance carrier that the midwife seeks to provide care that is consistent with best practice, is cognizant of the risk involved in this profession, and has taken reasonable steps to limit that risk.

A risk management plan is a helpful way to organize essential information about the various components needed to identify and manage risk in midwifery practice. The midwifery risk management plan should include practice policies and procedures that address topics such as the following (Greenwald, 2004):

- Written practice description
- Philosophy of practice
- Location(s) of practice
- Practice guidelines and standards
- The role and scope of practice for each midwife
- Medical record documentation standards
- Documentation forms that reflect care provided
- Informed consent policy and process
- Client autonomy in decision-making
- Provisions for practice coverage
- Indications for consultation or referral
- Collaborative practice relationships
- Plan for transfer of care or client when indicated
- Requirements for continuing education
- Education requirements for expanded scope of practice
- Peer review and outcomes-based evaluation of care
- Review process for client or practice-related complaints or concerns
- Licensing and professional practice issues as legally defined by state or professional organization
- Malpractice claims procedures

When Bad Things Happen

Midwives vary tremendously in the amount of risk they are willing to live with on a day-to-day basis. Some may prefer to work in settings where there is a physician available at all times, whereas others may practice in isolated settings where the nearest physician is miles away. Increased midwife autonomy may be associated with increased midwife risk, as can practicing in a setting that is antagonistic to midwives, regardless of their legal status.

Even with thorough documentation of excellent care and a healthy actively involved client, things can still go awry. Wherever there is life, there is also the possibility of death, illness, or injury. Most midwives encounter bad outcomes in caring for their clients from time to time in the course of their careers (Guidera et al., 2007). This is devastating to the client and her family but also to the midwife involved. Midwives' reactions after poor outcomes in practice can range from sorrow to departure from practice (Table 1-3).

Allow yourself time to grieve this event with your client and on your own, but also be prepared to take practical steps that protect your ability to continue to practice and to recover emotionally. Midwives have reported that formal debriefing with a counselor, attorney, midwife partners, or morbidity and mortality committee members have been helpful strategies to promote personal and professional recovery (McCool et al., 2007).

Review the chart with a midwife practice partner or your physician consultant—someone with legitimate rights to access the chart and the ability to evaluate the care. Some charts are automatically reviewed for certain key events in the hospital; for example, the occurrence of neonatal seizure or maternal death is discussed at a perinatal morbidity and mortality review. However, women's health care provided in the outpatient setting may not have such a review mechanism. It is important to extract the learning value from these difficult situations while maintaining client confidentiality.

Most malpractice suits in midwifery are initiated for poor neonatal outcomes from events such as shoulder dystocia or fetal distress, from misinterpretation of fetal heart rate tracings, or from delay in consultation (Angelini & Greenwald, 2005). If errors were made by you or your staff, it is best to be honest and compassionate with your client in a timely fashion. You can apologize without implying guilt or blame, such as "I am sorry this complication occurred" or "I am so sorry this happened to you." Continue providing such support to your client, just as you would before the event and document ongoing care and client response. It is always appropriate to share sympathy and sorrow with your client. Understand, however, that although midwives pride themselves on delivering excellent relationship-based care, this is only one of many considerations in a client's decision to take legal action.

ETHICAL MIDWIFERY PRACTICE

Ethical midwifery practice is based on a human rights framework (Thompson, 2004). This framework includes four foundational ethical principles:

1. Autonomy: The human right to personal independence and the capacity to make decisions and act on them

2. Justice: The human right to be treated fairly and with reasoned care

3. Beneficence: The human right to be treated with intent to do good

4. Nonmalfeasance: The human right to be treated with intent to avoid harm, the classic "First do no harm" directive attributed to Hippocrates

These guiding ethical principles are reflected in midwifery's philosophical tenets and have also been codified specifically for midwives by several midwifery organizations, including the ACNM, MANA, and the International Confederation of Midwives (MANA, 2006; Thompson & King, 2004).

For these ethical principles to have any meaning, they must be a touchstone for your practice decisions. Ethical problems are not always clear-cut issues. Sometimes, it is a matter of choosing between what is right and what is easy. There are ethical dilemmas inherent in midwifery care, and they are sometimes embedded in the simple day-to-day provision of care. An example of this is the client who says to you "I'll do whatever you think I should" after you provide a counseling session on birth control options (Narrigan, 2004). The reflective practitioner will examine and learn from decisions made

Table 1-3   Steps for Living With Bad Outcomes in Practice

DOS	DON'TS
Understand the emotional nature of this event for you and your client.	Do not alter the chart; however, a late entry is acceptable. Document it as such.
Continue to provide excellent midwifery care with good documentation, and take care of yourself physically and emotionally.	Do not discuss the details of the event with family and friends; however, do share your feelings to prevent emotional isolation so often associated with litigation.
Contact your malpractice insurance company for guidance in case a suit occurs.	Do not delay in honest communication with your client.
Know that you are not alone. All midwives experience poor outcomes during a lifetime of practice; many become involved in legal proceedings in the aftermath of a poor outcome.	

and actions taken in the clinical setting from an ethical perspective. Midwifery is a morally important endeavor that promotes women's optimal health, and the ethics of clinical care are worthy of your continued and thoughtful consideration.

EXEMPLARY MIDWIFERY PRACTICE

Optimal midwifery care occurs when the midwife is able to support the physiologic processes of birth and well-woman care while at the same time remaining vigilant for the unexpected (Kennedy, 2000). Remaining attuned to small details that might subtly indicate a significant change in maternal, fetal, or the well-woman's status provides the midwife with the opportunity for early identification of problems and prompt initiation of treatment geared toward improving outcomes. Midwifery encourages care that is individualized for each woman and each birth. Patience with the birth process is a hallmark of midwifery care. Midwives' compassionate and attentive care reinforces women's belief in their ability to give birth and care for themselves. By utilizing interventions and technology only when necessary, midwives bridge the chasm between medicine and traditional healing.

Exemplary midwives demonstrate professional integrity, honesty, compassion, and understanding. They are able to communicate effectively, remain open-minded and flexible, and provide care in a nonjudgmental manner. When these attributes are coupled with excellent clinical skills, they result in attentive and thorough assessments, excellent screening and preventive health counseling processes, and infinite patience with the process of labor and birth.

Finally, midwives provide personalized care that is tailored to the individual and her present circumstances. Regardless of clinical practice setting or educational background, midwives endeavor to create an environment that engenders mutual respect and focuses primarily on meeting the needs of the woman or mother and family. Recognition of individual variation is tempered by a thorough grounding in both normal and pathologic processes. This broad scope provides the midwife with a clear view of the continuum of health and allows more accurate assessment and personalization of care.

The midwife whose ideal is to provide exemplary midwifery care must actively create a balance between her professional life as a midwife and the needs and demands of her personal life. Time off to refresh and rejuvenate is as necessary to quality practice as is ongoing professional education. Personal relationships nourish the midwife and provide emotional sustenance. Each midwife must remain attentive to her own needs to bring her best to midwifery.

Midwives strive to provide exemplary midwifery and women's health care. This demands the development of excellent clinical skills and the determination and persistence to couple them with sound clinical judgment. Each midwife is called on, time and again, to make critical decisions and to act on them in a way that is appropriate for the setting in which she practices while demonstrating respect and honor for the uniqueness of each woman and family in her care.

Exemplary midwifery practice, according to Kennedy (2000), encompasses several key concepts. One of these concepts is the basic philosophy of midwifery and its active expression through the individual midwife's clinical practice. Each midwife's philosophy of care is reflected in her or his choice and use of healing modalities, the quality of her or his caring for and about women, and her or his support for midwifery as a profession. The midwife's underlying philosophy is brought to life through her or his clinical practice and professional involvement in midwifery. Throughout this book the driving philosophy is that of the ACNM (Box 1-2).

Box 1-2   Philosophy of the American College of Nurse-Midwives

We, the midwives of the American College of Nurse-Midwives, affirm the power and strength of women and the importance of their health in the well-being of families, communities, and nations. We believe in the basic human rights of all persons, recognizing that women often incur an undue burden of risk when these rights are violated.

We believe every person has a right to:

- Equitable, ethical, and accessible quality health care that promotes healing and health
- Health care that respects human dignity, individuality, and diversity among groups
- Complete and accurate information to make informed health care decisions
- Self-determination and active participation in health care decisions
- Involvement of a woman's designated family members, to the extent desired, in all health care experiences

We believe the best model of health care for a woman and her family:

- Promotes a continuous and compassionate partnership
- Acknowledges a person's life experiences and knowledge
- Includes individualized methods of care and healing guided by the best evidence available
- Involves therapeutic use of human presence and skillful communication

We honor the normalcy of women's life cycle events. We believe in:

- Watchful waiting and nonintervention in normal processes
- Appropriate use of interventions and technology for current or potential health problems
- Consultation, collaboration, and referral with other members of the health care team as needed to provide optimal health care

We affirm that midwifery care incorporates these qualities and that women's health care needs are well served through midwifery care.

Finally, we value formal education, lifelong individual learning, and the development and application of research to guide ethical and competent midwifery practice. These beliefs and values provide the foundation for commitment to individual and collective leadership at the community, state, national, and international level to improve the health of women and their families worldwide.

Source: American College of Nurse-Midwives [ACNM], 2004.

SUMMARY

Defining one's personal philosophy of midwifery care and expressing it in practice is one of the joys of midwifery. What constitutes "best care" for women, mothers, and infants is determined individually at the point of care with the woman herself and with standards of care and practice guidelines used as guides along the way. Clinical judgment is the heart and soul of midwifery care. A mindful approach to practice reduces client and midwife risk, improves outcomes, and fosters collaborative relationships. This provides the opportunity for the exemplary midwife to rest better at night and to continue a career of service to women and their families for decades.

WEB RESOURCES

Review of Systems form:
http://www.fammed.ouhsc.edu/forms/FMC_ROS_Form.pdf

American Cancer Society Guidelines for the Early Detection of Cancer
http://www.cancer.org/docroot/PED/content/PED_2_3X_ACS_Cancer_Detection_Guidelines_36.asp?sitearea=PED

National Institutes of Health: National High Blood Pressure Education Program
http://www.nhlbi.nih.gov/guidelines/hypertension/

National Institutes of Health: National Guidelines Clearinghouse
http://www.guideline.gov/index.aspx OR
http://www.ahrq.gov/clinic/gcpspu.htm

National Heart, Lung, and Blood Institute: Clinical Practice Guidelines
http://www.nhlbi.nih.gov/guidelines/

U.S. Preventive Services Task Force
http://www.ahrq.gov/clinic/uspstf/uspstopics.htm

REFERENCES

American Academy of Family Physicians. (2004). *Risk management and medical liability*. Retrieved January 4, 2008 from http://www.aafp.org/online/etc/medialib/aafp_org/documents/about/rap/curriculum/risk_management_and.Par.0001.File.tmp/riskmanagement.pdf

American College of Nurse-Midwives (ACNM). (2002). *Joint statement with the American College of Obstetricians and Gynecologists*. Silver Spring, MD: Author. Retrieved January 4, 2008 from http://www.midwife.org/siteFiles/position/Joint_Statement_05.pdf

American College of Nurse-Midwives (ACNM). (2004). *Philosophy of the American College of Nurse-Midwives*. Silver Spring, MD: Author. Retrieved January 4, 2008 from http://www.midwife.org/philosophy.cfm

American College of Nurse-Midwives (ACNM). (2007). *Core competencies for basic midwifery practice*. Silver Spring, MD: Author. Retrieved January 4, 2008 from http://www.midwife.org/siteFiles/descriptive/Core_Competencies_6_07_3.pdf

American Medical Association (AMA). (2004). *Current procedural terminology*. Chicago: Author.

Angelini, D., & Greenwald, L. (2005). Closed claims analysis of 65 medical malpractice cases involving nurse-midwives. *Journal of Midwifery & Women's Health*, 50, 454–460.

Farley, C. L. (2005). Midwifery's research heritage: a Delphi survey of midwife scholars. *Journal of Midwifery and Women's Health*, 50, 122–128.

Greenwald, L. (Ed.). (2004). *Perspectives on clinical risk management*. Boston: Risk Management Publications, ProMutual Group.

Guidera, M., McCool, W., Poell, J., & Stenson, M. (2007). *What to do if you are named in a lawsuit. The professional liability handbook*. In Professional Liability Resource Packet. Silver Spring, MD: American College of Nurse-Midwives. Retrieved 1/3/08 from: http://www.midwife.org/professional_liability.cfm

Hill, P. F., Lipson, J. G., & Meleis, A. I. (2003). *Caring for women cross-culturally*. Philadelphia: F.A. Davis.

Johnson, S. (2001). Documentation. In R. Carroll (Ed.). *Risk management handbook for health care organizations*. San Francisco: Jossey-Bass.

Kennedy, H. P. (2000). A model of exemplary midwifery practice: results of a Delphi study. *Journal of Midwifery & Women's Health*, 45, 4–19.

Lothian, J. A. (2004). Do not disturb: the importance of privacy in labor. *Journal of Perinatology Education*, 13:4–6. Retrieved January, 4, 2008 from http://www.pubmedcentral.nih.gov/articlerender.fcgi?artid=1595201

Lydon-Rochelle, M. T., Hodnett, E., Renfrew, M. J., & Lumley, J. (2003). A systematic approach for midwifery students: how to consider evidence-based research findings. *Journal of Midwifery and Women's Health*, 48, 273–277.

McCool, W., Guidera, M., Delaney, E., & Hakala, S. (2007). The role of litigation in the professional practice of midwives in the United States: results from a nationwide survey of certified nurse-midwives/certified midwives. *Journal of Midwifery and Women's Health*, 52, 458-464.

Midwives Alliance of North America [MANA]. (2006). *MANA statement of values and ethics*. Retrieved January 4, 2008 from http://www.mana.org/valuesethics.html

McFarlin, B. L., Gibson, M. H., O'Rear, J., & Harman, P. (1999). A national survey of herbal preparation use by nurse-midwives for labor stimulation: review of the literature and recommendations for practice. *Journal of Midwifery and Women's Health*, 44, 205–216.

Narrigan, D. (2004). Examining an ethical dilemma: a case study in clinical practice. *Journal of Midwifery & Women's Health*, 49, 243–249.

National Association for Healthcare Quality. (1998). *Guide to quality management* (pp. 44–45). Glenview, IL: Author.

Rozovsky, F. (2001). Informed consent as a loss control process. In R. Carroll (Ed.). *Risk management handbook for health care organizations.* San Francisco: Jossey-Bass.

Sackett, D. L., Richardson, W. S., Rosenberg, W., & Haynes, R. B. (1997). *Evidence-based medicine: how to practice and teach EBM.* New York: Churchill Livingstone.

Schon, D. A. (1983). *The reflective practitioner: how professionals think in action.* New York: Basic Books.

Slager, J. (2004). *Business Concepts for Health Care Providers.* Sudbury, MA: Jones & Bartlett.

Thompson, J. B. (2004). A human rights framework for midwifery care. *Journal of Midwifery & Women's Health, 49,* 175–181.

Thompson, J. B., & King, T. L. (2004). A code of ethics for midwives. *Journal of Midwifery & Women's Health, 49,* 263–265.

University of Washington School of Medicine. (1999). *What is informed consent?* Retrieved January 4, 2008 from http://depts.washington.edu/bioethx/topics/consent.html

Care of the Woman During Pregnancy

2

Prenatal care is a comprehensive ongoing program of care that addresses the biophysical, psychosocial, and educational needs of the pregnant woman and her family.

The content and structure of prenatal care follows a typical pattern of scheduled visits and tests, but this standard package of care can be easily modified to meet the needs and preferences of the women we serve. Prenatal care is an opportunity to deliver meaningful health care at a transformative time in a woman's life in the context of a continuing and nurturing relationship. We are privileged to witness and support the growth and development of the mother as well as the fetus.

The purpose of prenatal care is to provide primary preventive health care to all pregnant women and to identify that small, but significant, number of women whose pregnancy will deviate from the wide range of normal in a manner that may jeopardize maternal or fetal well-being. For those women with conditions that fall outside of normal variations, the midwife must be prepared to consult with, collaborate with, or refer to the appropriate specialist. For the pregnant client, an obstetrician or a perinatologist is the most common consultant needed, although pregnant women are susceptible to all the same ills and injuries as anyone else, so the services of other health care professionals, such as a dermatologist, endocrinologist, or physical therapist, may be required.

The basic components of the provision of prenatal care are included in the core competencies of midwifery practice. For further information, the midwife is encouraged to compare the standards for basic midwifery practice that have been developed by the American College of Nurse-Midwives, the Midwives Alliance of North America, and the International Confederation of Midwives. By reviewing the core documents of these organizations (all available online by accessing the respective organizations' Web sites), one can gain an understanding of the expected standards for midwifery practice in the United States. Additionally, each midwife must be aware of state and local regulations, resources, and standards of practice.

American College of Nurse-Midwives	http://www.midwife.org
Midwives Alliance of North America	http://www.mana.org
International Confederation of Midwives	http://www.internationalmidwives.org

Midwives are concerned with the structure, process, and outcomes of prenatal care and the intrinsic characteristics of the clients they serve. All these components are important in developing a model of care and service delivery that is responsive to women's needs and in ensuring ongoing quality assessment and improvement. The most typical model of prenatal care, recommended by the American College of Obstetricians and Gynecologists (ACOG), is care that is rendered by a provider or group of providers structured in 12 to 13 visits scheduled every 4 weeks until the 28th week of pregnancy, every 2 weeks until the 36th week of pregnancy, and then weekly until birth. Other models include a reduced visit schedule for low risk women, care provided by interdisciplinary health care teams, and group prenatal care (Rising et al., 2004; Walker et al., 2002).

Every woman has unique yet universal needs during pregnancy. It is a time of many changes and adjustments of a physical, psychological, and social nature. Caring for a woman during this time of transition can foster individual autonomy and enhance self-care practices. This may improve her ability to care for her child and to develop her strengths as a woman and a mother.

Many of the women we see are unfamiliar with the expectations of the health care system and need some guidance to navigate the system or to negotiate for care that is appropriate to their needs. Building a warm, caring, and professional relationship allows for mutual trust to develop. Trust fosters active maternal participation in health care decisions. A woman who trusts her midwife is more likely to accept the recommendations of the midwife if challenges or complications

occur. The midwife's ethical obligation, then, is to behave in a trustworthy manner by providing care during pregnancy that includes respecting each woman's individual desires in relation to the preferred type of health care provider, the amount of active participation in her care that she desires, her planned and preferred location of labor and birth, and the methods to access medical services should they be needed. Each midwife is responsible for outlining to the pregnant client the scope of her practice and usual parameters for prenatal, labor and birth, and postpartum care services.

The amount and types of testing performed during pregnancy should be determined by indications for testing or evaluation, current recommendations for practice, and discussion with the client regarding the risks, benefits, and alternatives to testing or evaluation processes. It is important to share information regarding costs of tests and procedures so she will be aware of any costs incurred. A method to clearly document a woman's decision to decline or refuse an offered or recommended test or procedure is an essential mechanism to have in place.

Maternal participation in prenatal care encourages self-determination and may enhance a woman's confidence to labor and give birth in a manner that helps her to feel safe and successful. The process of participation builds trust and fosters resilience in the face of unexpected or unfortunate events. Ongoing dialogue with the client demonstrates the multitude of potential situations and options that are possible in childbirth and encourages strength and flexibility on the part of both the mother to be and the midwife to deal with whatever circumstances come their way.

DIAGNOSIS OF PREGNANCY

Key Clinical Information

The diagnosis of pregnancy should be entertained when caring for any woman of childbearing age. Pregnancy is the most common cause of secondary amenorrhea in women in this life stage (Seller, 2007). Pregnancy signs and symptoms are classified as presumptive, those changes that the mother can perceive; probable, those changes that can be detected by the examiner; and positive, those changes that can be directly attributed to the fetus (Varney et al., 2004).

The diagnosis of pregnancy may be a welcome event or devastating news. Many women have mixed feelings about the changes that pregnancy will bring to their lives. Ambivalence is common as the newly pregnant woman adjusts her self-image to include a baby that is more an abstraction than a reality in the early days of pregnancy. The diagnosis of pregnancy should be shared in a private setting in a straightforward and kind manner. This allows the woman to express a wide range of emotions, and the midwife can then take her cues from the woman's response.

Client History and Chart Review:
Components of the History to Consider
(Varney et al., 2004)

- Reproductive history
  - Gravity, parity (G, P)
  - Last menstrual period
  - Method of birth control
  - Conception issues
    - Known or suspected date of conception
    - Assisted reproductive technologies or treatments
  - Symptoms of pregnancy
    - Breast tenderness
    - Fatigue
    - Fetal movement
    - Nausea and/or vomiting
    - Urinary frequency
  - Birth history

- Signs or symptoms of complications
  - Pain or cramping
  - Bleeding
  - Drugs or herbs taken since last menstrual period
- Relevant social history
  - Client intent and feelings about possible pregnancy
  - Information about the father of the baby
  - Support systems
- Relevant medical/surgical history
  - Allergies
  - Medications
  - Medical conditions
  - Surgeries
  - Previous sexually transmitted infections (STIs)
- Review of systems

Physical Examination:
Components of the Physical Exam to Consider

- Vital signs
- Skin changes
  - Darkening of pigmented skin
  - Vascular spiders
  - Palmar erythema
  - Striae
- Breast changes
  - Enlargement
  - Increased nodularity
  - Increased vascularity
- Abdominal examination
  - Fetal heart tones
  - Fundal height
  - Palpable fetal movement
  - Abdominal tenderness and consistency
- Pelvic evaluation
  - Uterine sizing
  - Consistency of uterus and cervix
  - Color of cervix
  - Cervical motion tenderness
  - Vaginal or cervical discharge
  - Adnexal tenderness

Clinical Impression:
Differential Diagnoses and Code Groups
to Consider
Additional suffix may apply (ICD9data.com, 2007;
Seller, 2007)

- Pregnancy examination or test, positive result
  (ICD-9 code V72.42)
- Also consider
  - Ectopic pregnancy (ICD-9 codes 633)
  - Other unwanted pregnancy (ICD-9 codes
    V22 and V61.7) (see Unplanned
    Pregnancy—Chapter 6)
  - Threatened abortion (ICD-9 codes 640)
  - Molar pregnancy (ICD-9 codes 630)
  - Blighted ovum (ICD-9 codes 631)
- Secondary amenorrhea (ICD-9 codes 626.0)
  (see Amenorrhea—Chapter 7)

Diagnostic Testing:
Diagnostic Tests and Procedures to Consider

- Urine or serum human chorionic gonadotropin
  (HCG)
- Quantitative β-HCG
- Abdominal or vaginal ultrasound

Providing Treatment:
Therapeutic Measures to Consider

- Prenatal or other vitamin supplement with
  folic acid
- Treatment of any underlying condition as
  indicated

Providing Treatment:
Alternative Measures to Consider

- Natural prenatal vitamin supplement
- Whole foods diet
- High folate foods
- Red raspberry leaf tea

Providing Support:
Education and Support Measures to Consider

- Pregnancy options counseling as indicated
  (Simmonds & Likis, 2005)

- Diet and nutrition counseling
- Prenatal care
  - Prenatal testing
  - Family involvement
- Practice
  - Providers
  - Medical affiliations
  - Billing arrangements
  - Birth options
    - Location(s)
  - Philosophy of care
  - Parent rights and responsibilities

Follow-up Care:
Follow-up Measures to Consider

- Document
  - Expected due date (EDD)
  - Relevant history
  - Clinical findings
  - Clinical impression
  - Discussion and client preferences
  - Midwifery plan of care
- Return for continued care
  - Between 6–12 weeks gestation for initial
    prenatal visit
  - As soon as possible if more than 12 weeks
    gestation
  - Prenatal testing as indicated and desired

Collaborative Practice:
Consider Consultation or Referral

- Maternity care services
  - Genetic counseling
  - Amniocentesis
  - Adoption services
  - Abortion services
  - Specialty care
- Social services
  - Pregnancy verification statement
    for various agencies, such as WIC,
    Medicaid
- For diagnosis or treatment outside the mid-
  wife's scope of practice

INITIAL EVALUATION OF THE PREGNANT WOMAN

Key Clinical Information

The initial evaluation of the pregnant woman provides the basis for ongoing prenatal care. Careful attention to client interaction, client history, and physical examination can help the midwife develop a comprehensive yet dynamic midwifery plan of care created with the client and alert the midwife to sensitive concerns that may require further investigation or follow-up over time. Gentle touch, coupled with an organized, systematic, yet unhurried manner, is ideal during the first visit. Careful documentation of all information is essential to allow for clear communication with other health care team members and to serve as a foundation of information for the busy midwife. This client encounter builds on the information obtained in the pregnancy diagnosis office visit. Some practices routinely separate the various activities and assessments done at the initial evaluation of the pregnant woman into two shorter office visits, because there is a lot to accomplish at this visit. This is a time intensive visit, but it is well worth the investment of time and energy to establish a good rapport with the pregnant woman and her family and to cocreate an optimal plan of care for this woman and her baby.

Client History and Chart Review:
Components of the History to Consider
(Varney et al., 2004)

- Cultural and demographic information
- OB/GYN history
  - Present pregnancy history
    - LMP, interval and flow
    - Signs and symptoms
  - G, P, pregnancy information, and complications
  - Gynecologic disorders or problems
  - Sexual history
  - Contraceptive history

- Health risk evaluation (see Evaluation of Health Risks in the Pregnant Woman)
- Past medical/surgical history
- Family history
- Social history
- Review of systems (ROS)

Physical Examination:
Components of the Physical Exam to Consider

- Vital signs
- Observation of general status
- Head, eyes, ears, nose, and throat (HEENT)
- Skin
  - Striae
  - Scars, tracks, or bruises
  - Body art, piercings, tattoos
- Cardiorespiratory system
- Breasts
- Abdomen
  - Fundal height
  - Fetal heart rate (FHR)
  - Fetal lie and position
- Gastrointestinal system
- Genitourinary system
  - Speculum examination
    - Vagina
    - Cervix
    - Collection of laboratory specimens
  - Bimanual examination
    - Uterine size, contour
    - Tenderness
    - Pelvimetry
  - Rectal examination as needed
- Musculoskeletal system
  - Varicosities

Clinical Impression:
Differential Diagnoses and Code Groups to Consider
Additional suffix may apply (ICD9data.com, 2007; Seller, 2000)

- Pregnancy, normal (ICD-9 codes V22)
- High risk pregnancy (ICD-9 codes V23)

- Secondary diagnoses related to other findings as indicated by
  - History
  - Physical examination
  - Diagnostic testing

Diagnostic Testing:
Diagnostic Tests and Procedures to Consider (Frye, 2007; Institute for Clinical Systems Improvement, 2006)
- Pregnancy testing
  - Urine or serum HCG
  - Quantitative β-HCG
- STI testing
  - Chlamydia and gonorrhea testing
  - Venereal Disease Research Laboratory (VDRL) or rapid plasma reagin (RPR)
  - Human immunodeficiency virus (HIV) testing
  - Hepatitis B surface antigen
- Pap smear with reflex human papilloma virus testing
- Hematology evaluation and titers
  - Hemoglobin and hematocrit or complete blood count (CBC)
  - Blood type, Rh factor, and antibody screen
  - Rubella titer
  - Varicella antibody screen
- Fetal and genetic testing
  - α-Fetoprotein testing
  - Ultrasound, vaginal or pelvic
    - Establish or confirm dates
    - Fetal viability
    - Fetal survey
- Urinalysis, with culture as indicated by history
- Group B strep culture at 35 to 37 weeks gestation (Centers for Disease Control and Prevention, 2002)
- For selected high risk populations or individuals, consider
  - Ultrasound for nuchal translucency
  - Amniocentesis or chorionic villus sampling
  - Cystic fibrosis testing
  - Thyroid-stimulating hormone

- Sickle cell screen or hemoglobin electrophoresis
- Blood lead screening
- One-hour glucose challenge test
- Wet prep for bacterial vaginosis, candidiasis, and trichomoniasis
- Tuberculosis testing: purified protein derivative (PPD)
- History of positive PPD or bacillus Calmette-Guérin (BCG) vaccine, consider chest x-ray

Providing Treatment:
Therapeutic Measures to Consider
- Prenatal vitamins with folic acid
- Continued or altered treatment of existing conditions in light of pregnancy diagnosis as indicated

Providing Treatment:
Alternative Measures to Consider (Frye, 1998)
- Regular mild to moderate exercise (ACOG, 2002)
- Adequate rest
- Stress management techniques
- Social support networks
- Whole foods diet
- Dietary sources of
  - Folate
  - Iron
  - Calcium
  - Fiber

Providing Support:
Education and Support Measures to Consider (Davis, 2004)
- Discussion regarding
  - Diet and activity recommendations
  - Danger signs and when to call
  - How to access care providers
  - Usual return visit schedule
  - Recommended prenatal visits
  - Recommended pregnancy, childbirth, and parenting classes
  - Recommended and optional prenatal testing

- Birth options
  - Location of birth
  - Water birth/hydrotherapy availability
  - Vaginal birth after cesarean (VBAC) counseling as needed
- Collaborative medical providers

Follow-up Care:
Follow-up Measures to Consider
- Document
  - Risk factors with plan for care
  - Informed consent as applicable
- Schedule return for prenatal visits
  - Every 4–6 weeks through 28–32 weeks
  - Every 2–3 weeks through 32–36 weeks
  - Weekly from 36 weeks to onset of labor
  - More frequent visits for women with risk factors
- Vaginal birth after cesarean (VBAC) or planned repeat cesarean section
  - ▽ Obtain and review operative notes to verify type of uterine incision
  - Surgical consultation

Collaborative Practice:
Consider Consultation or Referral
- OB/GYN services
  - Per practice standards
  - Genetic or other counseling
  - Other specialists as indicated by secondary diagnoses or findings
- For diagnosis or treatment outside the midwife's scope of practice

EVALUATION OF HEALTH RISKS IN THE PREGNANT WOMAN

Key Clinical Information

One of the important elements of prenatal care is the identification of health risks that may be modified or diminished by prompt diagnosis and treatment. Health risks may have the potential to affect the health of the mother, her unborn baby, or her newly born infant. Health risks may be related to

diet, social habits, genetic heritage, environmental exposures, and cultural or ethnic background and practices. Prenatal identification of health risks offers the opportunity to diagnose or treat actual or potential conditions or provide parents with information and support to help cope with unexpected outcomes.

Many risk factors for pregnant women are associated with habitual or addictive behaviors, such as dietary habits and smoking. The midwife needs to start tackling these modifiable behaviors with the client by assessing her readiness to change. The stages of change model (Connors et al., 2001) offers a framework to explore the client's readiness for behavior change and to suggest appropriate clinician actions designed to facilitate efforts toward positive changes. This model was originally applied in the area of substance abuse but has since been applied to other problem health behaviors. The interested reader is referred to http://www.doh.wa.gov/CFH/mch/documents/CessationFinal_122.pdf for the application of this model to smoking cessation. For those risk factors that cannot be modified, education, support, and planning to address potential problems are critical.

Client History and Chart Review:
Components of the History to Consider
- Maternal demographic information
  - Age
  - Partner status
  - Education
  - Socioeconomic status
  - Ethnic/racial background
  - Employment status
  - Religious preference
  - Sexual orientation
- Review of personal medical history
  - Diseases or health disorders
  - Medication use, over the counter or prescription
  - Surgeries

- Alternative therapies
  - Herbs
  - Homeopathy
  - Acupuncture
- OB/GYN history
  - Prior pregnancy conditions or complications
    - Prior pregnancy losses
    - Birth defects
    - Infertility
  - STIs
  - Previous gynecologic procedures
    - Loop electrosurgical excision procedure (LEEP)
    - Myomectomy
    - Hysterosalpingogram
- Review of family medical history
  - Ethnic heritage
  - Hereditary or genetic health conditions
  - Cultural health habits or conditions
- Pregnancy-related risks
  - Review of health habits
  - Smoking, alcohol, and/or drug use
  - Signs or symptoms of concern
- Nutritional status
  - Usual diet
  - Caffeine use (300 mg or less daily) (Christian & Brent, 2001)
  - Pica
- Physical activity
- Review of environmental exposures (Arnesen, 2006)
  - Cats or raw meat (toxoplasmosis)
  - Paint and pipes in older homes and various household items (lead)
  - Fish (mercury)
  - Soft cheeses, packaged meats (listeriosis)
  - Household cleaning chemicals
  - Occupational exposures
- Review of social situation and support
  - Presence of caring partner or support
  - Number and relationship of people in the home
  - Anticipated cultural practices during pregnancy

- Economic situation and resources
- Risk factors or signs of abuse
- Review of systems

Physical Examination:
Components of the Physical Exam to Consider
- Physical assessment, including
  - Vital signs
  - Weight
  - Height
    - Body mass index (BMI)
- Evaluate for evidence of
  - Illness
  - Malnutrition
  - Exhaustion
  - Abuse
- Skin examination for signs of
  - Needle tracks
  - Bruising
  - Burns
  - Petechia
  - Lesions
- Smell for signs of
  - Tobacco or alcohol use
  - Ketosis
  - General hygiene

Clinical Impression:
Differential Diagnoses and Code Groups
to Consider
Additional suffix may apply (ICD9data.com, 2007; Seller, 2000)
- Pregnancy, normal (ICD-9 codes V22)
- Pregnancy at risk (ICD-9 codes V23)
  - Health habits, specify
  - Genetic disorders
  - Maternal age
  - Health conditions, specify
  - Prior uterine or cervical surgery
  - Infection
  - Abuse
    - Physical
    - Sexual
    - Emotional

- Substance abuse
- Poor social support
- Occupational hazards
- Noncompliance (ICD-9 code V15.81), secondary to
  - Communication
  - Transportation
  - Limited resources
  - Psychological issues
  - Self-determination
  - Knowledge deficit
- Other diagnoses as noted

Diagnostic Testing:
Diagnostic Tests and Procedures to Consider
- Drug screening
- HIV testing
- Hepatitis B and C testing
- Sickle cell prep
- α-Fetoprotein, triple or quadruple screen
- Group B strep testing
- STI testing
- Ultrasound
  - Fetal anatomy
  - Nuchal translucency
- Amniocentesis
- Chorionic villus sampling

Providing Treatment:
Therapeutic Measures to Consider
- Prenatal or multivitamin with folic acid
- Brief behavioral therapy
  - Assess client readiness to change problem behavior in stages of change model
    - Precontemplation (not ready to change)
    - Contemplation (thinking about changing)
    - Preparation (ready to change)
    - Action (changed)
    - Maintenance (staying changed)
    - Relapse (back to previous problem behavior)

- Five As of smoking cessation: ask, advise, assess, assist, arrange (ACOG, 2005)
- Smoking cessation medications
  - Concerns with high risks and low effectiveness for nicotine replacement therapies and bupropion, use in pregnancy is discouraged (ACOG, 2005)
- Other medications or treatments based on diagnosis

Providing Treatment:
Alternative Measures to Consider
- Nutritional support
- Hypnosis to change health habits
- Other treatments based on diagnosis

Providing Support:
Education and Support Measures to Consider
- Allow private time to encourage disclosure
- Provide information about risks and benefits of
  - Current health behaviors
  - Prenatal tests
  - Testing options
  - Treatment options
- Genetic counseling
- Drug screening policy
- Social support services
  - Develop plan for safety (Little, 2000)
- Cultural support services
  - Translation services
- Diagnosis-related support groups

Follow-up Care:
Follow-up Measures to Consider
- Document
- Return visits
  - Frequency determined by
    - Client condition
    - Gestational age
  - Allow time to
    - Develop cooperative relationship
    - Observe for risk-related behaviors
  - Serial drug or STI testing as indicated

Collaborative Practice:
Consider Consultation or Referral

- Maternity care services
  - Genetic screening
  - Amniocentesis or chorionic villus sampling
  - OB/GYN consultation, collaboration or referral
- Medical service
  - As indicated for medical or specialty care
- Social service
  - As indicated by life-style and social indicators
  - Inpatient or outpatient drug rehabilitation program
  - Counseling or therapy
  - Women's shelter/safe house
- For diagnosis or treatment outside the midwife's scope of practice

ONGOING CARE OF THE PREGNANT WOMAN

Key Clinical Information

The routine prenatal visit is anything but routine for the pregnant woman. It is each woman's brief opportunity of having her needs met and her concerns addressed while at the same time being evaluated for the well-being of herself and her child. It provides an opportunity to look for subtle signs or symptoms that may indicate a deviation from normal. It is an opportunity for the midwife to develop the ongoing interaction that builds trust and understanding between patient and provider so that an optimal experience and outcome are achieved.

Prenatal care began in the early 1900s as a method to screen for signs and symptoms of preeclampsia. It has evolved into a platform for teaching and testing. Follow-up activities by the midwife are critical to fully realize the benefits of prenatal care: Follow-up on laboratory and test results, on behavioral changes, and on teaching demonstrates the value placed on these measures. The group prenatal care model capitalizes on the social support and compassion provided

by a cohort of peers—women from diverse backgrounds who meet on the common ground of childbearing.

Client History and Chart Review:
Components of the History to Consider
(Davis, 2004; Frye, 1998; Varney et al., 2004)

- Review relevant aspects of chart before client visit
- Interval history since last visit
  - Gestational age
  - Maternal well-being
    - Nutrition
    - Sleep
    - Activity
    - Bowel and bladder function
    - Signs or symptoms of
      - Preterm labor
      - Pregnancy-induced hypertension
      - Urinary tract infection
      - Vaginal bleeding or discharge
      - Exposure to infectious disease
  - Fetal movement
- Concerns
  - Questions
  - Plans related to pregnancy, labor, and birth

Physical Examination:
Components of the Physical Exam to Consider

- Blood pressure (BP), other vital signs as indicated
- Interval weight gain or loss
- Assessment of general well-being
- Abdominal examination
  - Fundal height
  - Fetal heart tones
  - Estimated fetal weight
  - Fetal lie, presentation, position, and variety
- Costovertebral angle (CVA) tenderness
- Examination of extremities for
  - Edema
  - Varicosities, phlebitis
  - Reflexes
- Additional components as indicated by history

Clinical Impression:
Differential Diagnoses and Code Groups
to Consider
Additional suffix may apply (ICD9data.com, 2007; Seller, 2000)

- Pregnancy
  - Low risk (ICD-9 codes V22)
  - At risk (ICD-9 codes V23), specify
- Additional diagnoses based on
  - History
  - Physical examination
  - Diagnostic testing

Diagnostic Testing:
Diagnostic Tests and Procedures
to Consider

- Dip urinalysis only for signs or symptoms of problems, not routinely (Institute for Clinical Systems Improvement, 2006)
- Urine culture for
  - History of asymptomatic bacteriuria
  - Sickle cell trait
  - History of pyelonephritis
  - Urinary symptoms
  - Positive dip urinalysis
    - Many bacteria
    - Positive nitrite with positive leukocytes
- Glucose challenge
  - First trimester
    - Previous gestational diabetic
    - High risk for gestational diabetes (see Gestational Diabetes—Chapter 3)
  - Twenty-four to 28 weeks gestation
    - Routine screen
    - Repeat testing in high risk women
- Blood type and antibody screen
  - Initial prenatal laboratory values
  - Twenty-four to 28 weeks for Rh-negative mothers
- Hematocrit and hemoglobin
  - Initial prenatal labs
  - Twenty-four to 28 weeks as needed
  - Every 4–6 weeks to evaluate iron replacement therapy

- Repeat STI testing as indicated
- Repeat wet prep as indicated
- Group B strep testing (Centers for Disease Control and Prevention, 2002)
  - Thirty-five to 37 weeks gestation
  - Signs or symptoms of preterm labor
- Ultrasound evaluation as indicated
  - Pregnancy dating
  - Genetic evaluation/amniocentesis
  - Fetal growth and development
  - Placental location
  - Biophysical profile
  - Amniotic fluid index
  - Cervical length
- Additional testing as indicated
  - CBC with reticulocytes, total iron binding capacity (TIBC), serum iron, serum ferritin
  - Thyroid-stimulating hormone, free T_4, thyroid antibodies (Weir & Farley, 2006)
  - Three-hour glucose tolerance testing
  - Fetal fibronectin
  - CBC with differential, renal and liver function studies, serum uric acid, 24-hour urine for protein
  - Other tests as indicated by findings

Providing Treatment:
Therapeutic Measures to Consider

- Prenatal vitamins with folic acid
- Iron supplementation (see Iron-Deficiency Anemia—Chapter 3)
  - Ferro-sequels 1–2 PO daily
  - Niferex 150 mg 1–2 PO daily
  - Ferrous gluconate 1–2 PO daily
  - Other supplement of choice
- Calcium supplements as needed, such as
  - Citracal: 200–400 mg BID
  - Tums: 500 mg one to two tablets daily
  - Os-cal: one tablet two to three times daily
  - Other supplement of choice
- Influenza vaccine in the fall for women who (ACOG, 2003a)
  - Currently have a chronic respiratory disorder (e.g., asthma, chronic bronchitis)

- Are in the second or third trimester of pregnancy October through March
- Immunization update if at significant risk or traveling abroad
- Preterm birth prevention for women with risk of preterm birth
  - Weekly progesterone (17p) shots beginning at 16–20 weeks until 36 weeks, still experimental, but showing promise (ACOG, 2003b)

Providing Treatment:
Alternative Measures to Consider

- Encourage appropriate weight gain through healthy varied diet
- Dietary sources of
  - Iron, see Appendix B-3
  - Folate
    - Deep-green leafy vegetables
    - Root vegetables
    - Orange juice
    - Whole grains
    - Nutritional yeast
    - Organ meats, lean beef
  - Calcium, see Appendices B-4 and B-5
- Third trimester herbal support (Weed, 1985)
  - Red raspberry leaf
  - Dandelion leaf
  - Nettle
  - Spirulina

Providing Support:
Education and Support Measures to Consider

- Pregnancy discussion
  - Planned schedule of prenatal visits
    - Offer group prenatal care if available
  - Expectations related to care
    - Client/family expectations
    - Midwife/practice expectations
  - Anticipated testing
  - Fee and payment information
- Health education
  - Midwife call system
    - When and how to call

- Importance of
  - Fetal movement
  - Nutrition and exercise
- Bowel and bladder function
- Feelings about pregnancy, birth, family
  - Relationship changes
  - Sexual relations in pregnancy
- Social services available
- Labor discussion
  - Preterm labor and birth education until 37 weeks
  - Planned location of birth
  - Preparation for labor
  - Signs and symptoms of labor
  - Anticipated labor care and birth options
    - Labor support
    - Pain relief
      - Hydrotherapy/water birth
      - Birth ball
      - Heated rice packs
      - Massage
      - Positioning
      - Acupressure
      - Medication options
    - Perineal support (see Perineal Massage—Chapter 4)
    - Episiotomy indicators
    - Transport/consult indicators
  - Physician coverage for needed care or emergencies
  - Anticipated infant care
    - Vitamin K options
    - Ophthalmic prophylaxis
    - Planned method of infant feeding
    - Transport indicators
    - Circumcision options
    - Newborn evaluation at home
  - Anticipated postpartum care
    - Based on location of birth
    - Cultural practices after birth
    - Planned help at home, resources
    - Postpartum method of birth control

- Anticipated visits for follow-up care
  - Home visits
  - Mother postpartum visits
  - Infant evaluation

Follow-up Care:
Follow-up Measures to Consider
- Review with client
  - Previously done laboratory results
  - Client education and expressed needs
  - Behavioral changes
  - Healthy life-style maintenance or improvement
    - Diet
    - Exercise/activity/rest
    - Stress management
- Midwifery plan of care
  - Identify
    - Alternate providers and/or location for birth
    - Client risk factors and anticipated management
    - Preferred newborn care provider(s)
  - Anticipated return visit schedule
    - Every 4–6 weeks until 28–32 weeks gestation
    - Every 2–3 weeks from 32–36 weeks gestation
    - Weekly from 36 weeks until birth occurs
    - More frequent visits as needed, specify indication
  - Informed consent or consultation, as indicated, for
    - Planned out-of-hospital birth
    - VBAC
    - Cesarean birth
    - Postpartum tubal ligation
- Document
  - Findings and update problem list
  - Discussions with client/family
  - Client preferences for labor and birth
  - Plan for continued care
  - Informed consents

Collaborative Practice:
Consider Consultation or Referral
- Health education
  - Pregnancy and/or childbirth education classes
  - Diabetes education and diet counseling for the gestational diabetic
  - Pregnancy yoga or exercise program
- Social services
- OB/GYN consultation, collaboration, or referral
  - Complications or problems during pregnancy
  - Surgical consultation
- Anesthesia services
  - Preoperative evaluation
- For diagnosis or treatment outside the midwife's scope of practice

CARE OF THE PREGNANT WOMAN WITH BACKACHE

Key Clinical Information

Backache is pain in the upper or lower back. It affects most pregnant women to some degree, whereas an estimated 15% will have severe back pain (Blackburn & Loper, 1992). As the pregnancy progresses a woman's center of gravity shifts and postural compensations are made—kyphosis of the cervical spine accommodating the growth and weight of the breasts and lordosis of the lumbar spine accommodating the distention of the abdomen. These changes combined with the hormonal influences that loosen ligaments and joints can lead to backache for the pregnant woman. Client posture, body mechanics, and muscle tone may affect the strain on the back from the growing belly.

Other causes of backache during pregnancy should not be dismissed without consideration, because this general symptom may be the only indication of preterm labor, pyelonephritis, or renal calculi. Additionally, back pathology, such as disc disease or muscle strains, should be considered when pain is severe or not ameliorated by typical treatments.

Client History and Chart Review:
Components of the History to Consider

- Gestational age
- Onset, duration, severity, and location of backache
- History of complaint
  - Precipitating event, if any
  - Timing of symptoms
  - Activities that exacerbate backache
  - Medications or self-help measures used and relief obtained
- Presence of other associated symptoms
  - Presence or absence of contractions
  - Urinary symptoms
    - Frequency
    - Flank pain
  - Presence of neurologic signs or symptoms
- Past medical history
  - Back injury or disease
  - Kidney stones or pyelonephritis
- Potential contributing factors
  - Body mechanics
  - Lifting at work or home
  - Physical abuse, trauma, or injury

Physical Examination:
Components of the Physical Exam
to Consider

- Vital signs, including weight
- Abdominal examination
  - Abdominal muscle tone
  - Uterine size
- Back examination
  - Mobility
  - Point tenderness
  - Posture, presence of lordosis, kyphosis, or scoliosis
  - CVA tenderness
  - Presence of muscle spasm
- Pelvic evaluation for
  - Backache accompanied by contractions
  - History suggestive of preterm labor
  - Evaluation of cervical status

- Evaluation of neurologic status
  - Muscle tone
  - Strength
  - Coordination
  - Reflexes
- Signs of physical abuse
  - Bruising
  - Burns
  - Partner presence for entire visit

Clinical Impression:
Differential Diagnoses and Code Groups
to Consider
Additional suffix may apply (ICD9data.com, 2007; Seller, 2000)

- Backache of pregnancy (ICD-9 codes 648)
- Muscle strain or sprain, lumbar (ICD-9 codes V22.2 and 847.2)
- Also consider
  - Pyelonephritis (ICD-9 codes V22.2, 590.10)
  - Renal calculi (ICD-9 codes V22.2 and 592.0)
  - Herniated disc (ICD-9 codes V22.2 and 722.10)
  - Irritable bowel syndrome (ICD-9 codes V22.2 and 564.1)
  - Rheumatoid arthritis (ICD-9 codes V22.2 and 714.0)

Diagnostic Testing:
Diagnostic Tests and Procedures to Consider

- Urinalysis
- Urine culture in the patient with a history of urinary tract infections
- Fetal/uterine monitoring
- Ultrasound of kidneys if renal calculi are suspected

Providing Treatment:
Therapeutic Measures to Consider

- Pain relief (Murphy, 2004)
  - Acetaminophen/aspirin
    - Alternate every 4 hours
    - Use for no more than 24–48 hours

- Naproxen/naproxen sodium
  - ◆ 200–375 mg every 8–12 hours
  - ◆ Pregnancy Category B
  - ◆ Avoid in late pregnancy
  - Ketoprofen (Orudis)
    - ◆ 75 mg TID
    - ◆ Pregnancy Category B
    - ◆ Avoid in late pregnancy
- Muscle spasm (Murphy, 2004)
  - Flexeril
    - ◆ 10 mg TID
    - ◆ Pregnancy Category B
- As appropriate for other confirmed diagnosis

Providing Treatment:
Alternative Measures to Consider
(Gladstar, 1993; Weed, 1985)
- Abdominal binder designed for pregnancy
- Ice to affected area followed by warm packs (moist heat, castor oil, vinegar)
- Massage with liniment rubs
  - Arnica
    - ◆ Infused oil for massage
  - Capsaicin salve or ointment
- Adequate calcium and magnesium intake
  - Calcium, see Appendices B-4 and B-5
  - Magnesium, see Appendix B-7
- Herbals
  - Chamomile tea
- Homeopathic
  - Arnica tablets

Providing Support:
Education and Support Measures to Consider
(Pennick & Young, 2007; Varney et al., 2004)
- Use of good body mechanics
  - Low-heeled shoes
  - Posture to minimize lordosis
  - Bend knees to lift using leg muscles
  - Avoid lifting with back
  - Avoid bending or turning from waist
- Planned back care program
  - Pelvic tilt
  - Stretching

- Swimming
- Yoga
- Supportive sleep environment
  - Firm mattress
  - Pillows between knees
- Mechanical support measures
  - Well-fitting supportive bra
  - Prenatal abdominal cradle
  - Lumbar support in chair/car
  - Footstool to raise knees above hips

Follow-up Care:
Follow-up Measures to Consider
- Document
- Notify adult protective services as needed for evidence of abuse (Little, 2000)
- Return for care
  - As scheduled for gestation
  - With worsening symptoms
    - ◆ Pain
    - ◆ Numbness or tingling
  - Signs of preterm labor
  - Urinary symptoms

Collaborative Practice:
Consider Consultation or Referral
- Acupuncture/acupressure therapy (Pennick & Young, 2007)
- Osteopathic manipulation
- Chiropractic manipulation (Pennick & Young, 2007)
- Physical therapy or physiatrist
  - For posture and lifting evaluation
  - For symptom management
  - For exercise training
  - For mobility aids
- OB/GYN consultation, collaboration, or referral
  - Persistent backache
  - Persistent backache with contractions
  - Development of fever and chills
  - Positive testing for kidney involvement
  - Presence of neurologic symptoms
- For diagnosis or treatment outside the midwife's scope of practice

CARE OF THE PREGNANT WOMAN WITH CONSTIPATION

Key Clinical Information

Constipation is a change in a person's normal bowel patterns to less frequent or more difficult defecation (Seller, 2000). It affects 11–30% of pregnant women (Blackburn & Loper, 1992). Constipation can occur or be exacerbated in pregnant women due to the decreased motility and increased water reabsorption in the intestine as well as pressure from the enlarged uterus. Prevention of constipation requires adequate intake of both fluid and fiber accompanied by physical activity to stimulate the bowels. Determining acceptable dietary sources of fiber for each client is essential. Candid discussion regarding frequency and consistency of bowel movements is an integral part of evaluation for this common malady.

Client History and Chart Review:
Components of the History to Consider

- Gestational age
- Onset of problem
- Bowel habits
    - Frequency and consistency of bowel movements
    - Straining
    - Passage of flatus
    - Remedies used and efficacy
- Other associated symptoms
    - Abdominal cramping with bowel movement
        - Nature of abdominal discomfort
        - Location, severity
        - Backache
        - Contractions
    - Presence of blood in the stool
- Potential contributing factors
    - Iron therapy
    - Inactivity
    - Inadequate fluid intake
    - Inadequate fiber intake
    - Narcotic use

- Past medical history
    - Abdominal surgeries (adhesions)
    - Pelvic inflammatory disease (PID)
    - Bowel disorders
    - Status of appendix

Physical Examination:
Components of the Physical Exam to Consider

- Vital signs, including temperature
- Abdominal examination
    - Auscultate bowel sounds in all four quadrants
    - Palpate for presence of abdominal pain
        - Location
        - Rebound
        - Guarding
- Pelvic examination
    - Palpate for hard stool in rectum
    - Cervical evaluation if cramping present
- Rectal examination as needed

Clinical Impression:
Differential Diagnoses and Code Groups to Consider
Additional suffix may apply (ICD9data.com, 2007; Seller, 2000)

- Constipation (ICD-9 codes V22.2 and 564.00)
- Appendicitis (ICD-9 codes V22.2 and 540–543)
- Irritable bowel syndrome (ICD-9 codes V22.2 and 564.1)
- Fecal impaction (ICD-9 codes V22.2 and 560.39)
- Intestinal obstruction (ICD-9 codes V22.2 and 560.30)
- Diverticulitis (ICD-9 codes V22.2 and 562.10)

Diagnostic Testing:
Diagnostic Tests and Procedures to Consider

- Urine for specific gravity
- CBC with differential
- Pelvic ultrasound

Providing Treatment:
Therapeutic Measures to Consider

- ⚠ Acute abdomen must be ruled out before treating constipation.

- Fiber therapy, such as (Murphy, 2004)
  - Citrucel: 1 Tbs in 8 oz fluid one to three times daily
  - Metamucil: 1 tsp in 8 oz fluid one to three times daily
  - FiberCon: 1 tab with 8 oz fluids one to four times daily
- Stool softeners, such as (Murphy, 2004)
  - Docusate sodium: 50–100 mg 1 PO QD or BID
  - Docusate calcium: 240 mg 1 PO QD
- Laxatives, such as (Murphy, 2004)
  - Senokot: 1 tablet at bedtime
  - Milk of magnesia
- Rectal treatments
  - Glycerin suppositories
  - Soapsuds enema
  - Fleet enema if stool impacted
- Irritable bowel with constipation (Murphy, 2004)
  - Zelnorm (Pregnancy Category B)

Providing Treatment:
Alternative Measures to Consider
- Increase fiber in diet
  - Dried fruits, prune juice
  - Whole grains, bran cereals, muffins
  - Uncooked vegetables, well chewed
  - Herbals
    - Psyllium seed 1 tsp TID (Foster, 1996)
    - Flaxseed meal, 2 Tbs daily with water (Walls, 2007)
- Increase fluid intake
  - 8 cups per day
  - Hot liquid in morning
    - Herbal teas
    - Decaffeinated coffee
    - Hot prune juice
- Increase physical activity
  - Brisk walk after hot drink
  - Follow by toileting
- Bowel retraining
  - Allow regular time for toileting
  - Follow natural urges

Providing Support:
Education and Support Measures
to Consider
- Walking helps stimulate natural peristalsis
- Fiber
  - Maintain adequate fiber intake
  - Helps to keep stool soft
  - Must be used with adequate fluid intake
- Stool softeners
  - Bring fluid to the stool to soften
  - Coat stool with surfactant to help move
- Laxatives
  - Stimulate peristalsis
  - Should be used with caution during pregnancy
  - May cause cramping
- Suppositories
  - Stimulate evacuation of lower bowel
  - May cause cramping
- Enemas
  - Flush the lower bowel
  - May cause cramping
- Life-style recommendations
  - Need for increased fiber and fluid
  - Need for activity to stimulate bowels
  - Hot drink in the morning may stimulate bowels
  - Need for time for toileting
- Warning signs of
  - Preterm labor
  - Acute abdomen

Follow-up Care:
Follow-up Measures to Consider
- Document
- Return for care
  - As scheduled for gestation
  - Return sooner if symptoms persist or worsen
- For emergency care
  - Symptoms of acute abdomen
  - Obstipation
  - Symptoms of preterm labor

Collaborative Practice:
Consider Consultation or Referral

- OB/GYN services
  - Threatened preterm labor
  - Positive occult blood in stool
  - Severe or persistent abdominal pain accompanied by
    - Fever
    - Abdominal rigidity or guarding
    - Obstipation
- For diagnosis or treatment outside the midwife's scope of practice

CARE OF THE PREGNANT WOMAN WITH DYSPNEA

Key Clinical Information

Dyspnea is an unpleasant sense of labored breathing, patient awareness of respiratory discomfort, or shortness of breath (Seller, 2000). It affects 60–70% of women during pregnancy, especially in the first or second trimester (Blackburn and Loper, 1992). Physiologic shortness of breath occurs in early pregnancy as the body adjusts to changes in carbon dioxide levels in the blood and its concomitant hyperventilation. Dyspnea again becomes common in the later stages of pregnancy as the uterus pushes against the diaphragm, reducing the functional residual volume of the lungs (Varney et al., 2004). Anemia, cardiac arrhythmias, and poor physical conditioning may also contribute to dyspnea during pregnancy. Additionally, anxiety or panic may precede or exacerbate the dyspneic episode. Evaluation of shortness of breath during pregnancy is necessary to determine whether it is physiologic or pathologic.

Client History and Chart Review:
Components of the History to Consider

- Gestational age
- Timing of onset, duration, and severity of symptoms
  - With activity or at rest
  - Supine or upright

- Self-help measures or medications used
- Other associated symptoms
  - Fever, chills
  - Cough, dry or productive
  - Syncope
  - Peripheral edema
  - Anxiety or panic symptoms
  - Palpitations
- Cardiopulmonary history
  - Asthma
  - Smoking tobacco or other substances
  - Environmental exposure to allergens, smoke, or fumes
  - Cardiac disorders and/or symptoms
- Review of systems

Physical Examination:
Components of the Physical Exam to Consider

- Vital signs
- Color
- Auscultation and percussion of the chest
  - Respiratory rate, depth, and volume
  - Cardiac rate and rhythm
  - Lung fields
  - Presence of abnormal breath sounds
- Observe for
  - Respiratory effort
  - Presence of cough, sputum
  - Signs of respiratory distress
  - Edema of the extremities

Clinical Impression:
Differential Diagnoses and Code Groups
to Consider

Additional suffix may apply (ICD9data.com, 2007; Seller, 2000)

- Physiologic shortness of breath of pregnancy
- Dyspnea related to
  - Exercise or exertion induced (ICD-9 codes V22.2 and 493.81)
  - Upper respiratory infection (ICD-9 codes V22.2 and 465.9)
  - Asthma (ICD-9 codes V22.2 and 493.90)

- Anemia (ICD-9 codes V22.2 and 648.23)
- Pulmonary embolism (ICD-9 code 673.03)
- Anxiety or panic disorder (ICD-9 codes V22.2 and 300)
- Other cardiovascular diseases (ICD-9 codes 648)
- Other respiratory disorders (ICD-9 codes V22.2 and 786)

Diagnostic Testing:
Diagnostic Tests and Procedures to Consider
- CBC with differential
- Sputum cultures
- Tuberculosis testing
- Chest x-ray
- Pulmonary function testing

Providing Treatment:
Therapeutic Measures to Consider
- Shortness of breath of pregnancy
  - Encourage calm, slow breathing
  - Lean forward or lie down
  - Raise arms to shoulder level
- Otherwise as indicated by diagnosis (see Respiratory Disorders—Chapter 8)

Providing Treatment:
Alternative Measures to Consider
- Stretch periodically
- Maintain good posture
- Maintain slow-paced physical activity
  - Walking
  - Yoga
  - Swimming
- Use pillows as needed for comfort while at rest

Providing Support:
Education and Support Measures to Consider
- Reassurance
- Review
  - Physiologic basis of shortness of breath
  - Deliberate intercostal breathing

- Comfort measures
  - Loose-fitting clothes
  - Rest periods
  - Avoid laying flat on back
- Warning signs
  - Flu-like symptoms
  - Productive cough
  - Chest pain, shortness of breath, diaphoresis
  - Anxiety
  - Palpitations

Follow-up Care:
Follow-up Measures to Consider
- Document
- Return for care
  - As scheduled for gestation
  - Sooner for
    - Presence of warning signs
    - Persistence or worsening of symptoms
    - As needed for support

Collaborative Practice:
Consider Consultation or Referral
- Medical service
  - Evidence of decompensation
  - History or symptoms of asthma
  - Evidence of respiratory infection or disorder
- Mental health service
  - Anxiety or panic attacks
- For diagnosis or treatment outside the midwife's scope of practice

CARE OF THE PREGNANT WOMAN WITH EDEMA

Key Clinical Information
Edema is abnormal accumulation of excess fluid in the intercellular tissue spaces, most commonly in dependent body parts, such as feet and ankles. Dependent edema is seen in 35–80% of pregnant women and becomes more common as pregnancy

progresses (Blackburn & Loper, 1992). Physiologic edema of pregnancy occurs secondary to fluid retention as the body works to increase and maintain adequate circulating fluid volume. Pressure of the pregnant uterus may cause venous stasis and force fluid out of the circulatory system and into the soft tissue.

Client History and Chart Review:
Components of the History to Consider
- Gestational age
- Diet history
- Recent medications
- Onset, location, duration, and severity of edema
  - Precipitating factors
  - Circadian variations in edema
  - Usual fluid intake and urination patterns
  - Self-help measures used and their effects
  - Other associated symptoms
- Symptoms of preeclampsia
- History of
  - Preeclampsia
  - Edema with pregnancy
  - Varicose veins
- Review of systems

Physical Examination:
Components of the Physical Exam
to Consider
- Vital signs, BP
- Note interval weight changes
- Note presence and pattern of edema
  - Diffuse or localized
  - Presence of pitting edema
  - Bilateral or unilateral
  - Facial, periorbital
- Examination of extremities
  - Deep tendon reflexes
  - Measurement of leg circumference
  - Varicosities
  - Signs of phlebitis: redness, tenderness, warmth
  - Signs of clothing constriction

Clinical Impression:
Differential Diagnoses and Code Groups
to Consider
Additional suffix may apply (ICD9data.com, 2007; Seller, 2000)
- Physiologic edema of pregnancy (ICD-9 code 646.13)
- Edema related to
  - Preeclampsia (ICD-9 codes 642)
  - Thrombophlebitis (ICD-9 codes 671)
  - Other cardiovascular diseases (ICD-9 codes 648)
  - Other renal disorders (ICD-9 codes V22.2 and 580–589)

Diagnostic Testing:
Diagnostic Tests and Procedures to Consider
- Office urinalysis
  - Proteinuria
  - Specific gravity
  - Appearance
- Preeclampsia laboratory values (see Preeclampsia—Chapter 3)

Providing Treatment:
Therapeutic Measures to Consider
- Rest 1 hour BID with feet higher than heart
  - Suggest elevating foot of bed for gentle overnight elevation
- Prescription support hose
  - Apply with legs elevated to maximize compression

Providing Treatment:
Alternative Measures to Consider
- Water immersion (Hartmann & Huch, 2005)
- Foot massage, reflexology
- Foot exercises
  - Draw the alphabet with your feet
- Herbal support for fluid balance, two to three cups of tea a day (Gladstar, 1993)
  - Parsley
  - Dandelion leaf
  - Stinging nettle (Foster, 1996)

Providing Support:
Education and Support Measures to Consider
- Provide information
  - Physiologic basis of edema in pregnancy
  - Warning signs
    - Preeclampsia
    - Phlebitis
- Self-help measures
  - Continue gentle physical activity
  - Rest, elevate extremities, pillow under right hip
  - Increase fluids
  - Add salt to diet to taste if low salt intake
  - Decrease dietary salt if high salt diet intake
- Avoid
  - Constrictive clothing
  - Diuretic medications, foods, or herbs

Follow-up Care:
Follow-up Measures to Consider
- Document
- Return for care
  - As scheduled for gestation
  - For increasing edema
  - Symptoms of preeclampsia or phlebitis

Collaborative Practice:
Consider Consultation or Referral
- OB/GYN services
  - Symptoms of preeclampsia
  - Severe progressive edema
  - Severe varicosities
  - Symptoms of phlebitis or thrombophlebitis
- For diagnosis or treatment outside the midwife's scope of practice

CARE OF THE PREGNANT WOMAN WITH EPISTAXIS

Key Clinical Information
Epistaxis is a nosebleed due to rupture of nasal blood vessels, which are richly supplied by the internal and external carotid arteries. Frequency of epistaxis is difficult to determine because most episodes resolve with self-treatment and are not reported; however, it is thought to occur more frequently during pregnancy. Although nosebleeds are rarely of a serious nature, most women are anxious about the blood loss and may require treatment if the bleeding does not stop promptly. Epistaxis may be the presenting symptom of labile hypertension. Inhaled drug use may elevate BP and lead to placental abruption or other hypertension-related complications of pregnancy.

Client History and Chart Review:
Components of the History to Consider
- Gestational age
- Onset, frequency, duration, and severity of bleeding
  - Precipitating factors or events
    - Allergies or upper respiratory tract infection
    - Use of inhaled drugs (e.g., cocaine, glue)
    - Use of anticoagulant or other medications
    - Trauma
  - Self-help measures used and efficacy
  - Typical nasal hygiene measures
  - Associated signs and symptoms
- Past medical history
  - Epistaxis
  - Bleeding disorder
- Family history
  - Bleeding disorder

Physical Examination:
Components of the Physical Exam to Consider
- Vital signs, BP
- Examination of nares for
  - Polyps
  - Trauma
  - Erosion
  - Inflammation
- Observation for bruising

Clinical Impression:
Differential Diagnoses and Code Groups
to Consider
Additional suffix may apply (ICD9data.com, 2007;
Seller, 2000)

- Epistaxis (ICD-9 codes V22.2 and 429.9), or secondary to
  - Hypertension (ICD-9 codes 642)
  - Nasal polyps (ICD-9 codes V22.2 and 471.9)
  - Inhalation drug use (ICD-9 codes 648)
  - Nasal trauma or injury (ICD-9 codes V22.2 and 959.09)
  - Coagulation defects (ICD-9 code 649)
  - Seasonal allergies (ICD-9 codes V22.2 and 477.0)
  - Upper respiratory tract infection (ICD-9 codes V22.2 and 465.9)

Diagnostic Testing:
Diagnostic Tests and Procedures to Consider

- Hematocrit and hemoglobin
  - Persistent, recurrent, copious flow
  - Signs or symptoms of anemia
- Serial BPs
- Drug screen

Providing Treatment:
Therapeutic Measures to Consider

- Normal saline nasal spray
- Pressure to nares

Providing Treatment:
Alternative Measures to Consider

- Herbal and dietary support:
  - Foods rich in vitamins A, C, and E
    - Deep-green leafy vegetables
    - Onions in diet
    - Parsley
    - Infusion of oat straw and nettle
- Treatment
  - Cold compresses of comfrey, yarrow, and/or mullein (Weed, 1985)
  - Plantain and yarrow ointment
  - Nettle or oat straw as teas

Providing Support:
Education and Support Measures
to Consider

- Provide information on
  - Physiologic basis for epistaxis
  - Nasal hygiene
    - Gentle clearing of nasal debris after bath or shower
  - Self-help measures
    - Avoid vigorous blowing or picking of nose
    - Use humidifier or vaporizer
    - Ice to bridge of nose to stop bleeding
    - Pinch bridge of nose to stop bleeding

Follow-up Care:
Follow-up Measures to Consider

- Document
- Return for care
  - As scheduled for gestation
  - For bleeding unresponsive to self-help measures

Collaborative Practice:
Consider Consultation or Referral

- Ear, nose, and throat (ENT) service
  - Electrocautery of bleeding vessel
  - Nasal polyps
- Medical service
  - Suspected bleeding disorder
- For diagnosis or treatment outside the midwife's scope of practice

CARE OF THE PREGNANT WOMAN WITH HEARTBURN

Key Clinical Information

Heartburn is a sensation of burning behind the breastbone that results from the backflow of stomach contents into the esophagus. Heartburn affects 30–70% of women at some point in pregnancy and affects 25% of women daily in their third trimester (Blackburn & Loper, 1992). The softening influence of the pregnancy hormone relaxin on the lower esophageal sphincter is one contributor to this increased incidence of heartburn in pregnancy. As pregnancy progresses, simple mechanical pressure also contributes to heartburn. Women with a history of gastroesophageal reflux disease may require treatment during pregnancy. Small meals and a bland diet are often helpful.

Client History and Chart Review:
Components of the History to Consider
- Gestational age
- Onset, frequency, timing, duration, and severity of symptoms
  - Common symptoms
    - ◆ Burning epigastric pain
    - ◆ Reflux
    - ◆ Belching, bloating
  - Precipitating factors or events
    - ◆ Foods
    - ◆ Anxiety
    - ◆ Positioning
  - Presence of symptoms before pregnancy
  - Usual diet
  - Self-help measures and efficacy

Physical Examination:
Components of the Physical Exam to Consider
- Vital signs
- Interval weight gain or loss
- Abdominal palpation
- Fundal height

Clinical Impression:
Differential Diagnoses and Code Groups to Consider
Additional suffix may apply (ICD9data.com, 2007; Seller, 2000)
- Physiologic heartburn of pregnancy
- Gastroesophageal reflux disease (ICD-9 codes V22.2 and 530.81)
- Hiatal hernia (ICD-9 codes V22.2 and 553.3)
- Gastritis (ICD-9 codes V22.2 and 535.0)
- Gallbladder disease (ICD-9 codes V22.2 and 574)

Diagnostic Testing:
Diagnostic Tests and Procedures to Consider
- Consult or refer if *Helicobacter pylori* testing is indicated; there are several noninvasive and invasive methods of testing

Providing Treatment:
Therapeutic Measures to Consider
- Antacid preparations such as
  - Tums
  - Gelusil
  - Amphojel
- Proton pump inhibitors (Pregnancy Category B) such as (Murphy, 2004)
  - Aciphex 20 mg QD
  - Nexium 20 mg QD
  - Prevacid 30 mg BID
- H_2 blockers (Pregnancy Category B)
  - Axid 150 mg PO BID
  - Pepcid 20 mg PO BID
  - Tagamet 300 mg PO QID
  - Zantac 150 mg PO BID

Providing Treatment:
Alternative Measures to Consider
- Herbal remedies (Weed, 1985)
  - Chamomile tea
  - Oat straw tea
  - Ginger tea or capsules
  - Papaya chewable tablets (Griffith, 2000)
  - Lemon balm tea
  - Slippery elm lozenges or capsules

Providing Support:
Education and Support Measures to Consider
- Information related to
  - Physiologic basis of heartburn
  - Warning signs
  - Comfort measures
    - ◆ Small frequent meals
    - ◆ Maintain good posture
    - ◆ Decrease intake of fatty or spicy foods
    - ◆ Take food and fluids separately
    - ◆ Elevate head of bed 10–30 degrees

Follow-up Care:
Follow-up Measures to Consider

- Document
- Return for care
  - As scheduled for gestation
  - Persistent reflux or abdominal pain
  - Indications for referral
    - Persistent severe reflux
    - Abdominal pain
    - Signs or symptoms of ulcer or perforation

Collaborative Practice:
Consider Consultation or Referral

- Medical or gastroenterology services
  - Severe symptoms unrelieved by treatment
  - For suspected or documented
    - *H. pylori* infection
    - Hiatal hernia
    - Gastroesophageal reflux disease (GERD)
    - Gastric ulcer or perforation
- For diagnosis or treatment outside the midwife's scope of practice

CARE OF THE PREGNANT WOMAN WITH HEMORRHOIDS

Key Clinical Information
Hemorrhoids are dilated veins of the hemorrhoidal plexus in the lower rectum. Hemorrhoids are considered common in pregnancy, but their prevalence in pregnancy is unknown. One study found 85% of women late in their second and third pregnancies had hemorrhoids (Gojnic et al., 2005). Symptoms include irritation, itching, pain, and bleeding. Hemorrhoids are internal when they occur inside the anal canal and external when they occur at the anal opening. Internal hemorrhoids are usually not painful unless they become ulcerated, infected, or project outside through the anus. The pressure of the pregnant uterus on pelvic vessels and constipation both aggravate hemorrhoids, causing bleeding, itching, and burning. Thrombosed hemorrhoids are extremely

painful and can require treatment with incision and drainage.

Client History and Chart Review:
Components of the History to Consider

- Gestational age
- Prior history of hemorrhoids
- Onset, duration, severity of symptoms
  - Presence of bleeding, pain, itching
  - Self-help measures used and efficacy
- Contributing factors
  - Toileting habits
  - Low-fiber diet
  - Constipation or diarrhea
  - Medications
    - Iron supplements
    - Stool softeners
    - Enemas

Physical Examination:
Components of the Physical Exam to Consider

- Examination and palpation of the rectum for presence of
  - Hemorrhoids
    - External
    - Internal
    - Strangulated
    - Thrombosed
- Anal lesions or masses
- Anal fissures

Clinical Impression:
Differential Diagnoses and Code Groups
to Consider
Additional suffix may apply (ICD9data.com, 2007; Seller, 2000)

- Hemorrhoids (ICD-9 code 671.83)
- Anal fissures (ICD-9 codes V22.2 and 565.0)
- Anal trauma (ICD-9 codes V22.2 and 863)
- Anal herpes (ICD-9 codes V22.2 and 569)
- Anal fistula (ICD-9 codes V22.2 and 565)
- Rectal polyp (ICD-9 codes V22.2 and 569)
- Rectal malignancy (ICD-9 codes 654)

Diagnostic Testing:
Diagnostic Tests and Procedures to Consider
- Stool for occult blood
- Herpes culture
- STI screen
- Anoscopy

Providing Treatment:
Therapeutic Measures to Consider
- AnaMantle HC: topical anesthetic and steroid
  - Pregnancy Category C
  - Apply BID for 7 days
- Anusol-HC: topical steroid in a soothing cream
  - Pregnancy Category C
  - Apply two to four times daily as needed
- Manual reduction of hemorrhoids

Providing Treatment:
Alternative Measures to Consider
- Herbal remedies (Weed, 1985)
  - Bilberry tablets or capsules TID
  - Horse chestnut tea, tincture or capsules
  - Nettle tea
- Herbal or warm water sitz baths
- Topical applications
  - Witch hazel compresses
  - Comfrey compresses
  - Epsom salt compresses
  - Plantain and yarrow ointment
  - Yellow dock root ointment
- Knee-chest position to promote drainage
- Homeopathic remedies
  - Hamamelis 30×
  - Arnica 30×

Providing Support:
Education and Support Measures to Consider
- Avoid
  - Straining at stool
  - Prolonged sitting on toilet
  - Constipation (see Care of the Pregnant Woman with Constipation)
- Ensure adequate fiber in diet
- Topical medication use
- Signs and symptoms necessitating return for care

Follow-up Care:
Follow-up Measures to Consider
- Document
- Return for care
  - As scheduled for gestation
  - As soon as possible for thrombosed hemorrhoids

Collaborative Practice:
Consider Consultation or Referral
- OB/GYN or surgical services
  - Evaluation of severe, strangulated, or bleeding hemorrhoids
  - Blood in stool with no evidence of hemorrhoids or rectal fissure
  - For incision and drainage of thrombosed hemorrhoids
- For diagnosis or treatment outside the midwife's scope of practice

CARE OF THE PREGNANT WOMAN WITH INSOMNIA

Key Clinical Information

Insomnia is difficulty in initiating or maintaining sleep and can include delays in falling asleep, poor quality of sleep, frequent awakening, and early morning wakefulness (Seller, 2000). Most women (66–94%) report alterations in their sleep patterns during pregnancy (Santiago et al., 2001). Chronic or acute sleep deprivation can significantly impair the pregnant woman's ability to function and her body's ability to regenerate and recover from daily stressors. Starting labor with severe sleep deprivation may result in early maternal exhaustion and dysfunctional labor patterns. Mood changes may be a primary cause or a result of sleep deprivation.

Client History and Chart Review:
Components of the History to Consider
- Gestational age
- Onset, duration, and severity of symptoms
  - Difficulty falling asleep
  - Wakefulness
  - Fitful sleep
  - Interruptions
    - Nocturia
    - Pain
    - Caretaking responsibilities
- Sleep habits
  - Sleep–wake patterns
    - Bedtime
    - Naps
  - Sleep partners
    - Intimate partner
    - Children
  - Total hours of sleep/24 hours
- Social issues
  - Emotional response to sleep deprivation
  - Caffeine intake and timing
  - Meal patterns and content
  - Work hours
  - Anxieties and concerns
  - Help and support
- Other related symptoms

Physical Examination:
Components of the Physical Exam
to Consider
- Assess for
  - Nutrition and hydration status
  - Evidence of sleep deprivation
  - Physical causes of sleep deprivation

Clinical Impression:
Differential Diagnoses and Code Groups
to Consider
Additional suffix may apply (ICD9data.com, 2007;
Seller, 2000)
- Insomnia (ICD-9 codes V22.2 and 780.52), or
  secondary to
  - Anxiety (ICD-9 code 648)

- Depression (ICD-9 code 648)
- Substance abuse (ICD-9 code 648)
- Other sleep disorders (ICD-9 codes V22.2
  and 327)

Diagnostic Testing:
Diagnostic Tests and Procedures to Consider
- Insomnia: diagnosed by self-report
- Other testing: as indicated by symptoms

Providing Treatment:
Therapeutic Measures to Consider
- ⚠ Use only when necessary
- For sleep (Murphy, 2004)
  - Ambien (Pregnancy Category B)
    - 5–10 mg at bedtime
  - Ambien CR (Pregnancy Category C)
    - 12.5 mg at bedtime
  - Lunesta (Pregnancy Category C)
    - 2 mg at bedtime
  - Benadryl (Pregnancy Category B)
    - 25–50 mg at bedtime
- For therapeutic sleep for false labor (see
  Prolonged First Stage Labor—Chapter 3)
  - Morphine sulfate
    - 10–15 mg IM
    - May combine with
      - Vistaril 25–50 mg, or
      - Phenergan 25–50 mg
    - Allows rest for 4–6 hours
    - May be reversed with Narcan as needed

Providing Treatment:
Alternative Measures to Consider
- Sleep environment
  - Darkened area
  - Sound dampened
  - Use of white noise (e.g., nature tapes, fan)
  - Comfort aids (e.g., blankets, pillows)
- Increase vitamin B intake
- Herbal remedies (Gladstar, 1993)
  - Chamomile tea
  - Valerian tincture or capsules
  - Hops tea or tincture (after 20 weeks gestation)

- Lemon balm tea
- Skullcap tincture
- Passion flower tea, tincture, or fluid extract tid
- Hydrotherapy
- Hypnotherapy
- Aromatherapy, add essential oils to warm bath water or diffuse in room air (England, 1994)
  - Lavender
  - Yling ylang
  - Geranium
- Massage of back, shoulders, and feet

Providing Support:
Education and Support Measures to Consider (Santiago et al., 2001)
- Information related to
  - Physiologic basis of insomnia
  - Other factors that may interfere with sleep
    - Work hours
    - Caretaking requirements
    - Small children
    - Elderly or ill parents/family
    - Sleep environment
    - Nighttime hunger
- Encourage a positive approach to this difficult problem
- Self-help measures
  - Nap during day to maintain rest
  - Warm bath before sleep
  - Warm milk or comfort foods
  - Massage
  - Extra pillows for support
  - Regular daily physical activity
  - Adequate nutrition
  - Limit fluids 2 hours before bedtime
  - Avoid or minimize caffeine
  - Reinforce abstinence from alcohol

Follow-up Care:
Follow-up Measures to Consider
- Document
- Return for care

- As scheduled for gestation
- Increased visits as needed for
  - Evaluation and monitoring of medication use
  - Emotional support

Collaborative Practice:
Consider for Consultation or Referral
- Sleep disorder center
- OB/GYN services
  - Maternal exhaustion
- Mental health services
  - Depression
  - Anxiety
- Social service
- For diagnosis or treatment outside the midwife's scope of practice

CARE OF THE PREGNANT WOMAN WITH LEG CRAMPS

Key Clinical Information

Leg cramps are intermittent painful muscle spasms of the lower leg muscles. A similar condition is restless leg syndrome, characterized by unpleasant sensations in the lower leg ranging from twitchy to burning to painful and accompanied by an urge to move the legs when at rest. Leg cramps are estimated to affect 45% of pregnant women, whereas restless leg syndrome is seen in 10–11% of pregnant women (Blackburn & Loper, 1992). Leg cramps are a common occurrence during pregnancy and may interfere with a woman's ability to sleep. They are more common during the nighttime hours. Cramping may be related to an imbalance of calcium and phosphorous metabolism or may be due to pressure of the enlarging uterus on pelvic blood vessels or nerves supplying the lower leg.

Client History and Chart Review:
Components of the History to Consider
- Gestational age
- Onset, frequency, duration, and severity of cramps

- Precipitating factors
- Self-help measures used and efficacy
- Calcium and magnesium intake
- Physical activity level
- Other associated symptoms

Physical Examination:
Components of the Physical Exam to Consider
- Vital signs
- Evaluate extremities for
  - Clonus
  - Muscle spasm
  - Varicosities
  - Homans' sign

Clinical Impression:
Differential Diagnoses and Code Groups
to Consider
Additional suffix may apply (ICD9data.com, 2007; Seller, 2000)
- Physiologic leg cramps (ICD-9 codes V22.2 and 728.85)
- Varicose veins (ICD-9 codes 671)
- Restless leg syndrome (ICD-9 codes V22.2 and 327.52)
- Thrombophlebitis (ICD-9 codes 671)
- Deep vein thrombosis (ICD-9 codes 671)
- Muscle strain (ICD-9 codes V22.2 and 729)

Diagnostic Testing:
Diagnostic Tests and Procedures to Consider
- Serial calf measurements
- Venous ultrasound
- Clotting studies

Providing Treatment:
Therapeutic Measures to Consider
- Calcium supplement
- Magnesium supplement

Providing Treatment:
Alternative Measures to Consider
- Dietary sources of calcium and magnesium, see Appendices B-4, B-5 and B-7

- Acupressure
  - Pressure to posterior mid-calf
  - Flex foot
- Homeopathic remedies
  - Calcarea phos. 30× TID or with acute symptoms
  - Calcarea carb. 30× TID or with acute symptoms
- Herbal remedies (Weed, 1985)
  - Raspberry leaf
  - Nettle
  - Dandelion

Providing Support:
Education and Support Measures to Consider
- Physiologic nature of leg cramps in pregnancy
- Self-help measures
  - Increase calcium and magnesium intake
  - Regular daily activity
    - Walking
    - Yoga
    - Swimming
  - Keep legs warm
  - When cramp occurs
    - Flex foot
    - Stretch heel away from body
    - Use homeopathic remedy every 15 minutes for two to four doses
- Warning signs
  - Increasing muscle spasms
  - Swelling, pain, or redness in leg

Follow-up Care:
Follow-up Measures to Consider
- Document
- Return for care
  - As scheduled for gestation
  - For persistent leg pain or warning signs

Collaborative Practice:
Consider Consultation or Referral
- Medical services
  - For nonpregnancy related cause of leg pain
  - Phlebitis

- ▪ Thrombophlebitis
- ▪ Deep vein thrombosis
- For diagnosis or treatment outside the midwife's scope of practice

CARE OF THE PREGNANT WOMAN WITH NAUSEA AND VOMITING

Key Clinical Information

Nausea is a subjective and unpleasant feeling in the abdomen associated with feeling ill and the urge to vomit. Vomiting is the expulsion of the stomach contents through the mouth as a result of involuntary muscle spasms. Nausea and vomiting in pregnancy is a self-limiting event that is experienced by 50–88% of pregnant women in Western cultures (Blackburn & Loper, 1992). Onset is typically at 5 weeks and resolution is most common at 12 weeks, although it persists to 14 weeks for 40%, to 16 weeks for 20%, and to 20 weeks for 10%. Although nausea and vomiting are considered a classic early pregnancy occurrence, they may cause significant dehydration and contribute to poor nutrition. In a few women the nausea and vomiting in pregnancy may continue throughout the pregnancy or may develop into hyperemesis gravidarum, characterized by severe unrelenting nausea and vomiting.

Client History and Chart Review:
Components of the History to Consider

- Gestational age
- Onset, duration, and severity of symptoms
  - ▪ Presence and frequency of vomiting
  - ▪ Symptoms of dehydration
  - ▪ Other associated symptoms
  - ▪ Self-help measures used and results
- Assess
  - ▪ Nutritional intake
  - ▪ Activity level
  - ▪ Bowel and bladder pattern
- Past medical history
  - ▪ Thyroid disorders
  - ▪ Eating disorders
- Review of systems

Physical Examination:
Components of the Physical Exam to Consider

- Vital signs
- Interval weight gain or loss
- Usual prenatal evaluation, including examination for
  - ▪ Overall appearance
    - ◆ Weight loss
    - ◆ Skin turgor
    - ◆ Self-care and hygiene
  - ▪ Abdominal examination
    - ◆ Fundal height for gestational age
    - ◆ Bowel sounds

Clinical Impression:
Differential Diagnoses and Code Groups to Consider
Additional suffix may apply (ICD9data.com, 2007; Seller, 2000)

- Physiologic nausea and vomiting of pregnancy (ICD-9 code 643.93)
- Also consider
  - ▪ Hyperemesis gravidarum (ICD-9 code 643.13)
  - ▪ Hydatidiform mole (ICD-9 codes 631)
  - ▪ Ectopic implantation (ICD-9 codes 633)
- Mental health conditions
  - ▪ Bulimia (ICD-9 codes V22.2 and 783.6)
  - ▪ Anxiety (ICD-9 codes 648)
  - ▪ Depression (ICD-9 codes 648)
- Other medical conditions, such as
  - ▪ Gallbladder disease (ICD-9 codes V22.2 and 574)
  - ▪ Pyelonephritis (ICD-9 codes V22.2 and 590)
  - ▪ Gastroenteritis (ICD-9 codes V22.2 and 535)

Diagnostic Testing:
Diagnostic Tests and Procedures to Consider

- Urine dipstick for ketones and glucose
- Urinalysis
- Blood urea nitrogen and electrolytes
- Serum albumin
- Thyroid-stimulating hormone
- Liver function testing
- CBC or white blood cell count

- Pelvic ultrasound
- Ultrasound of the gallbladder
- *H. pylori* testing

Providing Treatment:
Therapeutic Measures to Consider

⚠ Use caution with any medications used for treatment of nausea and vomiting in early pregnancy. Few medications have been demonstrated to be completely safe for the developing fetus.

- Treat conservatively, progressing as indicated by symptoms (Figure 2-1)
- IV hydration when indicated (Sinclair, 2004)
  - Hydration alone may resolve symptoms
  - Use balanced electrolyte solution, such as lactated Ringer's solution
  - 500-ml bolus to start
  - Titrate to maintain urinary specific gravity in normal range
- Vitamin B$_6$ (pyridoxine) (Sripramote and Lekhyananda, 2003)
  - 10–30 mg TID
  - Pregnancy Category A
- Meclizine HCl (Murphy, 2004)
  - 12.5 mg BID
  - Pregnancy Category B
- Metoclopramide (Reglan) (Murphy, 2004)
  - 5–10 mg PO 30 minutes before each meal and at bedtime
  - Pregnancy Category B
- Promethazine (Phenergan) (Murphy, 2004)
  - 25 mg PO every 8–12 hours
  - Pregnancy Category C
- Prochlorperazine (Compazine) (Murphy, 2004)
  - 5–10 mg PO/IM/slow IV every 3–6 hours
  - 15 mg spansule PO daily in AM
  - 10 mg spansule PO every 12 hours
  - Rectal 25 mg BID
  - Pregnancy Category C
  - Maximum daily dose 40 mg/day
- Ondansetron (Zofran) (Murphy, 2004)
  - 4–16 mg PO every 8 hours, as needed
  - Pregnancy Category B

Providing Treatment:
Alternative Measures to Consider

- Nutritional support
  - Ginger tea, tablets, capsules, or crystallized (Oates-Whitehead, 2004; Sripramote & Lekhyananda, 2003)
  - Peppermint tea
  - B vitamin foods (Weed, 1985)
    - Wheat germ
    - Molasses
    - Brewer's yeast
- Acupressure wristbands (Seabands) (Oates-Whitehead, 2004)

Providing Support:
Education and Support Measures to Consider

- Encourage
  - Small bland meals, primarily carbohydrates
  - Keep something in stomach (e.g., saltines, Cheerios)
  - Adequate fluids
  - Small bites or sips only
  - Use salt substitute (adds potassium)
  - Limit fat and increase protein
- Advise family of need for support
- Review when to call
  - For persistent vomiting
  - Symptoms of dehydration
  - Abdominal pain
  - Weakness, lethargy, confusion

Follow-up Care:
Follow-up Measures to Consider

- Document
- Return for care
  - As scheduled for gestation
  - As needed for worsening symptoms
  - Recommend hospital care for IV rehydration as needed

Collaborative Practice:
Consider Consultation or Referral

- Acupuncture therapy (Smith et al., 2002)

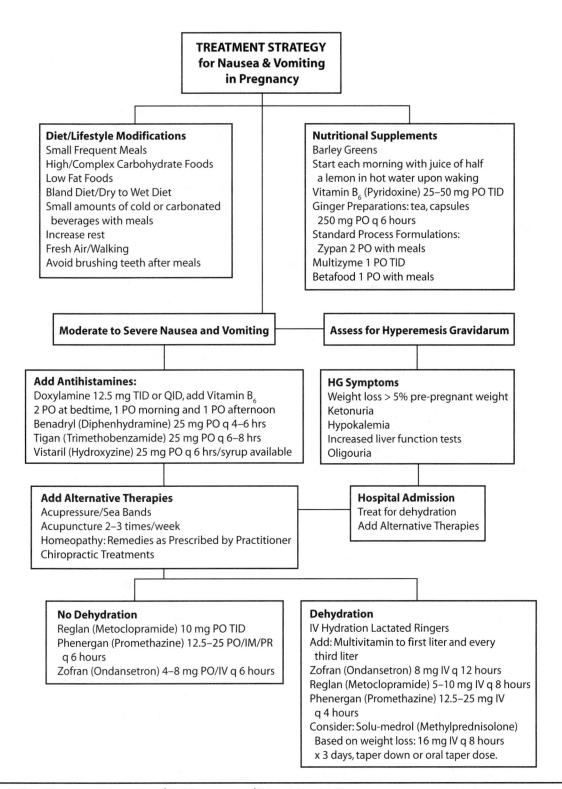

Figure 2-1   *Treatment Strategy for Nausea and Vomiting in Pregnancy*

Adapted from Association of Professors of Gynecology & Obstetrics Medical Education Foundation (2001) and ACOG (2004). Practice bulletin No. 52. Nausea and Vomiting of Pregnancy. In *2006 Compendium of selected publications.* Washington, DC: Author.

- OB/GYN services
  - Hyperemesis
  - Dehydration
  - Molar pregnancy
- For diagnosis or treatment outside the midwife's scope of practice

CARE OF THE PREGNANT WOMAN WITH PICA

Key Clinical Information

Pica is an eating disorder characterized by the ingestion of non-nutritive nonfood substances such as clay, starch, ice, and dirt. Pica is supported in some cultures and subcultures; for example, clay eating and starch eating are seen in the United States in some southern, rural, African-American communities, primarily among women and children (Ellis & Schnoes, 2006). Starch eating, in particular, is frequently started in pregnancy as a treatment of morning sickness. The prevalence of this practice is not known because pica is often undisclosed, unrecognized, and underreported. The nature and amount of ingested substances determine the health consequences of this behavior.

Client History and Chart Review:
Components of the History to Consider (Ellis & Schnoes, 2006)
- Gestational age
- Identify
  - Nonfood substances craved or consumed
  - 🌐 Cultural or ethnic expressions of pica
  - Social issues that may contribute to pica
    - Need for attention
    - Inadequate diet
    - 🌐 Cultural expectations
- Evaluate
  - Client's diet and nutritional resources
  - Use of vitamin and mineral supplements
  - Previous hematocrit and hemoglobin
  - Prior history of anemia

Physical Examination:
Components of the Physical Exam to Consider
- Vital signs
- Interval weight gain or loss
- Assess nutritional status
- Evaluate for symptoms of anemia
  - Color of mucous membranes
  - Capillary refill
  - Orthostatic hypotension
  - Elevated heart rate

Clinical Impression:
Differential Diagnoses and Code Groups to Consider
Additional suffix may apply (ICD9data.com, 2007)
- Pica (ICD-9 codes V22.2 and 307.52)
- Anemia (ICD-9 codes 648)
- Lead toxicity (ICD-9 codes V22.2 and 984)

Diagnostic Testing:
Diagnostic Tests and Procedures to Consider
- Hematocrit and hemoglobin
- Lead screening
- Anemia workup, see Anemia—Chapter 3

Providing Treatment:
Therapeutic Measures to Consider
- Iron replacement therapy if anemia present
- Multivitamin and mineral supplement

Providing Treatment:
Alternative Measures to Consider
- Iron rich foods, see Appendix B-3
- Sea vegetables, such as kelp, nori, wakame (high in iron and trace minerals)
- Red raspberry leaf tea

Providing Support:
Education and Support Measures to Consider
- Explore concerns about pica with client
  - Stress pica may interfere with good nutrition
  - Provide or arrange for nutritional education

- ▪ Encourage client to avoid nonfood items
    - ◆ 🔄 Try offering substitute items
- • Laundry starch, ice > frozen fruit pops
- • Clay > food-grade seaweed
- • Other acceptable nutritional items

Follow-up Care:
Follow-up Measures to Consider
- • Document
- • Return for care
    - ▪ As scheduled for gestation
    - ▪ Follow-up laboratory values as indicated
    - ▪ Inquire about continued pica practices

Collaborative Practice:
Consider Consultation or Referral
- • Diet counseling
- • Social services
    - ▪ WIC
    - ▪ Food stamps
    - ▪ Food bank
- • OB/GYN or Medical services
    - ▪ For severe pica accompanied by anemia
    - ▪ For elevated lead levels
- • For diagnosis or treatment outside the midwife's scope of practice

CARE OF THE PREGNANT WOMAN WITH ROUND LIGAMENT PAIN

Key Clinical Information

Round ligament pain is the unpleasant sensation that ranges from sharp knifelike pain to dull intermittent pain in the lower abdominal and inguinal areas of the pregnant woman. It is believed that virtually all pregnant women will experience this pain at some point in their pregnancy, so education and reassurance are important (Varney et al., 2004). Round ligament pain may be a frequent occurrence between 16 and 20 weeks gestation. It may mimic, or mask, more serious conditions, such as appendicitis or ovarian torsion. Round ligament pain may cause significant distress, especially in the athletic woman who continues to jog

or in women who have highly physical jobs such as waitresses or nurse's aides. An objective pain scale is recommended to assess and document client pain.

Client History and Chart Review:
Components of the History to Consider
- • Gestational age
- • Evaluation of the pain
    - ▪ Onset, location, severity, duration
    - ▪ Quality of the pain
        - ◆ Intermittent or constant
        - ◆ Sharp or dull
        - ◆ Exacerbating factors
    - ▪ Associated symptoms
        - ◆ Cramping
        - ◆ Backache
        - ◆ Nausea and vomiting
        - ◆ Change in bowel or bladder function
- • Relief measures used and efficacy
- • Activities of daily living
    - ▪ Employment activities

Physical Examination:
Components of the Physical Exam to Consider
- • Vital signs
- • Verify location of pain, observe and palpate area
- • Note posture and overall appearance
- • Abdominal examination
    - ▪ Palpate for tenderness
        - ◆ Note guarding
        - ◆ Rebound pain
        - ◆ Referred pain
    - ▪ Uterine examination
        - ◆ Fundal height
        - ◆ Fetal heart rate
        - ◆ Presence of contractions
        - ◆ Consistency and position of uterus
- • Pelvic examination
    - ▪ Cervical or vaginal discharge
    - ▪ Dilation and/or effacement
- • Evaluate for CVA tenderness

Clinical Impression:
Differential Diagnoses and Code Groups
to Consider
Additional suffix may apply (ICD9data.com, 2007;
Seller, 2000)

- Round ligament pain (ICD-9 codes V22.2 and 625.9)
- Also consider
  - Urinary tract infection (ICD-9 codes 646)
  - Ectopic pregnancy (ICD-9 codes 633)
  - Preterm labor (ICD-9 codes 644)
  - Placental abruption (ICD-9 codes 641)
  - Acute abdomen secondary to
    - Ovarian torsion (ICD-9 codes V22.2 and 620)
    - Renal calculi (ICD-9 codes V22.2 and 592)
    - Pyelonephritis (ICD-9 codes V22.2 and 590)
    - Appendicitis (ICD-9 codes V22.2 and 541)
    - Gallbladder disease (ICD-9 codes V22.2 and 574)
    - Pelvic inflammatory disease (ICD-9 codes V22.2 and 614.9)

Diagnostic Testing:
Diagnostic Tests and Procedures to Consider
- Urinalysis
- CBC, with differential
- Ultrasound evaluation
  - Pelvis
    - Uterus, ovaries, and tubes
    - Appendix
  - Abdomen
    - Kidneys, ureters, and bladder
    - Gallbladder

Providing Treatment:
Therapeutic Measures to Consider
- Maternity abdominal support or girdle
- Pain relief (Murphy, 2004)
  - Acetaminophen/aspirin
    - Alternate every 4 hours
    - Use for no more than 24–48 hours

Providing Treatment:
Alternative Measures to Consider
- Muscle strengthening and stretching
  - Yoga
  - Swimming
  - Prenatal exercise class
- Reflexology to waist and pelvic points
- Herbal remedies
  - Red raspberry leaf tea
  - Massage with arnica infused massage oil

Providing Support:
Education and Support Measures
to Consider
- Physiologic cause of round ligament pain
- Provide reassurance
- Self-help measures
  - Pelvic tilt
  - Slow graceful movements
  - Warm baths
  - Applying gentle heat to area
  - Positioning
    - Knees to abdomen
    - Bending toward pain to ease ligament
    - Side-lying with pillow under abdomen
  - Limit lifting and twisting
  - Ask for help as needed
- Warning signs
  - Onset of contractions
  - Persistent abdominal pain
  - Fever
  - Onset of nausea and vomiting
  - Vaginal bleeding or discharge
  - Pain with intercourse or bowel movement

Follow-up Care:
Follow-up Measures to Consider
- Document
- Return for care
  - As scheduled for gestation
  - As indicated by test results
  - With onset of warning signs

Collaborative Practice:
Consider Consultation or Referral

- Osteopathic or chiropractic manipulation
- OB/GYN services
  - Abdominal pain inconsistent with round ligament pain
  - Abnormal test results
- For diagnosis or treatment outside the midwife's scope of practice

CARE OF THE PREGNANT WOMAN WITH VARICOSE VEINS

Key Clinical Information

Varicose veins are distended veins with abnormal collections of blood caused by weak venous walls or improperly functioning venous valves. Varicosities develop in approximately 40% of pregnant women (Blackburn & Loper, 1992). Itching, swelling, or pain can accompany varicose veins, and they generally worsen as the pregnancy progresses and with each subsequent pregnancy. Care must be taken to avoid trauma to the vessels, which may result in hematoma formation, superficial phlebitis, or thrombophlebitis. Frequent rest periods with the feet elevated higher than the heart are essential for women with varicose veins. High quality support hose are helpful in easing the discomfort of significant lower limb varicosities. For women with vulvar varicosities, snug-fitting panties, bicycle shorts, or girdle may be needed to provide needed counterpressure.

Client History and Chart Review:
Components of the History
to Consider

- Gestational age
- Onset and location of varicose veins
  - Changes with pregnancy
  - Associated symptoms
    - Pain
    - Edema

- Redness
- Other associated symptoms
- Current relief measures and their effects
- Use of medications
  - Aspirin (acetylsalicylic acid)
  - Nonsteroidal anti-inflammatory drugs (NSAIDs)
- Past medical history
  - Varicose veins
  - Superficial phlebitis
  - Thrombophlebitis
- Activities of daily living
  - Employment activities

Physical Examination:
Components of the Physical Exam
to Consider

- Examination of varicosities
  - Location(s)
  - Number
  - Size
  - Severity
- Serial calf measurements
- Evaluate for symptoms of
  - Superficial phlebitis
    - Heat
    - Redness
    - Tenderness
  - Deep vein thrombosis
    - Pain
    - Positive Homans' sign
    - Leg edema

Clinical Impression:
Differential Diagnoses and Code Groups
to Consider
Additional suffix may apply (ICD9data.com, 2007; Seller, 2000)

- Varicose veins (ICD-9 code 671)
- Superficial phlebitis (ICD-9 code 671)
- Deep vein thrombosis (ICD-9 code 671)

Diagnostic Testing:
Diagnostic Tests and Procedures to Consider
- Serial calf measurements
- Testing for hemophilic disorders
- Clotting studies
- Ultrasound as indicated to rule out deep vein thrombosis

Providing Treatment:
Therapeutic Measures to Consider
- Support garments
  - Hosiery
    - Apply after elevating legs 10 minutes
    - Prescription hose may be needed
    - Wear daily
  - Foam pad to support vulvar varicosities
    - Use with close-fitting but nonconstricting undergarment
  - Maternity abdominal support to relieve pressure on pelvic veins
- Thromboprophylaxis
  - ◔ Women with a history of thrombosis or thrombophilia may be candidates for prophylactic treatment with low dose anticoagulants in pregnancy (ACOG, 2000)
- For symptoms of early superficial phlebitis
  - ◔ Consider use of broad spectrum antibiotic, such as Keflex

Providing Treatment:
Alternative Measures to Consider
- Onions in diet
- Herbal remedies
  - Bilberry tablets or capsules TID
    - Strengthens capillaries
    - Reduces platelet aggregation (Foster, 1996)
  - Nettle tea or tincture
    - Improves elasticity of vessels (Weed, 1985)
  - Horse chestnut tea, tincture or capsule
    - Strengthens capillaries (Weed, 1985)

- Positioning
  - Leg elevation above heart
  - Leg inversion (right-angle position)

Providing Support:
Education and Support Measures to Consider
- Encourage
  - Use and application of support hose
  - Rest with legs elevated
  - Regular mild exercise, especially walking or swimming
- Avoidance of
  - Constrictive clothing
  - Long periods of standing or sitting
- Medication instructions
- Warning signs
  - Persistent or worsening pain
  - Unilateral edema of extremity
  - Localized redness, heat, tenderness
  - Fever

Follow-up Care:
Follow-up Measures to Consider
- Document
- Return for care
  - As scheduled for gestation
  - Onset of warning signs
  - Four to 7 days for suspected early superficial phlebitis
  - Evaluate closely in early postpartum period

Collaborative Practice:
Consider Consultation or Referral
- OB/GYN services
  - For candidates for thromboprophylaxis (ACOG, 2000)
  - Severe vulvar varicosities
  - Suspected or confirmed
    - Phlebitis
    - Thrombophlebitis
- For diagnosis or treatment outside the midwife's scope of practice

REFERENCES

American College of Obstetricians and Gynecologists (ACOG). (2000). Practice bulletin number 19. Thromboembolism in pregnancy. In *2006 Compendium of selected publications* (pp. 961–970). Washington, DC: ACOG.

American College of Obstetricians and Gynecologists (ACOG). (2002). Committee opinion number 267. Exercise during pregnancy and the postpartum period. *Obstetrics and Gynecology, 99,* 171–173.

American College of Obstetricians and Gynecologists (ACOG). (2003a). Committee opinion number 282. Immunization during pregnancy. *Obstetrics and Gynecology,* 101, 207–212.

American College of Obstetricians and Gynecologists (ACOG). (2003b). Committee opinion number 291. Use of progesterone to reduce preterm birth. *Obstetrics and Gynecology,* 102, 1115–1116.

American College of Obstetricians and Gynecologists (ACOG). (2005). Committee opinion number 316. Smoking cessation during pregnancy. *Obstetrics and Gynecology,* 106, 883–888.

Arnesen, S. (2006). Environmental health information resources: healthy environments for healthy women and children. *Journal of Midwifery and Women's Health,* 51, 35–38.

Blackburn, S. T., & Loper, D. L. (1992). *Maternal, fetal and neonatal physiology: a clinical perspective.* Philadelphia: W.B. Saunders.

Centers for Disease Control and Prevention. (2002). Prevention of perinatal group B streptococcal disease. *Morbidity and Mortality Weekly Review 2002,* 51(RRII), 1–22. Retrieved January 4, 2007 from http://www.cdc.gov/mmwr/preview/mmwrhtml/rr5111a1.htm

Christian, M. S., & Brent, R. L. (2001). Teratogen update: evaluation of the reproductive and developmental risks of caffeine. *Teratology,* 64, 51–78.

Connors, G. J., Donovan, D. M., & DiClemente, C. C. (2001). *Substance abuse treatment and the stages of change.* New York: The Guilford Press.

Davis, E. (2004). *Hearts and hands: a midwife's guide to pregnancy and birth* (4th ed.). Berkeley, CA: Celestial Arts.

Ellis, C. R., & Schnoes, C. J. (2006). *Eating disorder: pica.* Retrieved January 4, 2008 from http://www.emedicine.com/PED/topic1798.htm

England, A. (1994). *Aromatherapy for mother and baby.* Rochester, VT: Healing Arts Press.

Foster, S. (1996). *Herbs for your health: a handy guide for knowing and using 50 common herbs.* Loveland, CO: Interweave Press.

Frye, A. (1998). *Holistic midwifery: a comprehensive textbook for midwives in homebirth practice, Vol. 1: care during pregnancy.* Portland, OR: Labrys Press.

Frye, A. (2007). *Understanding diagnostic tests in the childbearing year* (7th ed.). Portland, OR: Labrys Press.

Gojnic, M., Dugalic, V., Papic, M., Vidakovic, S., Milicevic, S., & Perulov, M. (2005). The significance of detailed examination of hemorrhoids during pregnancy. *Clinical Experience in Obstetrics and Gynecology,* 32, 183–184.

Gladstar, R. (1993). *Herbal healing for women.* New York: Simon and Schuster.

Griffith, H. W. (2000). *Healing herbs: the essential guide.* Tucson, AZ: Fisher Books.

Hartmann, S., & Huch, R. (2005). Response of pregnancy leg edema to a single immersion exercise session. *Acta Obstetrics and Gynecology Scandinavia,* 84, 1150–1153.

Institute for Clinical Systems Improvement (ICSI). (2006). *Routine prenatal care.* Bloomington, MN: Author. Retrieved January 4, 2008 from http://www.icsi.org/home/

Little, K. J. (2000). Screening for domestic violence: identifying, assisting, and empowering adult victims of abuse. *Postgraduate Medicine,* 108, 135–141. Retrieved January 4, 2008 from http://www.postgradmed.com/issues/2000/08_00/little.htm

Murphy, J. L. (Ed.). (2004). *Nurse practitioner's prescribing reference.* New York: Prescribing Reference.

Oates-Whitehead, R. (2004). Nausea and vomiting in early pregnancy. In F. Godlee (Ed.). *Clinical evidence concise* (pp. 392–394). London: BMJ Publishing Group.

Pennick, V. E., & Young, G. (2007). Interventions for preventing and treating pelvic and back pain in pregnancy. *Cochrane Database Systematic Review,* CD001139.

Rising, S. S., Kennedy, H. P., & Klima, C. S. (2004). Redesigning prenatal care through centering pregnancy. *Journal of Midwifery and Women's Health,* 49, 398–404.

Santiago, J. R., Nolledo, M. S., Kinsler, W., & Santiago, T. V. (2001). Sleep and sleep disorders in pregnancy. *Annals of Internal Medicine,* 134, 396–408. Retrieved January 4, 2008 from http://www.annals.org/cgi/reprint/134/5/396.pdf

Seller, R. H. (2000). *Differential diagnosis of common complaints* (4th ed.). Philadelphia: W.B. Saunders.

Simmonds, K. E., & Likis, F. E. (2005). Providing options counseling for women with unintended pregnancies. *Journal of Obstetric, Gynecologic and Neonatal Nursing, 34,* 373–379.

Sinclair, C. (2004). *A midwife's handbook.* St. Louis, MO: Saunders.

Smith, C., Crowther, C., & Beily, J. (2002). Acupuncture to treat nausea and vomiting in early pregnancy: a randomized controlled trial. *Birth, 29,* 1–9.

Sripramote, M., & Lekhyananda, N. (2003). A randomized comparison of ginger and vitamin B_6 in the treatment of nausea and vomiting of pregnancy. *Journal of the Medical Association of Thailand, 86,* 846–853.

Varney, H., Kriebs, J. M., & Gegor, C. L. (2004). *Varney's midwifery* (4th ed.). Sudbury, MA: Jones and Bartlett.

Walker, D. S., Day, S., Diroff, C., Lirette, H., McCully, L., Mooney-Hescott, C., et al. (2002). Reduced frequency prenatal visits in midwifery practice: attitudes and use. *Journal of Midwifery and Women's Health, 47,* 269–277.

Walls, D. (2007). *Natural families—healthy homes.* LaVergne, TN: Ingram Publishing Company.

Weed, S. (1985). *Wise woman herbal for the childbearing year.* Woodstock, NY: Ash Tree Publishing.

Weir, F., & Farley, C. L. (2006). Clinical controversies in screening for thyroid disorders in women during childbearing years. *Journal of Midwifery and Women's Health, 51,* 152–158.

BIBLIOGRAPHY

Briggs, G. G., Freeman, R. K., & Yaffe, S. J. (2005). *Drugs in pregnancy and lactation: a reference guide to fetal and neonatal risk* (7th ed.). Philadelphia: Lippincott, Williams & Wilkins.

Enkin, M., Keirce, M., Renfrew, M., Neilson, J., Crowther, C., Duley, L., et al. (2000). *A guide to effective care in pregnancy and childbirth* (3rd ed.). New York: Oxford University Press.

Fraser, D., & Cooper, M. (2003). *Textbook for midwives* (14th ed.). Edinburgh, Scotland: Churchill Livingstone.

Godlee, F. (Ed.). (2007). *Clinical evidence handbook.* London: BMJ Publishing Group.

Gordon, J. D., Rydfors, J. T., Druzin, M. L., Tadir, Y., El-Sayed, Y., Chan, J., et al. (2007). *Obstetrics, gynecology and infertility* (6th ed.). Glen Cove, NY: Scrub Hill Press.

Ickovics, J. R., Kershaw, T. S., Westdahl, C., Magriples, U., Massey, Z., Reynolds, H., et al. (2007). Group prenatal care and perinatal outcomes: a randomized controlled trial. *Obstetrics and Gynecology, 110,* 330–339.

Kirkham, C., Harris, S., & Grzybowski, S. (2005). Evidence-based prenatal care. Part I. General prenatal care and counseling issues. *American Family Physician, 71,* 1307–1316.

Low Dog, T., & Micozzi, M. (2005). *Women's health in complementary and integrative medicine: a clinical guide.* St. Louis, MO: Elsevier.

Morgan, G., & Hamilton, C. (2003). *Practice guidelines for obstetrics and gynecology.* Philadelphia: Lippincott-Raven.

National Institutes of Health. (1989). *Caring for our future: the content of prenatal care. A report of the Public Health Service Expert Panel on the Content of Prenatal Care.* Bethesda, MD: Author.

Scott, J. R., Gibbs, R. S., Karlan, B., & Haney, A. (2003). *Danforth's obstetrics and gynecology* (9th ed.). Philadelphia: Lippincott, Williams & Wilkins.

Soule, D., & Szwed, S. (2000). *The roots of healing: a woman's book of herbs.* Secaucus, NJ: Citadel Press.

U.S. Public Health Service. (2003). *Treating tobacco use and dependence—clinician's packet. A how-to guide for implementing the public health service clinical practice guideline.* Retrieved January 4, 2008 from http://www.surgeongeneral.gov/tobacco/clinpack.html

Ustianov, J. (2006). *Improving prenatal care in Vermont: a practice level toolkit and state guide.* Retrieved January 4, 2008 from https://www.med.uvm.edu/vchip/TB2+RL+3I.asp?SiteAreaID=669

Washington State Department of Health. (2002). *Smoking cessation during pregnancy: guidelines for intervention.* Olympia, WA: Author. Retrieved January 4, 2008 http://www.doh.wa.gov/CFH/mch/documents/CessationFinal_122.pdf

Care of the Pregnant Woman with Prenatal Variations

3

Prompt identification and treatment of prenatal variations that may result in harm to mother or baby ensures the best possible outcome.

The ability to anticipate problems in pregnancy is an essential component of skilled midwifery practice. Midwives must be steadfast in their belief that pregnancy is a normal physiologic condition while retaining a healthy respect for problems and complications that may develop (Ulrich, 2004). During optimal evaluation of potential or developing problems, the midwife actively engages the mother in decision-making regarding the options for care of herself and her unborn baby.

Among the hallmarks of midwifery care are advocacy for informed choice, shared decision-making, and the right to self-determination (American College of Nurse-Midwives, 2007). Although the mother may have no control over the development of problems during her pregnancy and may feel threatened when they occur, the midwife can offer her a sense of control by presenting options in the areas where client choice is possible. Respect for each woman's needs is especially important when an unexpected problem develops.

Many women look to their midwife to present a balanced view of the problem, diagnostic evaluation, and treatment process. Although many women may wish to be an active participant in all health care decisions, the expectation is that the midwife will clearly recommend a course of action. Recommendations are based on the midwife's judgment of what constitutes best care for the mother and fetus in light of the presenting problem. Occasionally, the midwife's recommendations may run contrary to either the mother's preferences or standard hospital-based expectations for obstetric care. A clear, focused, and confidently presented midwifery plan of care with rationale backed by evidence-based resources can be helpful in providing guidance to the client who hesitates at indicated obstetric intervention or in promoting understanding among providers in the medical setting where the midwife may feel pressured to intervene without clear indication. Midwifery care of problems in pregnancy forms a continuum from least intervention to most intervention. The skilled midwife may move along this continuum in either direction, understanding that appropriate medical or obstetric intervention in the presence of complication serves the mother's and baby's needs and is congruent with midwifery philosophy.

CARE OF THE PREGNANT WOMAN WITH IRON DEFICIENCY ANEMIA

Key Clinical Information

Iron deficiency anemia due to dietary deficiencies is the most common form of anemia in pregnant women (Varney et al., 2004). In developed countries, 20% of pregnant women have iron deficiency anemia, whereas in developing countries as many as 50% of pregnant women have this disorder (Rioux & LeBlanc, 2007; University of Maryland Medical Center, 2007). Anemia may affect the oxygenation of both mother and fetus and may result in diminished fetal growth, maternal exhaustion, and related complications, such as prematurity (Graves & Barger, 2001). Prompt diagnosis, treatment, and follow-up of anemia with attention to the overall nutritional status of the mother are critically important for fetal well-being and for optimizing maternal health before the onset of labor.

Client History and Chart Review:
Components of the History to Consider
- Gestational age
- Current hematocrit and hemoglobin
- Potential causes of anemia
  - Tobacco use
  - History of closely spaced pregnancies
  - Blood loss, heavy menses
  - Chronic illness
  - Malabsorption syndromes
  - Malignancy (Payton & White, 1995)
  - Risk for thalassemia or sickle cell
    - African descent
    - Mediterranean descent
    - Asian descent
- Presence of anemia-related symptoms
  - Fatigue
  - Dizziness
  - Headache

- Pica (eating nonfood items such as starch or clay)
- Dyspnea
- Palpitations or tachycardia (Engstrom & Sittler, 1994)
- Usual dietary patterns
  - General nutrition
  - Dietary iron sources
  - Prenatal vitamin use
  - Iron supplement use

Physical Examination:
Components of the Physical Exam to Consider
- Vital signs, including pulse and blood pressure (BP)
- Affect and energy level
- Pallor of skin and mucous membranes
- Brittle nails
- Examination for potential causes of anemia
  - Bruising
  - Bleeding

Clinical Impression:
Differential Diagnoses and Code Groups to Consider
Additional suffix may apply (ICD9data.com, 2007)
- Physiologic anemia of pregnancy (ICD-9 code 648.23)
- Iron deficiency anemia (ICD-9 codes V22.2 and 280)
- Other anemia
  - Pernicious (ICD-9 codes V22.2 and 281.0)
  - Hemolytic (ICD-9 codes V22.2 and 282)
  - Sickle cell (ICD-9 codes V22.2 and 282.60)
  - Thalassemia (ICD-9 codes V22.2 and 282.41)

Diagnostic Testing:
Diagnostic Tests and Procedures to Consider
- Complete blood count (CBC) with indices
  - Indices in simple iron deficiency anemia (Varney et al., 2004)
    - Microcytic
    - Hypochromic

- ◆ Serum ferritin is decreased
- ◆ Total iron binding capacity is increased
- Stool for occult blood, ova, and parasites
- See Table 3-1 for cut off hemoglobin and hematocrit values for diagnosis of anemia by weeks of pregnancy (CDC, 1998)

Providing Treatment:
Therapeutic Measures to Consider

- Iron replacement therapy for hemoglobin less than 11 or low serum ferritin (Rioux & LeBlanc, 2007; University of Maryland Medical Center, 2007)
  - ▪ 60–120 mg elemental iron daily
  - ▪ Iron salts such as
    - ◆ Ferrous sulfate (Feosol/Slow Fe)
      - ➤ 50–65 mg elemental iron
      - ➤ 1 PO BID
    - ◆ Ferrous gluconate (Fergon)
      - ➤ 27 mg elemental iron
      - ➤ 2 PO BID
    - ◆ Ferrous fumarate 200 mg (Chromagen)
      - ➤ 66 mg elemental iron
      - ➤ 1 PO BID
    - ◆ Polysaccharide iron complex (Niferex-150)
      - ➤ 150 mg elemental iron
      - ➤ One to two capsules PO daily (Murphy, 2004)

- ▪ Include vitamin C and folic acid
- ▪ Continue through 3 months postpartum
- IM or IV Imferon for severe or recalcitrant anemia
  - ▪ May cause anaphylactic reaction
  - ▪ 🚫 Use with caution and following consult

Providing Treatment:
Alternative Measures to Consider

- Floradix iron plus herbs liquid
  - ▪ 2 tsp BID
  - ▪ Vegetarian liquid formula
- High iron food sources (see Appendix B-3)
- Additional fiber to prevent constipation
- Chlorophyll, liquid or capsule
- Heme iron most easily absorbed
  - ▪ Meat
  - ▪ Poultry
  - ▪ Fish
- Non-heme iron
  - ▪ Egg yolk
  - ▪ Grains
  - ▪ Vegetables
- Cast iron cookware
  - ▪ Nonenamel surface
  - ▪ Adds elemental iron

Table 3-1   Cut Off Hemoglobin and Hematocrit Values for Diagnosis of Anemia by Weeks of Pregnancy

WEEK OF GESTATION	HEMOGLOBIN (G/DL)	HEMATOCRIT (%)
12	11.0	33.0
16	10.6	32.0
20–24	10.5	32.0
28	10.7	32.0
32	11.0	33.0
36	11.4	34.0
40	11.9	36.0

Source: Centers for Disease Control and Prevention. (1998). Recommendations to prevent and control iron deficiency in the United States. *Morbidity and Mortality Weekly Report, 47,* 1–25.

Providing Support:
Education and Support Measures
to Consider

- Physiologic nature of anemia in pregnancy
- Pica decreases iron absorption
- Iron supplementation recommendations
  - Dosages
  - Separate supplement from
    - Meals
    - Calcium intake
    - Fiber supplements
    - Other supplements (e.g., prenatal vitamins)
- For best absorption
  - Take with vitamin C or water
  - Take at bedtime
  - Avoid caffeine, black teas
- Common side effects include
  - Gastrointestinal upset, constipation, or diarrhea
  - Nausea
  - Heartburn (Engstrom & Sittler, 1994)

Follow-up Care:
Follow-up Measures to Consider

- Document
- List parameters for consultation
- Return for care
  - Repeat hematocrit and hemoglobin 4–6 weeks after initiating therapy
  - Add indices for persistent anemia

Collaborative Practice:
Consider Consultation or Referral

- Nutritional consult
- Social services
  - WIC
  - Food stamps
  - Local food pantry
  - Smoking cessation programs
- Medical consult
  - For abnormal indices or elevated serum ferritin

- For anemia resistant to conventional therapy
- For concern regarding cause of anemia
- For diagnosis outside the midwife's scope of practice

CARE OF THE PREGNANT WOMAN WITH FETAL DEMISE

Key Clinical Information

Early pregnancy loss before 22 weeks gestation is considered a spontaneous or missed abortion, whereas after 22 weeks gestation it is considered a fetal death (Varney et al., 2004). Fetal demise may occur at any stage of pregnancy. No matter when it occurs, a common response is for the mother to wonder what she did wrong. Emotional support and grief counseling may be helpful to parents. The cause of fetal demise is frequently unable to be determined. Some fetal or placental conditions are clearly incompatible with life, whereas other fetal loss may be related to maternal illness, heredity, or unknown factors. Genetic investigation and counseling may be useful for exploring potential causes of fetal demise (American College of Obstetricians and Gynecologists [ACOG], 2001a), particularly for the woman with a history of recurrent losses. Fetal demise is associated with an increased likelihood of maternal disseminated intravascular coagulation (DIC) (Lindsay & Azad, 2006).

Client History and Chart Review:
Components of the History to Consider

- Gestational age
- Regression of signs of pregnancy
  - Absence of fetal activity
  - Absence of fetal heart tones
  - Other associated signs and symptoms
- Previous human chorionic gonadotropin (HCG) results
- Precipitating event(s), if any
  - Idiopathic
  - Trauma/physical abuse
  - Substance abuse
- Medication and herb use

- Risk factors for stillbirth
  - Maternal age extremes
  - Multiple gestation
  - Body mass index (BMI) > 30
  - 🌐 Race: African-American risk twice that of whites
  - Maternal disorders, such as diabetes, hypertension, renal disease, lupus
- Review birth and surgical history

Physical Examination:
Components of the Physical Exam
to Consider
- Maternal vital signs
- Abdominal exam
  - Fundal height
  - Uterine tenderness
  - Absence of fetal heart tones
- Pelvic examination
  - Palpation of buckled fetal skull
  - Cervical status/Bishop's score

Clinical Impression:
Differential Diagnoses and Code Groups
to Consider
Additional suffix may apply (ICD9data.com, 2007)
- Intrauterine fetal demise
  - Early, before 22 weeks (ICD-9 codes 632)
  - Late, after 22 weeks (ICD-9 codes 656.4)
- Missed abortion (ICD-9 codes 632)
- Ectopic pregnancy (ICD-9 codes 633)
- Blighted ovum (ICD-9 codes 631)
- Pseudocyesis (ICD-9 code 300.11)

Diagnostic Testing:
Diagnostic Tests and Procedures to Consider
- Maternal blood work
  - CBC
  - Kleihauer-Betke
  - Hemoglobin A_{1c}
  - Rapid plasma reagin/Venereal Disease Research Laboratory
  - Serum/urine toxicology screen

- Weekly testing in expectant management
  - Prothrombin time, partial thromboplastin time
  - Fibrinogen, fibrin degradation products
  - Platelets
- Ultrasound
  - Absent fetal heart beat (verified by two examiners)
  - Overlapping of fetal cranial bones: Spalding's sign
  - Presence of gas in fetal abdomen: Robert's sign
- Fetal evaluation (ACOG, 2001a)
  - Cord blood
  - Placenta to pathology for gross and micro-scopic examination
  - Placental cultures
  - Fetal x-rays and autopsy with consent of parents
- Genetic testing with consent and if indicated (ACOG, 2001a)
  - Anomalies
  - Family history
  - Recurrent fetal losses

Providing Treatment:
Therapeutic Measures to Consider
(Belkin & Wilder, 2007)
- Expectant management
  - May be emotionally difficult
  - Increased risk of DIC after 3 weeks
  - Observe for onset of
    - Fever
    - DIC
    - Rupture of membranes (ROM) or labor
- Surgical Dilatation & Evacuation (D&E) in early pregnancy
- Induction of labor
  - Laminaria or Foley catheter
  - Prostin E_2 suppositories
  - Misoprostol 50–100 mg per vagina or PO if no uterine scar
  - Oxytocin drip after 32 weeks gestation

Providing Treatment:
Alternative Measures to Consider

- Natural remedies to stimulate labor
  - May not be effective before 32 weeks
  - Blue/black cohosh infusion or tincture
  - Castor oil
- Homeopathic caulophyllum 60×

Providing Support:
Education and Support Measures to Consider
(Belkin & Wilder, 2007)

- Cause of death if known
- Options for birth
  - Discussion regarding labor initiation
    - Maternal preferences
    - Parameters for consultation
    - Therapeutic measures to initiate labor
  - Location for birth
  - Anticipated course of events
- Care of the body
  - May vary with gestational age
  - Family time
  - Autopsy or testing
  - Burial, cremation, or hospital disposal
- Funeral or memorial service
- Postpartum period
  - Lochia
  - Lactation suppression
  - RhoGAM if needed
  - Rubella if needed
- Depression
  - Support groups and community resources
    - Review stages of grief

Follow-up Care:
Follow-up Measures to Consider

- Document
  - Maternal response
  - Course of labor and birth
  - Anomalies if any
  - Care and arrangements for the fetus
  - Placental disposition
  - Planned follow-up

- Follow-up care
  - Weeks 1–6
    - Phone, home, or office visit
    - Results of any testing
    - Evaluation of emotional status
  - Weeks 2–6
    - Postpartum check
    - Initiation of birth control as needed
    - Support

Collaborative Practice:
Consider Consultation or Referral

- For social support
  - Grief counseling
  - Support groups
- Medical/obstetric care
  - For fetal demise > 12 weeks gestation
  - For evidence of DIC
  - For mother who prefers surgical D&E in early pregnancy
  - For induction of labor as indicated by
    - Midwifery scope of practice
    - Maternal preference or condition
- For diagnosis outside the midwife's scope of practice

CARE OF THE PREGNANT WOMAN EXPOSED TO FIFTH'S DISEASE

Key Clinical Information

Fifth's disease, also known as erythema infectiosum, is caused by the parvovirus B19 (Goff, 2005). It is spread by droplet, most often in the springtime. Viremia occurs 7 days after inoculation and lasts 4 days. It is common for women who are school teachers to find that their students have Fifth's disease. Fortunately, most women contract Fifth's disease as children and are not at risk for primary infection during pregnancy. Parvovirus infection during pregnancy is considered to be a low risk for fetal morbidity; however, it may result in fetal hydrops, aplastic anemia, or intrauterine growth restriction (IUGR) (ACOG, 2000c).

Client History and Chart Review:
Components of the History to Consider
- Current gestation
- Blood type and Rh
- Rubella and rubeola titers
- Employment history
- History of recent outbreak with close contact
  - School teachers
  - Health care workers
- Symptoms of parvovirus infection
  - Rash
  - Fever
  - Malaise
  - Myalgia, arthralgia

Physical Examination:
Components of the Physical Exam to Consider
- Vital signs, including temperature
- Routine prenatal surveillance
- Evaluate for
  - Rash
    - Diffuse maculopapular rash
    - Trunk and extremities
    - Occurs 16 days postinoculation
    - 5 days postresolution of virus
  - Joint and muscle pain

Clinical Impression:
Differential Diagnoses and Code Groups
to Consider
Additional suffix may apply (ICD9data.com, 2007; Seller, 2000)
- Fifth's disease, erythema infectiosum (parvovirus B19) (ICD-9 codes V22.2 and 057.0)
- Other viral exanthema (ICD-9 codes V22.2 and 050–057)
- Allergic rash (ICD-9 codes V22.2 and 782)

Diagnostic Testing:
Diagnostic Tests and Procedures to Consider
- Serologic testing for parvovirus B19
  - Indicated for
    - Postexposure

- Positive clinical signs and symptoms
- Fetal nonimmune hydrops
  - Parvovirus B19 IgM and IgG
    - Positive IgM indicates recent infection
    - Positive IgG indicates current immunity; if nonimmune repeat in 3–4 weeks (ACOG, 2000c)
- α-Fetoprotein—as indicated by gestation
- Level II ultrasound
  - Fetal cardiac evaluation
  - Fetal hydrops

Providing Treatment:
Therapeutic Measures to Consider
- ⊗ No treatment available; however, heightened fetal surveillance is recommended if seroconversion occurs

Providing Treatment:
Alternative Measures to Consider
- For possible exposure consider
  - Rest
  - Stress reduction techniques
  - Immune support
    - Whole foods diet, avoiding processed foods

Providing Support:
Education and Support Measures to Consider
- Reassure: Most adults are immune
- Explain screening and management plan
- Warning signs to report
  - Rash
  - Decreased fetal movement
- Potential for fetal compromise with infection
  - May have no effect
  - Spontaneous abortion (SAB) in first trimester
  - Fetal death second trimester (3–6 weeks postmaternal infection)
  - Nonimmune hydrops
  - Severe anemia
  - Viral-induced cardiomyopathy

- May elevate α-fetoprotein
- No association of parvovirus B19 and birth defects

Follow-up Care:
Follow-up Measures to Consider
- Document
- Testing
  - Positive IgG: No further testing (immune)
  - Negative IgG: Repeat IgG in 3–4 weeks (Varney et al., 2004)
- Return for care
  - Two to 3 weeks postexposure
  - Onset of signs or symptoms
- Mother with acute illness
  - Follow for hydrops
    - Weekly ultrasound for 12 weeks
  - Provide emotional support

Collaborative Practice:
Consider Consultation or Referral
- OB/GYN services
  - Maternal infection with parvovirus B19
  - Fetus with evidence of
    - Cardiomyopathy
    - Hydrops
    - Anemia
- For diagnosis outside the midwife's scope of practice

CARE OF THE PREGNANT WOMAN WITH GESTATIONAL DIABETES

Key Clinical Information
Gestational diabetes occurs in 4–7% of all pregnant women in the United States (American Diabetes Association, 2003). It is defined as carbohydrate intolerance and increased insulin resistance first recognized in pregnancy (ACOG, 2001b). There is a significant increase in fetal malformations in pregnant women with persistently elevated glucose levels. This risk is noted to be higher for women with hemoglobin A_{Ic} levels that are elevated early in pregnancy compared with those pregnant women whose hemoglobin A_{Ic} levels are normal in spite of abnormal glucose metabolism.

It is especially important to enlist the participation of the mother when gestational diabetes presents. Daily attention to diet is imperative, with food sources providing excellent nutrition and a balance of proteins, fats, and complex carbohydrates. A food and blood glucose diary can be very helpful in making dietary recommendations that are culturally and financially reasonable.

Client History and Chart Review:
Components of the History to Consider
- Gestational age
- Identify risk factors for gestational diabetes
  - Maternal age > 25
  - BMI > 28 kg/m^2
  - Previous fasting blood sugar (FBS) 110–125 mg/dl
  - Suspected or documented previous gestational diabetes
    - Previous infant weighing > 4100 g
  - Previous unexplained fetal demise
  - Polyhydramnios
  - Previous birth of a child with a congenital anomaly
- Ethnic heritage
  - African
  - Alaskan native
  - Hispanic
  - Native American
  - South or East Asian
  - Pacific Islands
- History of polycystic ovarian syndrome
- Family history of diabetes in first-degree relative
- Symptoms of gestational diabetes
  - Glycosuria
  - Size larger than dates
  - Frequent urination
  - Intense thirst
  - Loss of energy

Physical Examination:
Components of the Physical Exam
to Consider

- Vital signs, including weight
- BMI
- Weight gain
- Monitor fundal heights
  - IUGR
  - Fetal macrosomia
  - Polyhydramnios

Clinical Impression:
Differential Diagnoses and Code Groups
to Consider

Additional suffix may apply (ICD9data.com, 2007)

- Gestational diabetes (ICD-9 codes 648.8)
- Disorders of carbohydrate metabolism and transport (ICD-9 codes 271)
- Diabetes mellitus (ICD-9 codes V22.2 and 250)
- Fetal macrosomia secondary to
  - Gestational diabetes (ICD-9 codes 775.0)
  - Constitutionally large fetus (ICD-9 codes 766.1)
- Polyhydramnios (ICD-9 codes 657.03)

Diagnostic Testing:
Diagnostic Tests and Procedures to Consider

- Dip urinalysis for glucose
- Screening women with risk factors
  - First visit or first trimester
  - 24–28 weeks
  - 34–36 weeks
  - Onset of
    - Glucosuria
    - Macrosomia
    - Polyhydramnios
    - Pregnancy-induced hypertension (PIH)
- Screening women without risk factors
  - 24–28 weeks
  - Testing with indications only
- Omitting screening is an option for women who meet all the following criteria; continue

screening for clinical signs of gestational diabetes (ACOG, 2001b)
  - Age < 25 years
  - Normal BMI before pregnancy
  - Member of an ethnic group with a low prevalence of gestational diabetes
  - No known diabetes in first-degree relatives
  - No history of abnormal glucose tolerance
  - No history of poor obstetric outcome
- Screening methods (Varney et al., 2004)
  - FBS
    - Value of > 126 mg/dl is diagnostic for gestational diabetes
  - One-hour glucose challenge test
    - Value of > 200 mg/dl is diagnostic of gestational diabetes
- If screen is elevated
  - Obtain 3-hour glucose tolerance test
  - Consider hemoglobin A_{1c} testing
- Diagnosis
  - Two or more elevated blood levels in 3-hour glucose tolerance test
- Maternal assessment
  - Hemoglobin A_{1c}
    - Normal range: 4.0–8.2%
    - Less than 6% preferable in pregnancy
  - Self-monitored blood glucose
    - All values within target range
    - Before meal and bedtime: 60–95 mg/dl
    - After meal
- Less than 120 mg/dl 2 hours after start of meal
- Less than 140 mg/dl 1 hour after start of meal
- Ultrasound for fetal anomalies, fetal growth

Providing Treatment:
Therapeutic Measures to Consider

- Regular exercise
- Dietary control
  - Caloric intake by weight, range from 1800 to 2400 kcal/day
    - Underweight (BMI < 22)—40 kcal/kg/day
    - Average weight (BMI 22–26)— 30 kcal/kg/day

Table 3-2   Screening and Diagnostic Testing for Gestational Diabetes

DOSE/TIME	PLASMA (G/DL)
Fasting: normal glucose metabolism	< 105
Fasting hyperglycemia	> 105 < 126
Diagnostic of gestational diabetes	
Fasting	≥ 126
Nonfasting	≥ 200
50-g glucose challenge test, 1 hr	≥ 130 or 140
100-g glucose tolerance test	
Fasting	≥ 95
1 hr	≥ 180
2 hr	≥ 155
3 hr	≥ 140

Source: American Diabetes Association. (2007). Standards of Medical Care in Diabetes—2007. *Diabetes Care;* 30: S4-41.

- ◆ Overweight (BMI 27–29)—24 kcal/kg/day
- ◆ Overweight (BMI > 30)—12–15 kcal/kg/day
- ■ Six small meals daily
  - ◆ Carbohydrates 55–60% of diet
  - ◆ Protein 12–20% of diet
  - ◆ Fat for the remainder (American Diabetes Association, 2003)
- • Medications
  - ■ Glyburide (Pregnancy Category B)
    - ◆ Use after organogenesis
    - ◆ Consult for use and dosage
  - ■ Metformin (Pregnancy Category B)
    - ◆ Clinical trial currently underway for use in gestational diabetes
    - ◆ ⚠ Await results on safety and efficacy before considering use
  - ■ Initiate insulin 2-hour postprandial glucose > 120 mg/dl (ACOG, 2001b)
    - ◆ Consult for use and dosages
    - ◆ Titrate to maintain glycemic control
- • FBS > 95 mg/dl
- • One-hour postprandial values > 130–140 mg/dl

Providing Treatment:
Alternative Measures to Consider
- • Macrobiotic or whole food diet
- • Cinnamon ¼ to ½ tsp daily (Hlebowicz et al. 2007)
- • Herbs
  - ■ Bilberry (Foster, 1996)
  - ■ Chicory
  - ■ Dandelion
  - ■ Nettle
  - ■ Red raspberry tea (Weed, 1985)

Providing Support: Education and Support
Measures to Consider
- • Risks and benefits of options for care
- • Diabetic education
  - ■ American Diabetes Association
    - ◆ 1-800-342-2383 or e-mail ask ADA@diabetes.org
    - ◆ American Diabetes Association publication number 4902-04, *Gestational Diabetes: What to Expect*, 4th edition

- Dietary control
  - ◆ Dietary recommendations for gestational diabetes
  - ◆ Physical activity recommendations
- Medication instruction, if used
- Daily home glucose monitoring (International Diabetes Center, 2003)
  - ◆ Meter with memory and log book
  - ◆ Six to seven times a day preferred until glycemic control established
    - ➤ Before and 1–2 hours after start of meals
    - ➤ Bedtime
  - ◆ Daily self-monitoring may be reduced once glycemic control established
    - ➤ Fasting
    - ➤ One to 2 hours after start of meals
- Warning signs and symptoms
  - ▲ Decreased fetal movement
  - Signs and symptom of hypoglycemia

Follow-up Care:
Follow-up Measures to Consider
- Document
- Prenatal follow-up
  - Maternal and fetal evaluation
  - Blood glucose follow-up
    - ◆ Evaluate results biweekly
    - ◆ Office or laboratory testing for validation of
      - ➤ Home monitoring results
      - ➤ Glycemic control
    - ◆ Medication use
- Fetal assessment
  - Fetal kick counts begin at 28 weeks
  - Ultrasound
    - ◆ 28–32 weeks: Begin serial ultrasound for
      - ➤ Asymmetric IUGR
      - ➤ Macrosomia
  - Non-stress test (NST) weekly beginning at 34 weeks
  - Biophysical profile (BPP)

- Labor plan
  - If well-controlled blood sugars and no other problems, can wait until 40 weeks to consider induction of labor (ACOG, 2001b)
  - 🕐 Consider induction before 40 weeks for
    - ◆ Client on insulin therapy
    - ◆ Fetal macrosomia
    - ◆ Poor or marginal control
    - ◆ Based on tests for fetal well-being
  - Plan birth at facility with newborn special care
    - ◆ Anticipate respiratory distress syndrome (RDS)
  - If the estimated fetal weight (EFW) > 4500 g, cesarean delivery may decrease the likelihood of brachial plexus injury in the infant (ACOG, 2001b)
  - Plan for pediatric care at birth
- Postpartum follow-up
  - FBS & 2-hour postprandial blood sugar for 7 days (International Diabetes Center, 2003)
    - ◆ Evaluate as soon as possible for diabetes mellitus with
      - ➤ FBS > 120 mg/dl, or
      - ➤ Two-hour postprandial blood sugar > 160 mg/dl
  - FBS at 6 weeks postpartum
  - More than 126 mg/dl diagnostic of diabetes mellitus

Collaborative Practice:
Consider Consultation or Referral
- Nutrition education and counseling
  - Referral to diabetic educator
- Social services, as indicated
- Medical, obstetric, or pediatric services
  - Referral to diabetic clinic for pregnant women
  - Gestational diabetic not controlled by diet
    - ◆ Initiation of insulin or glyburide
    - ◆ Ongoing medication dosage requirements

- Fetal macrosomia, IUGR, or anomalies
- Newborn care at birth
- For diagnosis outside the midwife's scope of practice

CARE OF THE PREGNANT WOMAN WITH HEPATITIS

Key Clinical Information

Hepatitis includes a range of viral illnesses that may be transmitted via blood or body fluids. Vertical transmission of hepatitis B, C, E, and G may occur to the fetus during pregnancy. Up to 90% of infants born to hepatitis B–infected mothers are infected without treatment shortly after birth (ACOG, 2007b). Infected infants may become chronic carriers or may develop significant illness. Infected women may present with acute illness, or they may be chronic carriers: asymptomatic but able to transmit infection (CDC, 2002).

Client History and Chart Review:
Components of the History to Consider

- Gestational age
- Immunization status—hepatitis B
- Potential exposure to hepatitis
  - Health care professional
  - IV drug use, shared needles
  - Sexual contacts
  - Presence of tattoos
  - Ingestion of raw shellfish
  - Hemodialysis patients
  - Blood or organ recipient before 1992
  - International travelers (Varney et al., 2004)
  - Day-care workers
  - Immigrants from
    - Asia
    - Africa
    - Pacific Islands
    - Haiti
- Presence, onset and duration, and severity of symptoms
  - Malaise and lethargy
  - Fever and chills
  - Right upper quadrant pain

- Jaundice
- Nausea and vomiting (CDC, 2002)

Physical Examination:
Components of the Physical Exam to Consider

- Vital signs, including weight
- Examine for evidence of jaundice
  - Skin
  - Mucous membranes
  - Sclera
- Palpate and percuss for
  - Liver margins
  - Splenomegaly
  - Right upper quadrant pain

Clinical Impression:
Differential Diagnoses and Code Groups
to Consider
Additional suffix may apply (ICD9data.com, 2007)

- Hepatitis B (ICD-9 codes V22.2 and 070.3)
- Hepatitis A (ICD-9 codes V22.2 and 070.1)
- Hepatitis C (ICD-9 codes V22.2 and 070.7)
- Cholestasis of pregnancy (ICD-9 codes V22.2 and 574)
- Cholelithiasis (ICD-9 codes V22.2 and 574)
- Other liver disorders in pregnancy (ICD-9 codes 646)

Diagnostic Testing:
Diagnostic Tests and Procedures to Consider

- Hepatitis B
  - Surface antibody; immunized individuals
  - Surface antigen; nonimmunized individuals
- Hepatitis profile, multiple antigen/antibody screen
- Liver function tests
  - Aspartate and alanine aminotransferases, SGOT (AST), SGPT (ALT), lactate dehydrogenase (LDH), bilirubin
  - Elevation occurs during acute phase (CDC, 2002)
- Ultrasound, right upper quadrant
  - Gallbladder (CDC, 2002)

Providing Treatment:
Therapeutic Measures to Consider
- Illness must run its course
- Supportive therapy for mother
- Consider immunization series
  - For at-risk noninfected women
  - May be used during pregnancy
  - Hepatitis B (Pregnancy Category C)
  - Hepatitis A (Pregnancy Category C)

Providing Treatment:
Alternative Measures to Consider
- Whole foods diet with minimum toxins
- Lemon water every morning
- Herbs
  - Milk thistle tea (Foster, 1996)
  - Dandelion tea, tincture or capsule
- Adequate rest

Providing Support:
Education and Support Measures to Consider
- Provide information about hepatitis
  - Transmission and prevention
  - Vaginal birth is recommended, cesarean for other indications only
  - Medication recommendations for infant
  - Breastfeeding
    - Not contraindicated for immunized infant
    - Not recommended for nonimmunized infant
- Discussion regarding
  - Options for care of self and infant
  - Location for birth
  - Parameters for referral

Follow-up Care:
Follow-up Measures to Consider
- Document
- Return for care
  - Per routine for carrier
  - Weekly for acute phase of infection
    - Periodic liver function tests
    - Fetal evaluation with acute illness

- Administer to infant born to hepatitis B–positive mother
  - Hepatitis B immune globulin
    - 0.5 ml IM in anterior thigh within 12 hours of birth
  - Hepatitis B vaccine
    - Engerix-B 10 μg/0.5 ml
    - Recombivax HB 5 μg/0.5 ml (Murphy, 2004)
    - IM in anterior thigh shortly after birth
    - Repeat in 1 and 6 months (CDC, 2002)

Collaborative Practice:
Consider Consultation or Referral
- Epidemiologic support
- Medical services
  - Acute hepatitis, any type
  - Hepatitis C to hepatitis specialist
- Pediatric care provider consult
  - Before birth
  - Collaborative plan for newborn care
- For diagnosis outside the midwife's scope of practice

CARE OF THE PREGNANT WOMAN WITH HERPES SIMPLEX VIRUS

Key Clinical Information
The prevalence of herpes simplex virus (HSV) has risen in the last several decades and poses an important health problem in pregnancy. Infection of the infant with HSV varies with the incidence of primary versus secondary infection (ACOG, 2007a). When primary genital HSV infection occurs during pregnancy, the perinatal transmission rate may be as high as 50%. This should be differentiated from a nonprimary genital infection with a first outbreak of lesions, which has a perinatal transmission rate of 33%. With secondary, or recurrent, genital HSV infection during pregnancy, the perinatal transmission rate diminishes to 0–3%. There are three categories of neonatal disease: localized disease of the skin, eye, and mouth; central nervous system disease; and disseminated disease. The mother may be asymptomatic in up to

70% of instances where the infant is infected (Emmons et al., 1997).

Client History and Chart Review:
Components of the History to Consider

- Gestational age
- Sexual history
- Previous history of
  - Genital or oral herpes
  - Other sexually transmitted infections (STIs)
- Duration and quality of present symptoms
  - Location and number of vesicular lesions
    - Oral
    - Genital
  - Symptoms
    - Pain
    - Tingling
    - Dysuria
- Primary infection associated with
  - Fever
  - Headache and photophobia
  - Malaise
  - Aseptic meningitis (CDC, 2002)

Physical Examination:
Components of the Physical Exam to Consider

- Vital signs, including temperature
- Usual prenatal evaluation
- Physical evaluation with emphasis on
  - Oral examination
  - Inguinal lymph nodes
    - Enlargement
    - Tenderness
  - External genitalia, buttocks, and pelvic region
  - Characteristic lesions
    - Vesicles
    - Shallow ulcers
- Speculum examination, as needed
  - Presence of other STI symptoms
  - Cervical discharge
  - Cervical or uterine motion tenderness

Clinical Impression:
Differential Diagnoses and Code Groups to Consider
Additional suffix may apply (ICD9data.com, 2007)

- HSV infection (ICD-9 codes 647)
- Other STI (ICD-9 codes 647.0–647.2)
- Genital trauma (ICD-9 codes V22.2 and 959.14)

Diagnostic Testing:
Diagnostic Tests and Procedures to Consider

- Culture lesions for HSV (Quest Diagnostics, n.d.)
- Consider serum testing for HSV antibody titer (CDC, 2002)
  - Documents primary vs. nonprimary first episode vs. recurrent infection
  - Repeat 7–10 days
  - Fourfold increase = primary infection (Fife et al., 2004)
- Other STI testing
  - With symptoms
  - As indicated by history

Providing Treatment:
Therapeutic Measures to Consider (ACOG, 2007a)

- Valtrex (valacyclovir hydrochloride)
  - Pregnancy Category B
  - Pregnancy registry 1-800-722-9292, extension 39437
  - Dose: 500 mg BID for 5 days
  - Begin medication within 24 hours of first symptom
  - For suppressive therapy at 36 weeks until birth
    - 500 mg PO daily (≤9 recurrences/year)
    - 250 mg PO BID (> 9 recurrences/year)
- Famvir (famciclovir)
  - Pregnancy Category B
  - Dose: 125 mg BID for 5 days
  - Begin medication within 6 hours of first symptom
  - For suppressive therapy at 36 weeks until birth
    - 250 mg PO BID

- Zovirax (Acyclovir)
  - Pregnancy Category C
  - Pregnancy registry 1-800-722-9292, extension 58465
  - Topical ointment 5%
    - Apply three times a day for 7 days
    - Initial outbreak
  - 200 mg PO five times a day for 10 days
  - Recurrent outbreak
    - 200 mg PO five times a day for 7 days
    - Repeat treatment as needed
  - Suppression or severe recurrent outbreaks
    - 400 mg PO BID for 6–12 months (CDC, 2002)
  - For suppressive therapy at 36 weeks until birth
    - 400 mg PO daily
- Acetaminophen (Tylenol) for pain relief

Providing Treatment:
Alternative Measures to Consider
- Lysine
  - 1000 mg PO BID for 3 months
  - Combine with vitamin C 500 mg
  - Begin with first sign of an outbreak
- Dietary recommendations
  - Include foods high in lysine
    - Brewer's yeast
    - Potatoes
    - Fish (Weed, 1985)
  - Avoid foods high in arginine
    - Chocolate, coffee, cola
    - Peanuts, cashews, pecans, almonds
    - Sunflower and sesame seeds
    - Peas and corn
    - Coconut
    - Gelatin
- Garlic, raw
  - Antiviral properties
  - Combine with sea vegetable for trace minerals (Weed, 1985)
- Lemon balm tea two to three cups daily

- Echinacea
  - Tea, tincture, tablets, or capsules
  - TID for 2 weeks
  - Some sources contraindicate internal use during pregnancy.
- Sitz bath or salve made with
  - Lemon balm
  - Calendula
  - Comfrey

Providing Support:
Education and Support Measures to Consider
- Information about HSV infection
  - CDC STI Hotline 1-800-227-8922
  - American Social Health Association www.ashastd.org
  - Potential effects for
    - Pregnancy
    - Anticipated location for birth
    - Newborn
    - Labor and birth plans
    - Potential for cesarean delivery
- Discussion regarding
  - Treatment options
  - Labor and birth options
  - Maternal preferences
  - Midwife recommendations
- Rest and comfort measures
  - With initial outbreak
  - To enhance immune response

Follow-up Care:
Follow-up Measures to Consider
- Document
- Return for care
  - Per routine with history of herpes
  - For culture with active lesion
  - Primary herpes
    - If symptoms persist > 10 days
    - Worsening symptoms
      - Stiff neck
      - Unremitting fever
      - Inability to urinate

- Labor care
    - Vaginal birth for no active lesion or no pro-dromal symptoms of vulvar pain or burning
        - Active lesion remote from genital region
            - Occlusive dressing applied
        - Limit cervical exams
        - Limit use of scalp electrode or intrauter-ine pressure catheter (IUPC)
    - Cesarean birth recommended for active genital lesion or prodromal symptoms of vulvar pain or burning
        - Before ROM
        - As soon as possible with premature rup-ture of membranes (PROM)
        - May delay with preterm premature rup-ture of membranes (PPROM) for steroid therapy
- Breastfeeding encouraged unless active lesion on the breast

Collaborative Practice:
Consider Consultation or Referral
- ☎ For symptoms of herpes meningitis
- For collaborative labor plan
    - Presence of active lesion
    - Potential for cesarean delivery
- For pediatric follow-up after HSV exposure (CDC, 2002)
- For diagnosis or treatment outside the mid-wife's scope of practice

CARE OF THE PREGNANT WOMAN WITH HUMAN IMMUNODEFICIENCY VIRUS

Key Clinical Information
Human immunodeficiency virus (HIV) testing is recommended for every pregnant woman with patient notification and consent. Many women feel threatened by the thought of HIV testing; it should be documented if HIV testing is declined. Many states require HIV-specific pretest counsel-ing and documentation of informed consent before test specimen collection. Early testing allows for prompt evaluation and the potential for antiretroviral medication, which can decrease the incidence of perinatal transmission of the infection from 13–30% to 2–8%. Vertical transmis-sion may be reduced in infants who reach term, are appropriate weight for gestation, and are born by cesarean. Women who are at risk for HIV infection may require additional testing during the pregnancy (Allen, 2001). Breastfeeding is con-traindicated where access to safe breast milk substitutes and clean water is assured (Clark & Fitzgerald, 2007).

Client History and Chart Review:
Components of the History to Consider
- Gestational age
- Gynecologic and sexual history
    - Previous HIV testing
    - Number of sexual partners
    - Self and/or partner(s)
        - Sexual practices
        - STIs
        - Substance abuse
            - IV drug use
            - Other substance use
        - Blood transfusions
    - Abnormal Pap smears
- History of opportunistic infections
    - Presence of current symptoms
        - Malaise
        - Fever
        - Cough
        - Skin lesions

Physical Examination:
Components of the Physical Exam to Consider
- Vital signs, including temperature
- Head, eyes, ears, nose & throat (HEENT)
    - Funduscopic exam
    - Oral examination for thrush or lesions
- Skin lesions
- Respiratory system
    - Cough
    - Adventitious breath sounds

- Shortness of breath
- Night sweats
- Liver margins
- Lymph nodes
  - Characteristics of enlarged nodes
  - Location(s) of enlarged nodes
- Pelvic examination
  - Internal or external lesions
  - Symptoms of STIs

Clinical Impression:
Differential Diagnoses and Code Groups
to Consider
Additional suffix may apply (ICD9data.com, 2007)
- HIV disease/acquired immunodeficiency syndrome (ICD-9 codes V22.2 and 042)
- Asymptomatic HIV infection status (ICD-9 codes V22.2 and V08)
- Other STI (ICD-9 codes 647.0–647.2)

Diagnostic Testing:
Diagnostic Tests and Procedures to Consider
- Rapid HIV test
- HIV enzyme-linked immunosorbent assay (ELISA) test
- HIV Western blot test
- CD4 and viral load every trimester

Providing Treatment:
Therapeutic Measures to Consider
- 🌐 New onset antiretroviral therapy
  - Delay onset until after first trimester unless needed for maternal health (Burdge et al., 2003)
    - Diminishes drug-related teratogenicity
    - Improve adherence once early nausea has passed (U.S. Public Health Service Task Force, 2004)
  - Use current facility guidelines for medication regimen
  - Management of side effects is important to maximize adherence
- Established antiretroviral therapy

- Modified antiretroviral treatment for perinatal prophylaxis
  - Intrapartum therapy
- Initiation of other therapies based on diagnosis

Providing Treatment:
Alternative Measures to Consider
- Supportive measures
- Most immune stimulating herbs not recommended
- Cautious use of herbals/homeopathic remedies for
  - Appetite stimulation
  - Skin integrity
  - Emotional and spiritual balance

Providing Support:
Education and Support Measures
to Consider
- Provide information, listening, and discussion regarding
  - HIV and acquired immunodeficiency syndrome (AIDS)
  - Prevention and transmission
  - Benefits of testing
  - Viral load evaluation and significance
    - Perinatal transmission
    - Potential effects on baby
  - Medication and treatment options
    - Antiretroviral medication (for self and/or baby)
      - Benefits
      - Risks
      - Side effects
      - Alternatives
- Life-style issues
  - Encourage
    - Abstinence, or
    - Consistent condom use
    - Avoid shared needles
  - Breastfeeding contraindicated where safe breast milk substitutes are available

Follow-up Care:
Follow-up Measures to Consider

- Document
- Informed consent for testing
- Laboratory results
- Maternal response to
  - Diagnosis
  - Treatment recommendations
- Discussions
  - Client preferences
  - Consultations and referrals
  - Anticipated location for birth
- Follow-up care
  - Coordinate testing with primary care provider/site
  - Pediatric consult for newborn care and follow-up
  - Register with the CDC Antiretroviral Pregnancy Registry
    - 800-258-4263
    - http://www.apregistry.com
  - Observe for side effects of medications
    - May cause hepatic toxicity
    - May mimic HELLP syndrome
- Return visits
  - As indicated by prenatal course and gestation
  - For support

Collaborative Practice:
Consider Consultation or Referral

- Social support services
  - Support groups
  - Mental health referrals
  - Victim advocacy groups
  - Clean needle programs
  - Substance abuse treatment options
- OB/GYN and medical services
  - For all newly diagnosed HIV-positive women
  - For coordination of antiretroviral regimen
  - For HIV-positive women with
    - Onset of infection

- Decrease in CD4 cell counts
- Significant medication side effects
- For diagnosis or treatment outside the midwife's scope of practice

CARE OF THE WOMAN WITH HYPERTENSIVE DISORDERS IN PREGNANCY

Key Clinical Information

In the United States hypertensive disorders are the most common cause of medical complications in pregnancy, affecting 6–8% of all pregnancies; they contribute significantly to maternal and neonatal morbidity and mortality (Saikul et al., 2006). Hypertension in pregnancy may be chronic (occurring before 20 weeks gestation and persisting beyond 42 days postpartum), may arise during pregnancy (gestational hypertension or preeclampsia), or may represent preeclampsia superimposed on chronic hypertension (National Heart, Lung, and Blood Institute, 2000). Severe hypertensive disorders may lead to complications such as eclampsia and HELLP. Differential diagnosis can be challenging because gestational hypertension may present with a varied array of symptoms. Onset of clinical signs and symptoms suggesting gestational hypertension and/or preeclampsia should always prompt careful evaluation to have the opportunity to institute early treatment. Laboratory testing is the most reliable way to assess a woman's potential for development of gestational hypertension. Treatment improves the likelihood of the pregnancy resulting in a healthy mother and healthy baby and increases the potential for a vaginal birth (National Heart, Lung, and Blood Institute, 2000).

Client History and Chart Review:
Components of the History to Consider

- Gestational age
- Presence, onset, and durations of symptoms (Table 3-3)

Table 3-3   Hypertensive Disorders of Pregnancy

HYPERTENSIVE DISORDER	SIGNS AND SYMPTOMS	CRITERIA FOR DIAGNOSIS
Chronic hypertension May be mild, moderate, or severe	Predates 20th week of pregnancy or persists beyond usual postpartum period. May have cardiac enlargement, vascular changes, renal insufficiency.	BP ≥ 140/90 mild/mod BP ≥ 170/110 severe Two or more BP elevations > 4 hr apart
Preeclampsia PIH, mild	Gestational age of ≥ 20 weeks Onset of: Elevated BP Proteinuria Elevated reflexes Fundal heights small for dates Elevated hemoglobin secondary to hemoconcentration Elevated serum uric acid (normal range 1.2–4.5 mg/dl)	Hypertension after 20 weeks: 1. Systolic ≥ 140 mm Hg, *or* 2. Diastolic ≥ 90 mm Hg 3. On two occasions ≥ 6 hr apart New onset proteinuria: 1. 1–2+ dip, on 2. Two specimens, in 3. Absence of UTI, *or* 4. ≥ 300 mg in 24-hr urine
Preeclampsia PIH, severe	Signs of mild PIH, plus 1. Clonus 2. Diminished renal function (elevated BUN, diminished urinary output, serum creatinine > 1.2 mg/dl, decreased creatine clearance) 3. Headache 4. Visual disturbances 5. Epigastric discomfort 6. IUGR and/or oligohydramnios by ultrasound May have onset of 1. HELLP syndrome 2. Eclampsia 3. Pulmonary edema	Hypertension: 1. Systolic ≥ 160 mm Hg 2. Diastolic ≥ 110 mm Hg 3. Two readings ≥ 6 hr apart Proteinuria: 1. New onset, or 2. 3–4+ dip 3. ≥ 5 g in 24-hr urine
Eclampsia	Grand mal seizure(s) Fetal distress Placental abruption	Gestational hypertension with seizure that is responsive to initiation of $MgSO_4$ therapy
HELLP Syndrome (HELLP = Hemolysis, Elevated Liver enzymes and Low Platelet count)	Epigastric pain General malaise Abnormal coagulation profile (low fibrinogen prolonged prothrombin time, prolonged partial prothrombin time)	Hemolysis of red blood cells Elevated liver enzymes (AST, ALT, LDH) Low platelets (< 100,000)

Sources: American College of Obstetricians and Gynecologists [ACOG]. (2001). Clinical management guidelines, number 29. Chronic Hypertension in Pregnancy. Washington, DC: The American College of Obstetricians and Gynecologists; American College of Obstetricians and Gynecologists [ACOG]. (2002). Clinical management guidelines, number 33. Diagnosis and Management of Preeclampsia and Eclampsia. Washington, DC: The American College of Obstetricians and Gynecologists; Varney, H., Kriebs, J. M., & Gegor, C. L. (2004). *Varney's midwifery* (4th ed.). Sudbury, MA: Jones and Bartlett.

- Evaluate for gestational hypertension risk factors (Wagner, 2004)
  - Primigravida (six to eight times risk)
  - Multipara with previous gestational hypertension or > 10 years since last child
  - Maternal age < 20 and > 35
  - Multiple gestations (five times risk)
  - Hydatidiform mole (10 times risk)
  - Fetal hydrops (10 times risk)
  - Preexisting medical disorders
    - Essential hypertension
    - Diabetes mellitus, especially with microvascular disease
    - Collagen vascular disease
    - Renal vascular disease
    - Morbid obesity
    - Antiphospholipid disease
    - Cardiovascular disease
    - Thrombophilias
    - Sickle cell disease
    - Dyslipidemia
  - Renal parenchymal disease
- African-American or Asian heritage
- Social factors that may contribute to gestational hypertension
  - Poor nutrition
  - Tobacco use
  - Alcohol use
  - Excessive sodium intake
  - Current vasoactive drug use
    - Nasal decongestants
    - Cocaine
- Family history of gestational hypertension

Physical Examination:
Components of the Physical Exam to Consider
- Vital signs, including BP and weight
- Weight: Patterns of gain
- BP evaluation
  - Two occasions > 4 hours apart
  - Allow a "rest" period after
    - Anxiety
    - Pain

- Smoking
- Exercise
  - Equipment of correct size should be used
  - Use same maternal position for each BP
  - Arm should be supported at level of the heart
- Evaluate extremities for
  - Presence or absence of edema
  - Deep tendon reflexes
- Abdominal examination
  - Fundal heights for evaluation of fetal growth
  - Liver margins
  - Epigastric pain
- Ophthalmic examination
  - Papilledema
  - Vessel narrowing
- Monitor pulmonary status

Clinical Impression:
Differential Diagnoses and Code Groups
to Consider
Additional suffix may apply (ICD9data.com, 2007)
- Gestational hypertension (PIH) (ICD-9 codes 642)
  - Preeclampsia, mild (ICD-9 code 642.43)
  - Preeclampsia, severe (ICD-9 code 642.53)
  - Eclampsia (ICD-9 code 642.63)
- Transient hypertension (ICD-9 code 642.33)
- Essential hypertension (ICD-9 code 642.03)
- PIH superimposed on chronic hypertension (ICD-9 code 642.73)
- HELLP syndrome (ICD-9 code 642.53)
- Elevated BP without diagnosis of hypertension (ICD-9 codes V22.2 and 796.2)

Diagnostic Testing:
Diagnostic Tests and Procedures to Consider
- Baseline gestational hypertension laboratory values
- Note: normal ranges may vary by laboratory
  - Urine analysis for protein by dip
  - Hematocrit (normal range 10.5–14 g/dl)

- Platelet count (normal range 130,000–400,000/ml)
- Liver function tests
  - ◆ Aspartate aminotransferase (AST/SGOT) (normal range 0–35 IU/L)
  - ◆ Alanine aminotransferase (ALT/SGPT) (normal range 5–35 IU/L)
  - ◆ Lactate dehydrogenase (LDH) (normal range 0–250 IU/L)
- Coagulation studies
  - Fibrinogen
  - Prothrombin time, partial thromboplastin time
- Renal function tests
  - Serum uric acid (normal range 1.2–4.5 mg/dl)
  - Serum albumin (normal range 2.5–4.5 g/dl)
  - Serum creatinine (normal range < 1.0 mg/dl)
  - Blood urea nitrogen (7–25 mg/dl)
  - 24-hour urine for protein and creatinine
    - ◆ Initiate based on symptoms, or
    - ◆ When dip urinalysis shows > 1+ protein
    - ◆ Analysis of the first 4 hours for protein-to-creatinine ratio of a 24-hour collection
      - ➤ ≥ 0.30 = highest accuracy for predictive of significant proteinuria (Saikul et al., 2006)
- Fetal evaluation
  - Fetal kick counts—daily
  - Non-stress test (NST) and biophysical profile (National Heart, Lung, and Blood Institute, 2000)
    - ◆ At diagnosis
    - ◆ Weekly
    - ◆ Biweekly for
      - ➤ Amniotic fluid index (AFI) ≤ (5 cm)
      - ➤ Estimated fetal weight (EFW) < 10th percentile for gestational age (GA)
    - ◆ Immediately with change in maternal condition (National Heart, Lung, and Blood Institute, 2000)

- Ultrasound (National Heart, Lung, and Blood Institute, 2000)
  - On diagnosis
  - Every 4 days to 3 weeks as indicated by maternal and fetal condition
    - ◆ Amniotic fluid index
    - ◆ Fetal growth evaluation

Providing Treatment:
Therapeutic Measures to Consider

- Increase calcium intake (1200–1500 mg daily) (Villar et al., 2006)
- Limit activity
- Low-dose aspirin therapy (Coomarasamy et al., 2003)
  - For women with
    - ◆ High risk of preeclampsia
    - ◆ Chronic hypertension
    - ◆ Diabetes mellitus
    - ◆ Renal disease
  - 50–150 mg daily at bedtime
- Consider hospitalization
  - Bed rest not possible at home
  - Progressive signs and symptoms
- Medications for sustained BP of
  - ≥ 160 mm Hg systolic, or
  - ≥ 105 mm Hg diastolic
  - Hydralazine (National Heart, Lung, and Blood Institute, 2000)
    - ◆ 5 mg IV or 10 mg IM
    - ◆ Repeat at 20-minute intervals until BP stable
    - ◆ Repeat as needed approximately every 3 hours
    - ◆ Change medication if no response by 20–30 mg
  - Labetalol
    - ◆ ⚠ Do not use in women with asthma or congestive heart failure
    - ◆ 20-mg IV bolus
    - ◆ May give 40 mg IV in 10 min, followed by
      - ➤ 80 mg IV for two doses
      - ➤ Maximum dose 220 mg

- ◆ Pregnancy Category C
- ■ Nifedipine
  - ◆ 10 mg PO
  - ◆ Repeat in 30 minutes
- • $MgSO_4$ therapy (Leeman et al., 2006)
  - ■ Four to 6-g bolus, slow IV
  - ■ Followed by 2 g/hr IV, or
  - ■ 5 g 50% $MgSO_4$ IM every 4 hours
  - ■ Titrated to renal output and reflexes
    - ◆ Monitor
      - ➤ BP
      - ➤ Therapeutic $MgSO_4$ level = 4–7 mg/dl
      - ➤ Reflexes
      - ➤ Intake and output
  - ■ Calcium gluconate at bedside
- • Avoid
  - ■ Angiotensin-converting enzyme inhibitors
  - ■ Angiotensin II receptor agonists
  - ■ Beta-blocker Atenolol
  - ■ Thiazide diuretics
- • Delivery if no improvement or condition worsens

Providing Treatment:
Alternative Measures to Consider
- • Balanced nutrition
  - ■ No salt restriction
  - ■ Whole foods diet
  - ■ Adequate protein intake
- • Chlorophyll, liquid or capsule
- • Cucumber, one daily
- • Hops tea, one cup a night in last month of pregnancy
- • Motherwort tea, tincture or capsule
- • Hawthorn berries (Foster, 1996)
  - ■ Best for chronic hypertension
  - ■ Infusion: one cup daily
  - ■ Tincture: 15 drops tid

Providing Support:
Education and Support Measures to Consider
- • Discussion with client and family regarding
  - ■ Gestational hypertension
  - ■ Treatment options and recommendations

- ■ Smoking cessation, as needed
- ■ Drug treatment plans, if indicated
- • Attention to
  - ■ Diet
  - ■ Rest
  - ■ Low impact exercise with mild gestational hypertension
- • Potential need for
  - ■ Hospitalization or more frequent prenatal visits
  - ■ OB/GYN consultation/referral
  - ■ Change in planned location for birth
  - ■ Pediatric care at birth
  - ■ Newborn special care after birth
- • ⚠ Indications for immediate care
  - ■ Epigastric pain
  - ■ Visual disturbance
  - ■ Severe headache

Follow-up Care:
Follow-up Measures to Consider
- • Document
  - ■ Serum $MgSO_4$ 4 hours after initiation of therapy
  - ■ List parameters for consultation and referral
  - ■ Update plan weekly or as indicated
- • Increased frequency of return visits
  - ■ Fetal surveillance testing
  - ■ Maternal evaluation/laboratory values
  - ■ Biweekly visits
  - ■ Consider hospitalization for
    - ◆ Noncompliant client
    - ◆ Progressive signs
- • Indications for delivery include
  - ■ Gestational age > 38 weeks
  - ■ Persistent or severe
    - ◆ Headache
    - ◆ Abdominal pain
  - ■ Abnormal liver function tests
  - ■ Rising serum creatinine
  - ■ Thrombocytopenia
  - ■ Pulmonary edema
  - ■ Eclampsia
  - ■ Abruptio placentae
  - ■ Oligohydramnios

- Nonreassuring fetal monitoring tracings
- IUGR noted by ultrasound
- Abnormal biophysical profile

Collaborative Practice:
Consider Consultation or Referral
- OB/GYN services
  - For chronic hypertension in pregnancy
  - With diagnosis or suspicion of preeclampsia or gestational hypertension
  - For any indications for delivery (see above)
- For diagnosis or treatment outside the midwife's scope of practice

CARE OF THE PREGNANT WOMAN WITH INADEQUATE WEIGHT GAIN

Key Clinical Information
Optimal weight gain during pregnancy is based on the woman's pre-pregnant BMI and age. Inadequate weight gain may indicate a number of medical problems. More commonly, however, inadequate nutrition is due to psychosocial issues, such as poverty, substance abuse, mental illness, or simply poor food choices. Women with a history of anorexia or bulimia may have difficulty maintaining adequate intake to support growth of a healthy baby (Peery, n.d.). Overweight women may require fewer calories during pregnancy while still demonstrating an adequate fundal growth pattern. Weight gain is a gross marker for the nutritional status of the mother, and it is a factor in body image issues for many women. A woman's body undergoes remarkable changes during pregnancy; she should be helped to appreciate the beauty of such changes. The focus of diet counseling should be on healthy food choices from a variety of whole foods in appropriate portions. In most cases, appropriate weight gain follows from a nutritious diet.

Client History and Chart Review:
Components of the History to Consider
- Age of client (Groth, 2007)
- Gestational age
- Review of gestational dating parameters

- Nutritional assessment
  - List what foods have been eaten in the past two days
  - Preferred diet and portion size
  - Food sources available
  - Use of enemas and laxatives
- Assessment for eating disorders
  - Do you ever eat in secret?
  - Are you satisfied with your eating habits; your body?
- Physical health issues
  - Activity level and general metabolic rate
  - Involvement in athletics
  - Presence of symptoms
    - Nausea and vomiting
    - Constipation, diarrhea
    - Abdominal pain
    - Pica
- Prior health history, such as
  - Presence of maternal illness or infection
  - Gastrointestinal and malabsorption disorders
  - Hyperthyroid
  - Hepatitis
  - Anemia
  - Malnutrition
  - Parity
- Emotional and spiritual health issues
  - Family and personal support for pregnancy
    - Education level
    - Social living conditions
    - Physical abuse
  - Stress levels and coping skills
    - Physical response to stress
    - Anorexia or bulimia
  - Other mental health issues
- Substance abuse

Physical Examination:
Components of the Physical Exam to Consider
- Vital signs, including height and weight
- BMI and weight distribution
  - Adult BMI charts for > 18 years old
  - Adolescent BMI-for-age charts for < 18 years old (CDC, 2007; Groth, 2007)

- Prepregnancy weight
- Interval gain
- Abdominal examination
  - Fundal height
    - For gestation
    - Fundal height growth curve
  - Bowel sounds
  - Palpation of abdomen
- Dental/oral evaluation
  - Caries
  - Abscess
- Evaluation of other symptoms

Clinical Impression:
Differential Diagnoses and Code Groups
to Consider
Additional suffix may apply (ICD9data.com, 2007)

- Short maternal stature, constitutional (ICD-9 codes V22.2 and 783.43)
- Small for gestational age baby (ICD-9 codes V22.2 and 764)
- Intrauterine fetal growth restriction (ICD-9 codes V22.2 and 764.9)
- Malnutrition, secondary to conditions such as
  - Homelessness (ICD-9 codes V22.2 and V60.0)
  - Poverty (ICD-9 codes V22.2 and V60.2)
  - Substance abuse (ICD-9 codes 648.33)
  - Physical abuse (ICD-9 codes V22.2 and 995.81)
    - Anorexia nervosa (ICD-9 codes V22.2 and 307.1)
    - Bulimia (ICD-9 codes V22.2 and 307.51)
  - Mental illness (ICD-9 codes V22.2 and 290–319)

Diagnostic Testing:
Diagnostic Tests and Procedures to Consider

- Calculate BMI specific recommended weight gain (CDC, 2007)
- Laboratory testing
  - PIH laboratory values
  - Toxicology if drug use suspected
  - Thyroid-stimulating hormone

- Serum albumin
- Hepatitis screen
- Fetal kick counts
- Ultrasound for
  - Gestational age
  - Interval fetal growth
  - Evidence of IUGR
  - Amniotic fluid index

Providing Treatment:
Therapeutic Measures to Consider

- Prenatal vitamin and mineral supplement 1 PO daily
- Diet and nutrition counseling
  - Normal weight women need 300 extra calories a day while pregnant
  - Daily calorie range from 1800 cal/day up to 2400 cal/day, depending on BMI
  - Explore suitable food choices
    - Adequate protein, fat, and carbohydrates
    - Culturally acceptable foods
    - Use of additional dietary supplements as needed
- Consider hospitalization for
  - Malnutrition
  - Anorexia or bulimia
  - Significant mental illness

Providing Treatment:
Alternative Measures to Consider

- Dietary supplements
  - Spirulina (Weed, 1985)
  - Smoothies
  - Energy bars
- Homeopathic pulsatilla
  - For persistent nausea
  - Intolerance of fatty foods (Smith, 1984)
- Herbal appetite stimulants
  - May be combined for flavor and effectiveness
  - Alfalfa 500 mg daily (avoid with lupus or allergies to pollen)

- Dandelion root tea one cup BID (avoid with history of gallstones)
- Hops tea one to two cups daily
- Chamomile tea one to two cups daily

Providing Support:
Education and Support Measures to Consider
- Provide information about
  - Weight gain and fetal growth pattern
  - Maternal and fetal nutrient needs from maternal diet
  - Anticipated weight gain for gestation
    - IUGR infants
    - Small for gestational age infants
    - Constitutionally small infants
- Fetal kick counts
- Warning signs, such as
  - ⚠ Decreased fetal motion
  - PIH signs and symptoms
- Potential effect on
  - Planned location for birth
  - Potential need for pediatric care at birth
- Importance of
  - Fundal/fetal growth over weight gain
  - Maternal and fetal well-being
  - Dietary needs during pregnancy
    - Small frequent meals
    - Balanced selection of food choices
    - Adequate caloric intake
- Excessive or rapid weight gain risks
  - Increased maternal insulin resistance
  - Postpartum or future obesity
- Provide support
  - Develop plan with client
  - Address client and family concerns

Follow-up Care:
Follow-up Measures to Consider
- Document
- Reevaluate weekly or biweekly for
  - Diet review
  - Interval fetal growth
  - Signs and symptoms of PIH

- Address client concerns and preferences
  - Nutritional counseling
  - Emotional issues
- Parameters for consultation or referral

Collaborative Practice:
Consider Consultation or Referral
- Nutritional counseling
  - Refer to dietician as needed
- Social service referral
  - Enroll in supplemental nutrition program, such as WIC program
  - Refer to local food assistance programs
- Obstetric/pediatric services
  - For persistent poor weight gain accompanied by
    - Lagging fetal growth
    - Asymmetric fetal growth
    - PIH
  - For transfer of care or change planned location of birth
- Medical services
  - Evidence of malnutrition
  - Suspected or documented
    - Mental health issues
    - Medical illness
- For diagnosis or treatment outside the midwife's scope of practice

CARE OF THE PREGNANT WOMAN WITH PRURITIC URTICARIAL PAPULES AND PLAQUES OF PREGNANCY

Key Clinical Information
Pruritic urticarial papules and plaques of pregnancy (PUPPP) is a form of urticaria that most commonly appears in the third trimester. These pruritic dermatoses typically erupt on the abdomen and may extend to the torso and extremities (Brzoza et al., 2007). It generally resolves within 6 weeks after birth of the infant. There are no systemic disorders associated with PUPPP; therefore treatment is aimed at relieving symptoms.

Client History and Chart Review:
Components of the History to Consider
- Gestational age
  - Most often primipara
  - Third trimester
- Onset, duration, and severity of symptoms
  - Pruritic papules often begin in striae (Brzoza et al., 2007)
    - May have small vesicles
    - Surrounded by narrow pale halo
    - Severe itching
  - Pattern of spread
    - Abdomen and striae
    - Periumbilical area not involved
    - Trunk and limbs
    - Face, palms, and soles spared
- Other associated signs and symptoms
- Presence of allergies
  - Medications
  - Exposure to topical irritants
- Exposure to viral infections
  - Immune titers as indicated
- Self-help remedies and their effects

Physical Examination:
Components of the Physical Exam
to Consider
- Vital signs, including temperature
- Abdominal distension
  - Striae gravidarum
- Location and appearance of lesions
  - Erythematous, edematous papules
  - Urticarial plaques
  - May form papulovesicular lesions
- Evaluate as needed for signs related to other differential diagnoses

Clinical Impression:
Differential Diagnoses and Code Groups
to Consider
Additional suffix may apply (ICD9data.com, 2007)
- PUPPP (ICD-9 codes 646.8)
- Scabies (ICD-9 codes V22.2 and 133.0)

- Allergic dermatitis (ICD-9 codes V22.2 and 692)
  - Drug or food reaction (ICD-9 codes V22.2 and 693)
  - Poison ivy (ICD-9 codes V22.2 and 692.6)
- Impetigo (ICD-9 codes V22.2 and 684)
- Viral exanthema (ICD-9 codes V22.2 and 050–057)
- Herpes gestationis (ICD-9 codes 646.8)
- Erythema multiforme (ICD-9 codes V22.2 and 695.1)
- Cholestasis of pregnancy (ICD-9 codes 646)

Diagnostic Testing:
Diagnostic Tests and Procedures to Consider
- Culture of vesicular lesions
  - Herpes
  - Impetigo
  - Scabies skin prep
- Immune titers as needed
  - Rubella
  - Rubeola
  - Varicella
- Liver function tests to evaluate for cholestasis
  - Alkaline phosphatase
  - Gamma-glutamyl transferase

Providing Treatment:
Therapeutic Measures to Consider
- Topical antipruritic lotions
  - Calamine or Caladryl (over the counter)
  - Doxepin HCl 5% cream (Pregnancy Category B)
- Oral antihistamines
  - Diphenhydramine HCl (Benadryl)
    - 25–50 mg every 4–6 hours
    - Pregnancy Category B in third trimester
  - Loratadine (Claritin)
    - 10 mg daily
    - Pregnancy Category B in third trimester
  - Cetirizine HCl (Zyrtec)
    - 5–10 mg daily
    - Pregnancy Category B in third trimester

- Hydroxyzine (Atarax)
  - 25–100 mg PO daily
  - Pregnancy Category C
- Topical corticosteroids
  - Pregnancy Category C
  - Rule out viral cause before using
    - Alclometasone dipropionate 0.05%
    - Aclovate cream or ointment
    - Hydrocortisone 1%
    - Cortisporin cream
    - Hytone cream, lotion, or ointment
    - Triamcinolone acetonide 0.025%, 0.1%, 0.5%
    - Aristocort cream
    - Kenalog cream, lotion, or ointment
- Oral steroid therapy
  - Prednisone 0.5–1 mg/kg/day PO
    - Use minimum effective dose
    - Taper off when symptoms abate
  - Pregnancy Category B
  - Use with caution in women with
    - Gestational diabetes
    - Hypertension (Murphy, 2004)

Providing Treatment:
Alternative Measures to Consider
- Topical relief of itching
  - Colloidal oatmeal baths
  - Calendula cream
  - Olive oil
  - Aloe gel
- Herbal support
  - Yellow dock root tea
  - Dandelion root tea
- Homeopathic support
  - Cantharis
  - Rhus tox
  - Urticaria

Providing Support:
Education and Support Measures to Consider
- PUPPP not associated with fetal jeopardy
- Call if symptoms persist or worsen

- Address client concerns
- Treatment options
- Medication instructions
  - Topical steroids
    - Apply thin film only
    - Do not cover or occlude
    - May be systemically absorbed
  - Oral steroids
    - Take as directed
    - Do not stop suddenly

Follow-up Care:
Follow-up Measures to Consider
- Document
- Return for care
  - Per routine for prenatal care
  - If symptoms worsen or additional symptoms develop

Collaborative Practice:
Consider Consultation or Referral
- Dermatology services
- For diagnosis or treatment outside the midwife's scope of practice

CARE OF THE PREGNANT WOMAN WHO IS RH NEGATIVE

Key Clinical Information
Rh alloimmunization or ABO incompatibility can have devastating results on both mother and baby. Infants are at risk when there is fetomaternal bleeding that initiates the process of Rh or ABO incompatibility or if the mother became sensitized previously after blood transfusion. This may result from an Rh-positive infant that is born to an Rh-negative mother, an infant with type A or B blood born to a mother with type O blood, an infant with type B or type AB blood born to a mother with type A blood, or an infant with type A or AB blood born to a mother with type B blood.

Often, the baby who is being carried when the fetomaternal bleed occurs may not have a problem, but the mother becomes sensitized. The problem manifests itself in a subsequent pregnancy when maternal antibodies attack the fetal blood. Alloimmunization may result in fetal hydrops, congestive heart failure, and fetal anemia (Sinclair, 2004). Adherence to established guidelines in the treatment of the Rh-negative mother significantly decreases the incidence of fetal hemolytic disease and its sequelae.

Client History and Chart Review:
Components of the History to Consider
- Gestational age
- Previous blood transfusions
- Prior obstetric history
  - Unexplained fetal losses
  - Stillbirth
  - Miscarriage
- Ectopic pregnancy
- Termination of pregnancy at > 8 weeks since last menstrual period
- Rh immune globulin indicated for unsensitized Rh-negative client with
  - Amniocentesis
  - Chorionic villus sampling
  - External version
  - Trauma, such as a car accident
  - Placenta previa
  - Abruptio placenta
  - Fetal death
  - Multiple gestation
  - Cesarean section
  - Twenty-eight weeks gestation prophylaxis if father of baby is Rh positive or his Rh status is unknown
  - Accidental transfusion of Rh-positive blood to an Rh-negative person

Physical Examination:
Components of the Physical Exam
to Consider
- Routine prenatal surveillance

Clinical Impression:
Differential Diagnoses and Code Groups
to Consider
Additional suffix may apply (ICD9data.com, 2007)
- Rh-negative mother (ICD-9 codes 656.13)
- Rh-sensitized mother (ICD-9 codes 656.13)
- ABO-sensitized mother (ICD-9 codes 656.23)

Diagnostic Testing:
Diagnostic Tests and Procedures to Consider
- Maternal—first prenatal and repeat at 24–28 weeks for Rh-negative mothers
  - Type and Rh factor
  - Antibody screen (indirect Coombs)
  - Antibody identification for positive antibody screen
  - Early RhIG after amniocentesis or threatened SAB may give positive titer at 24- to 28-week screen
- Maternal Test Results
  - Titer < 1:8 anti-D—Suggests passive immunity from RhIG
  - Titer > 1:8—Suggests active immunization due to Rh incompatibility
  - Rh(D) negative or type O mother
    - Plan to obtain cord blood at birth for analysis
    - Maternal/newborn follow-up postpartum

Providing Treatment:
Therapeutic Measures to Consider
- Offer Rh immune globulin (RhIG) (Pregnancy Category C)
  - Threatened or spontaneous miscarriage < 12 weeks, give 50 or 300 μg IM
  - Procedures or trauma, give 300 μg IM
  - Twenty-eight- to 36-week prophylaxis, give 300 μg IM with negative 28-week antibody screen
    - Consider redosing if pregnancy continues > 12 weeks from first dose

◆ If paternity is certain and father is Rh negative, antepartum prophylaxis is not needed (ACOG, 1999b).

▪ Postpartum, give 300 μg IM

   ◆ Provide to unsensitized Rh-negative mother with Rh-positive infant

   ◆ Give as soon as possible after birth, preferably within 72 hours postpartum

   ◆ Can be given up to 28 days postpartum for some benefit

   ◆ Adjust dose for large fetomaternal transfusion based on laboratory results

Providing Treatment:
Alternative Measures to Consider
- Maintain a healthy pregnancy and placenta
  ▪ Well-balanced diet
  ▪ Decrease or eliminate fluoride intake (may interfere with placental attachment)
  ▪ Ensure adequate trace mineral intake
- Limit invasive procedures
- Avoid traumatic placental delivery

Providing Support:
Education and Support Measures to Consider
- Provide information about
  ▪ Rh and blood type status
  ▪ Rh immune globulin
  ▪ Prophylaxis and desired result
  ▪ Potential risks with Rh immune globulin
    ◆ Transfusion-type adverse reactions
    ◆ Mercury sensitivity or reaction with RhoGAM
  ▪ Potential risks without Rh immune globulin
    ◆ Maternal sensitization
    ◆ Fetal hydrops or other complications with future pregnancy
    ◆ Difficulty cross-matching blood for woman in future (e.g., after accident or surgery)
    ◆ Potential for jaundice in infant due to Rh or ABO incompatibility

Follow-up Care:
Follow-up Measures to Consider
- Document
  ▪ Indication for RhIG
  ▪ Negative Rh and antibody status
  ▪ Client education, discussion, and preferences
- Observe for potential blood transfusion–type reactions
  ▪ Warmth at injection site
  ▪ Low-grade fever
  ▪ Flushing
  ▪ Chest or lumbar pain
  ▪ Poor clotting
- If mother is Rh(D) negative or type O
  ▪ Newborn
    ◆ Type and Rh
    ◆ Direct Coombs
    ◆ Bilirubin levels
  ▪ Maternal testing postpartum
    ◆ Type and Rh
    ◆ Antibody screen (indirect Coombs)
    ◆ Antibody ID for positive antibody screen
    ◆ Fetal red cell screen
- Kleihauer-Betke quantitative testing
  ▪ Determine volume of fetal blood in maternal system and dosage of RhIG to give mother
  ▪ Performed when high risk of fetomaternal hemorrhage exists
    ◆ Previa
    ◆ Abruption
    ◆ Abdominal trauma
    ◆ Hydrops
    ◆ Sinusoidal fetal heart rates (FHRs)
    ◆ Unexplained fetal demise

Collaborative Practice:
Consider Consultation or Referral
- For Rh-negative mother with positive antibody screen
- Evidence of large fetomaternal bleed

- Transfusion-type reactions
- For diagnosis or treatment outside the midwife's scope of practice

CARE OF THE PREGNANT WOMAN WITH SIZE–DATE DISCREPANCY

Key Clinical Information

Size alone is not an indication of a problem (ACOG, 2000b). Many infants may simply be constitutionally small or large. Maternal health habits and status play a role in the resiliency of the fetus. Size–date discrepancy has a multitude of potential contributing factors, with the most common causes including IUGR and gestational diabetes. Increased fetal surveillance and attention to maternal health help to prevent over- or under-intervention.

Client History and Chart Review:
Components of the History to Consider

- Review accuracy of last menstrual period and EDC
- Verify gestational age
  - Estimated date of conception
  - Size at first visit
  - Date of quickening
  - Early ultrasound report
- Obstetrics history
  - Review fundal growth curve
  - Hypertension
  - Gestational diabetes
  - Birth weights of prior infants
- Social history
  - Diet and weight gain pattern
  - Maternal activity patterns
  - Tobacco, alcohol, or drug use
  - Poverty
  - Psychosocial factors
    - Stress
    - Mental illness
    - Abuse
- Family history
  - Personal or family history of diabetes
  - Hypertension

- Other preexisting disease
- Ethnic norm for fetal weight
- Review of systems
  - Shortness of breath, palpitations
  - Signs or symptoms of illness
  - Fetal activity

Physical Examination:
Components of the Physical Exam
to Consider

- Vital signs, including BP and BMI
- Weight gain/loss and pattern
- General appearance and well-being
- Palpation of thyroid
- Cardiopulmonary evaluation
- Abdominal examination
  - Fundal height
  - Interval growth
  - Fetal lie
  - FHR
- Extremities
  - Reflexes
  - Edema
  - Physical evidence of substance abuse
- Pelvic examination
  - Station of presenting part
  - Evidence of ROM

Clinical Impression:
Differential Diagnoses and Code Groups
to Consider

Additional suffix may apply (ICD9data.com, 2007)

- Light for dates pregnancy (ICD-9 codes 656)
- Small for dates fetus (ICD-9 codes 764)
  - Intrauterine growth restriction (ICD-9 codes 764.9)
  - Small for gestational age (ICD-9 codes 764.0)
  - Constitutionally small infant (ICD-9 codes 783.43)
  - Oligohydramnios (ICD-9 codes 658.03)
- Congenital malformations (ICD-9 codes 740–759)

- Large for dates (ICD-9 codes 766.0)
  - Large for gestational age (ICD-9 codes 766.0)
  - Gestational or maternal diabetes (ICD-9 codes 648.0 or V22.2 and 250)
  - Multiple pregnancy (ICD-9 codes 651)
  - Polyhydramnios (ICD-9 codes 657.03)
  - Constitutionally large infant (ICD-9 codes 766.1)
  - Fibroid uterus (ICD-9 codes 654.1)
- Symmetric vs. asymmetric IUGR secondary to (ICD-9 codes 656.5)
  - Hypertension (ICD-9 codes 642)
  - Underlying maternal disease or infection (ICD-9 codes 640–649)
  - Poor nutrition (ICD-9 codes 648.9, V22.2 and 260–269)

Diagnostic Testing:
Diagnostic Tests and Procedures to Consider
- Dip urinalysis
- Urine toxicology
- Diabetes screen
- Maternal serum α-fetoprotein (may be elevated in early pregnancy)
- Maternal antiphospholipid antibody testing
- Maternal drug screen
- Symmetric IUGR
- Fetal karyotype
- Titers for
  - Toxoplasmosis
  - Cytomegalovirus
  - Herpes virus
- Preeclampsia laboratory profile
- Ultrasound evaluation
  - Verify singleton versus multiple pregnancy
  - Confirm estimated due date (EDD) by ultrasound parameters
  - Fetal anomaly study
  - Fetal growth—May be done serially
    - Schedule at least 3 weeks apart
    - Abdominal circumference
      - Decreased in asymmetric IUGR

- Umbilical arterial flow studies
  - AFI for oligo- or polyhydramnios
  - Placenta previa
  - Chronic placental abruption
  - Presence of uterine fibroids
- Fetal surveillance for IUGR
  - Begin as early as IUGR suspected
    - Weekly non-stress test (NST), biophysical profile (BPP)
    - Consider oxytocin challenge test (OCT) or contraction stress test (CST) if NST nonreactive
  - (Amniotic Fluid Index)—Weekly, should be > 6

Providing Treatment:
Therapeutic Measures to Consider
- Treat underlying medical condition(s), such as
  - Preeclampsia
  - Gestational diabetes
  - Infection
  - Anemia
- Substance abuse treatment
- IUGR
  - Decrease maternal activity
  - Left lateral position to elevated placental blood flow
  - Ensure adequate nutrition and oxygenation
  - Consider delivery if fetal compromise evident
- Macrosomia
  - Not an indication for induction (ACOG, 2000a)
  - Not a contraindication for vaginal birth after cesarean (VBAC)
  - Both ultrasound and clinical estimates of fetal weight are imprecise
  - Cesarean may be considered for
    - Estimated fetal weight of > 5000 g in nondiabetic mother
    - Estimated fetal weight of > 4500 g in diabetic mother

Providing Treatment:
Alternative Measures to Consider

- Whole foods diet
- Avoid substances that may affect placental efficiency, such as smoking or illegal drug use

Providing Support:
Education and Support Measures to Consider

- Provide information about
  - Implications for continued care
  - Options for treatment
  - Parameters for intervention
- Nutritional counseling and surveillance as needed
  - Evaluation of intake
  - Adequate hydration
  - Careful food choices for maximum nutrition
- Potential for
  - Serial evaluation of fetal well-being
  - Change in location or providers for birth
- Provide support
- Address client and family concerns

Follow-up Care:
Follow-up Measures to Consider

- Document
- Base midwifery plan on
  - Results of diagnostic testing
  - Discussions with client and family
  - Note indications for consultation or referral
- Anticipated follow-up
  - Serial fetal surveillance weekly or biweekly
  - Update plan weekly or as indicated
- Anticipate need for birth before term with
  - Positive OCT or CST
  - Oligohydramnios
  - Ultrasound documentation of limited cranial growth
- Large for gestational age infant, anticipate potential for
  - Shoulder dystocia
- Anticipate need for fetal/neonatal resuscitation
  - In utero
  - Postdelivery

Collaborative Practice:
Consider Consultation or Referral

- OB/GYN services
  - Prenatal consultation based on maternal and fetal condition
  - Documented IUGR
  - Potential referral to high-risk obstetrics service
  - For induction
  - For anticipated large for gestational age infant
  - As indicated or needed during labor and birth
- Pediatric services
  - Anticipated preterm infant
  - IUGR
  - Maternal diabetes
  - Anticipated newborn resuscitation
- Social services as indicated
  - Tobacco, drug, or alcohol (ETOH) use
  - Poor support systems
  - WIC, food stamps, local food assistance
- For diagnosis or treatment outside the midwife's scope of practice

CARE OF THE PREGNANT WOMAN WITH TOXOPLASMOSIS INFECTION

Key Clinical Information

Acute primary maternal infection with toxoplasmosis puts the unborn baby at risk for congenital toxoplasmosis infection. The risk of congenital fetal infection rises during pregnancy from 15% in the first trimester to 30% during the second trimester and peaks at 60% during the last trimester. Complications of maternal toxoplasmosis infection may include spontaneous abortion or miscarriage, fetal demise, fetal microcephaly, chorioretinitis, cerebral calcifications, and abnormalities of the cerebrospinal fluid (CDC, 2004). However, routine screening for toxoplasmosis in pregnancy is not currently recommended in the United States because disease prevalence is low (Pinard et al., 2003).

Client History and Chart Review:
Components of the History to Consider

- Gestational age
- Fetal activity
- Query regarding possible source of exposure (CDC, 2004)
  - Cat feces, fur, and bedding
  - Raw or rare meat
  - Soil or sand
  - Contaminated water or milk
- Onset, duration, and severity of symptoms
  - Fever
  - Exhaustion
  - Sore throat
  - Swollen lymph nodes
  - Other associated symptoms

Physical Examination:
Components of the Physical Exam
to Consider

- Vital signs, including temperature
- Evaluation for
  - Lymphadenopathy
  - Liver margins
- Fundal height growth

Clinical Impression:
Differential Diagnoses and Code Groups
to Consider

Additional suffix may apply (ICD9data.com, 2007)

- Toxoplasmosis (ICD-9 codes V22.2 and 130, 655)
- Mononucleosis (ICD-9 codes V22.2 and 075)
- Influenza (ICD-9 codes V22.2 and 487)
- Other viral illness (ICD-9 codes V22.2 and 042–079)

Diagnostic Testing:
Diagnostic Tests and Procedures to Consider

- Toxoplasmosis testing
  - Preconception as needed
  - Retest every trimester as needed
- Types of tests
  - IgG-Sabin-Feldman dye test

- IgM-Immunofluorescent antibody (IFA)
  - If titers exceed 1:512, recent acute infection is likely
- Possible exposure
  - IgG and IgM negative = no infection or previous exposure
  - IgG positive and IgM negative = previous infection/immunity
  - If both are positive = possible acute infection, repeat for rising titers
- Recheck IgM in 3 weeks
- If titers rising, acute infection likely

Providing Treatment:
Therapeutic Measures to Consider

- Maternal therapy per perinatologist or obstetrician
  - Spiramycin
  - Pyrimethamine, sulfadiazine, and folic acid

Providing Treatment:
Alternative Measures to Consider

- Immune support
  - Maintain quality diet
  - Rest
  - Echinacea
- Astragalus tea, tincture or capsule
- Emotional support and reassurance

Providing Support:
Education and Support Measures to Consider

- Prevention measures (CDC, 2004)
  - Avoid
    - Contact with cats, cat feces, and cat bedding
    - Travel to areas with endemic toxoplasmosis
    - Handling raw meat whenever possible
- Do practice
  - Careful hand washing with soap and water
  - Use of gloves when
    - Gardening
    - Cleaning litter or sandbox
    - Preparing raw meat

- Cook meat to at least 150°F
- Clean surfaces after processing raw meat
- Information and discussion about
  - Test results and diagnosis
  - Options for care
  - Recommendations for continued care
  - Optimal location for birth
  - Pediatric care for birth
  - Breastfeeding recommended

Follow-up Care:
Follow-up Measures to Consider
- Document
- Positive maternal titer
  - Ultrasound at 20–22 weeks for fetal anomalies
  - Serial ultrasounds as indicated
  - Percutaneous umbilical blood sampling (PUBS for fetal IgM and culture)
  - Evaluation of the newborn for congenital infection
- Return for care
  - Per prenatal routine
  - Provide ongoing support

Collaborative Practice:
Consider Consultation or Referral
- Diagnosis of acute toxoplasmosis, refer to
  - Perinatology
  - Genetic counseling
  - Counseling or support group
- For diagnosis or treatment outside the midwife's scope of practice

CARE OF THE PREGNANT WOMAN WITH URINARY TRACT INFECTION

Key Clinical Information
Urinary tract infection (UTI) during pregnancy may have a variety of presentations. Asymptomatic bacteriuria is common in pregnancy, and acute pyelonephritis occurs in up to 30% of women with previously untreated asymptomatic bacteriuria. Pyelonephritis is a serious complication for the woman and her fetus because she is more likely to experience premature delivery and give birth to a low birth weight baby. Simple cystitis may occur during pregnancy and can be extremely painful. Renal calculi may present as flank pain, accompanied by blood or leukocytes in the urine. UTIs may lead to renal damage, severe pain, and increased risk of preterm labor. Economic costs and impact on quality of life related to UTIs may be considerable (French, 2006).

Client History and Chart Review:
Components of the History to Consider
- Gestational age
- Current symptoms
  - Onset, duration, and severity
  - Dysuria, urgency, frequency, and burning
  - Fever, chills
  - Nausea, vomiting
  - Flank pain, back pain, suprapubic pain or heaviness
  - Colicky pain
  - Hematuria
  - Self-diagnosis in women with history of UTI
  - Symptoms of preterm labor
  - Other associated symptoms
- Review history related to
  - UTIs
  - Renal calculi
  - Recent urinary catheterization
  - Frequent intercourse, new partner
  - Voiding and fluid intake habits
  - Recent antibiotic therapy
  - Structural or functional abnormalities of the urinary tract
  - Intimate partner violence
  - Chronic conditions, such as sickle cell trait or disease, diabetes
  - Fetal movement (> 20 weeks gestation)

Physical Examination:
Components of the Physical Exam to Consider
- Vital signs, including temperature
- Evaluation of hygiene

- Abdominal evaluation
  - Fetal heart tone
  - Presence of contractions
  - Suprapubic tenderness
  - Guarding or rebound tenderness
  - Distended bladder
- Signs of renal involvement
  - Fever
  - Costovertebral angle (CVA) tenderness
- Pelvic examination
  - Evaluate cervical length, consistency, and dilation
  - Station of presenting part

Clinical Impression:
Differential Diagnoses and Code Groups to Consider
Additional suffix may apply (ICD9data.com, 2007)
- Urinary tract
  - Asymptomatic bacteriuria (ICD-9 codes 646.53)
  - Cystitis (ICD-9 codes V22.2 and 595)
  - Pyelonephritis (ICD-9 codes V22.2 and 590.10)
  - Renal calculi (ICD-9 codes V22.2 and 592.0)
- Pregnancy related
  - Preterm labor (ICD-9 codes 644.03)
  - Preeclampsia (ICD-9 codes 642)
  - Concealed abruption (ICD-9 codes 641)
  - Ectopic pregnancy (ICD-9 codes 633)
- Appendicitis (ICD-9 codes V22.2 and 541)
- STI (ICD-9 codes 647.0–647.2)

Diagnostic Testing:
Diagnostic Tests and Procedures to Consider
- Urinalysis
  - Dip (Rosenfeld, 1997)
    - Positive nitrites, first morning urine more accurate
    - Positive leukocytes, frequent false positives
    - Positive nitrites and positive leukocytes more predictive of UTI

- Microscopy
  - Blood (red blood cells)
  - Pyuria (white blood cells)
  - Bacteria
  - Casts
- Gram stain
  - Positive correlates with positive culture
- Urine culture and sensitivity indicated for
  - Positive urinalysis
  - History of UTI
  - Sickle trait
  - Diabetes
  - Chronic renal disease
  - Hypertension
  - Test of cure after treatment and every 6–12 weeks
- Urine culture findings
  - Less than 10,000 colonies
    - No infection
    - Treatment not indicated
  - Colonies of 25,000–100,000
    - Asymptomatic bacteriuria
    - Treatment indicated
  - More than 100,000 colonies
    - UTI if pathogenic bacteria
    - Contamination if mixed bacteria
    - Treat when UTI present
    - Check for sensitivity of bacteria to prescribed drug
- For complicated UTI (pyelonephritis, calculi)
  - CBC
  - Electrolytes
  - Blood urea nitrogen, creatinine
  - Renal ultrasound
  - Strain all urine
- Ultrasound to evaluate for
  - Maternal hydronephrosis
  - Calculi
  - Fetal status
- For recurrent UTI screen for
  - Group B strep
  - Sickle cell
  - Glucose-6-phosphate dehydrogenase (G6PD)

- Diabetes
- Kidney function
  - Blood urea nitrogen
  - Creatinine, 24-hour creatinine clearance
  - Total protein

Providing Treatment:
Therapeutic Measures to Consider
- Macrobid
  - Pregnancy Category B
  - Simple cystitis
    - 100 mg PO BID for 3 days (Sinclair, 2004)
  - Simple or recurrent UTI
    - 100 mg PO BID for 7–10 days
  - Suppressive therapy
    - 50–100 mg daily
  - ⚠ Do not use before 13 weeks or after 36 weeks gestation
  - ⚠ Do not use with G6PD anemia
- Ampicillin 500 mg
  - Pregnancy Category B
  - 1 PO QID for 7–10 days
- Sulfa trimethoprim DS
  - Pregnancy Category C
  - 1 (400/80 mg) PO BID for 7–10 days
  - ⚠ Do not use before 13 weeks or after 36 weeks gestation
  - ⚠ Do not use with G6PD anemia
- Keflex
  - Pregnancy Category B
  - 500 mg PO BID for 7–10 days, or
  - 250 mg PO QID for 7–10 days
- Pyridium, for dysuria
  - 200 mg TID after meals
  - Maximum six doses
  - Pregnancy Category B
- Pyelonephritis
  - Hospitalization
  - IV hydration
    - 200 ml/hr
    - Balanced electrolyte solution

- Antibiotics
  - IV Cefoxitin 1–2 g every 6 hours, or
  - Other cephalosporins
  - Change to PO when afebrile for 24 hours
- Pain control
  - Patient-controlled analgesic (PCA pump)
  - Demerol
  - Morphine

Providing Treatment:
Alternative Measures to Consider
- May be used in combination with antibiotics
- Herbals
  - Parsley tea
  - Concentrated cranberry tablets one to two tablets every 4–6 hours with fluid
- Homeopathic remedies
  - Aconitum (renal discomfort, fever, and chills)
  - Cantharis (painful urination, urgency, and frequency)

Providing Support:
Education and Support Measures to Consider
- Medication instructions
- Review warning signs of progression
  - Fever and chills
  - Flank pain
  - Urinary urgency, burning
  - Hematuria
  - Generalized abdominal pain
  - Nausea, vomiting, loss of appetite, inability to maintain hydration
- Review perineal hygiene
  - Void after intercourse
  - Blot after voiding
  - Wipe front to back after bowel movement
- When to call or come in for care
  - Symptoms
    - Do not resolve within 24 hours
    - Worsen
    - Recur
- Indications for
  - Hospitalization
  - Consult or referral

- Encourage
  - Increased frequency of voiding, every 1–2 hours while awake
  - Increased fluid intake
    - Water preferable
    - Cranberry juice/tea
    - One cup an hour while awake
  - Avoid
    - Caffeine
    - Excess vitamin C
    - Sugars

Follow-up Care:
Follow-up Measures to Consider
- Document
- Maternal surveillance
  - Observe for improvement
  - Change antibiotics based on sensitivities
  - Culture for test of cure
  - Urinalysis each visit for blood, nitrites, leukocytes
  - Culture each trimester
  - Suppressive therapy after two positive cultures
  - Observe for uterine contractions
  - Evaluate for cervical change
- Fetal surveillance
  - Monitor FHR and activity
- Hospital discharge after
  - Twenty-four hours on PO antibiotics
  - Afebrile
  - Calculi passed
  - No signs or symptoms of preterm labor

Collaborative Practice:
Consider Consultation or Referral
- OB/GYN services
  - Pyelonephritis
  - Renal calculi
  - Threatened preterm labor
- For diagnosis or treatment outside the midwife's scope of practice

CARE OF THE PREGNANT WOMAN WITH VAGINAL BLEEDING, FIRST TRIMESTER

Key Clinical Information

Although vaginal bleeding in the first trimester is a relatively common occurrence, affecting as many as 25% of women (Thorstensen, 2000), it must be considered serious until all potential abnormal causes have been effectively ruled out. The precipitating cause may not readily present itself and may take some investigation to identify. Serial evaluation of quantitative β-HCG levels may assist in evaluation, as may ultrasound. Ectopic pregnancy should always be considered. This emotionally difficult time is made more so by uncertainty and lack of effective treatments. The midwife must present a cautious prognosis while maintaining hope when this is warranted.

Client History and Chart Review:
Components of the History to Consider
- Onset, duration, and severity of bleeding
  - Color, amount, and characteristics of discharge
  - Precipitating events if any
  - Presence of cramping or abdominal pain
  - Fever or flulike symptoms
  - Presence or regression of pregnancy symptoms
  - Other associated symptoms
- Estimated gestational age
  - Last menstrual period
  - Date of conception if known
  - Ultrasound report if done
- Obstetric/gynecologic history
  - Gravida, para
  - Blood type and Rh
  - Risk factors for ectopic pregnancy
    - Pelvic inflammatory disease
    - Intrauterine device
    - Gynecologic surgery
    - STIs
  - Previous pregnancy losses

- History related to
  - Abnormal pap smears
  - STIs
  - Infertility
  - Cesarean birth
- Potential exposure to
  - STIs
  - Viral infections
  - Physical abuse or trauma

Physical Examination:
Components of the Physical Exam to Consider
- Vital signs, including temperature and orthostatic BP
- FHR as appropriate for gestation
- External genitalia for
  - Trauma
  - Lesions
  - Varicosities, hemorrhoids
  - Blood or discharge at introitus
- Speculum examination for
  - Blood or discharge from
    - Vaginal vault
    - Cervix
  - Visual cervical dilation
  - Presence of products of conception (POC) at os or in vaginal vault
  - Presence of erosion, polyps, or other cervical cause of bleeding
- Bimanual examination for
  - Cervical dilation
  - Uterine size for dates
  - Uterine tenderness
  - Presence of adnexal mass or pain

Clinical Impression:
Differential Diagnoses and Code Groups
to Consider
Additional suffix may apply (ICD9data.com, 2007)
- Implantation bleeding (ICD-9 codes 623.8)
- Spontaneous abortion (ICD-9 codes 634)
  - Threatened SAB (ICD-9 codes 640)
  - Inevitable SAB (ICD-9 codes 637)
  - Incomplete SAB (ICD-9 codes 637)

- Complete SAB (ICD-9 codes 637)
- Missed SAB (ICD-9 codes 637)
- Ectopic pregnancy (ICD-9 codes 633)
- Molar pregnancy (ICD-9 codes 630)
- Cervical bleeding (ICD-9 codes 626)
  - Cervicitis (ICD-9 codes 616.0)
  - Cervical polyps (ICD-9 codes 622.7)
  - Cervical trauma (ICD-9 codes 641.8)
  - Cervical cancer (ICD-9 codes V22.2 and 180)
- STI (ICD-9 codes 647.0–647.2)

Diagnostic Testing:
Diagnostic Tests and Procedures to Consider
- Serial quantitative β-HCG 48 hours apart
- Hematocrit and/or hemoglobin
- Type and Rh status
- Coagulation studies if missed abortion suspected
  - Prothrombin time
  - Partial prothrombin time
  - Fibrinogen level
  - Platelets
- Ultrasound for
  - Viability
  - Dating
  - Placenta previa or abruptio
  - Ectopic

Providing Treatment:
Therapeutic Measures to Consider
- Pelvic rest and watchful waiting
- Ⓡ Methotrexate for ectopic pregnancy
- Rh immune globulin for Rh-negative mother (see Care of the Woman Who Is Rh Negative)
- Iron replacement therapy for anemia (see Care of the Pregnant Woman with Iron Deficiency Anemia)
- Misoprostal for incomplete SAB < 13 weeks
  - 600–800 mg PO or vaginally
  - If PO not passed in 8–24 hours may repeat dose.

Providing Treatment:
Alternative Measures to Consider
- Await spontaneous resolution to SAB

	Table 3-4　　Anticipated β-HCG Levels	

WEEKS POST-LMP	ANTICIPATED HCG LEVEL (MIU/ML)
4	5–425
5	18–7350
6	1080–56,500
7–8	7650–230,000
9–12	25,700–288,000
13–16	13,500–253,000
17–24	4060–65,500

Source: Frye, A. (2007). *Understanding diagnostic tests in the childbearing year* (7th ed.). Portland, OR: Labrys Press.

- Encourage expulsion of products of conception with
  - Blue or black cohosh tincture
  - Homeopathic caulophyllum
- Promote healing after SAB
  - Homeopathic arnica
  - Rescue remedy
  - Herbal combinations which may include
    - Red raspberry leaf
    - Vitex berries
    - Black haw root
- Bleeding during pregnancy with rising HCG levels (Frye, 1998)
  - Red raspberry leaf
  - False unicorn root
  - Wild yam root
  - Cramp bark
  - Lemon balm

Providing Support:
Education and Support Measures to Consider
- Provide emotional support
- Discuss
  - Potential for miscarriage
  - Options for care
  - Expectant care
  - Tests available
  - Potential findings
  - RhIG for Rh-negative mother

- Threatened SAB
  - Pelvic rest
  - Avoid heavy lifting
  - Call if bleeding increases or is accompanied by pain
  - If awaiting spontaneous resolution of SAB at home, call or seek care immediately if
    - Heavy bleeding with pain for 1½ hours
    - Faintness or weakness
    - Adnexal pain
    - Fever
- After SAB
  - Abstain from intercourse for 2 weeks
  - Bleeding may last 7–10 days
  - Discuss birth control if desired
- Incomplete SAB
  - Provide information on options for care
- Before next pregnancy
  - Use multivitamin with folic acid daily
  - Improve nutrition if indicated
  - Avoid cigarettes, drugs, and alcohol

Follow-up Care:
Follow-up Measures to Consider
- Document
- ⚠ Rule out
  - Molar pregnancy
  - Choriocarcinoma
  - Ectopic pregnancy

- Incomplete SAB
- Follow β-HCG levels
  - Forty-eight to 96 hours if threatened SAB
  - Repeat every 3–5 days until
    - Clear regression
    - Appropriate increase
  - Four to 6 weeks post-SAB
- Ultrasound follow-up
  - No intrauterine pregnancy (IUP) seen on ultrasound
    - Serial HCG levels
    - Continued positive or elevated HCG
- ⚠ Suspect ectopic pregnancy
- Repeat ultrasound 2–7 days
  - Subchorionic bleed on ultrasound
    - Follow-up ultrasound for anomalies
    - Follow β-HCG levels
- After SAB
  - Examination in 2–4 weeks
  - Evaluate return to nonpregnant state
  - Assess emotional status
  - Initiate birth control if desired

Collaborative Practice:
Consider Consultation or Referral
- OB/GYN services
  - Ectopic pregnancy
  - No IUP seen on ultrasound
  - Molar pregnancy
  - Excessive bleeding
  - Dilatation and curettage as indicated or desired
  - Cervical lesion or suspected cervical cancer
- Genetic counseling
- Other referrals as needed
  - Pathology or genetic evaluation of products of conception (POC)
  - Evaluation for problems that can lead to SAB
    - Maternal disease (e.g., lupus, listeria, syphilis)
    - Congenital anomalies of the genital tract
    - Previous cervical surgery
    - Hormonal imbalances
    - Fibroids

- Social services
  - Mental health services
  - Grief counseling
- For diagnosis or treatment outside the midwife's scope of practice

CARE OF THE PREGNANT WOMAN WITH VAGINAL BLEEDING, THIRD TRIMESTER

Key Clinical Information

When a woman presents with vaginal bleeding in the third trimester, evaluation and stabilization of the mother and fetus are the immediate goals (Varney et al., 2004). There are benign causes for spotting or bleeding in the third trimester, such as postcoital spotting, postexamination spotting, vaginal or cervical infection or inflammation, and labor with bloody show. However, the midwife must be vigilant for signs and symptoms of placenta previa and abruption placenta. Bleeding is a frightening experience for the woman; the midwife's prompt attention and action are reassuring.

Client History and Chart Review:
Components of the History to Consider
- Onset, duration, and severity of bleeding
  - Color, amount, and characteristics of discharge
  - Precipitating events if any
  - Presence of contractions, abdominal pain or no pain
  - Other associated symptoms
- Recent examination or intercourse
- Recent trauma or strain
- Gestational age
  - Location of placenta on prior ultrasound if done
- Fetal activity
- Obstetric/gynecologic history (Varney et al., 2004)
  - Gravida para
  - Blood type and Rh
  - Risk factors for placenta previa
    - Multiparity
    - Maternal age > 35

- ◆ Previous placenta previa
- ◆ Previous uterine surgery, including cesarean section
- ◆ Multiple pregnancy
- ◆ Smoking
- ▪ Risk factors for abruptio placentae
  - ◆ Maternal hypertensive disorders
  - ◆ Advanced maternal age or parity
  - ◆ Poor nutritional status
  - ◆ Previous abruptio placentae
  - ◆ Chorioamnionitis
  - ◆ Smoking
  - ◆ External cephalic version
  - ◆ Sudden decrease in uterine volume (e.g., with spontaneous or artificial rupture of membranes (SROM or AROM)
  - ◆ Blunt abdominal trauma
  - ◆ Cocaine use, especially crack cocaine
- ▪ Physical abuse
- ▪ Trauma or injury

Physical Examination:
Components of the Physical Exam to Consider
- Vital signs
- FHR pattern
- Abdominal evaluation for
  - ▪ Uterine enlargement
  - ▪ Uterine pain
  - ▪ Board-like abdomen
- ⚠ No vaginal examination until placenta location known
- External genitalia for
  - ▪ Trauma
  - ▪ Lesions
  - ▪ Varicosities, hemorrhoids
  - ▪ Blood or discharge at introitus
- Speculum examination if no placenta previa for
  - ▪ Blood or discharge from
    - ◆ Vaginal vault
    - ◆ Cervix
  - ▪ Visual cervical dilation
  - ▪ Presence of erosion, polyps, or other cervical cause of bleeding

- Bimanual examination if no placenta previa for
  - ▪ Cervical dilation, effacement, station
  - ▪ Presenting part
  - ▪ Status of membranes

Clinical Impression:
Differential Diagnoses and Code Groups to Consider
Additional suffix may apply (ICD9data.com, 2007)
- Abruptio placentae (ICD-9 codes 641)
- Placenta previa (ICD-9 codes 641)
- Early labor (ICD-9 codes 644)
- Premature labor (ICD-9 codes 644)
- Bleeding, secondary to
  - ▪ Postcoital spotting (ICD-9 codes 641.9)
  - ▪ Postexamination spotting (ICD-9 codes 641.9)
  - ▪ Trauma (ICD-9 codes 641.8)
  - ▪ Cervicitis (ICD-9 codes 616.0)
- STI (ICD-9 codes 647.0–647.2)

Diagnostic Testing:
Diagnostic Tests and Procedures to Consider
- Ultrasound evaluation for previa, abruption, fetal status
- NST, BPP
- Type and Rh status
- CBC, hematocrit and/or hemoglobin
- Type and Rh status
- Coagulation studies
  - ▪ Prothrombin time
  - ▪ Partial prothrombin time
  - ▪ Fibrinogen level
  - ▪ Platelets

Providing Treatment:
Therapeutic Measures to Consider
- For benign spotting
  - ▪ Pelvic rest until spotting resolves
  - ▪ Treatment of underlying cause if known (e.g., bacterial vaginosis (BV))
  - ▪ Reassurance, review danger signs
- For labor at term or preterm
  - ▪ See Care of the Woman During Labor and Birth—Chapter 4

- 🕭 For placenta previa
  - If bleeding stops and fetal response reassuring
    - ◆ May go home on bed rest
    - ◆ Plan for emergency transport as needed
    - ◆ Plan for cesarean section at term
  - If bleeding continues and fetal response nonreassuring
    - ◆ Assemble surgical team and neonatal resuscitation team
    - ◆ Plan for emergency cesarean section
- 🕭 For abruptio placentae
  - If bleeding stops and fetal response reassuring
    - ◆ May cautiously induce or augment labor
    - ◆ Physician in house
  - If bleeding continues and fetal response nonreassuring
    - ◆ Assemble surgical team and neonatal resuscitation team
    - ◆ Plan for emergency cesarean section
- Rh immune globulin for Rh-negative mother (see Care of the Woman Who Is Rh Negative)
- Iron replacement therapy for anemia (see Care of the Pregnant Woman with Iron Deficiency Anemia)

Providing Treatment:
Alternative Measures to Consider
- No alternative treatments for placenta previa or abruptio placentae

Providing Support:
Education and Support Measures to Consider
- During emergency
  - Briefly explain nature of emergency
  - Keep client and family apprised of what is happening
  - Provide emotional support
- After emergency
  - Information about the emergency
  - Compassionate listening
- Education
  - Potential for recurrence in future pregnancies
  - Status and prognosis of the infant

Follow-up Care:
Follow-up Measures to Consider
- Document
- Rh immune globulin for Rh-negative mother
- Iron replacement therapy for anemia
- Postpartum
  - Examination in 1–4 weeks
  - Evaluate return to nonpregnant state
  - Assess emotional status
  - Initiate birth control if desired

Collaborative Practice:
Consider Consultation or Referral
- OB/GYN services
  - Placenta previa
  - Abruptio placentae
- For diagnosis or treatment outside the midwife's scope of practice

REFERENCES

Allen, D. (2001). CDC revised recommendations for HIV screening of pregnant women. *Morbidity and Mortality Weekly Report*, 50(RR19), 59–86.

American College of Nurse-Midwives. (2007). Hallmarks of midwifery care. In *Core competencies for basic midwifery practice*. Retrieved January 4, 2008 from http://www.acnm.org/siteFiles/descriptive/Core_Competencies__6_07.pdf

American College of Obstetricians and Gynecologists (ACOG). (1999a). Clinical management guidelines, number 8. *Management of herpes in pregnancy*. Washington, DC: Author.

American College of Obstetricians and Gynecologists (ACOG). (1999b). Clinical management guidelines, number 147. *Prevention of RhD alloimmunization*. Washington, DC: Author.

American College of Obstetricians and Gynecologists (ACOG). (2000a). Practice bulletin no. 22. *Fetal macrosomia*. Washington, DC: Author.

American College of Obstetricians and Gynecologists (ACOG). (2000b). Clinical management guidelines, no. 12. *Intrauterine growth restriction*. Washington, DC: Author.

American College of Obstetricians and Gynecologists (ACOG). (2000c). Practice bulletin no. 20. *Perinatal viral and parasitic infections*. Washington, DC: Author.

American College of Obstetricians and Gynecologists (ACOG). (2001a). Committee opinion 257. *Genetic evaluation of stillbirths and fetal deaths.* Washington, DC: Author.

American College of Obstetricians and Gynecologists (ACOG). (2001b). Practice bulletin no. 30. Gestational diabetes. *Obstetrics & Gynecology,* 98, 525–538.

American College of Obstetricians and Gynecologists (ACOG). (2007a). Clinical management guidelines for obstetrician-gynecologists. No. 82. Management of herpes in pregnancy. *Obstetrics & Gynecology,* 109, 1489–98.

American College of Obstetricians and Gynecologists (ACOG). (2007b). Practice bulletin no. 86. Viral hepatitis in pregnancy. *Obstetrics & Gynecology,* 110, 941–956.

American Diabetes Association. (2007). Standards of Medical Care in Diabetes—2007. *Diabetes Care,* 30, S4–41.

Belkin, T., & Wilder, J. (2007). Management option for women with midtrimester fetal loss: a case report. *Journal of Midwifery & Women's Health,* 52, 164–167.

Brzoza, Z., Kasperska-Zajac, A., Oles, E., & Rogala, B. (2007). Pruritic urticarial papules and plaques of pregnancy. *Journal of Midwifery & Women's Health,* 52, 44–48.

Burdge, D. R., Money, D. M., Forbes, J. C., Walmsley, S. L., Smaill, F. M., Boucher, M., et al. (2003). Canadian consensus guidelines for the care of HIV-positive pregnant women: putting recommendations into practice. *Canadian Medical Association Journal,* 168, 1671–1674.

Centers for Disease Control and Prevention (CDC). (1998). Recommendations to prevent and control iron deficiency in the United States. *Morbidity and Mortality Weekly Report,* 47, 1–25.

Centers for Disease Control and Prevention (CDC). (2002). Sexually transmitted diseases treatment guidelines (electronic version). *Morbidity and Mortality Weekly Report,* 51(RR-6).

Centers for Disease Control and Prevention (CDC). (2004). Parasites and health: toxoplasmosis. Retrieved January 4, 2008 from http://www.dpd.cdc.gov/DPDx/HTML/Search_Choices.htm

Centers for Disease Control and Prevention (CDC). (2007). Body mass index. Retrieved January 4, 2008 from http://www.cdc.gov/nccdphp/dnpa/bmi/index.htm

Clark, T., & Fitzgerald, L. (2007). Malaria, tuberculosis and HIV/AIDS. *Journal of Midwifery and Women's Health,* 52, e33–e35.

Coomarasamy, A., Honest, H., Papaioannou, S., Gee, H., & Saeed Khan, K. (2003). Aspirin for prevention of preeclampsia in women with historical risk factors: a systematic review. *Obstetrics & Gynecology,* 101, 1319–1332.

Emmons, L., Callahan, P., Gorman, P., & Snyder, M. (1997). Primary care management of common dermatologic disorders in women. *Journal of Nurse-Midwifery,* 42, 228–253.

Engstrom, J. L., & Sittler, C. P. (1994). Nurse-midwifery management of iron deficiency anemia during pregnancy. *Journal of Nurse-Midwifery,* 39, 20s–34s.

Fife, K. H., Bernstein, D. I., Tu, W., Zimet, G. D., Brady, R., Wu, J., et al. (2004). Predictors of herpes simplex virus type 2 antibody positivity among persons with no history of genital herpes. *Sexually Transmitted Diseases,* 31, 676–681.

Foster, S. (1996). *Herbs for your health.* Loveland, CO: Interweave Press.

French, L. (2006). Urinary tract infection in women. *Advanced Studies in Medicine,* 6, 24–29. Retrieved January 4, 2008 from http://www.jhasim.com/files/articlefiles/pdf/ASIM_Master_6_1_pFrench.pdf

Frye, A. (1998). *Holistic midwifery: a comprehensive textbook for midwives in homebirth practice, Vol. 1: Care during pregnancy.* Portland, OR: Labrys Press.

Frye, A. (2007). *Understanding diagnostic tests in the childbearing year* (7th ed.). Portland, OR: Labrys Press.

Goff, M. (2005). Parvovirus B19 in pregnancy. *Journal of Midwifery & Women's Health,* 50, 536–538.

Graves, B., & Barger, M. (2001). A conservative approach to iron supplementation during pregnancy. *Journal of Midwifery & Women's Health,* 46, 156–166.

Groth, S. (2007). Are the institute of medicine recommendations for gestational weight gain appropriate for adolescents? *Journal of Obstetric, Gynecologic, and Neonatal Nursing,* 36, 21–27.

Hlebowicz, J., Darwiche, G., Bjorgell, O., & Almer, L. (2007). Effect of cinnamon on post-prandial blood glucose, gastric emptying and satiety in healthy subjects. *American Journal of Clinical Nutrition,* 85, 1552–1556.

International Diabetes Center. (2003). *Gestational diabetes practice guidelines.* Minneapolis, MN: Author.

Leeman, L., Dresang, L., & Fontaine, P. (2006). *Medical complications in pregnancy. Advanced life support in obstetrics* (update). Retrieved January 4, 2008 from http://www.aafp.org/online/etc/medialib/aafp_org/documents/cme/courses/clin/also/chapterb.Par.0001.File.tmp/Chapter%20B.pdf

Lindsay, J., & Azad, S. (2006). Evaluation of fetal death. *E-medicine.* Retrieved January 4, 2008 from http://www.emedicine.com/med/topic3235.htm

Moise, K. J., & Brecher, M. E. (2004). Package insert for rhesus immune globulin. *Obstetrics & Gynecology,* 103, 998–999.

Murphy, J. L. (Ed.). (2004). *Nurse practitioner's prescribing reference.* New York: Prescribing Reference.

National Heart, Lung, and Blood Institute. (2000). *Working group on high blood pressure in pregnancy.* Retrieved

January 4, 2008 from http://www.nhlbi.nih.gov/guidelines/archives/hbp_preg/

Payton, R., & White, P. (1995). Primary care for women: assessment of hematological disorders. *Journal of Nurse Midwifery*, 40, 120–136.

Pinard, J. A., Leslie, N. S., & Irvine, P. I. (2003). Maternal serologic screening for toxoplasmosis. *Journal of Midwifery & Women's Health*, 48, 308–316.

Quest Diagnostics. (n.d.). *HerpeSelect*. Retrieved January 4, 2008 from http://www.questdiagnostics.com/hcp/topics/herpeselect/herpeselect.html?infectious

Rioux, F. M., & LeBlanc, C. P. (2007). Iron supplementation during pregnancy: what are the risks and benefits of current practice? *Applied Physiology, Nutrition and Metabolism*, 32, 282–288.

Rosenfeld, J. A. (1997). *Women's health in primary care*. Baltimore, MD: William & Wilkins.

Saikul, S., Wiriyasirivaj, B., & Charoenchinont, P. (2006). First 4-hour urinary protein-creatinine ratio for diagnosis of significant proteinuria in preeclampsia. *Journal Medical Association Thailand*, 89(Suppl. 4), S42–S46.

Sinclair, C. (2004). *A midwife's handbook*. St. Louis, MO: W.B. Saunders.

Smith, T. (1984). *A woman's guide to homeopathic medicine*. New York: Thorsons.

Thorstensen, K. A. (2000). Midwifery management of first trimester bleeding and early pregnancy loss. *Journal of Midwifery & Women's Health*, 45, 3481–497.

Ulrich, S. (2004). First birth stories of student midwives: keys to professional affective socialization. *Journal of Midwifery & Women's Health*, 49, 390–379.

University of Maryland Medical Center. (2007). *Anemia*. Retrieved on January 4, 2008 from http://www.umm.edu/patiented/articles/who_becomes_anemic_000057_2.htm

U.S. Public Health Service Task Force (2004). *Recommendations for use of antiretroviral drugs in pregnant HIV-1-infected women for maternal health and interventions to reduce perinatal HIV-1 transmission in the United States*. Washington, DC: Government Printing Office.

Varney, H., Kriebs, J. M., & Gegor, C. L. (2004). *Varney's midwifery* (4th ed.). Sudbury, MA: Jones and Bartlett.

Villar, J., Abdel-Aleem, H., Merialdi, M., Mathai, M., Ali, M., Zavaleta, N., et al. (2006). World Health Organization randomized trial of calcium supplementation among low calcium intake pregnant women. *American Journal of Obstetrics and Gynecology*. 194, 639–649. Retrieved January 4, 2008 from http://www.ncbi.nlm.nih.gov/sites/entrez?db=pubmed&uid=16522392&cmd=showdetailview&indexed=google

Wagner, L. K. (2004). Diagnosis and management of pre-eclampsia. *American Family Physician*, 70, 2317–2324.

Weed, S. (1985). *Wise woman herbal for the childbearing year*. Woodstock, NY: Ashtree.

BIBLIOGRAPHY

Briggs, G. G., Freeman, R. K., & Yaffe, S. J. (2005). *Drugs in pregnancy and lactation* (7th ed.). Philadelphia: Williams & Wilkins.

Enkin, M., Keirce, M., Renfrew, M., Neilson, J., Crowther, C., Duley, L., et al. (2000). *A guide to effective care in pregnancy and childbirth* (3rd ed.). New York: Oxford University Press.

Fennell, E. (1994). Urinary tract infections during pregnancy. *The Female Patient*, 19, 27–35.

Fraser, D., & Cooper, M. (2003). *Textbook for midwives* (14th ed.). Edinburgh, Scotland: Churchill Livingstone.

Gordon, J. D., Rydfors, J. T., Druzin, M. L., Tadir, Y., El-Sayed, Y., Chan, J., et al. (2007). *Obstetrics, gynecology and infertility* (6th ed.). Glen Cove, NY: Scrub Hill Press.

Morgan, G., & Hamilton, C. (2003). *Practice guidelines for obstetrics and gynecology*. Philadelphia: Lippincott-Raven.

Murray, M. (1998). Advanced fetal monitoring: antepartal and intrapartal assessment and intervention. Program presented in Milwaukee, Wisconsin, June.

Nolan, T. E. (1994). Chronic hypertension in pregnancy. *The Female Patient*, 19, 27–42.

Phelan, J. P. (1997). Intrauterine fetal resuscitation: betamimetics & amnioinfusion. Presented at Issues & Controversies in Perinatal Practice, Bangor, Maine, October.

Scott, J. R., Gibbs, R. S., Karlan, B., & Haney, A. (2003). *Danforth's obstetrics and gynecology* (9th ed.). Philadelphia: Lippincott, Williams & Wilkins.

Soule, D., & Szwed, S. (2000). *The roots of healing: a woman's book of herbs*. Secaucus, NJ: Citadel Press.

Speroff, L., & Fritz, M. A. (2004). *Clinical gynecologic endocrinology and infertility* (7th ed.). Philadelphia: Lippincott, Williams & Wilkins.

Care of the Woman During Labor and Birth

4

Continuous therapeutic presence at the side of women in active labor is a hallmark of midwifery care and remains the essence of being "with woman" in her time of greatest need.

Birth is a psychophysiologic event embedded in social processes. For many of the 4 million women who give birth in America every year, this event is normal, healthy, and a cause for celebration. Giving birth is an important developmental milestone in a woman's life, with influences on mother, child, and family that extend beyond the birth itself. The birth of a child is a marker event in a life history. Time is measured before children or after children. Women carry vivid memories of their birth experiences throughout their lives.

Women in labor are women at their most vulnerable, creative, and powerful moments. Women expend an incredible amount of energy in the process of laboring and bringing forth their children, but they also must be vigilant in protecting their birth experience, including the possible need to navigate the complexities of the health care system. Few women have the resources to attend to all these tasks at once. One reason many women choose midwifery care is to have a natural ally in their attempts to achieve the birth experience they desire during this formative and transitional time. Women from many cultures and all walks of life come to midwives for birth care. These women look to midwives for safe, compassionate, maternity care.

Midwifery care is distinguished from obstetric care by the belief that birth is fundamentally a normal process, as opposed to a pathologic process. This perspective makes all the difference in determining what women need during this time. However, midwives need to take care not to "normalize" conditions that are problematic. The natural dynamic and tension that exists between the two views of birth—normal versus pathologic—should be harnessed for the woman's benefit. Midwives remain an underutilized or nonexistent care provider in many American hospitals even today, although they consistently practice according to evidence and in a humane and cost-effective manner. Midwives should be part of every maternity care team and should be accessible to all women across America.

Expectations and standards for midwifery care vary geographically in the United States as well as by birth location. Familiarity with state, regional, and local standards for birth care can ease the way for negotiation when adopting an innovative or uncommon practice. Use of scientific resources is useful in developing midwifery policy, but it should not supersede the centuries of sound midwifery care that have served women so well. Nowhere in the life of a woman is individualized care more important than during labor and birth.

It is common wisdom among those who are "with woman" through the travails of labor and birth that confidence is an important asset to the birthing process. A confident woman, one who has faith in her ability to prevail no matter what circumstances she is given, calls forth the emotional stamina, positive attitude, and coping behaviors necessary for an optimal outcome. Midwives are privileged to support women in developing this belief in themselves, through wiping a brow, squeezing a hand, rubbing a back, or whispering "you are strong, you can do it".

INITIAL MIDWIFERY EVALUATION OF THE LABORING WOMAN

Key Clinical Information

Evaluation of the woman in labor encompasses not only physical evaluation of both mother and baby but also meticulous assessment of the woman's coping skills and strengths that she brings to the task of bringing forth her child. A comprehensive and accurate labor assessment forms the foundation for development of the midwifery plan of care and may provide critical information that influences the mother's care as labor progresses.

Client History and Chart Review:
Components of the History to Consider

- Verify last menstrual period (LMP), estimated date of conception (EDC), and anticipated gestational age

- Determine
  - Onset of labor
  - Frequency, length, duration of contractions
  - Status of membranes
    - Presence of meconium
  - Presence of bloody show
  - Recent nutritional intake
- Perform labor risk assessment
  - Current pregnancy course
  - Prenatal laboratory review
  - Group B streptococcus (GBS) status
  - Other risk factors
- Previous obstetric/gynecologic history
  - Length of previous labors
  - Size of previous infants
  - Previous use of anesthesia in labor
  - Previous problems in labor and birth
- Review past medical and surgical history
  - Allergies
  - Medication and herb use
  - Previous anesthesia
  - Surgical procedures
  - Chronic and acute illnesses
  - Injuries
- Social history
- Maternal and fetal well-being
  - Fetal activity patterns
  - Coping mechanisms for labor
    - Emotional status
    - Developmental status
    - Support people
  - Preferences for labor and birth
    - 🌐 Cultural practices
    - Support for labor
    - Birth plan
- Review of systems (ROS)
  - Genitourinary system
  - Respiratory system
  - Circulatory system
  - Gastrointestinal system
  - Nervous system
  - Musculoskeletal system

Physical Examination:
Components of the Physical Exam to Consider
- Maternal and fetal vital signs
- Abdominal examination
  - Contraction pattern: frequency, duration, strength
  - Evaluate fetus
    - Fetal lie, presentation, position, and variety
    - Fetal heart rate (FHR) and rhythm
      - Auscultation or electronic fetal monitoring (EFM)
      - Baseline heart rate
      - Beat-to-beat variability
      - Periodic changes
  - Estimated fetal weight (EFW)
- Pelvic examination
  - Determine presenting part
  - Dilation and effacement
  - Verify status of membranes
  - Station
  - Presence of bleeding or show
  - Assess external genitalia, perineum and pelvic floor
    - Presence of any lesions
    - Presence of female genital mutilation
- Presence of amniotic fluid
  - Nitrazine
  - Ferning
  - Meconium staining

- Extremities
  - Reflexes
  - Edema
- Preanesthesia considerations
  - Dentition
  - Airway
  - Cardiopulmonary status
  - Spine
- Evaluate additional body systems as indicated by
  - History
  - Client presentation
  - Physical examination findings
  - Diagnostic test results

Clinical Impression:
Differential Diagnoses and Code Groups to Consider
Additional suffix may apply (ICD9data.com, 2007)
- Braxton Hicks contractions (ICD-9 codes 644.1)
- False labor (ICD-9 codes 644.1)
- Onset of labor at term
  - Prolonged labor (ICD-9 codes 662)
  - Early labor, without delivery (ICD-9 codes 644)
  - Active labor, delivered (ICD-9 codes 650)
  - Premature rupture of membranes (PROM) before onset of labor (ICD-9 codes 658.1)

⊕ PRESENCE OF FEMALE GENITAL MUTILATION (FGM)

Inquire before initial exam

Maintain non-judgmental attitude

Note type of FGM present

　　Type I—partial or complete clitorectomy

　　Type II—clitorectomy and partial excision of labia minora

　　Type III—infibulation—excision and reapproximation of labia majora

　　Type IV—all other procedures not described here

Deinfibulation preferred prior to pregnancy, but may be done in second trimester.

Reinfibulation after delivery may be requested, but is not recommended.

Source: Braddy and Files, 2007.

Diagnostic Testing:
Diagnostic Tests and Procedures to Consider
- Testing is performed as indicated by
  - Client history
  - Active risk factors
  - Facility or practice standards
- Urinalysis
  - Dip for protein and glucose
  - Microscopic as needed
- Complete blood count (CBC)
- Type and screen/cross
- Other screening as indicated by history and physical
- Ultrasound
  - Fetal presentation
  - Amniotic fluid index (AFI)
  - Biophysical profile
  - Placental location and integrity

Providing Treatment:
Therapeutic Measures to Consider
- Expectant management
- As indicated by mother's history or facility protocol
  - Saline lock for venous access
  - IV fluids for hydration, or venous access
    - GBS antibiotic prophylaxis (see Care of the Woman with Group B Streptococcus)
    - Magnesium sulfate for pregnancy-induced hypertension (PIH) (see Care of the Woman with Pregnancy-Induced Hypertension in Labor)
    - Gestational diabetes on insulin (see Chapter 3, Care of the Pregnant Woman with Gestational Diabetes)
- Medications as indicated by
  - Maternal history
  - Fetal status

Providing Treatment:
Alternative Measures to Consider
- Watchful waiting
- Oral hydration and nutrition
- Ambulation

- Hydrotherapy
- Support people present

Providing Support:
Education and Support Measures to Consider
- Provide information about
  - Role of birth professionals
    - Labor evaluation process
    - Expected care during labor and birth
  - Hydration options
  - Activity options
  - Pain relief options
    - Nonpharmaceutical
    - Pharmaceutical
- Positions for birth
- Indications for
  - Artificial rupture of membranes
  - Internal examinations
  - Medications
- Provide progress updates
- Provide encouragement and support
- Provide information for shared decision-making

Follow-up Care:
Follow-up Measures to Consider
- Document admission history and physical
- Reevaluate for presence of progress
  - As indicated by maternal and fetal status
  - At least every 4–6 hours
  - Document in progress notes
- Monitor client responses to
  - Support people
  - Unfamiliar care providers
  - Labor progress and information
- Note
  - Anticipated progression
  - Anticipatory thinking
  - Consultations or referrals

Collaborative Practice:
Consider Consultation or Referral
- For diagnosis or treatment outside the midwife's scope of practice

CARE OF THE WOMAN IN FIRST-STAGE LABOR

Key Clinical Information

Ongoing evaluation of the woman in labor provides the midwife with necessary information for determining maternal and fetal well-being during labor. The range of progress during labor considered "normal" varies widely. The midwife plays a critical role in providing maternal support and reassurance while at the same time remaining vigilant for subtle variations in maternal or fetal condition that may indicate the presence of or potential for developing problems. Early identification of actual or potential problems allows problem-solving measures and treatments to be initiated promptly and proactively, with a goal of the best outcome possible for mother and baby in the given circumstances.

Client History and Chart Review:
Components of the History to Consider

- Chart review or verbal report
- Prior labor and birth history
  - Gravida, parity
  - LMP, EDC, gestational age
  - Prenatal course
  - Birth plan or preferences
- Interval history since admission, at least every 4–6 hours
  - Frequency, length, and duration of contractions
  - Pattern of labor
  - Status of membranes
  - Presence of bloody show
  - Recent fetal and maternal vital signs
  - Maternal coping ability
- Internal examination
  - When last assessed
  - Cervical dilation, effacement
  - Presenting part and station
  - Presence of pelvic pressure
- Deviations from anticipated labor course
- Initial midwifery plan of care

Physical Examination:
Components of the Physical Exam to Consider

- Maternal and fetal vital signs
  - Maternal blood pressure, pulse, respirations, and temperature
  - FHR pattern and variability
- Evaluation of fetal response to labor
  - Methods
    - Auscultation, using
      - Fetoscope
      - Doppler
    - Evaluate for 60 seconds
    - Evaluate during and after contraction
    - Electronic fetal monitoring
      - External fetal monitoring
        - Intermittent
        - Continuous
      - Internal scalp electrode
        - Not indicated for low-risk pregnancy
        - Direct electrocardiogram
        - For continuous assessment and evaluation of abnormal FHR patterns
    - Observation of fetal activity

MINIMUM FREQUENCY FOR INTERMITTENT AUSCULTATION OF FETAL HEART RATE IN LABOR (AMERICAN COLLEGE OF OBSTETRICIANS AND GYNECOLOGISTS [ACOG], 2005; VARNEY ET AL., 2004, P. 798)

Without risk factors
    Every 30 minutes in active labor
    Every 15 minutes in second stage
With risk factors
    Every 15 minutes in active labor after a contraction
    Every 5 minutes in second stage

- Note fetal heart tones (FHTs)
  - At least every 30 minutes
  - Immediately after ROM
  - After pain medication
    - At medication peak
  - With change in contraction pattern
  - As indicated by
    - Course of labor
    - Stage of labor
    - Previous FHR patterns
- Evaluation of maternal response to labor
  - Methods
    - Observation
    - Palpation of uterus
    - External tocotransducer
    - Intrauterine pressure catheter (IUPC)
  - Coping ability
    - Effectiveness of support people
    - Maternal response to labor
      - Cultural responses to labor
      - Maternal attitude and approach
      - Pain relief techniques and needs
  - Contraction pattern
    - Duration
    - Frequency
    - Strength
    - Maternal response
- Pelvic examination
  - Cervical dilation, effacement
  - Status of membranes
  - Presenting part
  - Station
  - Position
  - Reevaluate pelvimetry
  - Assess soft tissues for distensibility
- Urinary system
  - Bladder distension
  - Urine: protein and ketones
  - Output
- Hydration and nutrition
  - Fluid intake
  - Nutritive intake
  - Nausea and vomiting
  - Energy level

- Evaluate for changes in cervical status and/or fetal descent
  - ⚠ Less than four examinations decreases risk of post partum endometritis
  - With change in maternal behavior
  - Before administration of pain medication
  - With urge to push
  - As needed for ongoing evaluation of labor progress
- Additional assessments as indicated

Clinical Impression:
Differential Diagnoses and Code Groups to Consider
Additional suffix may apply (ICD9data.com, 2007)
- Progressive labor, with delivery (ICD-9 codes 650)
- Prolonged labor (ICD-9 codes 662)
- False labor (ICD-9 codes 644.1)
- Also consider
  - Abnormal FHR patterns (ICD-9 codes 656.3)
  - Maternal conditions, such as PIH (ICD-9 codes 630–677)
- Labor dystocia, secondary to
  - Cephalopelvic disproportion (ICD-9 codes 653.4)
  - Dysfunctional labor
    - Hypotonic (ICD-9 codes 661.2)
    - Hypertonic (ICD-9 codes 661.4)
    - Obstructed labor (ICD-9 codes 660)
  - Fetal position, such as
    - Persistent posterior presentation (ICD-9 codes 652)
    - Breech presentation (ICD-9 codes 652.2)
    - Face presentation (ICD-9 codes 652.4)

Diagnostic Testing:
Diagnostic Tests and Procedures to Consider
- Dip urine for protein and ketones
- Testing as indicated by
  - Labor progression and status
  - Developing maternal or fetal risk factors, such as
    - Preeclampsia
    - Suspected breech

◆ Obstructed labor
◆ Placental abruption

Providing Treatment:
Therapeutic Measures to Consider (WHO, 1996)
- False or prodromal labor
  - Reassurance
  - Medications (see Care of the Woman with Prolonged Latent-Phase Labor)
    - ◆ Morphine 10–20 mg IM, with
      - ➤ Vistaril 25 mg IM
      - ➤ Consider additional 10 mg MS if no sleep in 1–2 hours
- Hypertonic uterine dysfunction (spontaneous)
  - Reassurance
  - Hydration, PO or IV
  - Terbutaline 0.25 mg subcutaneous
  - Rest is essential
    - ◆ Morphine 10–20 mg IM as above
- Active management of labor
  - Augmentation of labor with oxytocin infusion (see Care of the Woman Undergoing Induction or Augmentation of Labor)
  - Amniotomy
- IV access as indicated
  - Client history
  - Facility standard
  - Consider saline lock versus continuous IV
  - Maintain IV start kit on hand for use as needed
- Sedatives, anxiolytics, and antiemetics
  - Vistaril 50 mg IM
    - ◆ Early or active labor
    - ◆ Causes sedation
    - ◆ Reduces anxiety
    - ◆ May combine with analgesic to potentiate effects
  - Phenergan 25–50 mg IM or IV
    - ◆ Use in early or active labor
    - ◆ Causes sedation
    - ◆ Reduces anxiety
    - ◆ Treats nausea and vomiting
    - ◆ May combine with analgesic to potentiate effects

- Analgesic medications (Sinclair, 2004)
  - May decrease newborn respiratory drive
  - May be reversed as needed with naloxone
    - ◆ ⚠ Use naloxone with caution with suspected narcotic addiction
    - ◆ Newborn dose 0.1 mg/kg IM, SQ, IV
    - ◆ Watch for rebound effect
  - Fentanyl
    - ◆ 50–100 mg IV every 1–2 hours
  - Stadol (butorphanol)
    - ◆ 1–2 mg IM every 3–4 hours
    - ◆ 0.5–2.0 mg IV every 1–3 hours
  - Nubain (nalbuphine)
    - ◆ 10–20 mg SQ or IM or IV every 1–2 hours
  - Demerol—active labor
    - ◆ 50–100 mg IM every 3–4 hours
    - ◆ 12.5–25 mg IV every 1–2 hours
- Regional anesthetic
  - Requires IV hydration
  - May decrease placental perfusion secondary to hypotension
  - Epidural
    - ◆ Continuous infusion possible
    - ◆ May diminish urge to push
  - Intrathecal
    - ◆ Generally one-time dose
    - ◆ Lasts 2–12 hours based on medications used
- Hydration
  - Oral fluid intake
  - IV fluids
- Consider IV access for the following conditions
  - Grand multiparity
  - Overdistended uterus (e.g., twins, polyhydramnios)
  - Oxytocin administration
  - History of postpartum hemorrhage
  - Maternal dehydration or exhaustion
  - Fetal distress with fatigued mother
  - Any condition requiring quick intravenous access (e.g., preeclampsia)
- Lactated Ringer's or similar balanced electrolyte solution
  - Fluid bolus of 300–1000 ml

- Before regional anesthesia
- To correct dehydration or volume depletion
  - Maintenance dose of 100–200 ml/hour
  - Titrate to urinary output
- Dysfunctional labor
  - IV oxytocin (see Care of the Woman Undergoing Induction or Augmentation of Labor)
  - Nipple stimulation
  - Enema
  - Artificial ROM if vertex well applied and station 0 or below
- Catheterize as needed for distended bladder if unable to void

Providing Treatment:
Alternative Measures to Consider
- Physiologic management of labor (Albers, 2007)
  - Watchful waiting
  - Onset of active labor at $\geq$ 4 cm
    - Send home for early labor, do not admit to hospital if low risk and < 4 cm
  - Allow broad time frame for progressive labor
  - Encourage
    - Gentle activity
    - Food and drink
    - Rest times
    - Music
    - Relaxation
    - Visualization
- Pain relief
  - Hydrotherapy
    - Shower
    - Tub
  - Acupressure
  - Hypnobirthing
  - Massage
    - Effleurage
    - Lower back
    - Neck and shoulders
  - Ice packs
  - Hot packs

- Frequent voiding
- Position changes
  - Encourage upright positions
  - Birth ball
  - Rocking chair
  - Hands and knees
  - Squatting
  - Side-lying
  - Walking
- Doula or support person

Providing Support:
Education and Support Measures
to Consider
- Active listening to maternal concerns
- Information and discussion regarding
  - Fetal and maternal well-being
  - The progress of labor
  - The process of labor
  - Any imposed limits, or medical therapies, with rationale
- Informed consent process for anticipated procedures
- Emotional support
  - Continuous presence of support people
  - Continuous presence of midwife in active labor or for problems
  - Familiar environment or objects
  - Reassurance of labor as normal physiologic process
- Encourage maternal control
  - Food and fluid as desired
  - Position changes as desired
  - Frequent voiding
  - Timing of maternal and fetal evaluation

Follow-up Care:
Follow-up Measures to Consider
- Document (see Chapter 1, Office Visit or Progress Note)
- Reevaluate every 1–4 hours in active labor
  - Anticipate labor progress
  - Notify additional personnel as indicated

Collaborative Practice:
Consider Consultation or Referral
- As indicated by collaborative practice agreements
- For diagnosis or treatment outside the midwife's scope of practice

CARE OF THE WOMAN IN SECOND-STAGE LABOR

Key Clinical Information

During the second stage of labor the fetus must traverse the bony confines of the birth canal before emerging from the womb. Fetal position at entry to the pelvis contributes to the duration and difficulty of second-stage labor. Prenatal evaluation of the internal pelvic diameters, known as *pelvimetry,* can be very useful in anticipating the course of second-stage labor and in offering suggestions for maternal positioning to facilitate fetal descent.

Encouraging the woman to listen to her body during pushing is a hallmark of midwifery care and promotes a quiet, calm, yet focused woman-centered atmosphere in the birth environment.

Client History and Chart Review:
Components of the History to Consider
- Documented pelvimetry
- EFW
- Review progress of first stage
  - Labor curve
  - Fetal presentation and position
  - Maternal positioning
  - Maternal attitude and coping
  - Analgesia or anesthesia
- Review progress of second stage
  - Length of second stage is variable
  - Second stage > 2 hours not an independent indication for delivery (Roberts, 2002)
  - Progressive second stage includes
    - Presence of effective contractions
    - Steady descent
    - Maternal and fetal well-being

- Previous obstetric history
  - Previous infants' weights
  - Second-stage length
  - Shoulder dystocia
  - Assisted delivery
    - Forceps
    - Vacuum extractor
    - Cesarean delivery

Physical Examination:
Components of the Physical Exam to Consider
- Abdominal examination
  - Evidence of fetal descent
    - Abdominal contour changes
    - Fetal position changes
    - Descent in location of FHT
- Pelvic examination
  - Verify complete dilation
  - Assess
    - Location of sutures
    - Flexion of fetal head
    - Fetal molding
    - Effectiveness of bearing down
    - Rate of descent
    - Caput formation
  - Bulging of perineum
- Fetal well-being
  - Frequent FHTs
  - FHR may decrease in midpelvis
  - Head compression may decrease FHR
    - FHR should return to > 100 between pushes
    - FHR < 90 anticipate resuscitation
- Determine maternal well-being
  - Vital signs
  - Assess hydration
  - Evaluate her energy level
  - Determine her coping ability
  - Assess for bladder distension
    - May cause second-stage obstruction
  - Perineal tissue elasticity
- Evaluate for signs or symptoms of
  - Lack of descent
  - Slow descent

- Caput formation
- Fetal distress
- Maternal exhaustion
- Perineal edema

Clinical Impression:
Differential Diagnoses and Code Groups
to Consider
Additional suffix may apply (ICD9data.com, 2007)
- Spontaneous vaginal birth (ICD-9 codes V27.0)
- Perineal injury
  - First-degree laceration (ICD-9 codes 664.0)
  - Second-degree laceration (ICD-9 codes 664.1)
  - Third-degree laceration (ICD-9 codes 664.2)
  - Fourth-degree laceration (ICD-9 codes 664.3)
  - Episiotomy (ICD-9 procedure codes 73.6)
- Also consider
  - Fetal distress (ICD-9 codes 656.3)
  - Precipitous birth (ICD-9 codes 661.3)
  - Meconium-stained fluid (ICD-9 codes 656.8)
  - Nuchal cord, state number of loops (ICD-9 codes 663.1)
  - True knot in cord, with compression (ICD-9 codes 663.2)
- Slowly progressive second stage, with
  - Asynclitic presentation (ICD-9 codes 652.9)
  - Persistent posterior presentation (ICD-9 codes 652.9)
  - Shoulder dystocia (ICD-9 codes 660.4)
- Failure of descent during second stage
  - Obstructed labor (ICD-9 codes 660)
  - Cephalopelvic disproportion (ICD-9 codes 653.4)

Diagnostic Testing:
Diagnostic Tests and Procedures to Consider
- Limited vaginal examinations for descent of presenting part

Providing Treatment:
Therapeutic Measures to Consider (WHO, 1996)
- Active management of second stage (Frigoletto et al., 1995; Peaceman & Socol, 1996)
  - Pushing with onset of full dilation
  - Prolonged controlled pushing

- Augmentation with oxytocin
- Episiotomy, restrict use to indications
- Assisted extension of fetal head with Ritgen manuever
- Manual rotation of shoulders
- Gentle traction for birth of infant
- Local or other anesthesia for
  - Episiotomy
  - Laceration repair as needed
- Catheterization if bladder distended and unable to void
- Assisted birth
  - Manual assistance (see Care of the Woman with Shoulder Dystocia)
  - Vacuum extraction (see Care of the Woman Undergoing Vacuum-Assisted Birth)
  - Manually reduce loose nuchal cord
- Clamping and cutting of the umbilical cord (WHO, 1998)
  - Before birth of the shoulders for tight nuchal cord
  - When cord has stopped pulsing (Mercer et al., 2007; Mercer & Skovgaard, 2002)
  - Immediately after birth
  - After birth of placenta
  - Family member may wish to cut cord
- Collect cord blood sample
  - For Rh-negative mother
  - Per facility or practice standard
  - As indicated by history
  - If sending specimen to cord blood bank
  - Consider cord blood gases in non-vigorous infants

SOMERSAULT MANEUVER (VARNEY ET AL., 2004)

Consider for nuchal cord with a bit of give to it
As shoulders deliver, gently push infant's head into mother's thighs
Keep infant's head next to mother's perineum as rest of body emerges
Infant somersaults out and cord is untangled from neck

Providing Treatment:
Alternative Measures to Consider

- Physiologic management of second stage (Roberts, 2002)
  - Onset of pushing with maternal urge
  - No prolonged pushing
  - No arbitrary time limits if mother and baby in good condition
  - Baby is born by mother's spontaneous expulsive efforts
  - Head is allowed to restitute spontaneously
  - Shoulders and body emerge spontaneously
  - Assistance may be provided at any point, as needed
- Positioning for second stage and birth
  - Semisitting
  - Left lateral
  - Squatting
  - Standing
  - Hands and knees
  - Birthing stool
  - Birthing tub
- Lithotomy position with feet braced
  - Flattens sacral spine
  - Opens midpelvis
  - Rotates symphysis anteriorly
  - Assists with
    - Persistent posterior
    - Slow descent
- Water birth
- Perineal management
  - Hot packs to perineum
  - Perineal massage
  - Perineal support
- Family participation in birth

Providing Support:
Education and Support Measures
to Consider

- Pushing
  - Allow for natural expulsive efforts
  - Direct pushing efforts when needed
  - Remind about pelvic pressure
  - Instruct when not to push

RECIPE FOR PERINEAL MASSAGE OIL

To use for prenatal or birth perineal massage
Place dried calendula petals and arnica leaves in slow cooker
Cover completely with cold pressed oil
Use wheat germ, apricot kernel, sweet almond, or olive oil
Simmer on low for 6 hours
Strain out herbs
Allow to cool
Add contents of one to two vitamin E capsules
Store in a dark glass jar out of direct sunlight
Use at room temperature or warmed in a hot pack

Source: Walls, 2007.

- Immediate care after birth
  - Discuss plan for newborn handling
    - Newborn to mother
    - Newborn to warming unit
    - Initial evaluation process for baby
    - Cord cutting
  - Remind about third stage

Follow-up Care:
Follow-up Measures to Consider

- Document (see Chapter 1, Delivery Note)
- Provide newborn resuscitation as indicated
- Evaluate perineal integrity
  - Note episiotomy or lacerations
    - Extent and location(s)
    - Repair, if necessary
      - Dermabond
      - Suture
      - Medications
  - Provide local anesthesia, as needed
  - Provide analgesia, as needed
- IV fluids
- Observe mother and newborn after birth for
  - Bonding
  - Breastfeeding
  - Maternal stability
  - Signs of third stage
- Provide for ongoing care postpartum

Collaborative Practice:
Consider Consultation or Referral

- OB/GYN on unit or on standby
  - Arrest of descent
  - Anticipated shoulder dystocia
  - Fetal distress
  - Repair of third- or fourth-degree lacerations
- Pediatrician or neonatologist, on unit or on standby
  - Fetal distress
  - Newborn resuscitation
  - Shoulder dystocia
- For diagnosis or treatment outside the midwife's scope of practice

CARE OF THE WOMAN IN THIRD-STAGE LABOR

Key Clinical Information

Birth of the placenta signals the end of labor and the beginning of the postpartum period. Significant blood loss may occur before or after the birth of the placenta. Active management of the third stage of labor consistently results in decreased maternal blood loss and is promoted in a joint statement by the International Confederation of Midwives and the International Federation of Gynaecology and Obstetrics (International Confederation of Midwives, 2003). Active management strategies typically include administration of a uterotonic drug within 2 minutes after the shoulders are born, and controlled traction of the umbilical cord in conjunction with uterine contractions, accompanied by counter traction on the uterus to prevent uterine inversion. Delayed cord clamping is compatible with active management of third stage labor. Current available evidence suggests that the key strategy in reducing hemorrhage is the prophylactic administration of a uterotonic drug, with synthetic oxytocin as the preferred medication (McDonald, 2007).

American midwives have been reluctant to embrace this evidence-based practice and generally have the luxury of practicing in resource-rich settings, with personnel and medications to treat hemorrhage easily available. However, hemorrhage remains the leading cause of maternal morbidity worldwide, and most hemorrhages occur in women with no risk factors.

Complete evaluation of the placenta should include manual palpation of the maternal surface and visual inspection of both sides of the placenta for areas of fragmentation, divots, or torn blood vessels that may indicate retained placental parts.

Client History and Chart Review:
Components of the History to Consider

- Previous obstetric history
- Risk factors for postpartum hemorrhage
  - Overdistended uterus
  - Large infant
  - Precipitous labor and birth
  - Prolonged first or second stage
  - Cervical manipulation
  - Anemia
- Course of labor and birth

Physical Examination:
Components of the Physical Exam to Consider

- Vital signs
- Evaluate for tears or lacerations
  - Vagina
  - Periurethral area
  - Rectum
  - Cervix
- Expectant management
  - Observe for placental separation
    - Lengthening cord
    - Globular fundus
    - Gush of blood
- Verify that placenta is intact (Varney et al., 2004)
  - Visual examination of maternal and fetal surfaces
  - Tactile examination of maternal surface
  - Cord insertion and vessel pattern
  - Look for gross pathologic changes
  - Examine for number of cord vessels (two arteries, one vein)

Clinical Impression:
Differential Diagnoses and Code Groups
to Consider
Additional suffix may apply (ICD9data.com, 2007)
- Normal spontaneous vaginal birth (ICD-9 codes 650)
- Third-stage labor with
  - Postpartum hemorrhage due to (ICD-9 codes 665–666)
    - Vaginal lacerations (ICD-9 codes 665.4)
    - Cervical lacerations (ICD-9 codes 665.3)
    - Uterine atony (ICD-9 codes 666.1)
    - Retained placental fragments (ICD-9 codes 666.2)
  - Retained placenta (ICD-9 codes 667.0)
    - Accreta (ICD-9 codes 667.0)
    - Percreta (ICD-9 codes 667.0)
    - Increta (ICD-9 codes 667.0)

Diagnostic Testing:
Diagnostic Tests and Procedures to Consider
- Placenta to pathology for evaluation (Hargitaib et al., 2004; Langston et al., 1997)
  - Maternal indications
    - Retained placenta
    - Abnormal gross placental examination
    - Placental abruption
    - Diabetes
    - Chronic hypertension or PIH
    - Preterm delivery (< 35 weeks)
    - Postterm delivery (> 42 weeks)
    - Unexplained fever
    - Previous poor obstetric history
    - No or minimal prenatal care
    - Substance abuse
    - Unexplained elevation of α-fetoprotein
  - Fetal indications
    - Stillbirth
    - Neonatal death
    - Multiple gestation
    - Intrauterine fetal growth restriction
    - Congenital anomalies
    - Hydrops fetalis
    - Admission to neonatal intensive care

- Low 5-minute Apgar (< 6)
- Umbilical artery pH (< 7.20)
- Meconium-stained fluid
- Polyhydramnios or oligohydramnios
- Fetal cord blood testing
  - Cord blood type and Rh
  - Cord blood gases

Providing Treatment:
Therapeutic Measures to Consider
- Cord care
  - Clamp and cut cord
  - Collect cord blood sample
- Physiologic management of third stage
  - Encourage infant to nurse at breast
  - Observe for signs of placental separation
    - May take up to 30 minutes
  - Once separation has been observed
    - Place one hand on symphysis to guard uterus
    - Use gentle traction on cord to guide placenta
    - Do not use excessive force on cord
  - After delivery of placenta
    - Evaluate firmness of uterus
    - Massage to firmness as needed
    - Nipple stimulation or breastfeeding for oxytocin release
    - Give oxytocin as needed for uterine atony
      - 10 units IM
      - 10–20 units in IV fluids
- Active management of third stage
  - Verify singleton infant
  - Early cord clamping not required (Miller et al., 2004)
  - Drain placental blood, reapply clamp
    - Reduces length of third stage (Brucker, 2001)
  - Uterotonic medication
    - With birth of anterior shoulder, or
    - After birth of entire infant
      - No prenatal ultrasound
      - Palpation of fundus to verify singleton fetus

- Assess for placental separation
- When placenta appears separated (Long, 2001)
  - Provide controlled cord traction
  - Guard uterus with one cupped hand
  - Push uterus toward maternal chest
  - Guide placenta down into vagina
- When placenta visible, guide to expel
  - Use ring forceps to twist trailing membranes into a "rope"
  - Tease membranes out as necessary
- Repair of episiotomy or lacerations
- Excessive bleeding (see Care of the Woman with Postpartum Hemorrhage)
  - Ensure IV access
  - Uterine atony
    - Fundal massage
    - Bimanual compression
    - Administer uterotonic medication
  - Lacerations
    - Locate source of bleeding
    - Clamp vessel
    - Pack as needed
    - Ensure prompt repair
  - Retained placenta or fragments
    - Perform manual exploration of uterus
    - Perform or arrange for manual removal of placenta
- Analgesic, as needed for
  - After pains
  - To facilitate laceration repair
- No signs of placental separation > 30 minutes
  - No bleeding
  - Assume abnormal implantation
  - Prepare for potential surgical removal of placenta

Providing Treatment:
Alternative Measures to Consider
- Infant to breast to stimulate uterine contractions
- Allow physiologic third stage
  - Gentle birth under maternal forces
  - Avoid clamping cord until pulsations stop

- Early breastfeeding
- No cord traction
- Maternal efforts for expulsion
- Allow up to 30 minutes for third stage if
  - No bleeding
  - No signs of separation
  - No maternal pain
- Herbal formulas to stimulate uterine contractions
  - Blue or black cohosh tincture
  - Shepherd's purse tincture (Weed, 1985)
- Leave cord intact until placenta births
- Comfrey compresses
- Homeopathic arnica 60×
- Allow placenta to come naturally
- Ice to perineum after birth

Providing Support:
Education and Support Measures to Consider
- Encourage mother–baby contact
- Encourage breastfeeding of baby
- Be gentle
- Provide information about
  - Third stage
  - Need for repair, if any
  - Interventions, if indicated
- Offer to show placenta, respect client request
  - Inquire if placenta is desired by family
- Show client firm fundus
- Advise to notify midwife or support staff if
  - Fundus boggy
  - Flow excessive
  - Concerns about baby

Follow-up Care:
Follow-up Measures to Consider
- Document (see Chapter 1, Delivery Note)
- Postpartum evaluation
  - One to 2 hours after birth or until stable
    - Vital signs
    - Fundal/flow checks
  - Evaluate maternal–infant bonding
- Follow-up evaluation within 12–24 hours

Collaborative Practice:
Consider Consultation or Referral

- For excessive bleeding uncontrolled by
  - Oxytocin, methylergonovine maleate (Methergine), or misoprostol (Cytotec)
  - Bimanual compression
- As needed for
  - Vaginal lacerations beyond the midwife's scope of practice
  - Rectal lacerations
  - Cervical lacerations
  - For suspected retained placental parts
    - For placenta that is undelivered > 30–60 minutes after birth of infant
    - Accompanied by significant vaginal bleeding
- For diagnosis or treatment outside the midwife's scope of practice

CARE OF THE WOMAN UNDERGOING AMNIOINFUSION

Key Clinical Information

During amnioinfusion, sterile fluid such as Ringer's lactate or normal saline is instilled into the uterine cavity via intrauterine catheter to replace or dilute amniotic fluid. Amnioinfusion is recognized as an effective way to reduce fetal risks associated with cord compression or oligohydramnios (Hofmeyr, 2004a,b,c) and may decrease the rate of cesarean delivery for fetal distress by decreasing the frequency and severity of variable decelerations and by improving umbilical cord pH (Paszkowski, 1994).

Amnioinfusion is not without risk. It has been associated with overdistension of the uterus, resulting in increased basal uterine tone and sudden deterioration of the FHR pattern (ACOG, 2006). ACOG no longer recommends amnioinfusion for meconium-stained amniotic fluid, because it does not decrease the rate of meconium aspiration syndrome or other respiratory disorders in the neonate (ACOG, 2006; Simpson, 2007).

Client History and Chart Review:
Components of the History to Consider

- LMP, EDC, gestational age
- Maternal vital signs, including temperature
- Cervical status
- Fetal presentation
- Status of membranes
- Indications for amnioinfusion
  - Low AFI/oligohydramnios
  - Presence of variable decelerations associated with cord compression
- Contraindications to amnioinfusion (Weismiller, 1998)
  - Presence of amnionitis
  - Polyhydramnios
  - Uterine hypertonus
  - Multiple gestation
  - Known uterine anomaly
  - Severe fetal distress
  - Nonvertex presentation
  - Fetal scalp pH < 7.20
  - Placental abruption or placenta previa

Physical Examination:
Components of the Physical Exam
to Consider

- Maternal vital signs, including temperature
- Vaginal examination
  - Status of membranes
    - Amniotomy must be performed if SROM has not occurred
  - Dilation, effacement, and station
    - Delivery should not be imminent
  - Verify presenting part
  - Place intrauterine pressure catheter
  - Place fetal scalp electrode if desired
- Abdominal examination
  - Verify singleton fetus in vertex lie
  - Evaluate FHR
    - Variable decelerations presenting before 8–9 cm associated with oligohydramnios
  - Evaluate for signs of amnionitis

Clinical Impression:
Differential Diagnoses and Code Groups
to Consider
Additional suffix may apply (ICD9data.com, 2007)
- Amnioinfusion for treatment of
  - Variable decelerations, secondary to (ICD-9 codes 656.3)
    - Oligohydramnios (ICD-9 codes 658.0)
    - Cord compression (ICD-9 codes 663.2)

Diagnostic Testing:
Diagnostic Tests and Procedures to Consider
- Preoperative laboratory tests
- Ultrasound
  - AFI before amnioinfusion
  - AFI after bolus

Providing Treatment:
Therapeutic Measures to Consider
- Insert intrauterine pressure catheter if not already in place
  - Use double-lumen IUPC if available
- Internal fetal scalp lead or external Doppler
- Procedure
  - Infuse sterile saline or Ringer's lactate into the intraamniotic space
  - Warmed solution not required
  - Bolus infusion
    - For treatment of variable decelerations
    - 250–600 ml at rate of 10–15 ml/min
    - Usual bolus ± 500 ml in 30 minutes
    - May follow with bolus of 250 ml after deceleration resolves
  - Continuous infusion (Weismiller, 1998)
    - May begin with 250-ml bolus
    - 10 ml/min for 1 hour
    - Maintenance rate of 3 ml/min
    - May take 20–30 minutes to see effect
- Management of fetal distress
  - Maternal position changes
  - Oxygen therapy
  - Terbutaline therapy
  - Emergency cesarean section

- ⚠ Do not delay preparations for cesarean delivery while performing amnioinfusion
- Assess uterine resting tone and FHT continuously

Providing Treatment:
Alternative Measures to Consider
- Watchful waiting
- Oligohydramnios
  - Maternal hydration
  - Left-lateral positioning
- Meconium-stained fluid
  - Assess for additional risk factors for fetal distress
- Variable decelerations
  - Maternal positioning to optimize FHR
  - Avoid stimulation of labor
  - Provide gentle birth environment
- Prepare for resuscitation of infant

Providing Support:
Education and Support Measures
to Consider
- Address concerns about infant
- Provide information to allow informed consent
- Address client and family concerns
- Risks, benefits, and alternatives
  - For indications benefits often outweigh risks
  - Safety and efficacy have been well documented
  - Elevated risk of endometritis/ chorioamnionitis (Tucker, 2004)
- Educate regarding client requirements
  - Positioning for procedure
  - Confined to bed postprocedure
- Continuous fetal and maternal monitoring

Follow-up Care:
Follow-up Measures to Consider
- Document (see Procedure Notes in Chapter 1)
- Observe for complications
  - Deterioration of FHR

- Uterine hypertonus
- Cord prolapse
- Uterine scar separation
- Amniotic fluid embolism
- Placental abruption
- Signs or symptoms of infection
- Monitor and document
  - Maternal and fetal response
  - Progress of labor

Collaborative Practice:
Consider Consultation or Referral
- OB/GYN services
  - With indication(s) for amnioinfusion
  - For potential surgical consult
  - For complications related to amnioinfusion
- Pediatric services
  - Fetal distress
  - Meconium aspiration syndrome
  - Newborn resuscitation
- For diagnosis or treatment outside the midwife's scope of practice

ASSISTING WITH CESAREAN SECTION

Key Clinical Information
Many midwives have expanded their clinical practice to include assisting with cesarean section and/or gynecologic surgery (American College of Nurse-Midwives [ACNM], 1998, 2006). By first assisting, the midwife may provide greater continuity of care to women and greater versatility within her clinical practice (Tharpe, 2007). First-assisting skills enhance the midwife's ability to perform perineal repairs when needed and lead to a greater appreciation of the complexities of the female body. Working with the surgeon provides an opportunity to develop another facet of the midwife's collaborative relationship.

Client History and Chart Review:
Components of the History to Consider
- Review current obstetric history
  - Prenatal laboratory values

- Admission laboratory values
- Course of labor/interval history
- Indication for cesarean section
  - Maternal
  - Fetal
  - Urgent versus scheduled
- Review past obstetric history
  - Previous cesarean sections
  - History of postpartum hemorrhage
- Medical history
  - Allergies
  - Medication or herb use
  - Medical conditions
    - Asthma
    - Cardiac dysfunction
    - Respiratory disorders
    - Scoliosis
  - Previous surgeries
    - Response to anesthesia
      - General
      - Regional
- Review of systems
- Social history
  - Support systems
  - Smoking
  - Alcohol or drug use
- Client concerns

Physical Examination:
Components of the Physical Exam
to Consider
- Maternal and fetal vital signs
- Admission physical, with focus on
  - Cardiopulmonary system
  - Gastrointestinal system
  - Fetal presentation, EFW
- Preoperative considerations
  - Maternal body mass index
  - Mobility of
    - Jaw
    - Neck
    - Back
  - Positioning limitations

Clinical Impression:
Differential Diagnoses and Code Groups
to Consider
Additional suffix may apply (ICD9data.com, 2007)

- Primary cesarean section (ICD-9 codes V30.01)
- Repeat cesarean section (ICD-9 codes V30.01)
  - After attempting vaginal birth after cesarean (VBAC) (ICD-9 codes V30.01)
  - Additional codes to document indication for cesarean section

Diagnostic Testing:
Diagnostic Tests and Procedures to Consider

- Preoperative laboratory tests (see Care of the Woman Undergoing Cesarean Delivery)
- Additional testing as indicated
  - Ultrasound localization of placenta
  - Coagulation studies

Providing Treatment:
Therapeutic Measures to Consider

- Ensure IV access and patency
- Ensure airway patency
- Assist with induction of general or regional anesthesia as needed
- Assist surgeon with (Tharpe, 2007)
  - Preparation
  - Draping
  - Retraction
  - Dissection
  - Suctioning
  - Extraction of infant and placenta
  - Clamping and cutting umbilical cord
  - Suctioning of infant as needed
  - Obtaining cord blood for laboratory tests
  - Hemostasis
  - Suturing
  - Stapling
- Procedure
  - Abdomen opened in layers
    - Skin
    - Subcutaneous fat
    - Fascia
    - Muscle
    - Peritoneum

- Bladder flap created
- Uterine incision made
  - Follow scalpel with suction
  - Rotate bladder blade to provide exposure
  - Incision extended with scissors or bluntly
- Rupture of membranes
- Remove bladder blade
- Head/buttocks delivered
  - Manually
  - Vacuum extractor
  - Piper forceps for after-coming head with breech
- Fundal pressure for birth of body
- Wipe or suction mouth and nares
- Clamp and cut cord
- Collect cord blood
- Administration of medications by anesthesia
  - Medications given after cord is clamped
  - Oxytocin
  - Antibiotics
  - Anxiolytics
  - Narcotics
  - Antiemetics
- Placenta
  - Spontaneous expulsion, associated with
    - Decreased risk infection
    - Decreased blood loss
  - Manual removal of placenta
    - Identification of attachment location
    - Opportunity to learn skill
  - Surgeon preference
- Uterus inspected and cleared of debris
- Uterus closed in layers
  - Assistant "follows" suture
  - Uterus exteriorized or left in situ
- Inspection of other organs: ovaries, tubes, appendix
  - Tubal ligation done at this point as indicated

Double-layer uterine closure recommended for future VBAC candidates (Bujold et al., 2002).

- Closure of layers per surgeon preference (Ethicon, 2004)
  - Assistant "follows" or sutures
- Sterile dressing applied

Providing Treatment:
Alternative Measures to Consider
- Allow/encourage support person(s)
  - Preoperative area
  - Holding area
  - Operating room
  - Post-anesthesia care unit (PACU)
- Encourage mother to hold baby after initial evaluation
- Allow support person(s) to care for infant until mother is able

Providing Support:
Education and Support Measures
to Consider
- Provide emotional support
- Advise client of routines related to
  - Anesthesia
  - Cesarean section procedure
  - Newborn care
  - Recovery room
  - Postoperative course
- Active listening to client and family concerns

Follow-up Care:
Follow-up Measures to Consider
(Tharpe, 2004)
- Document postoperative care provided
- Ensure adequate pain control
  - Long-acting spinal or epidural medications
  - Patient-controlled analgesia
  - IM narcotics
  - PO narcotics
  - PO nonsteroidal antiinflammatory drugs
- Postoperative laboratory tests: CBC or hematocrit and hemoglobin
- Physical examination
  - Vital signs
  - Reproductive system

- Cardiopulmonary system
  - Assess for signs or symptoms of
    - Anemia
    - Hypovolemia
  - Incentive spirometry
- Gastrointestinal system
  - Auscultate for bowel sounds
  - Note passage of flatus
  - Passage of stool
- Urinary system
  - Ensure voiding after catheter removal
  - Assess for
    - Urinary retention
    - Postvoid residual
    - Urinary tract infection
    - Bladder injury
    - Bladder spasm
- Assess for signs and symptoms of postoperative complications
  - Thrombus or embolism
  - Atelectasis
  - Infection
  - Ileus
  - Emotional difficulties
- Evaluate client's emotional response to
  - Events and procedure
  - Newborn
  - Parenting demands
- Evaluate for postpartum depression risk
- Other postoperative follow-up
  - Advance diet as tolerated
  - Ambulate when full sensation
  - Discontinue Foley when able to ambulate
  - Discontinue IV/saline lock when taking PO fluid well

Collaborative Practice:
Consider Consultation or Referral
- OB/GYN services
  - Presence of intraoperative or postoperative complications
  - For postoperative care per collaborative practice agreement
- For diagnosis or treatment outside the midwife's scope of practice

CARE OF THE WOMAN UNDERGOING CESAREAN DELIVERY

Key Clinical Information

In many settings the midwife cares for the woman whose child is delivered via cesarean section. Planned cesarean delivery may be due to previous cesarean section, a nonvertex presentation, or a placenta previa. Unplanned cesarean delivery may be due to failure to progress, significant fetal distress, or placental abruption. Midwives should discuss with all women the potential for cesarean section, the benefits when done for indications, and the risks inherent in the surgery and should quote their own practice statistics for their primary cesarean section rate and overall cesarean section rate so that women have a sense of how likely this event is under the care of this particular midwifery practice. The elective choice of cesarean section as a substitute for vaginal birth is not in the best interest of the woman or her child and is typically a fear-based response to perceptions of exaggerated danger and pressure from the provider (ACNM, 2005; Sakala & Corry, 2007). The mother who was anticipating an unmedicated birth or a planned birth center or home birth may need additional assistance in coping with the disappointment of the unexpected change in birth plans and in assimilating the procedure and its outcome. Any mother who undergoes cesarean delivery may have conflicting feelings about her labor and birth experience and can benefit from the midwife's gentle care.

Client History and Chart Review:
Components of the History to Consider
- See Assisting with Cesarean Section
- Indication for cesarean
- Client response to need for cesarean
- Complete maternity admission history
  - Obstetric/gynecologic history
  - Medical and surgical history
  - Review of systems
  - Laboratory values
  - Social history
- Interval labor history as applicable

Physical Examination:
Components of the Physical Exam to Consider
- Complete maternity admission physical
- Physical examination related to indication for cesarean

Clinical Impression:
Differential Diagnoses and Code Groups to Consider
Additional suffix may apply (ICD9data.com, 2007)
- Primary cesarean section (ICD-9 codes V30.01)
- Repeat cesarean section (ICD-9 codes V30.01)
  - After VBAC attempt (ICD-9 codes V30.01)
  - Additional codes to document indication for cesarean section

Diagnostic Testing:
Diagnostic Tests and Procedures to Consider
- Preoperative laboratory tests
  - Urinalysis
  - CBC with differential
  - Type and screen or type and cross
- Other necessary laboratory tests as indicated by maternal/fetal status
  - Fetal lung maturity assessment
  - Preeclampsia laboratory panel
  - Clotting studies
  - Antibody identification

Providing Treatment:
Therapeutic Measures to Consider
- NPO (6-hour minimum preferred)
- IV access and fluids
  - Lactated Ringer's, D-5 lactated Ringer's, normal saline or similar balanced electrolyte solution
  - 14–20 gauge IV catheter
  - Bolus of 500–1000 ml if regional anesthesia anticipated
  - Maintenance rate 100–150 ml/hr

- Foley catheter
  - May insert in
    - Labor and Delivery/admission unit
    - Holding area
    - After regional anesthesia
- Notify appropriate personnel of pending surgery
  - OB/GYN
  - Anesthesia
  - Nursing or operating room supervisor
  - Pediatrics
- Medications per anesthesia
- Maternal and fetal monitoring as indicated

Providing Treatment:
Alternative Measures to Consider

- Failure to progress is common cause of primary cesarean section (Lowe, 2007)
- Based on indication for cesarean consider
  - Watchful waiting
  - Pain management
  - Rest and nutrition
  - Augmentation of labor
  - VBAC
- Provide emotional support
  - Allow/encourage family or support person(s) in operating room
  - Engage mother in decision-making where possible

Providing Support:
Education and Support Measures
to Consider

- Obtain informed consent
  - Discuss indication(s) for cesarean delivery
  - Provide interpreter as necessary
  - Risks
    - Infection
    - Bleeding
    - Injury
      - Bowel or bladder
      - Fetus
      - Uterus
      - Blood loss

  - Benefits
    - Delivery in controlled environment
    - Expedited delivery
    - Cesarean section may decrease risk to mother or baby, based on indication for cesarean delivery
      - Breech/transverse lie
      - Cephalopelvic disproportion (CPD)
      - Severe PIH
      - Preterm fetus
  - Alternatives to procedure
    - Continued labor
    - Vaginal birth, based on indication(s)
- Discuss recommendations and process with family
  - Maternal participation in decision making may impact
    - Feelings about surgical delivery
    - Bonding with baby
    - Self-image as woman
- Considerations for client and family education
  - Time in operating room and post-anesthesia unit
  - If support person(s) may stay with mother
  - Expected care for baby after birth
- Anticipated postoperative care
- Provide emotional support related to
  - Indication for cesarean delivery
  - Change in
    - Birth plans
    - Birth attendant
    - Birth location

Follow-up Care:
Follow-up Measures to Consider

- Document
- Assist at surgery if qualified (see Assisting with Cesarean Section, above)
- Remain with client if possible during surgery
- Review experience with client postpartum
- Provide postoperative care as applicable
- Obtain operative note for records
  - Discuss future childbirth choices of VBAC or repeat cesarean

◆ Based on type of uterine incision

◆ Based on probability of recurrence of cesarean indication

Collaborative Practice:
Consider Consultation or Referral

• OB/GYN services
  ▪ Confirmed or suspected indication for cesarean delivery as indicated by
    ◆ Midwife scope of practice
    ◆ Practice setting
    ◆ Client preference
    ◆ Collaborative practice agreement
  ▪ Development of complications postoperatively
• Pediatric services
  ▪ Newborn care at birth
• Anesthesia service
  ▪ Preoperative evaluation
  ▪ Postoperative pain control, as needed
  ▪ Post-anesthesia complications
• For diagnosis or treatment outside the midwife's scope of practice

CARE OF THE WOMAN WITH CORD PROLAPSE

Key Clinical Information

Cord prolapse is a true clinical emergency. Unless compression is removed from the cord, the fetus will be deprived of oxygen and may suffer brain and organ damage. The midwife must elevate the presenting part off the umbilical cord while calling for immediate assistance (Varney et al., 2004). Emergency cesarean delivery is performed to save the infant's life. Placing the mother into the knee–chest position or Trendelenburg position may diminish or prevent cord compression. Cord prolapse occurs more commonly in women who have polyhydramnios, a fetal presentation other than vertex, or during spontaneous or artificial rupture of the membranes when the head or presenting part is not engaged in the pelvis.

Client History and Chart Review:
Components of the History to Consider

• LMP, EDC, gestational age
• ⚠ Identify risk factors for cord prolapse
  ▪ Polyhydramnios
  ▪ Multiple gestation
  ▪ Nonvertex presentation
  ▪ Compound presentation
  ▪ Recent intrapartum interventions
  ▪ Status of membranes
    ◆ Artificial ROM
    ◆ Spontaneous ROM
• Fetal heart rate
• Previously documented FHR
  ▪ FHR changes
  ▪ Maternal medical or obstetric problems

Physical Examination:
Components of the Physical Exam to Consider

• Diagnosis and prevention
  ▪ Avoid ROM unless presenting part is engaged
  ▪ Evaluate FHR after ROM
    ◆ Severe bradycardia = likely cord prolapse
    ◆ Severe FHR drop with resolution = potential occult cord or true knot in cord
• Abdominal examination
  ▪ Evaluation of fluid volume
  ▪ Determination of fetal lie and presentation
  ▪ Estimation of fetal weight
• Vaginal examination
  ▪ Determine presenting part(s)
  ▪ Feel for frank or occult cord (Varney et al., 2004)
    ◆ In vaginal fornices
    ◆ At cervical edge
    ◆ Through lower uterine segment
  ▪ Station, cervical dilation
• Risk for cord prolapse
  ▪ Floating presenting part
  ▪ Bulging bag of waters
  ▪ Ballooning or hourglass membranes

Clinical Impression:
Differential Diagnoses and Code Groups
to Consider
Additional suffix may apply (ICD9data.com, 2007)

- Cord prolapse (ICD-9 codes 663.0)
  - Occult (ICD-9 codes 663.0)
  - Frank (ICD-9 codes 663.0)
- Fetal distress due to cord compression (ICD-9 codes 656.3)

Diagnostic Testing:
Diagnostic Tests and Procedures to Consider

- Preoperative laboratory testing STAT if not obtained previously
- CBC
- Type and screen/cross

Providing Treatment:
Therapeutic Measures to Consider

- In presence of suspected occult cord prolapse
  - Discontinue any oxytocin if running
  - O_2 by mask at 6–8 liters
  - Positioning
    - Knee–chest position, or
    - Trendelenburg position with left lateral tilt
  - Elevation of presenting part off of cord
    - Manually
    - Insert Foley catheter
      - Instill 500 ml sterile saline into bladder to lift presenting part off cord
      - Clamp off catheter
      - Release clamp when prepped for cesarean
  - Cord care
    - Cover cord with warm saline-soaked gauze
    - Minimize manipulation to prevent cord spasm
    - Maintain elevation of presenting part off cord until delivery
  - Continuous evaluation of FHR

- Terbutaline
  - To decrease contractions and uterine tone
  - 0.25 mg SQ, or
  - 0.125–0.25 mg IV
- Prep for STAT cesarean section

Providing Treatment:
Alternative Measures to Consider

- Manually lift presenting part off the cord
  - Position mother left lateral Trendelenburg or knee–chest
  - Place entire hand in vagina
  - Lift presenting part out of pelvis
  - Evaluate for fetal response
    - Monitor FHR closely
  - Keep cord warm and moist
  - Maintain knee–chest or Trendelenburg position
  - Arrange for STAT surgical delivery, including transport if necessary

Providing Support:
Education and Support Measures to Consider

- Education
  - Include cord prolapse as a risk factor in
    - Vaginal breech birth
    - Polyhydramnios
- During emergency
  - Briefly explain nature of emergency
  - Keep client and family advised of what is happening
  - Provide emotional support
- After emergency
  - Compassionate listening
  - Information about the emergency

Follow-up Care:
Follow-up Measures to Consider

- After delivery
  - Document, as soon as possible after delivery
  - Provide client with information about events as applicable

- Encourage client to verbalize feelings, understanding
- Consider peer review
  - Overall case review
  - Learning experience
  - Maternal and fetal outcomes

Collaborative Practice:
Consider Consultation or Referral
- OB/GYN services
  - Conditions that may lead to cord prolapse
  - Suspected or confirmed cord prolapse
  - Fetal distress unresponsive to therapy
- Pediatric services
  - Fetal distress unresponsive to therapy
  - Newborn resuscitation
  - Newborn evaluation after emergency
- Social service
  - Counseling
  - Support group
- For diagnosis or treatment outside the midwife's scope of practice

CARE OF THE WOMAN WITH FAILURE TO PROGRESS IN LABOR

Key Clinical Information
"Failure to progress" is a catchall description. When labor does not progress, the suspected mechanism(s) should be clearly identified to systematically select the appropriate treatments. In some instances fetal size or positioning may slow the progression of labor, while the uterus works hard to literally push past the difficulty. Failure to progress is a common diagnosis that may have multiple components (Lowe, 2007). Delay in progression may be related to the effectiveness of uterine contractions, the size of the mother's pelvis in relation to the size of the fetus, fetal position (Hart & Walker, 2007) or anatomy, or psychosocial factors that inhibit labor progress. The challenge to the midwife is to identify and treat the specific component(s) causing the delay. Time and patience may be rewarded with slow but steady progress. When the uterus is not working efficiently, as in dysfunctional labor, augmentation of labor via oxytocin may help prevent prolonged labor and avoid unnecessary cesarean birth. Patience is essential because many women do not follow the average labor curve but need to find their own pace for labor and birth (Albers et al., 1996).

Client History and Chart Review:
Components of the History to Consider
- Gravida, parity
- LMP, EDC, gestational age
- Review of labor
  - Onset of labor
  - Progress of labor
  - Fetal response to labor
  - Maternal response to labor
  - Status of membranes
    - Color of fluid
    - Length of rupture
  - Oral intake of food or fluids
  - Positions used and results
  - Estimated fetal weight
  - Previous clinical evaluation of fetal lie
- Previous labor and delivery history
- Inquiry into potential barriers to labor progress
  - Cultural
  - Developmental
  - Emotional or social
  - Physical
    - Positioning
    - Hydration
    - Nutrition
    - Voiding

Physical Examination:
Components of the Physical Exam to Consider
- Maternal and fetal vital signs
- Evaluate for signs of exhaustion
  - Tachycardia
  - Ketonuria
  - Trembling
  - Lethargy

- Maternal attitude
  - Fear or anxiety
  - Tension
- Abdominal examination
  - Fetal lie, presentation, position
  - Estimated fetal weight
  - Signs of engagement
  - Uterine contractions: frequency, duration, intensity
  - Bladder distension
- Pelvic examination
  - Cervix
    - Dilation and effacement
    - Position
    - Edema or asymmetry of cervix
  - Presenting part
    - Verification of presenting part
    - Application to the cervix
    - Station
    - Asyncliticism
    - Caput formation
    - Molding
  - Assess pelvimetry
- Fetal vital signs
  - FHR short- and long-term variability
  - Fetal activity
  - Fetal response to stimulation

Clinical Impression:
Differential Diagnoses and Code Groups
to Consider
Additional suffix may apply (ICD9data.com, 2007)
- Slowly progressive labor (ICD-9 codes 662)
- Presence of a protraction disorder
  - Dilation (ICD-9 codes 662.0)
- Presence of an arrest disorder
  - Arrest of dilation (ICD-9 codes 662)
  - Prolonged second stage (ICD-9 codes 662)
- Secondary to
  - Dysfunctional labor (ICD-9 codes 661)
  - Cephalopelvic disproportion (ICD-9 codes 653)

- Fetal presentation or position (ICD-9 codes 652)
- Additional codes to document associated conditions

Diagnostic Testing:
Diagnostic Tests and Procedures
to Consider
- Urine for ketones
- Uterine pressure catheter to evaluate uterine contractions
- Preoperative laboratory tests with consideration for potential cesarean section

Providing Treatment:
Therapeutic Measures to Consider
- Watchful waiting
- Assess maternal environment for stress factors
  - Fear and pain
  - Light and noise
  - Dysfunctional family or staff members
- Hydration
  - PO clear liquids
  - IV bolus of 500 ml of solution suitable for labor
    - Maintain at 125–200 ml/hr
- Rest, if maternal and fetal status is stable
  - Consider morphine sulphate 10–20 mg IM in early labor
    - Have Narcan immediately available
  - Pain relief to facilitate rest/relaxation
- Clinical repositioning techniques
  - Manual flexion of vertex
  - Massage and stretch cervical lip over presenting part
  - Hip press to open midpelvis
- Active management of labor (Institute for Clinical Systems Improvement, 2004)
  - Oxytocin (see Care of the Woman Undergoing Induction or Augmentation of Labor)
  - Amniotomy
- Empty bladder

- Antibiotic prophylaxis
  - Not indicated with negative GBS
  - ROM > 18 hours or per facility recommendations
  - Maternal fever or elevated WBC

Providing Treatment:
Alternative Measures to Consider
- Watchful waiting
- Explore emotional issues that may interfere with labor
  - Fear
  - Previous trauma, such as rape, abortion
  - Family issues (e.g., gender of infant, history of abuse)
  - Deadlines related to
    - Labor management
    - Interventions
- Encourage position changes
  - Hands and knees
  - Side-lying
  - Walking
  - Rocking chair
  - Semisitting
- Empty bladder, bowels
- Hydrotherapy
  - Tub
  - Whirlpool
  - Shower
- Flat on back with knees flexed may encourage descent
  - Opens pelvic inlet
  - Flattens sacrum
  - Move upright once vertex descends
- Use upright positions once head enters pelvis
  - Squatting
  - Squatting bar
  - Birth stool
  - Standing
  - Sitting
    - Birth ball
    - Birth tub
    - Bed

- Chair
- Toilet
- If contractions slow secondary to fatigue
  - Mother and fetus are both stable
    - Sleep
    - Provide nutrition and hydration
    - Allow more time
    - Close monitoring of maternal and fetal well-being
- Stimulate contractions
  - Nipple stimulation
  - Herbal remedies (see Care of the Woman Undergoing Induction or Augmentation of Labor)

Providing Support:
Education and Support Measures
to Consider
- Discuss findings with client, family
  - Options available
  - Address client and family concerns
  - Formulate plan with patient
    - Potential need to transport if out-of-hospital
    - Recommendations for midwifery care
- Increased potential for augmentation with
  - Prolonged ROM
  - Dysfunctional labor
- Increased potential for cesarean with
  - Protracted active labor
  - Failure to descend
  - Maternal or fetal exhaustion

Follow-up Care:
Follow-up Measures to Consider
- Reassess
  - At least every 1–3 hours
  - After initiation of treatments
  - With maternal or fetal indication
- Update plan after each assessment
  - Maternal and fetal response
  - Interval change
  - Clinical impression

- Discussions with client and family
- Planned course of action

Collaborative Practice:
Criteria to Consider for Consultation
or Referral
- OB/GYN services
  - For persistently nonprogressive labor
  - Suspected CPD
  - Fetal malposition
  - For fetal or maternal distress
  - For transport
- Pediatric services
  - Nonreassuring FHR pattern
- For diagnosis or treatment outside the midwife's scope of practice

CARE OF THE WOMAN WITH GROUP B STREPTOCOCCUS

Key Clinical Information

On average 10–30% of women are colonized, either vaginally or rectally, with Group B Streptococcus (GBS) (Centers for Disease Control and Prevention [CDC], 2002, 2006). GBS may cause maternal urinary tract infection, amnionitis, postpartum endometritis, or wound infection. As many as 50% of infants born to colonized mothers may become colonized with GBS. Up to 4% of colonized infants develop significant complications related to GBS infection (CDC, 2006; Jolivet, 2002).

Early-onset GBS disease occurs in the presence of maternal colonization accompanied by additional risk factors associated with GBS disease. The rate of early-onset GBS disease has diminished significantly since the institution of antibiotic prophylaxis in the early 1990s. Late-onset GBS disease is defined as that which occurs between 1 week and several months of age. Late-onset GBS disease occurs in up to 20% of infants with GBS sepsis. Complications of neonatal GBS infection include meningitis, pneumonia, and sepsis. The associated newborn mortality rate for GBS disease in the 1990s was 4–6% (Schuchat, 1998).

Client History and Chart Review:
Components of the History to Consider
- Gravida, parity, EDC
- Review prenatal course
  - GBS cultures
    - Performed at 35–37 weeks
    - Rectovaginal
    - Urine
- Note documented discussions
  - GBS status
  - Antibiotic prophylaxis in labor
- GBS status unknown
  - Evaluate risk factors for risk-based management
- Identify risk factors associated with neonatal sepsis (CDC, 2002)
  - African-American women
  - Positive GBS culture
  - GBS bacteriuria in pregnancy
  - Previous infant with GBS sepsis
  - Previous amnionitis
  - Preterm PROM
  - Prolonged ROM
  - Maternal fever (> 38°C/100.4°F) in labor
  - Preterm birth/low birth weight
- Review labor course
  - Onset and progression of labor
  - Fetal and maternal vital signs
  - ROM
    - Odor and color
    - Anticipated time from ROM to birth

Physical Examination:
Components of the Physical Exam
to Consider
- Vital signs
- Usual maternal and fetal labor evaluation
- Evaluate for symptoms of chorioamnionitis
  - Febrile mother
  - Significant and persistent fetal tachycardia
  - Odor to amniotic fluid
  - Uterine tenderness (late sign)

- Observe newborn immediately after birth for symptoms of sepsis
  - Pallor and poor tone
  - Respiratory distress
  - Slow irregular pulse

Clinical Impression:
Differential Diagnoses and Code Groups
to Consider
Additional suffix may apply (ICD9data.com, 2007)
- GBS screening (ICD-9 codes V28.8)

Diagnostic Testing:
Diagnostic Tests and Procedures to Consider
- Obtain GBS culture at 35–37 weeks gestation
  - Distal vagina to rectum, through anal sphincter
    - If penicillin (PCN) allergic, note on laboratory slip and request culture and sensitivities
  - Self-collection an option for women (Tora & Dunn, 2000)
  - Use selective broth medium for GBS
  - Urine culture
- CBC with differential
- Cultures at delivery
  - No GBS results available
    - Amnion/placenta
    - Infant's axilla, groin, or ear fold

Providing Treatment:
Therapeutic Measures to Consider
- Follow current CDC recommendation (CDC, 2002)
- GBS negative—no treatment
- GBS unavailable
  - Use risk-based strategy
  - Offer antibiotics with anticipated
    - Delivery at < 37 weeks gestation
    - Intrapartum fever (> 38°C/100.4°F)
    - ROM > 18 hours
- GBS positive—offer treatment based on
  - Positive culture this pregnancy
  - Previous infant with GBS disease

- GBS bacteriuria in current pregnancy
- Labor onset at < 37 weeks gestation
- Local standards for risk factors
- Client preferences
- Intrapartum prophylaxis *not* required
  - Previous pregnancy with positive GBS culture
  - Planned cesarean without labor or ROM
  - Negative culture this pregnancy
  - Client preferences
- Allow time for two doses of antibiotics before delivery if possible
- Note antibiotic allergies
  - PCN allergy
    - Not at risk for anaphylaxis
      - Cefazolin 2 g IV followed by 1 g IV every 8 hours until birth
    - High risk for anaphylaxis
      - Clindamycin 900 mg IV every 8 hours until birth, *or*
      - Erythromycin 500 mg IV every 6 hours until birth, *or*
      - Vancomycin 1 g IV every 12 hours until birth
- Penicillin G
  - 5 million units IV followed by
  - 2.5 million units every 4 hours until birth
- Ampicillin
  - 2 g IV followed by
  - 1 g every 4 hours until birth
- Oral therapy for expectant management of PROM
  - Not included in current CDC recommendations
  - PROM < 37 weeks gestation
  - Begin at 18 hours ROM
    - Amoxicillin 500 mg PO TID
    - For PCN allergy
    - Clindamycin 300 mg PO every 6 hours
  - Client obtains temperature every 4–6 hours while awake
    - Call with temperature > 37.8°C

- Change to IV chemoprophylaxis
  - Onset of active labor
  - Temperature > 38°C

Providing Treatment:
Alternative Measures to Consider

- Expectant management
- Herbal remedies as prophylaxis
  - Astragalus root tea, tincture or capsule to build immunity
  - Echinacea for 2–3 weeks only, just before birth
  - Tea of lemon balm and oregano, two to three cups daily for several weeks
  - Raw garlic, no more than 1 clove per week, 2–3 weeks before birth
- Chlorhexidine vaginal wash (see box below)
- For clients on antibiotic prophylaxis
  - Replace bacteria in gut via
    - Acidophilus capsules
    - Live culture yogurt
- Immediate evaluation and treatment of symptomatic newborn

CHLOROHEXIDINE VAGINAL WASH

Chlorhexidine gluconate Hibiclens (4%) is available over the counter
Place 1 T Hibiclens in a measuring cup
Fill with water to 1 cup mark to yield a 0.25% solution
Apply as:
Vaginal flush
Use 200 cc in a douche bottle
Insert into vagina
Avoid inadvertent cervical insertion
Gently expel solution
Or
Vaginal wipe
Soak cotton gauze in the solution
Wrap around exam fingers
Wipe vaginal walls, labia, and perineum
Repeat every 6 hours, making new solution each time

Source: Ross, 2007.

Providing Support:
Education and Support Measures to Consider

- Discuss
  - Practice routine regarding GBS screening
  - Treatment options if GBS positive
- Provide information to allow informed decision-making
  - Current CDC recommendations
  - Risks and benefits of antibiotics
  - Individual risk for GBS disease in infant
  - Alternatives to current recommendations
- Provide information regarding neonatal sepsis
  - May occur from birth through 3 months
  - Seek care immediately if any symptoms develop
    - Lethargy
    - Pallor
    - Poor feeding
    - Fever
    - Abnormal cry (ACNM, 1997)

Follow-up Care:
Follow-up Measures to Consider

- Document all discussions
  - GBS culture results
  - Treatment plan options
  - Client preferences for care
  - Risk factors for GBS infection
- Schedule regular newborn assessment

Collaborative Practice:
Consider Consultation or Referral

- OB/GYN services
  - Women with intrapartum fever (> 38°C/100.4°F)
  - Women with positive GBS and preterm labor or PROM
  - Signs or symptoms of amnionitis
  - Transfer of care or birth location due to GBS status or symptoms
- Pediatric services
  - GBS-positive client with abnormal FHR pattern
  - Infant whose mothers have received antibiotics

- Newborn conditions
- Symptomatic infants
- For diagnosis or treatment outside the mid-wife's scope of practice

CARE OF THE WOMAN UNDERGOING INDUCTION OR AUGMENTATION OF LABOR

Key Clinical Information

Induction is the stimulation of the uterus by an external agent with the intent to start labor before the onset of spontaneous labor. *Augmentation* is the use of similar techniques to enhance uterine contractions after labor has started. Induction or augmentation of labor may be initiated for a wide variety of indications. Induction is used in cases when the fetus is believed to be safer outside the uterus than inside or for maternal indications or for both.

Practices vary tremendously toward the approach to induction and augmentation. Maternal involvement in the decision-making process is essential, because stimulation of labor may contribute to maternal feelings of failure or success based on maternal motivation and attitude toward the induction or augmentation process. Midwives must hold fast to the tenet of nonintervention in the absence of complication in the current milieu of rising elective induction rates.

Client History and Chart Review:
Components of the History to Consider
- Prenatal record review
  - LMP, EDC, gestational age
  - EFW
- Identify indication for induction
  - Maternal indication
    - ◆ Absolute indications
      - ➤ Chorioamnionitis
    - ◆ Relative indications
      - ➤ Preeclampsia/eclampsia
      - ➤ Chronic hypertension
      - ➤ Gestational diabetes
      - ➤ Maternal medical complications, such as diabetes or renal disease

- Fetal indications
  - ◆ Absolute indications
    - ➤ Chorioamnionitis
    - ➤ Nonreassuring FHTs
    - ➤ Intrauterine growth restriction
    - ➤ Isoimmunization
  - ◆ Relative indications
    - ➤ Post dates (> 42 weeks)
    - ➤ PROM
    - ➤ Positive GBS
    - ➤ Fetal macrosomia
    - ➤ Fetal demise
    - ➤ Previous stillbirth
    - ➤ Fetus with major congenital anomaly
    - ➤ Prolonged ROM
    - ➤ Other fetal risk in utero
  - Uteroplacental indications
    - ◆ Absolute indications
      - ➤ Placental abruption, partial and stable
    - ◆ Relative indications
      - ➤ Unexplained oligohydramnios
      - ➤ Placental insufficiency
- Identify indication for augmentation
  - Maternal indications
    - ➤ Nonprogressive labor
    - ➤ Insufficient contraction pattern
    - ➤ Maternal fever
    - ➤ Prolonged ROM
  - Fetal indications
    - ➤ Nonreassuring FHT
- Contraindications to induction or augmentation
  - Maternal contraindications
    - ◆ Absolute contraindications
      - ➤ Classical uterine incision
      - ➤ Active genital herpes
      - ➤ Serious chronic medical conditions
      - ➤ Pelvic structure abnormality
      - ➤ Invasive cervical cancer
    - ◆ Relative contraindications
      - ➤ Cervical carcinoma
      - ➤ Grand multiparity
      - ➤ Heart disease

- ➤ Severe maternal hypertension
- ➤ Uterine overdistension (secondary to polyhydramnios or multiple gestation)
- ■ Fetal contraindications
    - ◆ Absolute contraindications
        - ➤ Transverse/oblique lie
        - ➤ Extreme fetal compromise
    - ◆ Relative contraindications
        - ➤ Nonengaged presenting part
        - ➤ CPD
        - ➤ Malpresentation
        - ➤ Fetal macrosomia
- ■ Uteroplacental contraindications
    - ◆ Absolute contraindications
        - ➤ Cord prolapse
        - ➤ Placenta previa
        - ➤ Vasa previa
    - ◆ Relative contraindications
        - ➤ Low-lying placenta
        - ➤ Unexplained vaginal bleeding
        - ➤ Cord presentation
        - ➤ Myomectomy involving the uterine cavity
- • Misoprostol contraindications
    - ■ Previous uterine scar
    - ■ Asthma
- • Obtain labor admission history or review interval labor history

Physical Examination:
Components of the Physical Exam to Consider
- • Maternal and fetal vital signs
- • Assess fetal and maternal well-being
    - ■ Contraction status
    - ■ Frequency, duration, strength
        - ◆ Palpation
        - ◆ External or internal monitoring
- • Pelvic examination
    - ■ Bishop's score (6 or more is considered favorable for induction, see Table 4-1 below)
    - ■ Pelvimetry to rule out CPD
    - ■ Cervical status
        - ◆ Effacement
        - ◆ Dilation
        - ◆ Consistency
    - ■ Status of membranes
    - ■ Descent of presenting part

Clinical Impression:
Differential Diagnoses and Code Groups to Consider
Additional suffix may apply (ICD9data.com, 2007)
- • Induction of labor, secondary to
    - ■ PROM (ICD-9 codes 658.1)
    - ■ Preeclampsia (ICD-9 codes 642.4)
    - ■ Postterm pregnancy ($\geq$ 42 weeks) (ICD-9 codes 645)

Table 4-1 Bishop's Score				
	0	1	2	3
Dilation	0	1–2 cm	3–4 cm	5–6 cm
Effacement	0–30%	40–50%	60–70%	80+%
Station	−3	−2	−1/0	+1/+2
Consistency	Firm	Medium	Soft	N/A
Position	Posterior	Mid-position	Anterior	N/A

N/A, not applicable.
Source: Bishop, E. H. (1964). Pelvic scoring for elective induction. *Obstetrics and Gynecology, 24,* 267.

- Maternal diabetes mellitus (ICD-9 codes 648.0 or 250)
- Maternal medical problems (ICD-9 codes 640–649)
- Intrauterine fetal growth restriction (ICD-9 codes 656.5)
- Fetal demise (ICD-9 codes 656.4)
- Augmentation of labor, secondary to
  - Dysfunctional labor (ICD-9 codes 661)
  - Uterine inertia (ICD-9 codes 661.2)

Diagnostic Testing:
Diagnostic Tests and Procedures
to Consider
- Fetal evaluation
  - Non-Stress Test (NST)/Contraction Stress Test (CST)
  - Biophysical profile
  - AFI
  - Fetal kick counts
- Fetal surveillance
  - Intermittent auscultation for FHR
  - Continuous fetal monitoring
- Preoperative laboratory tests
  - CBC
  - Urinalysis
  - Type and screen (or red-topped tube to hold)
  - Other laboratory tests as indicated

Providing Treatment:
Therapeutic Measures to Consider
- Cervical-ripening agents (Summers, 1997)
  - Prostin E_2
    - Prepidil
    - Cervidil
    - Hospital compounded Prostin E_2 gel 2–6 mg
  - Misoprostol (may result in induction)
    - Off-label use
    - ⚠ Informed consent recommended
    - Maximum recommended dose, 25 micrograms
    - PO or in posterior vaginal fornix
    - Repeat doses every 3–6 hours

- Laminaria
- Foley catheter balloon
  - Place inside internal os
  - Fill with 30 ml fluid
  - Tape to client's thigh
- Induction/augmentation
  - Amniotomy
  - Oxytocin infusion
    - 10 units oxytocin/1000 ml IV solution such as lactated Ringer's
    - Titrate until contraction pattern of every 3 minutes
    - Rates vary, examples include
      - 0.5 to 2 mU/min
      - Increase 1–2 mU/min every 15–60 minutes
    - Maximum dose 20–40 mU/min
- Potential complications
  - Overstimulation of the uterus
  - Fetal distress
  - Under-dosing and maternal exhaustion
  - Water intoxication (oxytocin)

Providing Treatment:
Alternative Measures to Consider
- Repeated antepartum fetal surveillance
- Encourage patient waiting in woman, family and provider
- Cervical ripening/initiation of labor (Summers, 1997)
  - Nipple stimulation
  - Sexual intercourse
  - Castor oil 2–4 oz PO
  - Stripping of membranes
  - Herbs
    - Evening primrose oil, apply to cervix or take orally
    - Red raspberry tea every 1–2 hours in labor
  - Homeopathic remedies
    - Caulophyllum 60× (Weed, 1985)
    - Cimicifuga
    - Pulsatilla

Providing Support:
Education and Support Measures to Consider
- Outline recommendations for care
  - Indication for induction or augmentation
  - Obtain informed consent
  - Client/family preferences
- Potential for
  - Transport if out-of-hospital
  - IV access
  - Fetal monitoring
- Potential restrictions with induction/augmentation
  - NPO
  - Clear liquids
  - IV oxytocin
  - Electronic fetal monitoring
  - Limited mobility
  - Operative assistance at birth
    - Vacuum extraction
    - Forceps
    - Cesarean section
- Provide support

Follow-up Care:
Follow-up Measures to Consider
- Document
- Address client preferences
- Evaluate maternal/fetal status at regular intervals
  - Evaluate for progress
  - Per indication for induction/augmentation
  - Update plan after each evaluation
- Ensure access to emergency services as needed
- Encourage client to express feelings and concerns

Collaborative Practice:
Consider Consultation or Referral
- OB/GYN services
  - Before induction or ripening per collaborative practice agreement
  - Women requiring cesarean section or other assisted birth
  - As needed for transport

- Pediatric services
  - For evidence or suspicion of fetal compromise
- For diagnosis or treatment outside the midwife's scope of practice

CARE OF THE WOMAN WITH MECONIUM-STAINED AMNIOTIC FLUID

Key Clinical Information

Meconium-stained amniotic fluid occurs in approximately 7–22% of all pregnancies (Fraser et al., 2005), with increasing frequency in advancing gestational age (Varney et al., 2004). Although it is more common in the postterm pregnancy, it can also occur before term (Hernandez et al., 1993). Meconium-stained amniotic fluid is theorized to be the result of either an acute or chronic hypoxic event leading to relaxation of the fetal anal sphincter, allowing meconium to be released into the amniotic fluid.

Meconium aspiration syndrome affects 1.7–35.8% of infants born with meconium staining of the amniotic fluid (Fraser et al., 2005). Meconium aspiration syndrome may occur when the fetus born through meconium-stained fluid breathes meconium into the lungs, but it occurs more often in utero in the already compromised fetus. The initiation of amnioinfusion in labor and suctioning of the infant's nares, mouth, and pharynx on the perineum are not effective measures to prevent meconium aspiration syndrome (Fraser et al., 2005; Vain et al., 2004; Xu et al., 2007). Meconium-stained amniotic fluid is an indication to step up fetal surveillance for signs of fetal distress and to be prepared for intrauterine and extrauterine resuscitation.

Client History and Chart Review:
Components of the History
to Consider
- Verify EDC, gestational age
- Assess fetal well-being
  - Reassuring FHR pattern
  - Patterns of fetal activity

- Characteristics of meconium in fluid
  - Thin
  - Moderate
  - Thick
  - Particulate
- Risk factors for meconium aspiration syndrome (Hernandez et al., 1993; Wiswell et al., 2000)
  - Maternal factors
    - Less than five prenatal visits
    - Oligohydramnios
    - Term or postterm pregnancy
  - Labor risk factors
    - Consistency of meconium
    - Abnormal FHR patterns
    - Precipitous birth
    - Cesarean delivery
  - Fetal factors
    - Advancing gestational age (> 42 weeks)
    - Apgar < 7 (1 or 5 minutes)

Physical Examination:
Components of the Physical Exam to Consider
- Abdominal examination
  - FHT in relation to contractions
  - Fetal movement
  - Fluid adequacy (thick meconium may indicate oligohydramnios)
  - Frequency, duration, and strength of contractions
  - Fetal lie, presentation (meconium common with breech)
- Pelvic examination
  - Cervical status
  - Confirmation of presentation
  - Station of presenting part
  - Amnioscopy offers
    - Visualization of fluid through intact membranes
    - Ability to maintain intact membranes
    - Information for earlier decision making regarding
      - Additional personnel for birth
      - Transport in utero, as indicated

Clinical Impression:
Differential Diagnoses and Code Groups
to Consider
Additional suffix may apply (ICD9data.com, 2007)
- Meconium-stained amniotic fluid (ICD-9 codes 656.8)
- Meconium noted at birth, affecting infant (ICD-9 codes 763.84)
- Fetal distress (ICD-9 codes 656.3)

Diagnostic Testing:
Diagnostic Tests and Procedures
to Consider
- Amnioscopy for early evaluation of fluid color
- Evaluation of fetal well-being
  - Intermittent auscultation
    - Follow "with risk factors" minimum timing (Varney et al., 2004)
      - Every 15 minutes in active labor after a contraction
      - Every 5 minutes in second stage
  - Electronic fetal monitor
    - External
    - Internal
- Ultrasound
  - AFI
  - Fetal presentation
- Preoperative laboratory tests
  - Nonreassuring FHR pattern
  - Arrest of dilation or descent
  - Per facility standard

Providing Treatment:
Therapeutic Measures to Consider
- Amnioinfusion (see Care of the Woman Undergoing Amnioinfusion) for meconium-stained fluid with
  - Low AFI/oligohydramnios
  - Presence of variable decelerations associated with cord compression
- Prepare for potential outcomes (Figure 4-1)
  - Vigorous newborn receives routine care

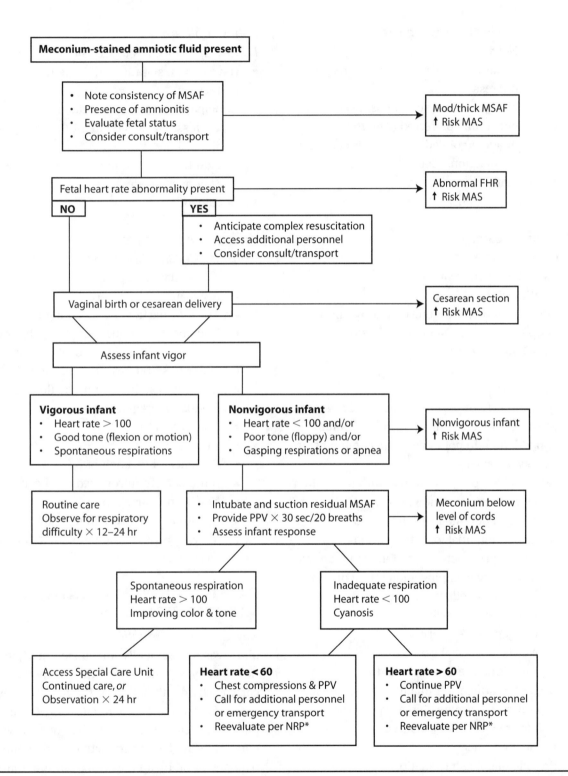

Figure 4-1 *Meconium Algorithm*

Source: American Heart Association & American Academy of Pediatrics. (2006). Neonatal Resuscitation Program recommendations. In *Textbook of neonatal resuscitation* (5th ed.). Elk Grove, IL: American Academy of Pediatrics.

- Suctioning for newborns who are
  - Not vigorous
  - Initially vigorous but develop respiratory distress
  - Intubation and suction using endotracheal tube preferred (American Academy of Pediatrics/American Heart Association, 2000)
- Neonatal resuscitation
- Neonatal transport

Providing Treatment:
Alternative Measures to Consider
- Expectant management
- Gentle birth
- Suctioning method determined by midwife scope of practice, such as DeLee or Res-Q-Vac

Providing Support:
Education and Support Measures to Consider
- Most healthy term infants with meconium-stained fluid do not develop meconium aspiration syndrome
- Advise client of potential risk with meconium
  - Meconium aspiration syndrome
  - Trauma potential with intubation
- Advise of potential for interventions
  - Transport if out-of-hospital birth planned
  - Immediate clamping and cutting of cord for handoff to pediatric team
  - Intubation of newborn
  - Oxygen for newborn
  - Newborn special care
  - Antibiotic therapy for infant
- Lack of treatment for infant with meconium aspiration syndrome increases risk for
  - Severe respiratory disorders
  - Newborn death
- Provide ongoing information
  - In labor
  - At birth
  - If newborn needs special care

Follow-up Care:
Follow-up Measures to Consider
- Have all resuscitation equipment on hand and tested
- Anticipate newborn condition at birth
  - Professional skilled in intubation present if possible
  - Additional personnel for newborn resuscitation, as needed
- Document

Collaborative Practice:
Consider Consultation or Referral
- OB/GYN services
  - Abnormal FHR patterns
  - Thick or particulate meconium
  - Documented or suspected oligohydramnios
  - For change in planned location of birth
- Consider hospital birth in presence of
  - Meconium-stained amniotic fluid, and
  - Postdates pregnancy, or
  - Abnormal FHR pattern
- Pediatric services
  - Presence of meconium
  - Anticipate compromised newborn
  - Newborn resuscitation
  - Respiratory distress in neonate
- For diagnosis or treatment outside the midwife's scope of practice

CARE OF THE WOMAN WITH MULTIPLE GESTATION

Key Clinical Information
Midwives occasionally diagnose multiple gestation in any setting where they provide prenatal care. Early identification of the multiple gestation provides an opportunity to address potential complications before they arise. Midwives provide prenatal care and labor and birth care to women with twin gestation in some settings. In the home birth setting the midwife assumes the responsibility for advising parents of the increased risk of adverse outcomes with multiple pregnancy when birth

occurs in the home (ACOG, 2004c; Mehl-Medrona & Medrona, 1997). Regardless of planned birth location, the midwife must have a means to provide access to obstetric or pediatric care if it is indicated. Incidence of multiple gestation has increased by 65% in the case of twin pregnancies and by 500% in triplet and higher order pregnancies, largely due to assisted reproductive technologies (ACOG, 2004c). Multifetal pregnancy is associated with increased risk for preterm labor, preterm ROM, intrauterine fetal growth restriction, twin-to-twin transfusion, and perinatal death (Sinclair, 2004). Maternal morbidity and health care costs are significantly higher in women with multifetal pregnancies (ACOG, 2004c).

Client History and Chart Review:
Components of the History to Consider
- LMP, EDC, gestational age
- Contributing factors for multiple gestation
  - Family history of multiples
  - Personal history of multiples
  - Use of fertility drugs
  - In vitro fertilization or other assisted reproductive technologies (ACOG, 2004c)
- History suggestive of multiple gestation
  - Fundal growth pattern
  - Size larger than dates by examination
  - Fetal motion not detected by 18–20 weeks size
  - Elevated α-fetoprotein results
- Multiple pregnancy complications
  - Increased incidence of
    - Fetal anomalies
    - Spontaneous abortion
    - Fetal demise
    - Preeclampsia
    - Preterm labor
      - Uterine irritability
      - Cervical changes
      - Preterm PROM
    - Polyhydramnios
    - Placental abruption

- Other pregnancy considerations
  - Rh status
  - Medical conditions
- Social support
  - Nutrition status
  - Working or living conditions
  - Response to multiple gestation

Physical Examination:
Components of the Physical Exam to Consider
- Interval weight gain
- Abdominal examination
  - Interval fundal growth pattern
  - Size larger than dates on two or more occasions
  - Multiple small parts felt on palpation
  - Two fetal hearts heard simultaneously at different rates via Doppler or fetoscope
- Pelvic examination
  - Cervical length and dilation

Clinical Impression:
Differential Diagnoses and Code Groups to Consider
Additional suffix may apply (ICD9data.com, 2007)
- Multiple gestation (ICD-9 codes 651)
  - Twins (ICD-9 codes 651.0)
  - Triplets (ICD-9 codes 651.1)
  - Quadruplets (ICD-9 codes 651.2)
  - Other multiple pregnancy (ICD-9 codes 651.8)

Diagnostic Testing:
Diagnostic Tests and Procedures to Consider
- Maternal serum α-fetoprotein
- Amniocentesis
- Ultrasound evaluation for
  - Gestational age
  - Presence of multiple gestation
  - Presence of anomalies
  - Placenta(s) and membranes
    - Monochorionic
    - Dichorionic, diamniotic

- Fetal gender(s)
- Interval growth
- Cervical evaluation
  - Width
  - Length
  - Funneling
- Antepartum surveillance
  - Perform in situations as indicated in single-ton pregnancy (ACOG, 2004c)
  - For complications of multiple gestation, such as
    - Intrauterine growth restriction
    - Abnormal AFI
    - Discordant fetal growth
    - PIH
    - Fetal anomalies
    - Monoamniotic twins
  - Nonstress testing
  - Biophysical profile

Providing Treatment:
Therapeutic Measures to Consider
- Not recommended (ACOG, 2004c)
  - Cervical cerclage
  - Bed rest
  - Hospitalization
  - Home uterine activity monitoring
- Selective fetal termination
  - Common consideration with in vitro fertilization
  - Poses ethical dilemmas
- Treat
  - Preterm labor (see Care of the Woman with Preterm Labor)
  - Preterm ROM (see Care of the Woman with Premature Rupture of the Membranes)
  - Preeclampsia (see Preeclampsia in Chapter 1)
- Delivery should occur by 40 weeks
- Vertex–vertex twins
  - Anticipate vaginal birth
  - Second twin may require time to be born
  - Cesarean delivery for same indications with singleton birth (ACOG, 2004c)

- Vertex–nonvertex twins
  - Consider vaginal birth for second twin over 1500 g
  - Consider cesarean delivery based on
    - Fetal weight under 1500 g
    - Maternal preference
    - Clinician skill and experience
- Nonvertex first twin
  - Cesarean delivery is usual
  - Vaginal delivery of nonvertex first twin has not been studied
  - Potential for locked twins with breech–vertex twins
- Ongoing evaluation of second fetus after first birth
  - Ultrasound
  - Electronic fetal monitoring
  - Close observation for complications
    - Cord prolapse
    - Placental abruption
    - Abnormal FHR pattern (ACOG, 2004c)
  - Stimulation or augmentation of labor as needed
    - Oxytocin
    - Amniotomy
  - For deteriorating fetal status
    - Internal podalic version as needed
    - Breech extraction
    - Cesarean delivery of second twin

Providing Treatment:
Alternative Measures to Consider
- Diagnosis of twins via clinical examination
- Out-of-hospital birth
  - Uncomplicated multiple gestation
  - Maternal preference
  - Informed choice considerations
  - Risk factors for individual
  - Midwife skill and experience
  - Distance/time to emergency care
- Multiple births hold increased risk regardless of birth location (Mehl-Medrona & Medrona, 1997)

- Poor outcomes at home birth may damage home birth
- Freedom of choice includes ready access to care as needed
- In-hospital birth
  - Vaginal birth
  - Birth room
  - Minimum of people
  - Opportunity to meet staff beforehand
  - Negotiation of preferences
  - Ability to see and touch babies immediately
  - Care provided in family's presence
  - Rooming-in and breastfeeding fostered
- Cesarean delivery
  - Support people present
  - Ability to see and touch babies immediately, if stable
  - Care provided in family's presence
  - Rooming-in and breastfeeding fostered

Providing Support:
Education and Support Measures
to Consider
- Discussion and education regarding multiple gestation
  - Anticipated care during pregnancy
  - Information on testing or surveillance
    - Procedures
    - Results
    - Implications
    - Options and recommendations
- Active listening to client
  - Individual needs
  - Preferences
  - Collaborative planning of care
  - Options for high-risk care as indicated

Follow-up Care:
Follow-up Measures to Consider
- Document
- Increased frequency of prenatal visits
  - By gestational age
  - As indicated by results of testing

- In presence of any complicating factors
- As term approaches (third trimester)
- Identification of risk factors
  - Problem list
  - Update plan as changes occur
- Labor, anticipate potential complications
  - Preterm labor (see Care of the Woman with Preterm Labor)
  - Preterm ROM (see Care of the Woman with Premature Rupture of the Membranes)
  - Uterine inertia
  - Placental abruption
  - Postpartum hemorrhage

Collaborative Practice:
Consider Consultation or Referral
- OB/GYN services
  - For all multiple pregnancies per midwife scope of practice
  - For multiple gestation with complications
    - Maternal complications
    - Fetal complications
  - Triplet or greater multiple pregnancy
  - Maternal preference
- Pediatric services
  - Presence of prenatal complications
  - Immediate newborn care at birth
- Social service
  - Mothers of twins support group
  - Grief support group for pregnancy losses
  - Other support services
- For diagnosis or treatment outside the midwife's scope of practice

CARE OF THE WOMAN WITH A NONVERTEX PRESENTATION

Key Clinical Information
Breech presentation is the most common nonvertex presentation, occurring in 3–4% of term singleton pregnancies. Breech and other nonvertex presentations carry an increased risk of complications, such as cord prolapse and fetal injury, over a vertex presentation. Specific prenatal techniques,

such as hands and knees position with pelvic rocking, the Webster chiropractic technique, moxibustion, auricular plaster therapy, and acupuncture, used during the prenatal period can prevent or reverse common fetal malpositions and malpresentations (Andrews & Andrews, 2004; Guangfeng & Hongjin, 1989; Habek et al., 2003; Pistolese, 2002). These alternative therapies are evidence-based strategies that can aid in optimal fetal alignment for birth. However, they are underutilized because they are either unknown or poorly understood by most women and their care providers.

ACOG recommends external version to convert breech or transverse lie to vertex presentation to decrease the risks associated with nonvertex presentations and avoid unnecessary cesarean delivery (ACOG, 2000b). Current recommendations include offering planned cesarean to women with term breech infants in an attempt to decrease perinatal morbidity and mortality (Hannah & Hannah, 2000). Planned cesarean for nonvertex presentation does not apply to women who refuse surgical delivery, women whose birth is imminent at the time of diagnosis, or women whose second twin is a nonvertex presentation.

Client History and Chart Review:
Components of the History to Consider
- LMP, EDC
- Previous maternity history
  - Previous breech births
  - Previous birth weights of children
  - Presence of uterine scars
- Contraindications for vaginal breech birth
  - Inexperienced birth attendant
  - Maternal preference
  - Birth attendant preference
  - Suspected CPD
  - Large infant
  - Nonreassuring FHR patterns
  - Maternal or fetal complications
  - Previous
    - Shoulder dystocia
    - Dysfunctional labor
    - Protracted labor

- Current pregnancy history
  - Methods of dating pregnancy
  - Current gestation
  - Rh status
  - Placental location
  - Presence of labor
- Contributing factors to nonvertex presentation
  - Polyhydramnios
  - Lax abdominal muscle tone
  - Multiparity
  - Prematurity
  - Multiple gestation
  - Placenta previa
  - Hydrocephalus
  - Fetal or uterine anomalies (Varney et al., 2004)

Physical Examination:
Components of the Physical Exam
to Consider
- Diagnosis of nonvertex presentation
  - Abdominal examination
    - Leopold's maneuvers
    - Determine fetal presentation, lie, and variety
    - Estimate fetal weight
    - Note abdominal muscle tone
    - Uterine tone
    - FHR and location
- Pelvic examination
  - Clinical pelvimetry
  - Cervical status
    - Palpation of presenting part through cervix or lower uterine segment
    - Determine fetal presentation, lie, and variety
    - Estimate fetal weight

Clinical Impression:
Differential Diagnoses and Code Groups
to Consider
Additional suffix may apply (ICD9data.com, 2007)
- Pregnancy, nonvertex presentation (ICD-9 codes 652)
  - Breech (ICD-9 codes 652.2)

- Transverse (ICD-9 codes 652.3)
- Face or brow (ICD-9 codes 652.4)

Diagnostic Testing:
Diagnostic Tests and Procedures
to Consider
- Ultrasound
  - Confirmation of fetal position
  - Evaluation of placental position
  - Version may be performed under ultrasound guidance
- External cephalic version
  - Fetal evaluation
    - Preprocedure
    - During and postprocedure
    - Continuous fetal monitoring
    - NST and/or Biophysical Profile (BPP)
  - Maternal
    - IV access
    - Preoperative laboratory tests

Providing Treatment:
Therapeutic Measures to Consider
- External cephalic version (ACOG, 2000b)
  - Success rates of 35–86%
  - More successful in
    - Multiparous women
    - Transverse or oblique lie
  - Use of tocolytics
    - For nulliparous women
    - For all women
  - Rh immune globulin for Rh-negative women
  - Ready access to emergency cesarean delivery
- Method, after fetal evaluation
  - Have client empty bladder (Frye, 1998)
  - Client relaxes with knees bent and supported
  - Abdominal muscles must be relaxed
  - Attempt forward roll using gentle steady pressure
  - Lift breech from pelvis
  - Encourage head toward pelvis with gentle pressure and flexion

- Attempt backward roll if forward roll not successful
- Two practitioners may work together to encourage fetus to turn
- Stop in the presence of
  - Fetal bradycardia
  - Maternal pain
  - Vaginal bleeding
  - Rupture of membranes
  - Unsuccessful version
  - Successful version
- Vaginal breech birth
  - More successful in women with
    - Adequate pelvis
    - Previous vaginal birth
    - Skilled birth attendant
  - Higher risk of perinatal complications versus
    - Vaginal vertex birth postversion
    - Planned cesarean delivery

Providing Treatment:
Alternative Measures to Consider
- Breech tilt position
  - Perform 5 minutes three to four times daily
  - Hips higher than head on tilt board
  - Music at maternal feet to encourage fetus to turn
- Hands and knees with or without pelvic rocking (Andrews & Andrews, 2004)
- Moxibustion (Cardini & Weixin, 1998; Frye, 1998)
  - Burn moxa cone 15 minutes daily
  - Place at outer corner of little toe nailbed
- Homeopathic pulsatilla (Frye, 1998)
  - Potency: 200C
  - One dose TID
  - Use with breech tilt
- Acupuncture (Habek et al., 2003)
- Auricular plaster therapy (Guangfeng & Hongjin, 1989)
  - Acupuncture needle used to locate sensitive spots on auricle of ear
  - Seed of *Vacarria segetalis* fixed tightly to ear at these points
  - Cover with a piece of plaster

Providing Support:
Education and Support Measures to Consider
- Provide information on risks, benefits, and availability of
  - Vaginal breech birth
  - External cephalic version
  - Planned cesarean delivery
- Obtain informed consent for planned birth or procedure
  - Perinatal risk with planned vaginal breech ≈ 5%
  - Perinatal risk with planned cesarean for breech ≈ 1.6% (ACOG, 2004d)
  - Perinatal risk includes
    - Fetal injury or death
    - Neonatal injury or death
  - Maternal risk deemed equivalent for cesarean section versus vaginal breech
- Encourage questions regarding options
- Consider maternal preferences in jointly determining plan for care

Follow-up Care:
Follow-up Measures to Consider
- Document
- Reconfirm
  - Fetal position before birth
  - Maternal preference for planned birth or procedure
- Persistent breech
  - Repeat version attempt
  - Reconsider vaginal breech or planned cesarean
- Document
  - All discussions
  - Informed consent/informed choice
  - Maternal preferences for care
- For planned vaginal breech birth
  - Plan access to emergency care
  - Estimate fetal weight
  - Plan for birth
    - Number and type and skill of birth attendants

- Presence of resuscitation team for newborn
- Plan for emergency care
- Procedure for vaginal breech birth (El Halta, 1996)
  - Evaluate fetal well-being frequently
  - Allow lull between first- and second-stage labor
    - Mother may have urge to push before full dilation
    - Avoid head entrapment by ensuring full dilation
  - Keep "hands off" infant and perineum
    - Allow infant to stretch tissues slowly
    - Avoid stimulation of infant
  - Allow infant to birth to above umbilicus
    - At this point cord compression is likely
    - *Gently* pull down a loop of cord
  - Encourage maternal pushing
    - Keep infant in anterior position
    - Allow infant to birth until nape of neck can be seen
    - ⚠ Do not pull on infant
    - Arms and legs may need gentle assistance to be born
  - To birth face and head
    - Wrap infant's body in warm towel
    - Head may be guided into pelvis with gentle rotation of body
    - Assistant provides suprapubic pressure
    - Gently swing infant onto mother's abdomen
    - As face appears, suction mouth and nose
    - Keep infant warm as head molds and is born
  - If birth does not occur promptly
    - Cut episiotomy

➤ Use Ritgen maneuver as needed

➤ ⚠ Do not pull on infant; severe injury may result

Collaborative Practice:
Consider Consultation or Referral

- Chiropractic care
  - Webster technique for turning breech (Pistolese, 2002)
- OB/GYN services
  - For persistent nonvertex presentation
  - For cesarean delivery
    - For failed version
    - Maternal preference
    - For nonvertex presentations
    - Contraindications to vaginal breech birth
- Pediatric service
  - For newborn care after vaginal breech birth
- For diagnosis or treatment outside the midwife's scope of practice

CARE OF THE WOMAN WITH POSTPARTUM HEMORRHAGE

Key Clinical Information

Postpartum hemorrhage is defined as a blood loss of greater than 500 ml at delivery or within the first 24 hours after vaginal birth (Varney et al., 2004). Postpartum hemorrhage is a leading cause of maternal mortality worldwide. The anemia that results from hemorrhage may be a significant contributor to delayed postpartum healing and predispose to infection. Hemorrhage may be the primary indicator of retained placental tissue, uterine fatigue, significant lacerations, or disorders of coagulation. The primary cause of postpartum hemorrhage is uterine atony (Long, 2001). Length of time to placental delivery increases the risk of postpartum hemorrhage; at more than 30 minutes the risk of postpartum hemorrhage triples. Active management of the third stage of labor is an evidence-based strategy that reduces postpartum hemorrhage (Simpson, 2007).

Client History and Chart Review:
Components of the History to Consider

- Past obstetric history
  - Prior history of postpartum hemorrhage
  - Parity
    - Nulliparous
    - Grand multiparity
  - Cesarean section
  - Prior history of retained placenta
- Course of labor
  - Gestational age
  - Hematocrit and hemoglobin at onset of labor
  - Effectiveness of uterine contractions
  - Length of each stage
  - Oxytocin administration
  - Placental delivery and status
  - Genital tract laceration
- Risk factors for hemorrhage
  - 🌐 Ethnic history
    - Asian
    - Hispanic
  - Preterm delivery
  - Precipitous labor and birth
  - Overdistension of the uterus
    - Fetal macrosomia
    - Polyhydramnios
    - Multiple gestation
  - Prolonged third stage (Simpson, 2007)
  - PIH, HELLP syndrome
    - $MgSO_4$ use
    - Low platelets
  - Operative delivery
    - Vacuum extraction
    - Forceps
    - Uterine manipulation (i.e., version)
  - Placenta previa or abruption
  - Chorioamnionitis
  - Fetal demise
  - Disseminated intravascular coagulation (DIC)
- Medical history
  - Bleeding disorders
  - Asthma (avoid Prostin)
  - Hypertension (avoid Methergine)

Physical Examination:
Components of the Physical Exam to Consider
- Evaluate cause of bleeding
  - Uterine atony
  - Lacerations
  - Retained placenta or fragments
  - Coagulopathy
- Evaluate bladder, empty as needed
- Evaluate for shock (EBL > 500 ml)
  - Rapid thready pulse
  - Rapid shallow respirations
  - Pale clammy skin and mucous membranes
  - Anxiety or lack of affect
- Placenta undelivered
  - Evaluate the uterus for placental separation
    - Uterus globular, firm
    - Fundus rises and is mobile
    - Cord lengthens
    - Brandt-Andrews maneuver (see box below)
  - Assess for lacerations
- Placenta delivered
  - Examine placenta for completeness
  - Evaluate the uterus for atony
    - If atony present
      - Massage fundus
      - Bimanual compression
      - Consider retained placental or membrane fragments
  - If no atony
    - Evaluate for traumatic source of bleeding
      - Cervical lacerations
      - Vaginal lacerations
      - Uterine rupture

MODIFIED BRANDT-ANDREWS MANEUVER

Hold umbilical cord taut with clamp in one hand

Press downward just above maternal symphysis with other hand

If cord retracts, the placenta is not yet separated

If cord lengthens, the placenta has separated

Source: Varney et al., 2004.

Clinical Impression:
Differential Diagnoses and Code Groups to Consider
Additional suffix may apply (ICD9data.com, 2007)
- Postpartum hemorrhage, secondary to (ICD-9 codes 666)
  - Uterine atony (ICD-9 codes 666.1)
  - Genital tract laceration(s) (ICD-9 codes 664–665)
  - Retained placental tissue (ICD-9 codes 666.2)
  - Clotting disorders (ICD-9 codes 649.3)

Diagnostic Testing:
Diagnostic Tests and Procedures to Consider
- CBC
- Hematocrit and hemoglobin
- Platelets
- Type and cross-match
- Preeclampsia laboratory panel (see Care of the Woman with Pregnancy-Induced Hypertension in Labor)
- Coagulation studies
  - Prothrombin time, partial thromboplastin time
  - Fibrinogen
- Ultrasound evaluation for
  - Retained placental tissue
  - Hematoma formation

Providing Treatment:
Therapeutic Measures to Consider
- Preventive measures
  - Controlled birth of infant to minimize tissue trauma
  - Physiologic management of third stage
    - Clients without risk factors for postpartum hemorrhage
  - Active management of third stage (see Care of the Woman in Third-Stage Labor)
    - Clients with risk factors for postpartum hemorrhage, *or*
    - All clients
  - Massage uterus until firm once placenta born
  - Encourage breastfeeding and skin contact with infant

- Postpartum hemorrhage placenta in situ
  - Bleeding indicates partial separation
  - Manual exploration and removal may be necessary
    - Do not pull on cord
    - Procedure for manual removal
      - Insert sterile gloved hand into vagina
      - Follow cord to placenta
      - Move hand laterally to find edge
      - Wedge fingertips under leading edge of placenta
      - Shear placenta off uterine wall using short strokes
      - Remove placenta
      - Treat for postpartum hemorrhage with placenta delivered
      - Potential need for follow-up dilation and curettage (D&C)
- Postpartum hemorrhage with placenta delivered, assess
  - Placenta for completeness
  - Tissues for lacerations
  - Maternal vital signs
- Perform bimanual compression
  - If uterus fails to contract well
  - Decreases blood supply to large uterine vessels
  - Will not diminish bleeding due to lacerations
  - Technique
    - One hand in vagina against lower uterine segment
      - Form into fist in anterior fornix
    - Second hand on abdomen
      - Cup posterior wall of uterus
    - Bring hands firmly together
      - Uterus will be compressed between hands
      - Maintain steady pressure until bleeding controlled
      - Order uterotonic medications (Varney et al., 2004)

- Medications
  - Pitocin 10 units IM or 20–40 units/1000 ml IV fluids
    - Preferred first-line therapy
  - Misoprostol (Cytotec) (Lokugamage et al., 2001; Walraven et al., 2004)
    - 200–800 micrograms rectally
    - Thermostable uterotonic agent
    - Low incidence of side effects
    - Onset of action rapid
    - Half-life (oral) is 20–40 min (Rx Med, n.d.)
  - Methergine 0.2 mg IM (Murphy, 2004)
    - May follow with 0.2 mg PO every 6 hours
    - Indicated for persistent boggy uterus
    - Avoid in client with hypertension
  - Hemabate 250 mg IM
    - Significant side effects
    - Not preferred first-line therapy
  - Prostin 15 M, 0.25 mg IM
- IV therapy
  - Large-bore catheter(s)
  - D-5 lactated Ringer's, lactated Ringer's, Normosol, or other similar solution
  - 10 units oxytocin/500 ml IV fluids
  - Run rapidly until atony subsides
  - Use second IV as needed for fluid replacement
- 🕿 Uterine exploration for retained placental tissue
  - May need D&C under anesthesia
- Replacement blood transfusion
  - For estimated blood loss of > 1000 ml or signs of shock
  - Blood products
    - Whole blood
    - Packed red blood cells
    - Other blood components as indicated
- 🕿 For shock
  - Additional IV access
  - O_2 by mask
  - Trendelenburg or shock position
  - Foley catheter
  - Monitor intake and output closely

- 🕐 Extreme bleeding
  - Packing
    - Deep vaginal or cervical lacerations
    - While awaiting surgical repair
  - ⚠ Aortic compression
    - Emergency measure while awaiting surgical care
  - Surgical control of bleeding
    - Repair of lacerations
    - Suture ligature of bleeding vessels
    - Dilation and evacuation of retained placenta fragments
    - Hysterectomy or uterine artery ligation in extreme cases

Providing Treatment:
Alternative Measures to Consider
- Preventives
  - Nettle or alfalfa leaf infusion (Weed, 1985)
    - Given during pregnancy
    - Immediately after birth of baby
  - Motherwort tincture
- Treatment of hemorrhage due to atony
  - Shepherd's purse tincture (Soule & Szwed, 2000)
  - Tincture of
    - Blue cohosh
    - Shepherd's purse
  - Breast stimulation
  - Homeopathic
    - Caulophyllum
    - Arnica
    - Rescue remedy

Providing Support:
Education and Support Measures to Consider
- Discuss and arrange transport if out-of-hospital
- After resolution of hemorrhage discuss
  - Occurrence of hemorrhage
  - If symptomatic, call for help before arising
  - Take iron replacement therapy as directed
    - Dietary sources
    - Supplements

- Rest and adequate nutrition are essential for healing
- Reinforce signs and symptoms of infection
  - How to recognize
  - When and how to call
- Active listening

Follow-up Care:
Follow-up Measures to Consider
- Document findings, treatment, client response
- Observe for
  - Persistent bleeding
  - Signs of hypovolemia or anemia
    - Weakness
    - Dyspnea
    - Syncope
- CBC/hematocrit and hemoglobin
  - First postpartum day
  - Repeat if bleeding continues
  - 4–6 week check

Collaborative Practice:
Consider Consultation or Referral
- OB/GYN services
  - Hemorrhage that does not respond
    - Immediately to treatment
    - As expected with appropriate treatment
  - Signs and symptoms of shock
  - For transport from out of hospital
  - For suspicion of
    - Retained placental fragments
    - Severe vaginal lacerations or hematomas
    - Cervical lacerations
    - Uterine rupture
- For diagnosis or treatment outside the midwife's scope of practice

Each 500 ml of blood lost roughly translates to a drop of 1 g in the hemoglobin level (Blackburn & Loper, 1992).

CARE OF THE WOMAN WITH POSTTERM PREGNANCY

Key Clinical Information

Postterm pregnancy is defined as pregnancy that has exceeded 42 completed weeks. Approximately 7% of women have postterm pregnancies. ACOG recommends beginning fetal surveillance between 41 and 42 weeks (ACOG, 2004b). Women with an unfavorable cervix and postterm pregnancy can be managed expectantly. Induction may be indicated for either maternal or fetal indications but not simply for 42 weeks gestation. Perinatal morbidity and mortality increase as gestational age advances (Hart, 2002).

Client History and Chart Review:
Components of the History to Consider

- Assess EDC using multiple parameters
  - LMP
  - Conception date if known
  - First positive pregnancy test
  - Uterine size at first visit
  - Initial FHR
    - Fetoscope or stethoscope 18–20 weeks
    - Doppler 10–14 weeks
  - Quickening
  - Fundal height at umbilicus at 20 weeks
  - Early or mid-pregnancy ultrasound
- Postdates risk assessment
  - Fetal macrosomia
  - Fetal postmaturity syndrome
  - Oligohydramnios
  - Meconium aspiration syndrome
- Review history for additional factors that may prolong pregnancy
  - Adrenal hyperplasia
  - Maternal psychosocial stresses
  - Certain fetal anomalies
- Assess
  - Ongoing nutrition
  - Fetal activity and changes
  - Contraction patterns
  - Maternal concerns and state of mind

Physical Examination:
Components of the Physical Exam to Consider

- Vital signs
- Weight
- Abdominal examination
  - Fetal presentation, position, lie, and variety
  - Fetal flexion and engagement
  - EFW
  - Palpate for
    - Fluid adequacy
    - Presence of contractions
- Pelvic examination
  - Calculate Bishop's score
  - Verify presenting part
  - Reassess pelvimetry

Clinical Impression:
Differential Diagnoses and Code Groups to Consider
Additional suffix may apply (ICD9data.com, 2007)

- Prolonged pregnancy ($\geq$ 42 weeks) (ICD-9 codes 645.2)
- Term pregnancy ($>$ 37 and $<$ 42 weeks) (ICD-9 codes 650)

Diagnostic Testing:
Diagnostic Tests and Procedures to Consider

- Fetal surveillance
  - Daily fetal kick counts
  - Nonstress test
    - Weekly
    - Biweekly
  - Biophysical profile
    - Weekly
    - Biweekly
  - AFI as separate indicator
  - Contraction stress testing (ACOG, 2004b)

Providing Treatment:
Therapeutic Measures to Consider

- Watchful waiting; requires
  - Close observation of maternal and fetal well-being

- Informed choice
- Willingness to intervene as needed
- Cervical ripening (see Care of the Woman Undergoing Induction or Augmentation of Labor)
  - No demonstrated benefit over expectant care for healthy mother and fetus (ACOG, 2004b)
  - As indicated by maternal or fetal status
    - Preeclampsia
    - Gestational diabetes
    - Nonreassuring fetal surveillance
  - Generally followed by induction of labor
- Induction (see Care of the Woman Undergoing Induction or Augmentation of Labor)
  - As indicated by maternal or fetal status

Providing Treatment:
Alternative Measures to Consider
- Watchful waiting (see previous section)
- Alternative measures for cervical ripening/induction (see Care of the Woman Undergoing Induction or Augmentation of Labor)

Providing Support:
Education and Support Measures to Consider
- Discuss potential risks and benefits of
  - Expectant management
  - Interventions
- Review or teach
  - Postdates is after 42 weeks
  - Fetal kick count
  - Process of labor
  - When to call
- Discuss labor options
  - Obtain informed consent
  - Expectant care
  - Elective intervention
  - Indicated intervention
  - Any potential change in location or anticipated care for labor and birth
- Listen to and note client and family
  - Preferences
  - Concerns

Follow-up Care:
Follow-up Measures to Consider
- Fetal surveillance
  - Schedule to evaluate fetal status every 4–7 days
  - Review results promptly
- Document ongoing plan
- Anticipate potential for complications (ACOG, 2004b)
  - Meconium-stained amniotic fluid
  - Shoulder dystocia
  - Postpartum hemorrhage
  - Elevated chance of cesarean
  - Newborn respiratory distress

Collaborative Practice:
Consider Consultation or Referral
- OB/GYN services
  - Pregnancy after 42 weeks
  - Nonreassuring fetal testing
  - Concerns regarding reasons for postterm status
  - Change in location of birth due to fetal status/postdates
- Pediatric services
  - Anticipatory for postdates infant
  - As indicated by
    - Nonreassuring fetal surveillance
    - Meconium-stained amniotic fluid
    - Shoulder dystocia
    - Cesarean delivery
    - Newborn respiratory distress
- For diagnosis or treatment outside the midwife's scope of practice

CARE OF THE WOMAN WITH PREGNANCY-INDUCED HYPERTENSION IN LABOR

Key Clinical Information
Approximately 5–7% of pregnant women develop gestational hypertension, preeclampsia, or pregnancy induced hypertensive disorders (PIH) (see Chapter 3, Care of the Pregnant Woman with Hyper-

tensive Disorders in Pregnancy). Prompt identification of PIH offers the opportunity for early treatment, which may increase the likelihood of vaginal birth and decrease the potential for maternal or fetal harm (Livingston et al., 2003). The woman who presents with preeclampsia during labor may initially appear to be fine; therefore systematic evaluation for PIH is warranted in all women with *any* clinical indicators suggestive of PIH (Roberts, 1994).

⚠ PIH frequently causes elevations in maternal blood pressure, urinary protein, serum uric acid, and liver function tests. The maternal circulating blood volume is diminished, resulting in hypovolemia in spite of generalized peripheral edema. Placental and renal blood flow is frequently diminished. Platelets may fall well below the normal range. HELLP syndrome is associated with a greater incidence of maternal morbidity, including a greater incidence of seizures, epigastric pain, nausea and vomiting, significant proteinuria, and stillbirth (Martin et al., 1999). Severe preeclampsia may result in maternal or perinatal death (Chandrasekhar & Datta, 2002). Seizures may be the first sign of PIH and may occur 24–48 hours postpartum (Katz et al., 2000).

Client History and Chart Review:
Components of the History to Consider

- Prenatal history
  - EDC, LMP
  - Review of preeclampsia laboratory values if previously obtained
  - Vasoactive drug use (e.g., nasal decongestants, cocaine)
- Labor history, as applicable
- Maternal blood pressure
  - During pregnancy
  - During evaluation
- Presence and onset of symptoms
  - Symptoms of end-organ involvement
    - Persistent severe headache
    - Epigastric pain
    - Visual disturbance

- Evaluate for PIH risk factors
  - History of essential hypertension
  - Hydatidiform mole (10 times the risk)
  - Fetal hydrops (10 times the risk)
  - Primigravida (6–8 times the risk)
  - Hypertension in previous pregnancy, other than first
  - Diabetes
  - Collagen vascular disease
  - Persistent nausea and vomiting
  - Renal vascular disease
  - Renal parenchymal disease
  - Multiple gestation (5 times the risk)
  - 🌐 African-American and other minority women
  - Ages < 20 and > 35 years
- Other complicating medical factors
- Family history

Physical Examination:
Components of the Physical Exam to Consider

- 🔻 Serial blood pressure readings
  - Intact equipment of correct size should be used
  - Use same maternal position for each blood pressure
  - Arm should be supported at level of the heart
- Evaluation for pitting edema
  - Face
  - Hands
  - Feet and lower legs
- Deep tendon reflexes
  - Patellar, Achilles tendon
  - 3+ or clonus indicates central nervous system irritability
- Optic fundi for evidence of edema or hemorrhage
- Evaluate pulmonary status
- Evaluate fetal status
- Pelvic examination, as indicated
  - Bishop's scope before induction
  - Labor progress

Clinical Impression:
Differential Diagnoses and Code Groups
to Consider
Additional suffix may apply (ICD9data.com, 2007)

- Gestational hypertension (PIH) (ICD-9 codes 642)
  - Preeclampsia, mild (ICD-9 codes 642.4)
  - Preeclampsia, severe (ICD-9 codes 642.5)
  - Eclampsia (ICD-9 codes 642.6)
- Transient hypertension (ICD-9 codes 642.3)
- Essential hypertension (ICD-9 codes 642.0)
- PIH superimposed on chronic hypertension (ICD-9 codes 642.7)
- HELLP syndrome (ICD-9 codes 642.5)
- Elevated blood pressure without diagnosis of hypertension (ICD-9 codes 796.2)

Diagnostic Testing:
Diagnostic Tests and Procedures to Consider

- Baseline preeclampsia/preoperative laboratory panel
  - Urinalysis

MILD PREECLAMPSIA (ACOG, 2002B)

Blood pressure of 140/90 to 159/109

Proteinuria of 0.3 g or higher in a 24-hour urine specimen

SEVERE PREECLAMPSIA (ACOG, 2002B)

Blood pressure of 160/110 or higher

Proteinuria of 5 g or higher in a 24-hour urine specimen

Oliguria

Cerebral or visual disturbances

Pulmonary edema or cyanosis

Epigastric or right upper quadrant pain

Impaired liver function

Thrombocytopenia

Fetal growth restriction

- CBC w/differential
  - Platelet count (normal range, 130,000–400,000/ml)
  - Elevated hematocrit may indicate severity of hypovolemia
- Serum uric acid (normal range, 1.2–4.5 mg/dl)
- Type and screen or cross-match
- Renal function testing
  - Blood urea nitrogen
  - Creatinine (normal range, < 1.0 mg/dl)
- Liver function testing
- Coagulation studies, in presence of
  - Abnormal liver function tests
  - Abruptio placenta (Frye, 1998)
- Fetal surveillance
  - Biophysical profile
  - Amniotic fluid index
- Fetal monitoring, observe for
  - Decreased beat-to-beat variability
  - Pattern of late decelerations

Providing Treatment:
Therapeutic Measures to Consider

- Expectant management
  - Preferred for gestation < 34 weeks
  - Bed rest with sedation as needed
  - Monitoring of blood pressure, weight, reflexes
  - Serial fetal surveillance
  - Serial preeclampsia laboratory tests
  - Medications as indicated below
- Active management
  - Expedite delivery
  - Steroids to promote fetal lung maturity as needed
  - IV access and fluids
  - Route of birth dictated by
    - Maternal and fetal condition
      - Preterm fetus may do best with cesarean delivery
      - Prompt delivery is indicated for eclamptic mother
      - $MgSO_4$ may slow labor/induction (ACOG, 2002b)

- Anesthesia concerns
  - ➤ Prompt cesarean section may be preferred
  - ➤ Labile blood pressure may contraindicate regional anesthesia
  - ➤ Edema may make endotracheal intubation more difficult
- Medications
  - MgSO$_4$, anticonvulsant
    - 4–6 g IV bolus followed by 2 g/hr
    - Titrate to renal output, reflexes (ACOG, 2002b)
    - Have calcium gluconate immediately available at bedside
  - Oxytocin induction or augmentation of labor as necessary
  - Antihypertensive medications
    - Limited benefit
    - Used to regulate labile blood pressure
      - ➤ 170/110 to 130/90 optimum
      - ➤ Monitor intake and output
        - ▶ Hourly intake and output
        - ▶ NPO
        - ▶ Foley catheter
        - ▶ IV fluids on pump

Providing Treatment:
Alternative Measures to Consider
- Expectant management
  - Quiet dark room
  - Rest in left lateral position
  - Support people present or available
  - Provide calm atmosphere of caring and safety
- Homeopathic rescue remedy to pulse points

Providing Support:
Education and Support Measures to Consider
- Provide information about
  - Diagnosis
  - Options for care
  - Symptom recognition
  - Anticipated course of events
    - Need for calm and quiet

- Discussion regarding potential for
  - Change in birth plans
  - Medical interventions
  - Initiation of labor
  - Newborn special care
- Address client and family concerns
- Client/family to notify if additional symptoms develop, such as
  - Epigastric pain
  - Scotomata
  - Visual disturbance
  - Severe headache

Follow-up Care:
Follow-up Measures to Consider
- Follow vital signs/reflexes/symptoms
  - At least every 2–4 hours
  - Follow for 24–48 hours postpartum
- Repeat preeclampsia or HELLP laboratory tests
- Document

Collaborative Practice:
Consider Consultation or Referral
- OB/GYN services
  - Suspected or confirmed preeclampsia
  - For women requiring transport due to PIH
  - For women with PIH who appear unstable
- Pediatric services
  - For presence at birth when maternal PIH present
  - Fetal status, such as
    - Preterm birth
    - Nonreassuring FHR patterns
- For diagnosis or treatment outside the midwife's scope of practice

CARE OF THE WOMAN WITH PRETERM LABOR

Key Clinical Information
Preterm labor is defined as the onset of regular uterine contractions in a woman who is between 20 and 37 weeks gestation, who in addition has either spontaneous ROM or progressive cervical change (ACOG, 2003). It is the second leading cause of

neonatal mortality in the United States, occurring in approximately 10% of pregnancies (Reedy, 2007; Sinclair, 2004; Tucker et al., 1991). Many women who have preterm contractions do not in fact go into preterm labor. Differentiation of preterm labor from preterm contractions can be challenging and stressful, especially for the midwife practicing in a rural area where perinatal services are limited or require substantial travel time. The combination of positive fetal fibronectin (fFN) testing and cervical length less than 25 mm is a strong predictor of impending preterm delivery (ACOG, 2003; Reedy, 2007).

Client History and Chart Review:
Components of the History to Consider
- EDC confirmation
  - LMP, menstrual cycles
  - Ultrasound dating
  - β-Human chorionic gonadotropin results
- Determination of labor status
- Signs and symptoms of preterm labor
- Onset and duration of symptoms
- Precipitating factors
  - Sexual activity within 96 hours (see fFN, below)
  - Prolonged standing, heavy lifting
  - Stress, trauma
  - Vaginal bleeding
- Signs and symptoms may be vague
  - Mild or severe cramping
  - Dull backache
  - Suprapubic or pelvic pressure
  - Loose stools
  - Increased or "different" vaginal discharge
- History or symptoms of infection, such as
  - Urinary tract infections or asymptomatic bacteriuria
  - Vaginal infections or sexually transmitted infections
  - GBS
- Assess risk factors for preterm birth
  - Adolescent pregnancy
  - Advanced maternal age
  - Prepregnant body mass index < 19.8

- Cervical cone biopsy
- Poverty
- Multiple gestation
- Tobacco use
- Prior history of preterm birth
- Intrauterine growth retardation
- Uterine anomalies
- Previous determinations of cervical status
  - Length
  - Consistency
  - Funneling

Physical Examination:
Components of the Physical Exam to Consider
- Maternal and fetal vital signs
- Abdominal examination
  - Presence of contractions
  - Uterine tenderness
  - Fetal heart rate
  - Estimated fetal weight for gestational age
  - Fetal presentation, position, lie
  - Costovertebral angle (CVA) tenderness
- Pelvic examination
  - Sterile speculum exam for specimen collection
    - Fetal fibronectin fFN
    - GBS culture
    - Wet preparation
    - Chlamydia/gonorrhea
    - Specimen for ferning
  - Cervical change from baseline
  - Status of membranes
  - Vaginal discharge
- Evaluation for complications of pregnancy which would favor delivery over tocolysis

Clinical Impression:
Differential Diagnoses and Code Groups to Consider
Additional suffix may apply (ICD9data.com, 2007)
- Preterm labor (ICD-9 codes 644.2)
- False preterm labor (ICD-9 codes 644.0)
- Multiple gestation (ICD-9 codes 651)
- Pyelonephritis (ICD-9 codes V22 and 590.10)

- Renal calculi (ICD-9 codes V22 and 592.0)
- Abruptio placentae (ICD-9 codes 641.2)
- Gastritis (ICD-9 codes V22 and 535.0)
- Appendicitis (ICD-9 codes 648.9)
- Urinary tract infection (ICD-9 codes 646.6)
- Intrauterine fetal growth restriction (ICD-9 codes 656.5)

Diagnostic Testing:
Diagnostic Tests and Procedures to Consider
- Laboratory tests
  - fFN
    - Collect before digital examination
    - Recent sexual activity or blood may affect results
  - GBS
  - Chlamydia
  - Gonorrhea
  - Wet preparation
  - Ferning, Nitrazine testing if spontaneous ROM suspected
  - STAT urinalysis, C & S
  - CBC with differential smear
  - Additional laboratory tests as indicated by client history and presentation
- Ultrasound—based on symptoms and gestational age
  - Cervical length and funneling
    - Length > 40 mm = low risk
    - Length 40–26 mm = moderate risk
    - Length < 26 mm = high risk
  - Determination of approximate gestational age
  - Verify number of fetuses
  - Placental location and status
  - AFI, biophysical profile
  - Guidance for amniocentesis
- Amniocentesis for fetal surfactant and lecithin/sphingomyelin (L/S) ratio

Providing Treatment:
Therapeutic Measures to Consider
- Rest
  - Stop work, avoid lifting

- Refrain from sexual arousal and intercourse
- Stop breastfeeding or other breast stimulation
- Hydration—IV or PO
- Tocolytic medication
  - Use before 34 weeks gestation
  - Dilation less than 4 cm
  - 🐾 Medications to consider with collaborating physician (ACOG, 2003)
- Calcium channel blockers (ACOG, 2003; Byrne & Morrison, 2004)
  - Prolonged pregnancy ≥ 48 hours
  - Less severe side effect profile than β agonists
    - May cause hypotension
    - Avoid in client with liver disease
  - Nifedipine 5–10 mg SL every 15 minutes (Sinclair, 2004)
    - May repeat for 4 doses
    - Maintenance 10–20 mg PO every 4–6 hours
- β Agonists
  - Significant side-effect profile
  - Decrease dose for maternal heart rate ≥ 130 beats/min
  - Begin with IV dosing
  - Change to PO
    - Labor stopped for 12–24 hours
    - 30 minutes before stopping IV dosing
  - Terbutaline
    - IV 2.5 mg/min—increase in 2.5-mg increments
    - Increase every 20 minutes based on effect
    - Maximum dose 20 mg/min
    - SQ dose 0.25 mg every 3 hours
    - PO dose 2.5–5.0 mg every 4–6 hours
  - Ritodrine
    - IV dose 0.05–0.35 mg/min
    - PO dose 20 mg every 2–4 hours (ACOG, 2003)
- Magnesium sulfate
  - 40 g in 100–500 ml
  - 4–6 g loading dose
  - 2–4 g/hr maintenance

- Indomethacin (Moses, 2004)
  - Only used before 32 weeks
    - May cause premature closure of ductus arteriosis
  - Loading dose 50 mg PO
  - Maintenance dose 25 mg PO every 4 hours
  - Maximum dosing period 48 hours
- Corticosteroid use (ACOG, 2002a)
  - Use between 24 and 34 weeks gestation
  - Maximum benefit 1–7 days postdosing
  - Betamethasone—two doses
    - 12 mg IM every 24 hours, or
  - Dexamethasone—four doses
    - 6 mg IM every 12 hours
- Selective cesarean for very preterm infant(s)

Providing Treatment:
Alternative Measures to Consider
- Observe for preterm contractions versus preterm labor
- Alternative therapies:
  - Black Haw tea, tincture, or capsule
  - Valerian root tincture, *or*
  - Skullcap tincture, *or*
  - Cramp bark and wild yam tincture (1:1)
    - ½ dropperful TID (Frye, 1998)
- Assess overall nutritional status, supplement with
  - Calcium citrate 1000 mg daily
  - Magnesium 500 mg daily

Providing Support:
Education and Support Measures to Consider
- Threatened preterm labor
  - Limit activity, stop work, arrange for household help
  - Avoid sexual arousal or activity
  - Call if symptoms resume or increase
  - Daily fetal kick counts
  - Encourage smoking cessation, improvement of nutrition as applicable
- Progressive preterm labor
  - Discuss
    - Best care in circumstances
    - Anticipated events for preterm birth

- Neonatal care for gestational age
- Encourage family and social support involvement

Follow-up Care:
Follow-up Measures to Consider
- Document
  - Symptoms
  - Cervical changes
  - Fetal well-being
  - Treatment and education
  - Client response
- Threatened preterm labor
  - Negative cervical change and negative fFN (Reedy, 2007)
    - Standard prenatal care
    - Reassurance
    - fFN every 2 weeks
    - Sooner if symptoms persist or increase
    - Consider serial ultrasound evaluation based on findings
      - Fetal surveillance
      - Cervical length
    - Follow as high risk for preterm birth
  - Negative cervical change and positive fFN (Reedy, 2007)
    - Comfort measures
    - Education of woman and family
    - Weekly office visits
    - fFN every 2 weeks
    - Sooner if symptoms persist or increase
    - Consider home monitoring
    - Consider antenatal corticosteroids
    - Consider serial ultrasound evaluation based on findings
      - Fetal surveillance
      - Cervical length
    - Follow as high risk for preterm birth
  - Positive cervical change and positive fFN (Reedy, 2007)
    - Consult OB/GYN or perinatologist
    - Antenatal corticosteroids
    - Tocolysis in hospital

- ◆ Activity restriction
- ◆ Consider home monitoring
- Preterm labor and birth
  - Preterm infant care options locally or regionally
  - Consider transfer of care to perinatal specialist
- Provide support and reassurance
- Connect with community resources for assistance as indicated
  - Breastfeeding support
  - "Preemie" clothing
  - Rides to neonatal special care unit

Collaborative Practice:
Criteria to Consider for Consultation
or Referral
- OB/GYN or perinatal services
  - For suspected preterm labor
  - Confirmed preterm labor
- Consider transfer, as applicable, to
  - Hospital care
  - Regional perinatal care center
- Pediatric services
  - For presence at birth
  - For follow-up of premature newborn
- Social Service
  - Social support services
  - Parents of "preemies" support groups
  - Grief counseling as needed
- For diagnosis or treatment outside the midwife's scope of practice

CARE OF THE WOMAN WITH PROLONGED LATENT-PHASE LABOR

Key Clinical Information
The latent phase of labor is considered to be prolonged when it exceeds approximately 20 hours in nullipara or 14 hours in multipara from the onset of regular contractions to the onset of active labor (3–4 cm dilation). However, labor frequently does not have a discrete beginning (Greulich & Tarrant, 2007), and the recall of the laboring woman can get lost in the excitement or fear of the moment.

Progressive cervical change is the hallmark of labor; persistent uterine contractions in the absence of cervical change should not be considered labor and should be treated as preparation for labor. Maternal fatigue caused by persistent irregular contractions can have a profound impact on the woman's labor energy levels and may influence the clinician to intervene when labor has not yet begun in earnest.

Client History and Chart Review:
Components of the History to Consider
- LMP, EDC
- Gravida, parity, gestational age
- Previous labor patterns in multipara
- Current contraction pattern
  - Onset of contractions
    - ◆ Intermittent contractions
    - ◆ Presence of regular contractions
    - ◆ Associated cervical change
  - Maternal response to contractions
  - Status of membranes
  - Associated factors and symptoms
    - ◆ Increase in vaginal discharge
    - ◆ Mucous plug
    - ◆ Spotting
    - ◆ Recent intercourse or orgasm
    - ◆ Use of alternative uterotonics
- Maternal and fetal well-being
  - Sleep, rest, and activity
  - Nutrition and fluid intake
  - Fetal activity

Physical Examination:
Components of the Physical Exam
to Consider
- Fetal vital signs and well-being
  - FHT
  - Fetal movement
- Maternal well-being
  - Vital signs, including temperature
  - Abdominal examination
    - ◆ EFW
    - ◆ Fetal presentation and position

- Pelvic examination for progressive changes in
  - Cervical effacement
  - Cervical dilation
  - Descent of presenting part
  - Status of membranes
  - Pelvimetry
- Assess hydration
  - Urine output, color, specific gravity
  - Skin turgor
- Signs of decreased coping ability
  - Excessive anxiety
  - Fear
  - Tension
- Evaluate for signs of exhaustion

Clinical Impression:
Differential Diagnoses and Code Groups to Consider
Additional suffix may apply (ICD9data.com, 2007)

- Prolonged prodromal labor (ICD-9 codes 662.0)
  - False labor (ICD-9 codes 644.1)
- Dysfunctional labor (ICD-9 codes 661)
  - Uterine inertia (ICD-9 codes 661.0)
  - Malpresentation or malposition of the fetus (ICD-9 codes 652)
  - Obstructed labor (ICD-9 codes 660)

Diagnostic Testing:
Diagnostic Tests and Procedures to Consider

- Fetal evaluation
  - NST
  - Fetal kick counts
  - Amniotic fluid color if ROM
  - Biophysical profile (BPP)/Amniotic fluid index (AFI) as indicated
- Maternal evaluation
  - Urine for specific gravity
  - Evaluation of contractions
    - Palpation
    - External electronic monitoring
    - Intrauterine pressure catheter (IUPC) if membranes ruptured
- Preoperative laboratory tests if concerned about CPD

Providing Treatment:
Therapeutic Measures to Consider

- Discharge home from unit (Greulich & Tarrant, 2007)
  - Instructions for rest, hydration, and nourishment
  - Return for active labor
  - Otherwise keep next prenatal appointment
- Therapeutic rest
  - May stop contractions due to uterine irritability
  - Allows rest and restoration
    - Benadryl 50 mg PO
    - Ambien 10 mg PO
    - Morphine sulfate 10–20 mg IM or SQ (with or without Vistaril 50 mg IM)
    - Vistaril 50–75 mg IM
    - Demerol 25–50 mg IM (with or without Phenergan 25 mg)
- Hydration, oral or IV
- Stimulation of labor
  - Oxytocin stimulation
  - Artificial ROM

Providing Treatment:
Alternative Measures to Consider

- Watchful waiting (Greulich & Tarrant, 2007)
- Provide safe environment to allow for
  - Rest, including intermittent naps
  - Hydration and adequate nutrition
- Warm bath/hydrotherapy
- Massage
- Strong chamomile or hops tea to facilitate rest (Foster, 1996)
- Position changes to facilitate optimal fetal positioning
- Labor stimulation
  - Membrane sweeping
  - Sexual intercourse or orgasm
  - Nipple stimulation
  - Enemas
  - Castor oil
    - 2–4 oz PO
    - Repeat in 1–2 hours if necessary

- ▪ Homeopathic caulophyllum 60×
- ▪ Evening primrose oil
  - ◆ Apply directly to the cervix or take orally

Providing Support:
Education and Support Measures to Consider
- Listen to maternal concerns
  - ▪ Explore fears related to labor, birth, parenting
  - ▪ Provide reassurance
- Work to provide a safe-feeling birth environment
- Discuss options with woman and her significant other(s)
  - ▪ Review stages of labor
  - ▪ Rest
  - ▪ Stimulation of contractions
  - ▪ Potential change in birth plans
    - ◆ Location
    - ◆ Provider(s)

Follow-up Care:
Follow-up Measures to Consider
- Document
- Update documentation after each evaluation
- Reevaluate every 1–2 hours for
  - ▪ Response to therapy
  - ▪ Progressive labor signs
    - ◆ Strength and duration of contractions
    - ◆ Application of presenting part to cervix
    - ◆ Dilation and descent
    - ◆ Positioning of fetal vertex
    - ◆ Status of membranes
  - ▪ Developing maternal and fetal complications
    - ◆ Hourglass membranes
    - ◆ Caput formation
    - ◆ Swelling of cervix
    - ◆ Maternal exhaustion
    - ◆ Obstructed labor
    - ◆ Infection
    - ◆ Fetal distress
- If therapeutic rest is not successful
  - ▪ Consider stimulation of labor
  - ▪ Reevaluate potential causes

- If progress does not occur evaluate for evidence of
  - ▪ Ineffective uterine contraction
  - ▪ Suboptimal fetal presentation or position
  - ▪ Fetopelvic disproportion

Collaborative Practice:
Consider Consultation or Referral
- OB/GYN services
  - ▪ Diagnosis of prolonged latent phase
  - ▪ Lack of successful response to therapy
  - ▪ As needed for change of birth location
- For diagnosis or treatment outside the midwife's scope of practice

CARE OF THE WOMAN WITH PREMATURE RUPTURE OF MEMBRANES

Key Clinical Information
Premature rupture of membranes (PROM) is defined as the rupture of membranes that happens before the onset of labor, occurring in about 8% of term pregnancies (Marowitz & Jordan, 2007). Ninety percent of women with PROM enter labor by 24 hours post-ROM. When there is greater than 24 hours between ROM and delivery of the infant, prolonged ROM is said to occur. Preterm PROM is ROM that occurs before term. Complications of PROM include complications related to preterm birth after PROM, fetal distress related to cord compression, and fetal infection. Maternal complications include maternal intra-amniotic infection, increased risk of cesarean delivery, and postpartum endometritis (ACOG, 1998; Varney et al., 2004).

Client History and Chart Review:
Components of the History to Consider
- LMP, EDC, gestational age
- Relevant prenatal and maternity history
  - ▪ GBS status
  - ▪ Complications of current or previous pregnancy
  - ▪ Previous PROM
  - ▪ Sexually transmitted infection test results

- Current signs and symptoms
  - Onset of symptoms
  - Duration of symptoms
  - Amount, color, consistency of vaginal leakage
  - Last sexual activity
  - Presence of warning signs
    - Fever or chills
    - Palpitations
    - Uterine tenderness
    - Flank tenderness
- Presence of risk factors for PROM (Varney et al., 2004)
  - Nonvertex presentation
  - Previous pregnancy with PROM
  - Chorioamnionitis
  - Polyhydramnios
  - Multiple gestation
  - Vaginal GBS or other pathogenic vaginal flora
  - Smoking > ½ pack per day
  - Nutritional deficiencies
  - Family history of PROM
  - Cervical procedure
    - Loop electrocautery excision procedure (LEEP)
    - Conization
    - Cryosurgery
  - Occupational fatigue in nulliparas

Physical Examination:
Components of the Physical Exam to Consider
- Vital signs with temperature every 1–2 hours
  - Maternal fever (temperature > 32.2°C [99°F])
  - Maternal or fetal tachycardia (maternal heart rate > 100, FHR > 160)
- Abdominal examination
  - Amniotic fluid volume/ballottement
  - Presence of contractions
  - EFW
  - Determine fetal presentation, lie
  - Frequent evaluation of FHR
  - Palpation for uterine tenderness
- Sterile speculum examination
  - Visualization of leakage of amniotic fluid
  - Visualization of cervix

- Collection of specimen(s) for examination
  - Ferning
  - Nitrazine
  - GBS culture or screen
- Sterile digital vaginal examination (defer until labor begins)
  - Cervical dilation
  - Effacement
  - Station
  - Confirm presentation
  - Rule out cord prolapse

Clinical Impression:
Differential Diagnoses and Code Groups
to Consider
Additional suffix may apply (ICD9data.com, 2007)
- Premature rupture of membranes (ICD-9 codes 658.1)
- Urinary incontinence (ICD-9 codes 625.6)
- Urinary tract infection (ICD-9 codes 646.6)
- Increased vaginal secretions due to
  - Pregnancy (ICD-9 codes V72)
  - Vaginitis (ICD-9 codes 616)
  - Sexually transmitted infection (ICD-9 codes V22 and 099, 647.0–647.2)

Diagnostic Testing:
Diagnostic Tests and Procedures
to Consider
- Vaginal fluid evaluation
  - Nitrazine or pH testing (pH 7.0–7.7)
  - Ferning
  - Wet prep and KOH
- Cultures as indicated
  - If expectant management planned
    - GBS culture of vagina and rectum
    - Chlamydia/gonorrhea status
- Ultrasound evaluation
  - Oligohydramnios/AFI
  - Biophysical profile
  - Guidance for amniocentesis
- Amniocentesis for fetal pulmonary maturity testing

- CBC with differential
  - Maternal leukocytosis (WBC > 16,000 with no labor)
- Urine for urinalysis and culture & sensitivity (C & S)
  - Clean catch
  - Straight catheter specimen
- Fetal surveillance
  - NST if > 32 weeks gestation
  - Daily fetal movement counts
  - Biophysical profile/AFI

Providing Treatment:
Therapeutic Measures to Consider
- Bed rest recommended for
  - Nonvertex presentation
  - Preterm PROM
- Antibiotic prophylaxis (see Care of the Woman with Group B Streptococcus)
- Expectant management based on gestational age (ACOG, 1998)
  - Term
    - Labor and birth occur within 28 hours in 95% of cases
    - Observation of 24–72 hours acceptable per ACOG (1998)
    - Avoid digital examinations until labor well established
    - Induction of labor (see Care of the Woman Undergoing Induction or Augmentation of Labor)
  - Preterm with no additional complications
    - Conservative management preferred
    - Birth generally occurs within 7 days
    - Glucocorticoids to enhance fetal lung maturity
    - Tocolysis (rarely)
    - Transport to center with newborn special care

Providing Treatment:
Alternative Measures to Consider
- Watchful waiting
  - No internal examinations
  - Temperature every 2 hours

- Daily CBC
- Adequate hydration and nutrition
- Await onset of labor
- Stimulation of labor with natural remedies (see Care of the Woman Undergoing Induction or Augmentation of Labor)

Providing Support:
Education and Support Measures to Consider
- Discuss significance of PROM
  - Anticipated fetal outcome for gestational age
  - Anticipated newborn care
  - Risks and benefits of options for care
  - Maternal risk with PROM
    - Ascending intrauterine infection
    - Increased incidence of intervention
  - Fetal risks with PROM
    - Umbilical cord compression
    - Ascending or preexisting infection
  - Potential need for medical care
  - Potential for change in
    - Birth plan
    - Location of birth
    - Birth attendant
- Signs and symptoms of
  - Chorioamnionitis
  - Neonatal sepsis
  - Postpartum endometritis

Follow-up Care:
Follow-up Measures to Consider
- Review and document results of
  - Maternal testing
  - Fetal surveillance
    - Fetal kick counts
    - NST
    - Biophysical profile
    - Serial AFI
    - FHR
      - Intermittent auscultation of FHT
      - Continuous fetal monitoring
      - Cervical ripening or induction of labor (see Care of the Woman

Undergoing Induction or Augmentation of Labor)

- ▪ Essential if amnionitis suspected
- ▪ ROM > 24–72 hours
- • Reassess for signs or symptoms of complications
  - ▪ Maternal fever
  - ▪ Abdominal tenderness
  - ▪ Nonreassuring FHT patterns
    - ◆ Tachycardia
    - ◆ Bradycardia
    - ◆ Late or severe variable decelerations
    - ◆ Decreased variability
- • Update plan as changes occur
- • Expedite birth if
  - ▪ Symptoms of infection develop
  - ▪ Fetal compromise occurs
  - ▪ Maternal preference
- • Evaluate postpartum for
  - ▪ Endometritis
  - ▪ Other infection
  - ▪ Newborn sepsis
- • Offer time for discussion and processing
  - ▪ Labor and birth events
  - ▪ Outcomes
  - ▪ Potential effect on future pregnancies

Collaborative Practice:
Consider Consultation or Referral

- • OB/GYN services
  - ▪ Confirmed PROM with
    - ◆ Delay in onset of labor
    - ◆ Signs or symptoms of
      - ➤ Infection
      - ➤ Cord prolapse
      - ➤ Fetal compromise
- • Pediatric services
  - ▪ Onset of labor with fetal or maternal infection
  - ▪ For birth as indicated by fetal status
  - ▪ Newborn evaluation after prolonged ROM
- • For diagnosis or treatment outside the midwife's scope of practice

CARE OF THE WOMAN WITH SHOULDER DYSTOCIA

Key Clinical Information

Midwives and other maternity care providers consider shoulder dystocia to be one of the most frightening complications they encounter (Ramirez & Frye, 2004). Shoulder dystocia is defined as occurring when the fetal shoulders fail to deliver despite routine maneuvers (Naef & Martin, 1995). It is associated with significant fetal and maternal morbidity, perinatal mortality, and costly litigation. The incidence of shoulder dystocia is reported to be less than 0.6–1.4% (ACOG, 2002c; Jevitt, 2005). The potentially profound adverse effects of shoulder dystocia require all obstetric care providers to be quick to diagnose and respond to this condition. It only takes 4–5 minutes from birth of the head to birth of the shoulders before severe acidosis, fetal injury, and death can occur (Basket, 2002).

This uncommon obstetric emergency requires the midwife to be skilled in rapid identification of shoulder dystocia and specific interventions to remediate this situation. Mental preparedness includes knowing when to notify additional members of the obstetric team, which may include midwives, OB/GYN physicians, maternity and pediatric nurses, pediatricians, and anesthesiologists, for immediate action. Nearly half of all shoulder dystocia occurs in infants who weigh less than 4000 g, so it is not the infant's size alone that creates the difficulty. Rather, it is the fit of this particular infant through the pelvis of this particular mother. Studies have been unable to reliably predict which mothers and infants will be at risk for shoulder dystocia (ACOG, 2002c).

Shoulder dystocia may be anticipated with a long second stage and the presence of the "turtle sign" after the head emerges. The head extends with difficulty, and the chin remains snug against the perineum. Restitution does not occur. The shoulders may be wedged in the pelvis—referred to as "tight shoulders"—or they may be impacted above the pelvic brim. Prompt identification of shoulder dystocia should result in the rapid initiation of systematic maneuvers to deliver the infant. Shoulder dystocia may result in significant damage to the infant, such as brachial plexus injury, fracture of the clavicle, hypoxia, or death. Traction on the infant has been associated with increased risk of newborn injury (Varney et al., 2004).

Client History and Chart Review:
Components of the History to Consider
- LMP, EDC, gestational age
- Maternal height/weight
- Documented clinical pelvimetry
- Potential risk factors for shoulder dystocia
  - Maternal diabetes
  - History of large infants
  - Maternal obesity
  - Postdate pregnancy
  - Large fetus, by palpation or ultrasound
  - History of prior difficult delivery
  - History of prior shoulder dystocia
  - CPD (ACOG, 2002c)
  - Dysfunctional labor
  - Prolonged second stage

Physical Examination:
Components of the Physical Exam to Consider
- Abdominal examination in labor
  - Fetal presentation and position
  - Flexion of head at pelvic brim
  - Estimate fetal weight with onset of labor
- Pelvic examination(s) during labor
  - Progression of cervical dilation
  - Rate of descent
  - Maternal tissue elasticity
  - Pelvimetry
- At delivery
  - Slow progression of extension
  - Retraction of head ("turtle sign")
  - Failure to restitute
  - Suffusion, discoloration of infant's face
  - Need for one or more maneuvers to deliver infant

Clinical Impression:
Differential Diagnoses and Code Groups
to Consider
Additional suffix may apply (ICD9data.com, 2007)
- Shoulder dystocia (ICD-9 codes 660.4)
- Short cord (ICD-9 codes 663.4)
- Fetal anomaly (ICD-9 codes 760–779)

Diagnostic Testing:
Diagnostic Tests and Procedures to Consider
- Ultrasound for EFW
  - Can be inaccurate by > 1–2 lbs
  - Size is often not the issue
- Preoperative laboratory tests

Providing Treatment:
Therapeutic Measures to Consider
- Engage mother in cooperating
- Mother on back
  - McRoberts maneuver (knees to shoulders)
    - Advantages
      - Alters angle of inclination of symphysis
      - Flattens sacrum
      - Gives midwife most room to work
      - Reduces amount of traction required to effect birth
      - May decrease traction-related fetal injury
    - Disadvantages
      - Requires two assistants
  - Request firm suprapubic pressure
- Encourage maternal pushing efforts
- Attempt birth
  - With gentle traction on head
  - If descent occurs, assist with birth
    - Fingers on both shoulders
    - Maintain arms in close contact with trunk
- If birth does not occur
  - Stop maternal pushing efforts
  - With dominant hand in vagina check position of shoulders
    - Place hand on infant's back

- ◆ Palpate anterior axillary crease
  - ➤ ⚠ Do *not* pull with fingers in axilla
  - ➤ Use firm traction on the suprascapular bones to
    - ❭ Decrease the bisacromial diameter
    - ❭ Attempt rotation of anterior shoulder into pelvis
      - ★ Use firm gentle pressure
      - ★ Rotate infant's back toward symphysis
      - ★ Rotate shoulders into the oblique
    - ❭ As anterior shoulder rotates
    - ❭ Move client to hands and knees as needed
    - ❭ Maintain infant's position
    - ❭ Use gentle outward traction
    - ❭ This should bring posterior shoulder into the pelvis
      - ★ Deliver posterior arm as needed
    - ❭ Encourage maternal pushing efforts
      - ★ "Walk" shoulders out using both hands
      - ★ Traction on suprascapular bones
      - ★ Keep arms close to body
      - ★ Use gentle firm outward traction
    - ❭ Rotate infant manually from side to side
      - ★ Back always moving anteriorly
      - ★ "Corkscrew" the body out (Woods screw maneuver)
- • Mother on hands and knees for birth
  - ▪ Flex legs so belly rests on legs
  - ▪ Knees to shoulders
  - ▪ Deliver posterior arm first
- • Tub birth
  - ▪ Have mother stand and lean over tub
    - ◆ This may release impaction

- ▪ Assist as you would for mother on hands and knees, or
- ▪ Have mother exit tub
  - ◆ Move to hands and knees, or McRoberts maneuver
  - ◆ Continue as above
- • For severe unrelieved shoulder dystocia, consider
  - ▪ Alternative positioning
  - ▪ ☏ Call for STAT obstetric and pediatric assistance
  - ▪ Fracture of clavicle
  - ▪ Empty bladder with straight catheter
  - ▪ Enlarge or cut episiotomy
  - ▪ Rule out other causes of dystocia
    - ◆ Direct palpation of pelvic contents
    - ◆ Fetal anomalies
    - ◆ Extremely short cord
  - ▪ Zavenelli maneuver (ACOG, 2002c; Varney et al., 2004)
    - ◆ Replacement of head in vagina
    - ◆ Reverse process of extension
    - ◆ Follow with immediate cesarean section
- • Prepare for
  - ▪ Full neonatal resuscitation (American Academy of Pediatrics/American Heart Association, 2006)
  - ▪ Immediate postpartum hemorrhage
- • Cesarean section for documented macrosomia
- • Consider cesarean delivery with EFW
  - ◆ Over 5000 g in normoglycemic mothers
  - ◆ Over 4500 g in diabetic mothers (ACOG, 2002c)
  - ◆ ⚠ All methods of estimating fetal weights are imprecise (ACOG, 2002c)

Providing Treatment:
Alternative Measures to Consider
- • Gaskin maneuver (Bruner et al., 1998)
  - ▪ Rotate mother to hands and knees
  - ▪ Rotate in direction infant is facing
  - ▪ Alters pelvic geometry

- Advantages
  - ◆ Position change may resolve impaction
  - ◆ Gravity may facilitate delivery
- Disadvantages
  - ◆ Cannot use suprapubic pressure
  - ◆ Limited access to infant
  - ◆ May exaggerate impaction
- Squatting
  - Advantages
    - ◆ Position change may resolve impaction
    - ◆ Results in a wider pubic (outlet) angle
  - Disadvantages
    - ◆ Cannot use suprapubic pressure
    - ◆ May decrease inlet dimensions
    - ◆ Limited access to infant

Providing Support:
Education and Support Measures to Consider

- Discuss potential for difficult birth with mother who has
  - Documented macrosomia
  - EFW more than 1 lb larger than largest previous infant
- Follow-up after birth with discussion
  - Regarding care given
  - Infant well-being
  - Maternal feelings about
    - ◆ Complications
    - ◆ Interventions
    - ◆ Outcomes
    - ◆ Labor and birth
- Review signs of
  - Postpartum endometritis
  - Postpartum depression

Follow-up Care:
Follow-up Measures to Consider

- Immediately after birth
  - Provide newborn resuscitation as necessary
  - Evaluate infant for birth injury
  - Observe for postpartum hemorrhage after delivery
  - Evaluate for maternal injury

- Document
  - ⚠ Birth details in delivery note
    - ◆ Physical findings at birth
    - ◆ Identification of shoulder dystocia
    - ◆ Maneuvers used and their effects
    - ◆ Note injury to mother or infant
    - ◆ Note movement of infant's arms
  - Consultations requested during birth
- Seek opportunity for peer support
  - Peer review (nondiscoverable)
  - Case presentation or discussion
  - Informal support

Collaborative Practice:
Consider Consultation or Referral

- OB/GYN services (Sinclair, 2004; Varney et al., 2004)
  - Potential for shoulder dystocia anticipated
  - Diagnosis of shoulder dystocia
- Pediatric service
  - In anticipation of neonatal resuscitation
  - For newborn evaluation after difficult birth
- For diagnosis or treatment outside the midwife's scope of practice

CARE OF THE WOMAN UNDERGOING VACUUM-ASSISTED BIRTH

Key Clinical Information

Vacuum-assisted birth carries with it significant risks to mother and baby and increases liability for the midwife (ACOG, 2000a; Clark, 2005). The benefits of using the vacuum extractor to aid in the birth of the infant should clearly outweigh the potential risks associated with this procedure. Midwives who assist with birth using outlet vacuum extraction should be educated and trained in indications and contraindications, techniques, and complications associated with the use of the device.

Client History and Chart Review:
Components of the History to Consider

- Verify LMP, EDC, and term gestation

- Relevant prenatal and obstetric history
  - Progress of labor, including second stage
  - Fetal and maternal response to labor
  - Review pelvimetry
- Presence of any contraindications to vacuum-assisted birth (ACNM, 2003)
  - Weak or infrequent uterine contraction
  - Vertex not well engaged
  - CPD
  - Premature infant ($<$ 37 weeks)
  - Suspected macrosomia
  - Nonvertex presentation
  - Uncooperative client
  - Poor expulsive effort
- Indications for vacuum-assisted birth (ACOG, 2000a)
  - Prolonged second stage
    - $>$ 3 hours for nullipara
    - $>$ 2 hours for multipara
  - Nonreassuring FHR pattern
  - Maternal exhaustion
    - Not indicated for midwife exhaustion (Clark, 2005)

Physical Examination:
Components of the Physical Exam
to Consider
- Abdominal examination
  - Fetal lie, presentation, position
  - EFW
  - Presence of adequate, effective, regular contractions
- Pelvic examination
  - Dilation must be complete
  - Station
    - Vertex visible at introitus = outlet delivery
    - +2 station = midforceps delivery
  - Physician management recommended
  - Vacuum extraction versus forceps versus cesarean section
  - Presence of caput or marked molding
  - Increases risk of fetal trauma
  - Assess fetal presentation and position

Clinical Impression:
Differential Diagnoses and Code Groups
to Consider
Additional suffix may apply (ICD9data.com, 2007)
- Vacuum-assisted birth for
  - Prolonged second stage (ICD-9 codes 662.2)
  - Fetal distress (ICD-9 codes 656.3)
  - Maternal exhaustion (ICD-9 codes 669.8)

Diagnostic Testing:
Diagnostic Tests and Procedures to Consider
- Preoperative laboratory tests
- Evaluate effectiveness of uterine contractions
  - Palpation
  - Electronic fetal monitoring
- Evaluate fetal response via FHR
  - Auscultation
  - Electronic fetal monitoring

Providing Treatment:
Therapeutic Measures to Consider
- Oxytocin stimulation to improve contractions
- Vacuum-assisted birth procedure
  - Empty bladder and rectum
  - Consider local anesthesia
  - Consider episiotomy
    - May increase risk of third- or fourth-degree laceration
    - Mediolateral episiotomy may give more room
  - Verify position of vertex
  - Apply vacuum cup to posterior fontanel
  - Verify that no maternal tissues are under cup rim
    - Request suction
  - 4 in Hg or 100 mm Hg between contractions
  - 15–23 in Hg or 500 mm Hg with contractions

Do not allow vacuum to remain at maximum levels for more than 10 accrued minutes

Do not follow failed vacuum with forceps attempt: success rate low, morbidity rate high

- Apply gentle steady traction
  - With contractions only
  - Follow curve of Carus
- ⚠ Discontinue attempts to assist birth with vacuum if
  - Cup disengages three times
  - Scalp trauma visible after cup disengages
  - No progress after three attempts at traction
  - 15–30 minutes with no success
  - Birth has not occurred within 10 accrued minutes of maximum suction

Providing Treatment:
Alternative Measures to Consider
- Assess for maternal and fetal well-being
  - Be patient
  - Allow rest period
  - Provide for adequate hydration and nutrition
- Continue maternal pushing efforts
  - Encourage voiding
  - Push only with urge
- Vigilant assessment of maternal and fetal status
  - Vital signs
  - Fetal descent
- Position changes
  - Side-lying
  - McRoberts position
  - Lithotomy with leg support
    - Feet should push against fixed object
    - Arms should pull
    - Back should be as flat as possible
    - Use of squatting bar helpful
  - Squatting
  - Birthing stool
  - Hands and knees
  - Floating in birthing tub

Providing Support:
Education and Support Measures to Consider
- ▽ Discuss with client and family
  - Concerns related to slow progress
  - Options for care
  - Recommendations and indications

- Vacuum-assisted birth procedure
  - Discuss risks and benefits with client
    - Risk of fetal trauma
      - Cephalohematoma
      - Intracranial trauma
      - Shoulder dystocia
      - Ecchymosis, abrasions (ACOG, 2000a)
    - Risk of maternal trauma
      - Third- or fourth-degree laceration
      - Sulcus tears
      - Possible need for cesarean birth
    - Benefits
      - Vaginal birth of infant
      - Faster than forceps or cesarean section
      - Less risk of fetal trauma than forceps
  - Depends on skill of operator and force used
    - May decrease need for cesarean section

Follow-up Care:
Follow-up Measures to Consider
- Prepare for potential
  - Shoulder dystocia
  - Postpartum hemorrhage
  - Third- or fourth-degree laceration
  - Newborn injury
  - Newborn resuscitation
- Document (see Procedure Note in Chapter 1)
- Evaluate for maternal or neonatal injury
  - Examine vagina carefully for lacerations
  - Examine infant carefully for injury
- Discuss birth with mother and family
  - Allow exploration of feelings
  - Review indications for assisted birth

Collaborative Practice:
Criteria to Consider for Consultation
or Referral
- OB/GYN services
  - Indications for vacuum extraction
  - Maternal indications, cesarean section may be necessary

- Pediatric services
  - Fetal distress
  - Fetal injury
  - For evaluation of delayed signs of injury
- For diagnosis or treatment outside the midwife's scope of practice

CARE OF THE WOMAN DURING VAGINAL BIRTH AFTER CESAREAN

Key Clinical Information

Vaginal birth after cesarean (VBAC) provides carefully selected women with an alternative to surgical delivery of their infant. Successful VBAC results in significant benefits and fewer risks for women and infants than repeat cesarean birth. Midwives are qualified to care for women planning VBAC if appropriate arrangements for medical consultation and emergency care are in place (ACNM, 2000). Application of the midwifery model of care increases successful VBAC rates and decreases primary cesarean section rates and the need for subsequent VBAC.

Uterine ruptures following cesarean occur at a documented rate of approximately 0.5–1%. This rate is increased in women with a single-layer uterine closure, two or more previous cesarean births, an interdelivery interval of 24 months or less, history of postoperative fever or infection, and labor augmented or induced with oxytocin (Shipp, 1999). When uterine rupture does occur, outcomes are improved with the immediate availability of skilled surgical services.

Client History and Chart Review: Components of the History to Consider

- ▽ Obtain operative records for previous cesarean section
  - Indication for primary cesarean section
  - Gestational age with prior cesarean section
  - Type of uterine incision
  - Type of uterine closure
  - Postoperative course (Ethicon, 2004)
- Review current pregnancy course

- Positive predictors for the VBAC candidate
  - Nonrepeating cause
  - Client motivated for vaginal birth
  - Previous vaginal birth
  - Vertex presentation
  - Bishop's score > 4
  - Two-layer uterine closure
  - No history of postoperative fever or infection
  - Maternal age < 30
  - 24+ months since previous cesarean section
  - Spontaneous onset of labor
  - Progressive labor
- Contraindication to VBAC
  - Classical or midline uterine incision
- Negative predictors for the VBAC candidate
  - Nonvertex presentation of infant
  - Two or more previous cesareans
  - Single-layer uterine closure
  - Maternal age > 30
  - Less than 18 months since previous cesarean section
  - Nonprogressive labor (ACOG, 2004a)

Physical Examination: Components of the Physical Exam to Consider

- Comprehensive labor evaluation
  - Clinical pelvimetry with history of cephalopelvic disproportion (CPD) or failure to progress (FTP)
  - Estimated fetal weight (EFW)
  - Presentation, position, engagement
  - Maternal and fetal vital signs
- Reevaluate progress at frequent intervals
- Maternal and fetal response to labor
  - Contraction pattern
  - Cervical change
    - ◆ > 4 cm has > 86% success rate of VBAC
    - ◆ > 75% effaced has 81% success rate of VBAC (King, 2004)
  - Fetal descent

- Signs of uterine rupture
  - Fetal bradycardia or non-reassuring FHR
  - Maternal tachycardia
  - Abdominal pain may or may not be present (ACOG, 2004a)

Clinical Impression:
Differential Diagnoses and Code Groups
to Consider
Additional suffix may apply (ICD9data.com, 2007)
- VBAC candidate (ICD-9 codes 654.2)
- Cesarean section (ICD-9 codes 669.7)

Diagnostic Testing:
Diagnostic Tests and Procedures
to Consider
- Preoperative laboratory tests
  - CBC
  - Type and screen
- Continuous observation of maternal and fetal status
  - 1:1 nurse or midwife care with auscultation or
  - External fetal monitor or
  - Internal fetal monitor

Providing Treatment:
Therapeutic Measures to Consider
- Evaluate for onset of progressive labor
- Provide a supportive labor and birthing environment
- Limit invasive examinations or procedures
- Oral intake
  - NPO
  - Ice chips
  - Clear liquids
- IV access
  - Saline lock
  - Lactated Ringers at 125 cc per hour
- Maternal and fetal evaluation of well-being
- Medications
  - ⚠ Cytotec contraindicated for use with scarred uterus

- Oxytocin as indicated
  - May facilitate vaginal birth due to uterine inertia
  - Overstimulation may increase risk of rupture (ACOG, 2004a)
  - Pain relief as needed (see Care of the Woman in First-Stage Labor)

Providing Treatment:
Alternative Measures to Consider
- Facilitate physiologic labor
  - Ambulation
  - Hydrotherapy
  - Positioning
  - Doula support
  - Adequate hydration and nutrition
- Foster maternal autonomy
  - Provide a supportive labor environment

Providing Support:
Education and Support Measures to Consider
- 📋 Discuss options with client and family
  - VBAC versus repeat cesarean section
  - Surgical coverage options
  - Location(s) for birth
  - Options for labor care and support
- Obtain signed informed consent
  - Success rate 60–80% (ACOG, 2004a)
  - Risk of catastrophic uterine rupture
    - Low transverse uterine incision 0.19–0.8% (Varney et al., 2004)
    - Higher with any other type of incision
    - Risk of maternal or fetal death with catastrophic rupture
  - Risks, benefits, and alternatives to VBAC
  - Discussion regarding facility/practice parameters for VBAC
- Anticipated care of VBAC women in labor
  - Labor procedures (e.g., IV, laboratory tests)
  - Average length of time for urgent cesarean section
    - At facility
    - If transport required

Follow-up Care:
Follow-up Measures to Consider

- Consult OB/GYN of client choice prenatally
- Uterine scar dehiscence or rupture
  - May result in fetal and/or maternal death
  - May occur in labor or during birth
  - Access surgical services immediately
  - Ensure IV access
    - Provide fluid replacement
    - Order blood
  - Treat shock
- ⚠ Document
  - Review of previous cesarean section operative notes
  - Discussions with client and family
  - Client preference
  - Informed choice and consent
  - Treatment of complications
  - Consultations
- Update notes frequently, especially in labor

Collaborative Practice:
Criteria to Consider for Consultation or Referral

- OB/GYN services
  - Previous incision that is not low transverse
  - Planned repeat cesarean section
  - Planned VBAC
  - STAT for client in labor with
    - Symptoms of uterine rupture
      - Nonreassuring fetal status is the most common indication of uterine rupture (King, 2004)
    - Evidence of developing dystocia or obstruction
    - Demand for repeat cesarean section
- Pediatric services
  - Nonreassuring FHR
- For diagnosis or treatment outside the midwife's scope of practice

REFERENCES

Albers, L. (2007). The evidence for physiologic management of the active phase of the first stage of labor. *Journal of Midwifery & Women's Health*, 52, 207–215.

Albers, L., Schiff, M., & Gorwoda, J. G. (1996). The length of active labor in normal pregnancies. *Obstetrics & Gynecology*, 87, 355–359.

American Academy of Pediatrics/American Heart Association. (2006). *Textbook of neonatal resuscitation* (5th ed.). Elk Grove, IL: American Academy of Pediatrics.

American College of Nurse-Midwives (ACNM). (1997). Clinical bulletin no. 2. Early-onset group B strep infection in newborns: prevention and prophylaxis. *Journal of Nurse-Midwifery*, 42, 403–408.

American College of Nurse-Midwives (ACNM). (1998). *Position statement: The certified nurse-midwife/certified midwife as first assistant at surgery*. Washington, DC: Author.

American College of Nurse-Midwives (ACNM). (2000). *Position statement: Vaginal birth after cesarean delivery*. Washington, DC: Author.

American College of Nurse-Midwives (ACNM). (2003). *Vacuum assisted birth in midwifery practice* (2nd ed.). Washington, DC: Author.

American College of Nurse-Midwives (ACNM). (2005). *Position statement: Elective primary cesarean section*. Washington, DC: Author.

American College of Nurse-Midwives (ACNM). (2006). *The midwife as surgical first assistant handbook*. Washington, DC: Author.

American College of Obstetricians and Gynecologists (ACOG). (1998). Practice bulletin #1: Premature rupture of membranes. In *2006 compendium of selected publications*. Washington, DC: Author.

American College of Obstetricians and Gynecologists (ACOG). (2000a). Practice bulletin #17: Operative vaginal delivery. In *2006 compendium of selected publications*. Washington, DC: Author.

American College of Obstetricians and Gynecologists (ACOG). (2000b). Practice bulletin #13: External cephalic version. In *2006 compendium of selected publications*. Washington, DC: Author.

American College of Obstetricians and Gynecologists (ACOG). (2002a). Committee opinion #273: Antenatal corticosteroid therapy for fetal maturation. In *2006 compendium of selected publications*. Washington, DC: Author.

American College of Obstetricians and Gynecologists (ACOG). (2002b). Practice bulletin #33: Diagnosis and management of pre-eclampsia and eclampsia. In *2006 compendium of selected publications*. Washington, DC: Author.

American College of Obstetricians and Gynecologists (ACOG). (2002c). Practice bulletin #40: Shoulder dystocia. In *2006 compendium of selected publications.* Washington, DC: Author.

American College of Obstetricians and Gynecologists (ACOG). (2003). Practice bulletin #43: Management of preterm labor. In *2006 compendium of selected publications.* Washington, DC: Author.

American College of Obstetricians and Gynecologists (ACOG). (2004a). Practice bulletin #54: Vaginal birth after cesarean. In *2006 compendium of selected publications.* Washington, DC: Author.

American College of Obstetricians and Gynecologists (ACOG). (2004b). Practice Bulletin #55: Management of post-term pregnancy. In *2006 compendium of selected publications.* Washington, DC: Author.

American College of Obstetricians and Gynecologists (ACOG). (2004c). Education bulletin #56: Multiple gestation: complicated twin, triplet, and high-order multifetal pregnancy. In *2006 compendium of selected publications.* Washington, DC: Author.

American College of Obstetricians and Gynecologists (ACOG). (2004d). Committee opinion #265: Mode of singleton breech delivery. In *2006 compendium of selected publications.* Washington, DC: Author.

American College of Obstetricians and Gynecologists (ACOG). (2005). Practice bulletin #70: Intrapartum fetal heart rate monitoring. In *2006 compendium of selected publications.* Washington, DC: Author.

American College of Obstetricians and Gynecologists (ACOG). (2006). Committee opinion #346: Amnio-infusion does not prevent meconium aspiration syndrome. Washington, DC: Author.

Andrews, C., & Andrews, E. (2004). Physical theory as a basis for successful rotation of fetal malpositions and conversion of fetal malpresentations. *Biological Research for Nursing,* 6(2).

Basket, T. F. (2002). Shoulder dystocia, best practice and research. *Clinical Obstetrics and Gynecology,* 16, 57–68.

Blackburn, S. T., & Loper, D. L. (1992). *Maternal, fetal and neonatal physiology: a clinical perspective.* Philadelphia: W. B. Saunders.

Bishop, E. H. (1964). Pelvic scoring for elective induction. *Obstetrics and Gynecology,* 24, 267.

Braddy, C. M., & Files, J. A. (2007). Female genital mutilation: cultural awareness and clinical considerations. *Journal of Midwifery & Women's Health,* 52, 158–163.

Brucker, M. C. (2001). Management of the third stage of labor: an evidence-based approach. *Journal of Midwifery & Women's Health,* 46, 381–392.

Bruner, J., Drummond, S., Meenan, A. L., & Gaskin, I. M. (1998). The all fours maneuver for reducing shoulder dystocia. *Journal of Reproductive Medicine,* 43, 439–443.

Bujold, E., Bujold, C., Hamilton, E. F., Harel, F., & Gauthier, R. J. (2002). The impact of single-layer or double-layer closure on uterine rupture. *American Journal of Obstetrics and Gynecology,* 186, 1326–1330.

Byrne, B., & Morrison, J. (2004). Preterm birth. In F. Godlee (Ed.). *Clinical evidence concise* (pp. 392–394). London: BMJ.

Cardini, F., & Weixin, H. (1998). Moxibustion for correction of breech presentation: a randomized controlled trial. *Journal of the American Medical Association,* 1580–1584.

Centers for Disease Control and Prevention (CDC). (2006). *Group B streptococcal disease: hospitals and healthcare providers, summary.* Retrieved January 15, 2008, from http://www.cdc.gov/groupbstrep/hospitals/hospitals_guidelines_summary.htm

Chandrasekhar, S., & Datta, S. (2002). Anesthetic management of the pre-eclamptic parturient. In *Current reviews for nurse anesthetists.* Fort Lauderdale, FL: Frank Moya Continuing Education Programs.

Clark, P. A. (2005). Use of the vacuum extractor by midwives—what has changed in the last decade? *Journal of Midwifery & Women's Health,* 50, 517–524.

El Halta, V. (1996). Normalizing the breech delivery. *Midwifery Today,* 38, 22–24, 41.

Ethicon. (2004). *Wound closure manual.* Retrieved January 15, 2008, from http://www.jnjgateway.com/public/NLDUT/Wound_Closure_Manual1.pdf

Foster, S. (1996). *Herbs for your health.* Loveland, CO: Interweave Press.

Fraser, W., Hofmeyr, J., Lede, R., & Faron, G. (2005). Amnioinfusion for the prevention of meconium aspiration syndrome (Electronic version). *The New England Journal of Medicine,* 353, 909–918.

Frigoletto, F. D. Jr., Lieberman, E., Lang, J. M., Cohen, A., Barss, V., Ringer, S., et al. (1995). A clinical trial of active management of labor. *New England Journal of Medicine,* 333, 745–750.

Frye, A. (1998). *Holistic midwifery.* Portland, OR: Labrys Press.

Greulich, B., & Tarrant, B. (2007). The latent phase of labor: diagnosis and management. *Journal of Midwifery & Women's Health,* 52, 190–198.

Guangfeng, Q., & Hongjin, T. (1989). 413 Cases of abnormal fetal position corrected by auricular plaster therapy. *Journal of Traditional Chinese Medicine,* 9, 235–237.

Habek, D., Habek, J., & Jagust, M. (2003). Acupuncture conversion of fetal breech presentation. *Fetal Diagnosis and Therapy,* 18, 418–421.

Hannah, M. E., & Hannah, W. J. (2000). Planned cesarean section versus planned vaginal birth for breech presentation at term: a randomized multicenter trial. *Lancet,* 356, 1375–1383.

Hargitaib, B., Marton, T., & Cox, P. M. (2004). Best practice no. 178: Examination of the human placenta. *Journal of Clinical Pathology*, 57, 785–792.

Hart, G. (2002). Induction and circular logic. *Midwifery Today*, 63, 24–26, 66.

Hart, J., & Walker, A. (2007). Management of occiput posterior. *Journal of Midwifery & Women's Health*, 52, 508–513.

Hernandez, C., Little, B. B., Dax, J. S., Gilstrap, L. C., & Rosenfield, C. R. (1993). Prediction of the severity of meconium aspiration syndrome. *American Journal of Obstetrics & Gynecology*, 169, 61–70.

Hofmeyr, G. J. (2004a). Amnioinfusion for meconium-stained liquor in labour. The Cochrane Library, Issue 2, 2004.

Hofmeyr, G. J. (2004b). Amnioinfusion for preterm rupture of membranes. The Cochrane Library, Issue 2, 2004.

Hofmeyr, G. J. (2004c). Amnioinfusion for umbilical cord compression in labour. The Cochrane Library, Issue 2, 2004.

Institute for Clinical Systems Improvement. (2004). *Prevention, diagnosis and treatment of failure to progress in obstetrical labor.* Bloomington, MN: Author.

International Confederation of Midwives. (2003). *Management of the third stage of labour to prevent post-partum haemorrhage.* Retrieved on January 15, 2008 from http://www.internationalmidwives.org/index.php?module=ContentExpress&func=display&ceid=54&bid=32&btitle=Focus%20on...&meid=50

Jevitt, C. M. (2005). Shoulder dystocia: etiology, common risk factors, and management. *Journal of Midwifery & Women's Health*, 50, 485–497.

Jolivet, R. R. (2002). Early-onset neonatal group B streptococcal infection: 2002 guidelines for prevention. *Journal of Midwifery & Women's Health*, 47, 435–446.

Katz. V. L., Farmer, R., & Kuller, J. A. (2000). Pre-eclampsia into eclampsia: toward a new paradigm. *American Journal of Obstetrics & Gynecology*, 182, 1389–1396.

King, T. (2004). Vaginal birth after previous cesarean section (Electronic version). *Journal of Midwifery & Women's Health,* 49, 68–75.

Langston, C., Kaplan, C., Macpherson, T., Manci, E., Peevy, K., Clark, B., et al. (1997). Practice guideline for examination of the placenta: developed by the Placental Pathology Practice Guideline Development Task Force of the College of American Pathologists. *Archives of Pathology and Laboratory Medicine*, 121, 449–476.

Livingston, J. C., Livingston, L. W., Ramsey, R., Mabie, B. C., & Sibai, B. M. (2003). Magnesium sulfate in women with mild pre-eclampsia: a randomized controlled trial. *Obstetrics & Gynecology*, 101, 217–226.

Lokugamage, A. U., Sullivan, K. R., Niculescu, I., Tigere, P., Onyangunga, F., El Refaey, H., et al. (2001). A randomized study comparing rectally administered misoprostol versus syntometrine combined with an oxytocin infusion for the cessation of primary post partum hemorrhage. *Acta Obstetricia et Gynecologica Scandinavica*, 80, 835–839.

Long, P. (2001). Safe management of third stage labor: a technical report based on review of the current literature. In C. L. Farley (Ed.). *Final projects database.* Philadelphia University.

Lowe, N. K. (2007). A review of factors associated with dystocia and cesarean section in nulliparous women. *Journal of Midwifery & Women's Health*, 52, 216–228.

Marowitz, A., & Jordan, R. (2007). Midwifery management of prelabor rupture of membranes at term. *Journal of Midwifery & Women's Health*, 52, 199–206.

Martin, J. N., Jr., Rinehart, B. K., May, W. L., Magann, E. F., Terrone, D. A., & Blake, P. G. (1999). The spectrum of severe pre-eclampsia: a comparative analysis of HELLP syndrome classification. *American Journal of Obstetrics & Gynecology,* 180, 1373–1384.

McDonald, S. (2007). Management of the third stage of labor. *Journal of Midwifery & Women's Health*, 52, 254–261.

Mehl-Medrona, L., & Medrona, M. M. (1997). Physician- and midwife-attended home births: effects of breech, twin, and post-dates outcome data on mortality rates. *Journal of Nurse-Midwifery*, 42, 91–98.

Mercer, J. S., Erickson-Owens, D. A., Graves, B., & Haley, M. M. (2007). Evidence-based practice for the fetal to newborn transition. *Journal of Midwifery & Women's Health*, 52, 262–272.

Mercer, J. S., & Skovgaard, R. L. (2002). Delayed cord clamping. Neonatal transitional physiology: a new paradigm. *Journal of Perinatal & Neonatal Nursing*, 15, 56–75.

Miller, S., Lester, F., & Hensleigh, P. (2004). Prevention & treatment of PP hemorrhage: new advances for low-resource settings. *Journal of Midwifery & Women's Health,* 49, 283–292.

Moses, S. (2004). *Indomethacin.* Retrieved November 18, 2007 from http://www.fpnotebook.com/PHA37.htm

Murphy, J. L. (Ed.). (2004). *Nurse practitioner's prescribing reference.* New York: Prescribing Reference.

Naef, R. W., & Martin, J. N. (1995). Emergent management of shoulder dystocia. *Obstetric and Gynecology Clinics of North America,* 22, 247–259.

Paszkowski, T. (1994). Amnioinfusion: a review. *Journal of Reproductive Medicine,* 39, 588–594.

Peaceman, A. M., & Socol, M. L. (1996). Active management of labor. *American Journal of Obstetrics & Gynecology,* 175, 363–368.

Pistolese, R. (2002). The Webster technique: a chiropractic technique with obstetric implications. *Journal of Manipulative and Physiological Therapeutics,* 25, E1–E9.

Ramirez, N., & Frye, J. (2004). Shoulder dystocia: an evidence-based clinical practice guideline. In Farley, C. L. (Ed.). *Final projects database.* Philadelphia University.

Reedy, N. J. (2007). Born too soon: the continuing challenge of preterm labor and birth in the United States. *Journal of Midwifery & Women's Health,* 52, 281–290.

Roberts, J. (1994). Current perspectives on pre-eclampsia. *Journal of Nurse-Midwifery,* 39, 70–90.

Roberts, J. (2002). The push for evidence: management of the second stage. *Journal of Midwifery & Women's Health,* 47, 2–15.

Ross, S. (2007). Chlorhexidine as an alternative treatment for prevention of group B streptococcal disease. *Midwifery Today,* 82, 42–43.

Rx Med (n.d.) *Cyotec.* Retrieved March 1, 2008 from http://www.xmed.com/b.main/b2.pharmaceutical/b2.prescribe.html

Sakala, C., & Corry, M. P. (2007). Listening to Mothers II reveals maternity care quality chasm. *Journal of Midwifery & Women's Health,* 52, 183–185.

Schuchat, A. (1998). Epidemiology of group B streptococcal disease in the United States: shifting paradigms. *Clinical Microbiology Reviews,* 11, 497–513.

Shipp, T. D. (1999). Intrapartum rupture and dehiscence in patients with prior lower uterine segments vertical and transverse incisions. *Obstetrics & Gynecology,* 94, 735–740.

Simpson, K. R. (2007). Intrauterine resuscitation during labor: review of current methods and supportive evidence. *Journal of Midwifery & Women's Health,* 52, 229–237.

Sinclair, C. (2004). *A midwife's handbook.* St. Louis, MO: W.B. Saunders.

Soule, D., & Szwed, S. (2000). *The roots of healing: a woman's book of herbs.* Secaucus, NJ: Citadel Press.

Summers, L. (1997). Methods of cervical ripening and labor induction. *Journal of Nurse-Midwifery,* 42, 71–83.

Tharpe, N. (2004). Holistic evaluation of healing after cesarean birth. *Midwifery Today,* 72, 46–47.

Tharpe, N. (2007). First assisting in obstetrics: a primer for women's healthcare professionals. *Journal of Perinatal and Neonatal Nursing,* 21, 30–38.

Tora, P., & Dunn, J. (2000). Self-collection of antepartum anogenital group B streptococcus cultures. *Journal of the American Board of Family Practice,* 13, 107–110.

Tucker, J. M., Goldenberg, R. L., Davis, R. O., Copper, R. L., Winkler, C. L., & Hauth, J. C. (1991). Etiologies of preterm birth in an indigent population: is prevention a logical expectation? *Obstetrics & Gynecology,* 77, 343–348.

Tucker, M. (2004, July 1). Expert opinion backs two indications for amnioinfusion. *OB-GYN News.*

Vain, N. E., Szyld, E. G., Prudent, L. M., Wiswell, T. E., Aguillar, A. M., & Vivas, N. I. (2004). Oropharyngeal and nasopharyngeal suctioning of meconium-stained neonates before delivery of their shoulders: a multicenter randomized controlled trial (Electronic version). *Lancet,* 364, 597–602.

Varney, H., Kriebs, J. M., & Gegor, C. L. (2004). *Varney's midwifery* (4th ed.). Sudbury, MA: Jones and Bartlett.

Walls, D. (2007). Natural Families—Healthy Homes. LaVergne, TN: Ingram Publishing Company.

Walraven, G., Dampha, Y., Bittaye, B., Sowe, M., & Hofmeyr, J. (2004). Misoprostol in the treatment of postpartum haemorrhage in addition to routine management: a placebo randomised controlled trial. *British Journal of Obstetrics & Gynaecology,* 111, 1014–1017.

Weed, S. (1985). *Wise woman herbal for the childbearing year.* Woodstock, NY: Ashtree.

Weismiller, D. G. (1998). Transcervical amnioinfusion. *American Family Physician,* 57, 504–512.

Wiswell, T. E., Gannon, C. M., Jacob, J., Goldsmith, L., Szyld, E., Weiss, L., et al. (2000). Delivery room management of the apparently vigorous meconium-stained neonate: results of the multicenter, international collaborative trial. *Pediatrics,* 105, 1–7.

Wood, C. L. (1994). Meconium-stained amniotic fluid. *Journal of Nurse-Midwifery,* 39, 106s–109s.

World Health Organization. (1996). *Care in normal birth: a practical guide. Report of a technical working group.* Geneva, Switzerland: Author.

World Health Organization. (1998). *Care of the umbilical cord: a review of the evidence.* Retrieved January 15, 2008 from http://www.who.int/reproductive-health/publications/MSM_98_4/MSM_98_4_chapter2.en.html

Xu, H., Hofmeyr, J., Roy, C., & Fraser, W. D. (2007). Intrapartum amnioinfusion for meconium-stained amniotic fluid: a systematic review of random controlled trials (Electronic version). *British Journal of Obstetrics and Gynaecology,* 114, 383–390.

Yoder, B. (1994). Meconium-stained amniotic fluid and respiratory complications: impact of selective tracheal suction. *Obstetrics & Gynecology,* 83, 77–84.

BIBLIOGRAPHY

Briggs, G. G., Freeman, R. K., & Yaffe, S. J. (2005). *Drugs in pregnancy and lactation* (7th ed.). Philadelphia: Lippincott, Williams & Wilkins.

Enkin, M., Keirce, M., Renfrew, M., Neilson, J., Crowther, C., Duley, L., et al. (2000). *A guide to effective care in pregnancy and childbirth* (3rd ed.). New York: Oxford University Press.

Fraser, D., & Cooper, M. (2003). *Textbook for midwives* (14th ed.). Edinburgh, Scotland: Churchill Livingstone.

Frye, A. (2007). *Understanding diagnostic tests in the childbearing year* (7th ed.). Portland, OR: Labrys Press.

Gordon, J. D., Rydfors, J. T., Druzin, M. L., Tadir, Y., El-Sayed, Y., Chan, J., et al. (2007). *Obstetrics, gynecology and infertility* (6th ed.). Glen Cove, NY: Scrub Hill Press.

Morgan, G., & Hamilton, C. (2003). *Practice guidelines for obstetrics and gynecology*. Philadelphia: Lippincott-Raven.

Murphy, J. L. (Ed.). (2004). *Nurse practitioner's prescribing reference*. New York: Prescribing Reference.

Murray, M., Heulsmann, G., Romo, P. (2007). Essentials of fetal monitoring (3rd ed). New York: Springer Publishing LLC.

Scott, J. R., Gibbs, R. S., Karlan, B., & Haney, A. (2003). *Danforth's obstetrics and gynecology* (9th ed.). Philadelphia: Lippincott, Williams & Wilkins.

Smith, T. (1984). *A woman's guide to homeopathic medicine*. New York: Thorsons.

Speroff, L., & Fritz, M. A. (2004). *Clinical gynecologic endocrinology and infertility* (7th ed.). Philadelphia: Lippincott, Williams & Wilkins.

Sweet, B. R. (Ed.). (1997). *Mayes' midwifery* (12th ed.). London: Bailliere Tindall.

Care of the Infant and Mother After Birth

5

The extrauterine transition for the infant and the postpartum recovery for the mother are enhanced both physiologically and emotionally when the mother and baby are kept together as an inseparable dyad.

The baby's birth signals a time of immense changes when both mother and infant are particularly vulnerable to disruption. The newly born infant must make the transition from the intrauterine environment, where nutritional and respiratory needs are met through the umbilicus, to the outside environment, where the infant must initiate breathing and suckling to survive. Temperature regulation requires the infant adapt to the environment as it changes. Maternal–infant interaction is an essential part of this process. Skin-to-skin contact provides the newborn with warmth, the comfort of the familiar sounds of the maternal heartbeat and gastrointestinal tract, and the tactile stimulation of touch. Fostering mother–baby bonding is an integral part of midwifery practice. Supportive care allows the mother and baby to focus on each other as they adapt under the watchful eye of the skilled midwife.

The postpartum period highlights cultural practices and beliefs about birth and the newborn. For the midwife practicing in a multicultural environment, it provides a wonderful opportunity to explore nurturing in its many forms. Infant feeding and bonding influence each woman's self-image and her view of herself as competent to meet the challenges and tasks that parenting brings. Changes in intimate relationships are common, because the infant takes up time and physical as well as emotional energy. Concerns about fertility resurface, providing another opportunity to explore women's health within the context of individual women's lives. Ongoing evaluation for postpartum depression, effective infant feeding, and variations from the norm allows early intervention to reduce sequelae of potential complications that may result in harm to mother or baby. The guidelines in this section are presented in the order in which they would be used if needed, with acute conditions taking first priority.

CARE OF THE INFANT: NEWBORN RESUSCITATION

Key Clinical Information

Most infants born into a midwife's hands begin to breathe with nothing more required than gentle supportive care. Occasionally, however, some newly born infants need assistance to successfully make the transition to life outside the womb. Maintaining the umbilical cord intact during resuscitation may provide a secondary source of oxygen to the baby as well as necessary volume expansion (Mercer & Skovaard, 2002).

The most effective method of evaluating the newborn's pulse is by auscultation of the infant's chest with a stethoscope. Low neonatal blood pressure, or spasm of the cord secondary to cord palpation or tension, may inhibit cord blood flow and limit oxygenation via cord pulsation. As neonatal blood pressure improves with resuscitative measures, umbilical cord pulsation and blood flow frequently resume, enhancing resuscitative efforts through the sounds and heart rate may be assessed simultaneously.

⚠ To maintain the skills required for newborn resuscitation, the midwife must perform them on a regular basis. Ideally, resuscitation drills are performed regularly and documented in the midwife's continuing education log.

Client History and Chart Review: Components of the History to Consider

- Presence of risk factors for fetal asphyxia (American Academy of Pediatrics [AAP] and American Heart Association [AHA], 2006)
  - Cord factors, such as
    - Cord prolapse
    - Cord compression
  - Placental factors, such as
    - Placental abruption
    - Placental insufficiency
    - Placenta previa
  - Maternal factors, such as
    - Vascular disease
    - Hypoxia
    - Hypertension
    - Hypotension
    - Uterine hyperstimulation
    - Maternal narcotic use in labor
  - Fetal factors, such as
    - Prematurity
    - Meconium aspiration
    - Forceps or vacuum-assisted delivery
    - Malpresentation
    - Shoulder dystocia
- Causes of respiratory distress include
  - Hyaline membrane disease
  - Persistent pulmonary hypertension
  - Sepsis
  - Fetal isoimmunization
  - Choanal atresia
  - Diaphragmatic hernia

Physical Examination: Components of the Physical Exam to Consider

- Evaluate for (AAP & AHA, 2006)
  - Gestational age
  - Presence of meconium
  - Respirations
  - Muscle tone
- Evaluate respirations
  - Normal rate 40–60/min
  - May be irregular
  - No abdominal retractions
  - No grunting, gasping, or wheezing
- Evaluate heart rate
  - Normal rate 120–160 beats/min
  - Regular rate and rhythm
- Evaluate color
  - Should pink easily with respirations
  - Cyanosis of hands and feet is common
  - Pallor indicates poor perfusion due to
    - Volume depletion, or
    - Inadequate blood pressure
  - Central cyanosis indicates
    - Current adequate perfusion, with
    - Hypoxia

- Meconium present
  - Assess vigor
    - Muscle tone
    - Respirations
    - Heart rate

Clinical Impression:
Differential Diagnoses and Code Groups
to Consider
Additional suffix may apply (ICD9data.com, 2007)

- Acute inadequate ventilation and/or cardiac output
  - Fetus or newborn affected by complications of placenta cord and membranes (ICD-9 codes 762)
  - Fetus or newborn affected by other complications of labor and delivery (ICD-9 codes 763)
  - Birth trauma (ICD-9 codes 767)
  - Intrauterine hypoxia and birth asphyxia (ICD-9 codes 768)
  - Respiratory distress syndrome in newborn (ICD-9 codes 769)
  - Other respiratory conditions of fetus and newborn (ICD-9 codes 770)
- Newborn resuscitation procedure codes include
  - Assisted ventilation
    - < 30 minutes
    - > 30 minutes
  - Chest compressions
- Insertion of
  - Endotracheal intubation
  - Orogastric tube
  - Oral airway

Diagnostic Testing:
Diagnostic Tests and Procedures to Consider
(AAP & AHA, 2006)

- Endotracheal intubation
  - Nonvigorous infant, with meconium
    - Evaluate for meconium below cords
    - Suctioning of trachea
  - For ventilation and medication administration

- Laboratory testing
  - Cord blood gases
  - Hematocrit
  - Blood glucose
  - Chest x-ray

Providing Treatment:
Therapeutic Measures to Consider
(AAP & AHA, 2006)

- Nonvigorous infant with meconium
  - Suction before any stimulation
  - Use method appropriate for scope of practice
  - Proceed with ventilation as needed
- Basic steps, no meconium
  - Prevent heat loss
    - Place on warm surface
      - Maternal abdomen
      - Radiant warmer
    - Dry
    - Remove wet linen
  - Open airway
    - Position
    - Suction as needed
      - Gently use bulb suction
      - Avoid causing vagal response
  - Tactile stimulation
    - Flick or tap soles
    - Rub back
- Positive pressure ventilation (PPV) with room air or oxygen, for newborns with
  - Absent or weak respiratory efforts
  - Heart rate < 100 beats/min
  - Persistent central cyanosis
- Chest compressions
  - After 30 seconds PPV
  - Infants with heart rate < 60
  - Call for additional assistance
- Free-flow O_2 as indicated by
  - Respiratory effort
  - Color
- Epinephrine 1:10,000
  - Newborns with heart rate < 60 beats/min, after
    - 30 seconds PPV, and
    - 30 seconds PPV and chest compressions

- Stimulates cardiac contraction and rate
- Causes peripheral vasoconstriction
- Dose: 0.1–0.3 ml/kg
  - Route: endotracheal tube or IV
  - Give rapidly
  - Heart rate should improve within 30 seconds

Providing Treatment:
Alternative Measures to Consider
- Maintain intact umbilical cord
  - If cord is pulsing, infant is getting oxygen
  - Cord pulses with infant's heart rate
  - Avoid traction or pressure on cord
- Head-down position facilitates drainage of fluids
- Encourage infant to be present through
  - 🌐 Prayer and visualization
  - Talking to infant
  - Physical touch
- PPV using room air (Davis et al., 2004)
- Application of homeopathic remedies (e.g., Rescue Remedy) to pulse points is considered safe
- ⚠️ Oral administration of any medication, homeopathic, or herbal remedy may cause aspiration and further compromise infant.

Providing Support:
Education and Support Measures to Consider
- Discuss care of infant with parents as time allows
- Provide information about
  - Indication for resuscitation
  - Plan for ongoing infant care
  - Tests or treatments
  - Specialty care
- Listen to parents' concerns and fears
- Provide information about support groups or services as indicated

Follow-up Care:
Follow-up Measures to Consider
- 🔻 Document resuscitation
  - Indication for resuscitation
  - Respiratory effort, heart rate, color, tone

- Sequence of events
  - Resuscitation techniques used
  - Procedures or medication
  - Infant response
- Consultations
- Plan for continued care
- 📞 Notify appropriate personnel that infant required resuscitation
  - Infant should be evaluated promptly based on
    - Resuscitation measures required
    - Condition after resuscitation
    - Parent or midwife preferences
- Postresuscitation care
  - Based on length and extent of resuscitation
  - Evaluate newborn frequently for 24 hours
    - Vital signs: temperature, pulse, respirations, blood pressure
    - Color
    - Activity
    - Oxygen saturation
  - 📞 Transport of newborn, as indicated, from
    - Community hospital
    - Birth center
    - Home birth

Collaborative Practice:
Consider Consultation or Referral
- OB/GYN service
  - As indicated during labor and birth
- Pediatric service
  - For anticipated need of neonatal resuscitation
  - For infant who
    - Does not improve rapidly with PPV
    - Requires chest compressions
    - Has signs or symptoms that may indicate organ damage, such as (AAP & AHA, 2006)
      - Vital signs outside of accepted range
      - Respiratory distress
      - Difficulty with temperature regulation
      - Persistent cyanosis or pallor
      - Seizures or apnea
      - Abnormal tone or activity

➤ Diminished urinary output

➤ Feeding difficulties

- For diagnosis or treatment outside the mid-wife's scope of practice

CARE OF THE INFANT: INITIAL EVALUATION AND EXAMINATION OF THE NEWBORN

Key Clinical Information

The initial examination of the newborn serves to assess the effectiveness of the neonate's transition from the total support provided within the womb to healthy adaptation as a newborn. The evaluation provides the midwife with an opportunity to identify newborn characteristics and variations that may impact the newborn's ability to make this transition successfully or may require ongoing care by a pediatric health care professional.

Client History and Chart Review:
Components of the History to Consider
(American College of Medical Genetics,
1999; McHugh, 2004a)

- Labor and birth information
  - Duration of labor
  - Drug or medication exposure
  - Presentation and mode of delivery
  - Complications, such as
    - Cesarean birth
    - Vacuum extractor
    - Fetal distress
    - Meconium-stained fluid
  - Infant's condition at birth
  - Resuscitation measures, if any
  - Evaluation of placenta
- Neonatal course
  - Apparent gestational age
  - Apgar scores
  - Birth weight for gestational age
  - General newborn well-being
  - Activity
  - Feeding
  - Bladder and bowel function
  - Significant events or findings since birth

- Maternal history
  - Genetic disorders
  - Medical conditions, such as
    - Sickle cell
    - Hepatitis
    - Human immunodeficiency virus (HIV)/acquired immunodeficiency syndrome
    - Sexually transmitted infections
    - Thyroid
    - Diabetes
  - Contributing pregnancy history
    - Onset of prenatal care
    - Use of drugs, tobacco, and/or alcohol
    - Pregnancy complications
    - Duration of pregnancy

Physical Examination:
Components of the Physical Exam to Consider
(American College of Medical Genetics, 1999;
McHugh, 2004a)

- Assessment of gestational age using physical parameters
  - Length, weight, and head circumference
  - Additional measurements when indicated
- General appearance
  - Tone, posture, positioning
  - Alertness, vigor, color
  - Respiratory effort
  - Body proportion and symmetry
- Skin
  - Vernix, lanugo
  - Pigmentation patterns
  - Lesions, bruising or peeling
- Head
  - Shape, symmetry, fontanelles
  - Molding, caput, cephalohematoma
  - Hair patterning and location of hair whorls
  - Eyes
    - Pupils
    - Palpebral fissure inclination and length
    - Red reflex
    - Position, size, shape of orbits
    - Color of iris and sclera

- ◆ Subconjunctival hemorrhage
- ◆ Conjunctivitis
- ■ Ears
  - ◆ Location, rotation, configuration, and size
  - ◆ Patency
  - ◆ Position and shape
  - ◆ Presence of periauricular sinus or skin tags
  - ◆ Hearing
- ■ Nose
  - ◆ Shape
  - ◆ Patency of nares
  - ◆ Presence of flaring
- ■ Mouth
  - ◆ Configuration of upper lip, palate, and tongue
  - ◆ Shape and symmetry of lower jaw
  - ◆ Assessment of suck and swallow
- ■ Neck
  - ◆ Location of posterior hairline
  - ◆ Presence of sinus tract, torticollis, or webbing
- • Chest and trunk
  - ■ Shape and symmetry
  - ■ Nipples and breast buds
    - ◆ Location
    - ◆ Accessory nipples
  - ■ Cardiopulmonary system
    - ◆ Respiratory effort and breath sounds
    - ◆ Heart rate and rhythm
    - ◆ Murmurs, pulses
  - ■ Abdomen
    - ◆ Number of cord vessels
    - ◆ Muscle tone
    - ◆ Presence of bowel sounds (> 1 hour after birth)
    - ◆ Palpation for
      - ➤ Hernia, umbilical or inguinal
      - ➤ Enlarged organs or masses
  - ■ Back
    - ◆ Symmetry
    - ◆ Presence of dimple or hair tuft in intergluteal cleft
- • Genitalia
  - ■ Size, appearance, presence of ambiguity

- ■ Female
  - ◆ Configuration
  - ◆ Edema
  - ◆ Discharge
- ■ Male
  - ◆ Position of urinary meatus
  - ◆ Descent of testes in scrotum
- ■ Anus: location and patency
- • Extremities
  - ■ Proportion, appearance, range of motion
  - ■ Number of digits, presence of nails
  - ■ Pulses: femoral, brachial
  - ■ Creases: palmar, phalangeal and flexion
- • Neurologic
  - ■ Tone, response, alertness
  - ■ Reflexes: rooting, Moro, Babinski

Clinical Impression:
Differential Diagnoses and Code Groups
to Consider
Additional suffix or CPT code may apply
(ICD9data.com, 2007; American Academy of
Family Physicians, 2006)

- • Hospital-based history and physical examination (H&P) for the normal newborn (ICD-9 codes V30)
- • Out-of-hospital H&P for the normal newborn (ICD-9 code V30.2)
- • Same day H&P and discharge for the normal newborn (ICD-9 codes V30)
- • Newborn morbidity or mortality related to
  - ■ Maternal conditions that may be unrelated to present pregnancy (ICD-9 codes 760)
  - ■ Maternal complications of pregnancy (ICD-9 codes 761)
  - ■ Complications of placenta cord and membranes (ICD-9 codes 762)
  - ■ Other complications of labor and delivery (ICD-9 codes 763)
  - ■ Other perinatal conditions, such as (ICD-9 codes 764–779)
    - ◆ Postterm and high birth weight (ICD-9 codes 766)

- Birth trauma (ICD-9 codes 767)
- Respiratory distress syndrome in newborn (ICD-9 codes 769)

Diagnostic Testing:
Diagnostic Tests and Procedures to Consider (McHugh, 2004a)
- Cord blood gases
- Cord blood studies (Rh, ABO)
- Glucose, heel stick (normal value > 45 mg/dL)
- Hematocrit (normal value, 45–65%)
- Total bilirubin (normal value < 13 mg/dL)
- Screening recommendations (March of Dimes, 2006)
  - Metabolic disorders
  - Fatty acid oxidation disorders
  - Sickle cell diseases
  - Cystic fibrosis
  - Hearing impairment
  - Other disorders
    - Congenital hypothyroidism
    - Biotinidase deficiency
    - Congenital adrenal hyperplasia
    - Classical galactosemia
- Sexually transmitted infection testing
  - RPR, VDRL
  - HIV
  - Herpes simplex (HSV)
  - Hepatitis B
- Conjunctivitis
  - Gram stain of eye exudate
  - Culture of eye exudate for gonorrhea/chlamydia (GC/CT) and/or herpes simplex virus (HSV)

Providing Treatment:
Therapeutic Measures to Consider
- Infant bath
  - 🌀 Verify parent's cultural preferences for bathing of infant
- Vitamin K_1 (AAP, 2003)
  - Injection: AquaMEPHYTON (phytonadione)
    - 0.5–1 mg IM within 1 hour of birth

- Prophylactic ophthalmic treatment (Centers for Disease Control and Prevention, 2006a)
  - Erythromycin ophthalmic ointment: 0.5% for one dose
  - Tetracycline ophthalmic ointment: 1% for one dose
  - Silver nitrate solution 1% for one dose
- Hepatitis B (Centers for Disease Control and Prevention, 2005)
  - Vaccine prophylaxis (HBsAg-negative mother)
    - Begin soon after birth
    - Three dose series: 0–1, 1–2, and 6–18 months
    - May delay first dose up to 1 month
  - HBIG (see Care of the Woman with Hepatitis, Chapter 7)
- Phototherapy for hyperbilirubinemia

Providing Treatment:
Alternative Measures to Consider
- Defer infant bath or have parent give bath
- Defer vitamin K
  - Incidence of hemorrhagic disease without vitamin K ranges from 0.25% to 1.7% (AAP, 2003)
  - May occur in breast-fed infants who do not receive vitamin K
  - Vitamin K is concentrated in colostrum and hind milk
  - Formula-fed infants get significant vitamin K from cow's milk formula
- Oral vitamin K
  - Konakion MM, mixed micellular preparation (Clark & James, 1995)
    - 2 mg PO within 1 hour of birth, followed by
    - Additional dose at 7 and 30 days of age
  - AquaMEPHYTON (Canadian Pediatric Society and College of Family Physicians of Canada, 2004)
    - 2 mg PO at first feeding, followed by
    - Additional doses at 2–4 and 6–8 weeks

- Defer erythromycin ophthalmic ointment
  - Negative maternal GC/CT results
  - Culture and treat if conjunctivitis occurs
  - Use plain water wash, as needed

Providing Support:
Education and Support Measures to Consider
- Discuss physical findings
  - Range of normal
  - Potential or actual concerns
  - Signs and symptoms to watch for
  - Purpose of testing and/or medications
- Encourage questions
- Engage parents in decision-making
- Discuss options for care
  - Well-baby care providers
  - Recommended treatments
  - Anticipated results/benefits
  - Risks/side effects
  - Alternatives
- Anticipatory guidance for parenting of newborn
  - Expected feeding and activity levels
  - Evaluation of adequate hydration
  - Common patterns of voiding and stooling
  - Planned follow-up for well-baby care
  - When/how to contact pediatric care provider
  - Warning signs (McHugh, 2004b)
    - Poor feeding
    - Lethargy
    - Irritability
    - Jaundice
    - Dehydration
    - Fever
    - Poor color
    - Vomiting

Follow-up Care:
Follow-up Measures to Consider
- Daily evaluation first 2–3 days of life
  - Observation of feeding
    - Determine suck/swallow
    - Note latch if breastfeeding
    - Maternal–infant interaction

- Document
  - Findings
  - Discussions
  - Recommendations and referrals
  - Plan for continued newborn care
- Weight check at 1 to 2 weeks
- Recheck of variations from normal

Collaborative Practice:
Consider Consultation or Referral
- Pediatric service
  - If newborn evaluation is not included in midwife's practice
- Variations, such as (McHugh, 2004b)
  - Presence of anomalies
  - Evidence of infection
  - Hyperbilirubinemia
  - Other conditions not within the range of normal or expected findings
- Lactation consultant
  - Breastfeeding difficulties
- Social services
  - Need for infant supplies or car seat
- For diagnosis or treatment outside the midwife's scope of practice

CARE OF THE INFANT: ASSESSMENT OF THE NEWBORN FOR DEVIATIONS FROM NORMAL

Key Clinical Information

Midwives strive to improve the health and well-being of each mother and baby through the provision of excellent midwifery care. The midwife is alert to noteworthy maternal and/or perinatal history and is observant for subtle signs or symptoms in the newborn that may indicate a need for gentle assistance or medical intervention. Although most babies born to healthy mothers are themselves healthy, the midwife must consider whether newborn variations represent the wide range of normal or indicate the presence of a condition requiring further evaluation by a clinician skilled in evaluation and care of the newly born infant.

Client History and Chart Review:
Components of the History to Consider
(American College of Medical Genetics, 1999;
McHugh 2004a)

- Maternal medical history
  - Age
  - Illnesses
  - Medications
- Social factors
- Prenatal history
  - Maternal reproductive history
  - Gravida, para, and pregnancy outcomes
  - Preconception folate intake
  - Fetal activity during pregnancy
  - Genetic testing or screening
  - Prenatal test results
  - Complications of pregnancy
    - Drug, alcohol, or tobacco use
    - Teratogenic or environmental exposures
    - Maternal disease or illness, such as
      - Group B streptococcal infection (GBS)
      - Herpes
      - Diabetes
      - Epilepsy
      - HIV
      - Viral and parasitic infections
- Family history (three generations, as applicable)
  - Ethnic background
  - Consanguinity
  - Genetic testing
  - Conditions such as
    - Reproductive losses or infertility
    - Cerebral palsy or mental retardation
    - Congenital anomalies
    - Genetic disorders
- Perinatal history
  - Estimated gestational age
  - Labor and birth events
    - Duration
    - Drug or medication exposure
    - Presentation and mode of delivery
    - Abnormal fetal heart rate patterns

- Complications at birth, such as
  - Presence of meconium
  - Endotracheal intubation or suctioning
  - Instrument or surgical birth
  - Shoulder dystocia
- Infant's condition at birth
  - Apgar scores
  - Resuscitation
  - Evidence of birth trauma
  - Description and disposition of placenta
- Neonatal course
  - Postresuscitation status
  - Birth weight for gestational age
  - Feeding difficulties
  - Complications or unusual findings
  - Laboratory test results
  - Review symptoms since birth
    - Type of symptom(s)
    - Onset
    - Duration
    - Severity
    - Treatments and infant response

Physical Examination:
Components of the Physical Exam to Consider
(McHugh, 2004b; Varney et al., 2004)

- ⚠ Signs and symptoms suggesting need for further evaluation
  - Respirations
    - Presence of apnea
    - Grunting or gasping
    - Rate < 30 or > 60
  - Heart rate and rhythm
    - Bradycardia < 100 beats/min
    - Tachycardia > 170 beats/min
    - Cardiac instability
  - Temperature instability
  - Color
    - Pallor
    - Cyanosis
    - Rubor
    - Jaundice

- ◆ Before 24 hours—most likely pathologic
- ◆ After 24 hours—most likely physiologic
- ▪ Muscle tone and activity level
  - ◆ Poor muscle tone, flaccidity
  - ◆ Poor feeding
  - ◆ Lethargy, poor response to stimulation
  - ◆ Irritability
  - ◆ Hyperactivity
  - ◆ Seizures
  - ◆ Failure to move an extremity
- ▪ Gastrointestinal adaptation
  - ◆ Vomiting
  - ◆ Diarrhea
  - ◆ Abdominal distension
- ▪ Presence of congenital anomalies
- ▪ Presence of birth-related injuries, such as
  - ◆ Cephalohematoma
  - ◆ Brachial plexus injury
  - ◆ Pneumothorax
  - ◆ Fractured rib or clavicle
  - ◆ Subgaleal hemorrhage after vacuum extraction
- ▪ Unusual behavior or findings
- ▪ 🕭 Arrange for comprehensive newborn assessment

Clinical Impression:
Differential Diagnoses and Code Groups to Consider
Additional suffix may apply (ICD9data.com, 2007)
- Perinatal disorders relating to
  - ▪ Family history (ICD-9 codes V17.2–V19.8)
  - ▪ Congenital anomalies, including genetic disorders (ICD-9 codes 740–759)
  - ▪ Maternal conditions (ICD-9 codes 760–763)
  - ▪ Intrauterine growth retardation (ICD-9 codes 764)
  - ▪ Gestational age and birth weight (ICD-9 codes 765–766)
  - ▪ Birth trauma (ICD-9 codes 767)
  - ▪ Intrauterine hypoxia and birth asphyxia (ICD-9 codes 768)

- ▪ Respiratory distress syndrome (ICD-9 codes 769)
- ▪ Other respiratory conditions (ICD-9 codes 770)
- ▪ Infection (ICD-9 codes 771)
- ▪ Hemorrhage (ICD-9 codes 772)
- ▪ Hemolytic disease (ICD-9 codes 773)
- ▪ Jaundice (ICD-9 codes 774)
- ▪ Endocrine and metabolic disturbances (ICD-9 codes 775)
- ▪ Hematologic disorders (ICD-9 codes 776)
- ▪ Digestive system disorders (ICD-9 codes 777)
- ▪ Integument and temperature regulation disorders (ICD-9 codes 778)
- ▪ Other perinatal conditions (ICD-9 codes 779)

Diagnostic Testing:
Diagnostic Tests and Procedures to Consider
- 🕭 As indicated by infant presentation, and
- Appropriate for midwife's scope of practice

Providing Treatment:
Therapeutic Measures to Consider
- Provide neutral thermal environment
  - ▪ Skin-to-skin on mother
  - ▪ On warmed resuscitation unit
  - ▪ Cloth-wrapped hot water bottle for transport
- Provide O2 as needed for cyanosis (AAP & AHA, 2006)
  - ▪ Blow-by or mask
  - ▪ Positive pressure ventilation (PPV)
- As indicated by diagnosis, such as
  - ▪ Phototherapy
  - ▪ Antibiotics

Providing Treatment:
Alternative Measures to Consider
- Home phototherapy: lights or sunlight
- Homeopathic Rescue Remedy to pulse points
- 🕭 Prayer and acceptance of infant as perfect being
- Other remedies as indicated by infant's condition or presentation

Providing Support:
Education and Support Measures to Consider
(American College of Medical Genetics, 1999)

- 🌐 Offer interpreter as needed for ethnocultural and language differences
- Maintain a caring nonjudgmental environment
  - Provide support to parents during
    - ◆ Newborn workup
    - ◆ Diagnosis
    - ◆ Treatment
  - Assist, as desired by family, to ensure
    - ◆ Privacy
    - ◆ Autonomy
    - ◆ Inclusion of additional family members, clergy
  - Provide acknowledgment of and support during
    - ◆ Times of uncertainty
    - ◆ Grieving process
- Infant with mild condition
  - Provide information regarding
    - ◆ Warning signs and symptoms of condition
    - ◆ Who to contact if symptoms develop
    - ◆ How to contact infant's health care professional
- Infant with significant illness or abnormality
  - Provide factual information, as appropriate, regarding
    - ◆ Working diagnosis
    - ◆ Planned diagnostic workup
    - ◆ Anticipated prognosis
    - ◆ Treatment plan and priorities
    - ◆ Recurrence risks
    - ◆ Resources

Follow-up Care:
Follow-up Measures to Consider

- Reevaluate infant
  - To establish baseline or note change
  - If uncertain regarding normalcy of condition
- Documentation
  - Annotated history and physical
  - Diagnostic test results

- Plan for continued care
- Consultations and referrals
- Summarize discussions

Collaborative Practice:
Consider Consultation or Referral

- Pediatric service
  - Neonate with signs or symptoms of
    - ◆ Illness
    - ◆ Injury
    - ◆ Anomaly
    - ◆ Unusual behavior or findings
  - Newborn transport or transfer care of infant as indicated by problem
- Resources
  - Social service assistance during acute phase
    - ◆ Family adjustment
    - ◆ Housing and support services
    - ◆ Health interpretation and advocacy
  - Long-term needs
    - ◆ Early intervention
    - ◆ Support groups
    - ◆ Psychosocial services
- For diagnosis or treatment outside the midwife's scope of practice

CARE OF THE INFANT: BREASTFEEDING

Key Clinical Information

Human milk is the ideal food for newborns. Breast milk is a dynamic biologically active food source that provides nutritional and immunologic factors for optimal infant health, growth, and brain and organ development. Exclusive breast milk feedings in the first 4 months of life foster antibody formation to environmental pathogens and support immune system development. Breast-fed infants demonstrate earlier and healthier colonization of the gut, which may contribute to decreased incidence of allergies, in particular to large proteins such as in cow's milk (Walker, 2006).

The process of breastfeeding fosters maternal–infant interaction and bonding. The close contact between mother and baby during breastfeeding results in enhanced feelings of security and benefits future social development. However, many factors influence a mother's decision as to how she will feed her infant. Social and cultural factors influence a woman's decision on infant feeding. The need to return to full-time work may limit the opportunity to exclusively breastfeed. Many women pump breast milk or use commercial formulas to feed their infants when they are not available to breastfeed. Women with a history of sexual abuse or neglect may not wish for the stimulation of the baby suckling at breast.

Evidence shows that breastfeeding during the baby's first 2–4 months of life has a long-lasting positive impact on the baby's future health (Walker, 2006). Prenatally, all patients should be given information on the benefits of breastfeeding to both mother and infant. Referral to a breastfeeding class is helpful for information on initiating and maintaining lactation.

Client History and Chart Review: Components of the History to Consider (Walker, 2006)

- Maternal
  - Age
  - Prenatal history
    - Medications
    - Attendance at childbirth classes
  - Labor and birth history
    - Medications and interventions
      - Analgesics and anesthetics
      - Oxytocin
      - Intravenous fluids
      - Magnesium sulfate
      - Instrument delivery
    - Maternal/newborn separation
  - Obstetric/gynecologic history
    - Pregnancy and breastfeeding history
    - Length of breastfeeding
    - Contraceptive preference
  - Psychosocial assessment
    - Nutrition patterns
      - Adequacy
      - Eating disorders
    - Physical activity level
    - Alcohol, tobacco, or drug use
    - Sexual abuse
  - Review of systems
- Family history
  - Food allergies
- Newborn
  - Birth weight
  - Breastfeeding efforts
    - Early breastfeeding
    - Suck/swallow
    - Intensity and duration of breastfeeding
    - Weight loss/gain
    - Frequency of feeds
    - Need for assistance with feeding
  - Sleep/wake patterns
  - Elimination
    - Passage of meconium
    - Number of voids per day
    - Number of stools per day
- Supplementation
  - Indications for supplementation
    - Geographic separation of mother and baby
    - Maternal medications incompatible with nursing
    - Insufficient milk supply in baby who nurses well
    - Maternal conditions, such as
      - Psychosis
      - Eclampsia
      - Varicella-zoster
      - Breast cancer
    - Infant conditions, such as
      - Inability to effectively suck and swallow
      - Hypoglycemia
      - Weight loss greater than 7–10%
      - Illness or anomalies that prevent effective nursing
- Conditions that may impact breastfeeding
  - Low birth weight
  - Congenital anomalies, such as
    - Cleft palate
    - Pierre-Robin syndrome
    - Choanal atresia

- Disorders, such as
  - Respiratory distress
  - Down syndrome
  - Cerebral palsy
  - Congenital heart defects
  - Phenylketonuria
  - Galactosemia
- Contraindications to breastfeeding (Centers for Disease Control and Prevention, 2007)
  - Infants with the metabolic disorder galactosemia
  - Maternal
    - Illicit drug use
    - HIV infection
    - Human T-cell lymphotropic virus infection
    - Untreated active tuberculosis
    - Antiretroviral medication
    - Cancer chemotherapy
    - Therapy with radioactive compounds (temporary)

Physical Examination:
Components of the Physical Exam to Consider
(Walker, 2006)

- Infant
  - Weight, vital signs
  - Structural evaluation
    - Tongue
    - Jaw
    - Lips and cheeks
    - Palate
    - Airway
  - Reflexes
    - Rooting
    - Suck
    - Swallow
    - Gag
- Maternal
  - Nipples and areola
    - Erect, inverted, or flat
    - Size
    - Presence of
      - Cracks or fissures
      - Blisters
      - Pain

- Breasts
  - Colostrum or milk present
  - Engorgement
  - Masses
  - Axilla
  - Pain
- Breastfeeding assessment
  - Maternal readiness
    - Attentiveness to infant cues
    - Ability to hold and examine breast
    - Ability to position infant for effective feeding
    - Maternal let-down
  - Infant feeding
    - Rooting
    - Effective latch
      - Tongue curved around areola
      - Complete seal with lips
      - No smacking sounds
    - Effective feeding
      - Sustained bursts of sucking
      - Audible and/or visible swallowing
      - Coordination of suck, swallow, and breathing
      - Colostrum/milk clearly present
  - Postfeeding observations
    - Infant appears satisfied
    - Maternal breasts softer
    - Pre- and postfeed weights

Clinical Impression:
Differential Diagnoses and Code Groups
to Consider
Additional suffix may apply (AAP, n.d.
ICD9data.com, 2007)

- Maternal
  - Cracked nipple (ICD-9 codes 676.1)
  - Engorgement of breasts (ICD-9 codes 676.2)
  - Nonpurulent mastitis (ICD-9 codes 675.2)
  - Other disorders of lactation (ICD-9 codes 676.8)
  - Retracted nipple (ICD-9 codes 676.0)
  - Suppressed lactation (ICD-9 codes 676.5)
  - Unspecified disorder of lactation (ICD-9 codes 676.9)

- Newborn
  - Abnormal loss of weight (ICD-9 codes 783.21)
  - Abnormal tongue position (ICD-9 codes 750.1)
  - Cleft palate/lip (ICD-9 codes 749)
  - Dysphagia (ICD-9 codes 787.2)
  - Failure to thrive (ICD-9 codes 784.4)
  - Infant feeding difficulty (ICD-9 codes 783.3)
  - Feeding problems in newborn (ICD-9 codes 779.3)
  - Neonatal candida infection (ICD-9 codes 771.7)
  - Suck reflex abnormal (ICD-9 codes 796.1)

Diagnostic Testing:
Diagnostic Tests and Procedures to Consider
- Total serum bilirubin
- Blood glucose
- Metabolic screen

Providing Treatment:
Therapeutic Measures to Consider (Walker, 2006)
- Breast pump
- Nipple shield
- Tube feeding device
  - Lact-Aid
- Engorgement pain relief
  - Serrapeptase (enzyme)
- Plugged ducts
  - Oral lecithin 15 ml daily

Providing Treatment:
Alternative Measures to Consider
- Rest and tender loving care
  - Mother and baby remain together
  - Family support
  - Postpartum doula
- Herbal remedies that support breast milk production (Laurence, 1998–2007)
  - Fenugreek
  - Blessed thistle
  - Fennel (seed or root only)

- Herbs to avoid while nursing (Straus, 2003)
  - Black cohosh
  - Buckthorn
  - Cascada sagrada
  - Kava kava
  - Sage
  - Senna
  - Wintergreen
- Sore nipples, apply
  - Expressed milk, allow to dry
  - Cool tea bag compresses

Providing Support:
Education and Support Measures to Consider
- Provide age-appropriate information
- Encourage good nutrition and health habits
  - Ample fluids
  - Well-balanced food choices
  - Avoid alcohol, drugs, and tobacco
- Breastfeeding basics
  - First breastfeeding within 60 minutes of birth
  - Keep newborn skin-to-skin with mother until first feeding completed
  - Limit stressors
  - Feed 8–12 times a day
  - Nursing positions
    - Cradle hold
    - Cross cradle
    - Football
    - Side-lying
  - Assess for swallowing
  - Hand expression or pumping
- In the first postpartum days
  - Mother and baby remain together
  - Encourage unlimited on-demand feedings
  - Assure mother of adequacy of colostrum for all newborn nutritional needs
  - Assess for correct latch
    - Wide gape of the mouth
    - Latch far back on the areola
    - Mother feels a tugging sensation
    - Audible swallowing of colostrum

- Observe for adequate output
- Troubleshooting
  - Newborn irritability
    - Swaddle infant
    - Dim lights
    - Create quiet peaceful environment
  - Difficulty with latch
    - Feed at first infant cues
    - Position facing mother
    - Infant brought to breast
    - Colostrum at nipple
    - Gentle traction on chin
    - Nipple shield
  - Sleepy infant
    - Keep baby with mother
    - Feed at first infant cues
    - Unwrap and gently stimulate infant
    - Avoid distractions for infant
    - Offer breast frequently
  - Engorgement
    - Nurse frequently
    - Pump or express as needed
    - Cool packs for comfort
    - Cabbage leaves
  - Low milk supply
    - Nurse frequently
    - Rest
  - Plugged ducts
    - Warm compresses
    - Gentle massage during feedings
  - Breast infection (see Care of the Mother: Mastitis)
- Maternal benefits of breastfeeding
  - Decreased blood loss after delivery
  - Enhanced maternal/infant bonding
  - Stimulates uterine involution
  - Reduced fertility while exclusively breastfeeding
  - Fosters maternal weight loss postpartum
- Menstrual cycle and function
  - Breastfeeding and amenorrhea
  - Return to fertility
  - Contraceptive options

Follow-up Care:
Follow-up Measures to Consider (AAP, n.d.)
- Document
  - Breastfeeding assessment
  - Observation of feeding
- Three to 5 days of age
  - Assess ability of the infant to
    - Remain hydrated
      - Six to eight wet diapers in 24 hours
      - Three to four stools in 24 hours
    - Maintain growth consistent with age
    - Show appropriate physical activity for age
    - Stimulate adequate milk production
  - Observe for signs of feeding difficulty
    - Weight loss/gain
    - Dehydration
    - Jaundice
- Continued follow-up for infants with
  - Jaundice
  - Persistent dark stool or urine
  - Ineffective milk transfer
  - Infrequent feeding
  - Weight loss > 7%
  - Formula supplementation
- As indicated for routine well-infant care

Collaborative Practice:
Criteria to Consider for Consultation or Referral
- Pediatric care provider
  - Infant with significant problems affecting ability to feed, such as
    - Congenital anomalies
    - Infection
    - Metabolic disorders
- Lactation consultant (Walker, 2006)
  - Early or persistent feeding difficulties
  - Maternal request
  - Flat or inverted nipples
  - Prior breast surgery
  - Nursing multiples
  - Preterm infant(s)

- Infant with congenital anomalies or health issues
- Maternal or infant health issues that temporarily prevent breastfeeding
- OB/GYN service or gynecologic endocrinologist
  - Dysfunctional lactogenesis
  - Mastitis or breast abscess
- Mental health service
  - Depression
  - Eating disorder
- Nutritionist
- For diagnosis or treatment outside the midwife's scope of practice

CARE OF THE INFANT: NEONATAL CIRCUMCISION

Key Clinical Information

Medical societies around the world recommend against elective circumcision, which is the surgical removal of all or part of the foreskin of the penis without evidence of disease or disorder (Circumcision Information and Resource Pages, 2007). Evidence demonstrates no clear medical value of nontherapeutic or elective newborn circumcision (American Academy of Family Physicians, 2001; AAP, 1999; College of Physicians and Surgeons of British Columbia, 2007). Elective circumcision is ideally performed exclusively for religious, cultural, or ethnic reasons.

The American College of Obstetricians and Gynecologists (2001) recommends that parents be provided with "accurate and impartial information" as part of the informed choice process for circumcision. Prenatal discussion allows parents time to thoughtfully weigh the risks of the procedure against the putative potential benefits. There is insufficient evidence to demonstrate that the limited potential for long-term medical benefit related to circumcision are greater than the risks of pain, infection, injury, and bleeding that are the most common complications of this procedure. Noninvasive measures exist that may be more effec-

tive to reduce or prevent the diseases or disorders that circumcision may occasionally prevent (American Academy of Family Physicians, 2001; AAP, 1999; College of Physicians and Surgeons of British Columbia, 2007).

The midwife who chooses to include circumcision in her or his practice for religious, cultural, or ethnic reasons is obligated to learn and perform the procedure under expert guidance until skilled at the procedure and must perform an adequate number of procedures annually to maintain competence. Use of analgesia and/or local anesthesia is recommended for circumcision to minimize the stress to the infant during the procedure (American College of Obstetricians and Gynecologists, 2001).

Client History and Chart Review:
Components of the History to Consider
(Lowenstein, 2004)
- Review infant record
  - Neonatal course since birth
    - Temperature stability
    - Feeding and voiding
    - Physical examination results
  - Vitamin K administration
    - Oral vitamin K requires up to three doses before full effectiveness
  - Demonstrated voiding since birth
- Contraindications to circumcision
  - Hypospadias
  - Abnormality of the penis
  - Medically unstable infant
  - Parents decline procedure

Physical Examination:
Components of the Physical Exam to Consider
- Vital signs, including temperature
- Examination of the penis
  - Evaluate for hypospadias before procedure
  - Evaluate redundancy of foreskin
  - Identify landmarks for penile block if used

Clinical Impression:
Differential Diagnoses and Code Groups to Consider
Additional suffix or procedure code may apply
(ICD9data.com, 2007)

- Elective or ritual circumcision (ICD-9 codes V50.2)

Diagnostic Testing:
Diagnostic Tests and Procedures to Consider

- As indicated to ensure infant's stability before procedure

Providing Treatment:
Therapeutic Measures to Consider

- Maintain intact foreskin
- Circumcise later in life if and when indicated

Providing Treatment:
Alternative Measures to Consider

- Nontherapeutic or ritual circumcision
  - Remove only very tip of foreskin
  - Remove entire foreskin
- Circumcision technique
  - Obtain informed consent
  - Prepare equipment
    - Gomco clamp
    - Plastibell clamp
    - Mogen clamp
- Provide for pain relief (AAP, 1999)
  - EMLA cream
  - Dorsal penile block
  - Subcutaneous ring block
  - Parental presence
  - Swaddling
  - Analgesics
- Perform procedure (Lowenstein, 2004)
  - 🌐 Honor religious or ethnic circumcision rituals
  - Strict aseptic technique
  - Use preferred method (Varney et al., 2004)
  - Observe for, and treat, active bleeding

- Apply petroleum jelly gauze or other nonadherent dressing
- Comfort baby and return to mother and family

Providing Support:
Education and Support Measures to Consider

- Provide information for informed consent (American Academy of Family Physicians, 2001; AAP, 1999)
  - Decision is personal and subjective
    - Procedure is not essential to child's well-being
    - Parents have no obligation to consent to circumcision
    - Parents determine what is in the "best interest" of the infant
      - Religious, cultural, ethnic considerations
      - Future sexual and psychological considerations
      - Child's right to body integrity
  - Risks associated with circumcision
    - Pain
    - Bleeding
    - Infection
    - Injury
    - Complication rate 0.2–0.6%
  - Potential benefits of circumcision
    - Decreased incidence of infrequent conditions
      - Urinary tract infections
      - Penile cancer
      - Sexually transmitted infection transmission
    - Number needed to treat based on diagnosis (Christakis et al., 2000)
      - 100 circumcisions to prevent 1 urinary tract infection
      - 909 circumcisions to prevent 1 penile cancer
    - Good hygiene and safe sex practices reduce these risks

- Provide education to parents
  - Care of infant with intact foreskin (Sinclair, 2004)
    - Keep diaper area clean
    - Do not retract foreskin
    - If redness or irritation occurs
      - Flush area with clear water
      - Allow to air dry if possible
      - Apply diaper ointment to glans
  - Care of infant postcircumcision (Lowenstein, 2004)
    - Crying is common with first voids
    - Head of penis may be quite red
    - Swelling just under the glans is normal
    - A blood clot may form at incision site
    - Pink or yellow serous drainage may occur
    - Instruct in care of circumcised penis
    - Call with signs or symptoms of complications
      - Active bleeding
      - Infection at incision site
      - Fever
      - Lack of urination within 12–24 hours after circumcision

Follow-up Care:
Follow-up Measures to Consider
- Document, as indicated
  - Discussions
  - Informed consent process
  - Parents' decision
  - Procedure (see Procedure Note, Chapter One)
  - Postprocedure findings
- Observe for potential complications
  - 12–24 hours postprocedure
  - At follow-up visit(s)
    - Bleeding
    - Infection or inflammation
    - Urinary retention
    - Tissue trauma or necrosis
    - Cosmetic results

- Criteria for release from care
  - Infant stable and feeding
  - Bleeding minimal
  - Voiding has occurred

Collaborative Practice:
Consider Consultation or Referral
- Mohel/mohelet for Jewish families
  - For information and opinion about circumcision
  - To perform circumcision
- Pediatric service
  - Infant with congenital defects of the genitals
  - To perform circumcision
- OB/GYN service
  - To perform circumcision
- For diagnosis or treatment outside the midwife's scope of practice

CARE OF THE INFANT: WELL-BABY CARE

Key Clinical Information
The midwife who provides well-baby care after the immediate newborn period forms collaborative relationships with other infant care professionals, such as pediatricians, pediatric nurse practitioners, and family physicians, who provide medical care or evaluation during times of illness, injury, or deviations from the norm. Routine well-baby care includes periodic screening to assess the infant's health status, growth and development, behavior, and family functioning. Group visits are effective for anticipatory guidance and support during the challenges of parenting and for update of immunizations. The midwife facilitates "best care" for the infant through information, education, and support for parents, while evaluating the well-being and safety of the child.

Client History and Chart Review:
Components of the History to Consider
(McHugh, 2004a; University of Arizona, 2005)
- Indication for present evaluation
  - Routine care
  - Problem-oriented care

- Significant perinatal or interim history
  - Pregnancy history
    - Maternal illness
    - Sexually transmitted infection exposure
    - Substance abuse
    - Isoimmunization
  - Gestational age at birth
- Current patterns of behavior
  - Activity and interaction
  - Sleep/wake patterns
  - Feeding method and efforts
  - Elimination patterns
  - Developmental milestones
  - Cognitive/linguistic development
  - Social/emotional development
- Assess
  - Family strengths
  - Parental observations and concerns
  - Parent–child interaction
    - Eye contact
    - Comfort seeking
    - Tone of voice
- Variations from expected well-baby course
  - Significant findings or events since last visit
  - Social or developmental delay
  - Infection or injury
- Immunization status
- Review of systems

Physical Examination:
Components of the Physical Exam
to Consider
(University of Arizona, 2005)
- Vital signs
- Growth parameters
  - Head circumference
  - Chest circumference
  - Height/weight
  - Growth pattern
- General appearance
  - Alertness
  - Muscle tone and activity

- Nutrition
- Response to environment
- Skin
  - Color and turgor
  - Rashes or lesions
  - Bruises or signs of abuse
- Head, Eyes, Ears, Nose and Throat (HEENT)
  - Fontanels: size and shape
  - Tracking movements of eyes
  - Suck and swallow
  - Tympanic membranes
  - Lymph nodes
- Chest and back
  - Shape and symmetry
  - Heart rate and rhythm
  - Breath sounds
- Abdomen
  - Size and shape
  - Palpation of organs
  - Bowel sounds
  - Muscle tone and integrity
  - Hernias
- Extremities
  - Strength
  - Flexibility and mobility
  - Femoral pulses
- Genitalia and anus
- Neurologic evaluation
  - Reflexes
  - Motor function
- Assessment for signs of illness or injury (McHugh, 2004b)
  - Fever
  - Skin tone variations
    - Pallor
    - Cyanosis
    - Ruddiness
    - Jaundice
    - Rash
  - Cardiopulmonary
    - Heart rate or rhythm abnormalities
    - Respiratory difficulty or wheezing

- Neurologic
  - Jitteriness or irritability
  - Bulging or sunken fontanels
  - Unusual sounding cry
- Musculoskeletal
  - Poor muscle tone
  - Hip clicks or laxity
- Gastrointestinal
  - Feeding difficulties
  - Abdominal distension
  - Absence of voiding or stooling
- Indications of abuse or neglect
  - Injuries, burns, or bruises
  - Malnutrition
  - Poor hygiene
  - Behavioral disorders

Clinical Impression:
Differential Diagnoses and Code Groups
to Consider
Additional suffix may apply (ICD9data.com, 2007)

- Well-baby care (ICD-9 codes V20.2)
- Acute conjunctivitis (ICD-9 codes 372.0)
- Otitis media (ICD-9 codes 382.0)
- Developmental delay (ICD-9 codes 783.4)
- Hearing screening (CPT code 92587)
- Child abuse (ICD-9 codes 995.5)

Diagnostic Testing:
Diagnostic Tests and Procedures to Consider

- Hematocrit
- Lead testing
- Developmental screening
- Hearing screening
- Vision testing
- Oral evaluation
- Other laboratory values or tests as indicated

Providing Treatment:
Therapeutic Measures to Consider

- Childhood immunizations (Centers for Disease Control and Prevention, 2006b)
  - Hepatitis B immunization: three (HepB) doses
  - Rotavirus: three (Rota) doses

- Diphtheria, tetanus, acellular pertussis: five (DTaP) doses
- Haemophilus influenza type b: four (Hib) doses
- Pneumococcal: four doses
- Oral polio/inactivated polio vaccine: four (OPV/IPV) doses
- Influenza: one dose annually
- Measles, mumps, rubella: two (MMR) doses
- Varicella: two doses
- Hepatitis A: two doses
- Treatment for underlying disease or illness
  - Antibiotics
  - Congenital hypothyroid treatment
  - Other treatments as indicated

Providing Treatment:
Alternative Measures to Consider

- Nutritional supplementation
  - Lact-Aid if breastfeeding
  - Goat's milk, fresh, raw
  - Homemade infant formula
  - Commercial infant formula
- Immunizations
  - Delay in onset of immunizations
  - Lower initial dose of immunizations
  - No immunizations
  - Information on vaccine safety
    - http://www.cdc.gov/od/science/iso/about_iso.htm
- Oral vitamin K: follow-up doses at 1- and 4-week visits

Providing Support:
Education and Support Measures to Consider

- Provide information on anticipated
  - Growth and development
  - Behaviors
  - Developmental milestones
- Diet and nutrition recommendations
  - Breastfeeding
  - Formulas

- Primary feeding method
- Supplementation
- Solid foods
- Signs and symptoms of concern
  - Warning signs
  - When to call with concerns
  - How to call in off-hours
- Routine for well-infant care
  - Schedule of visits
  - Immunization recommendations
  - Encourage parental participation in decision-making
  - Provide rationale for recommendations
  - Discuss alternatives
  - Provide access to additional resources as needed

Follow-up Care:
Follow-up Measures to Consider
- Document
  - Findings, especially any variations from normal
  - Plot growth on appropriate charts
  - Discussions with parents
  - Plan for continued care
  - Consultations or referrals
- Well-child examination schedule (Green & Palfrey, 2002)
  - 1 week
  - 1 month
  - Every 2 months from 2 to 6 months
  - Every 3 months from 6 to 18 months
  - Every 6 months from 18 to 24 months
  - Annually 2–5 years
  - ⚠ Report adverse vaccine reactions
    - Vaccine Adverse Event Reporting System form
    - Online http://www.vaers.hhs.gov
    - Telephone 1-800-822-7967

Collaborative Practice:
Consider Consultation or Referral
- Pediatric care provider
  - For routine well-child care

- In the presence of
  - Variations from normal
  - Illness
  - Injury
- For diagnosis or treatment outside the midwife's scope of practice

CARE OF THE MOTHER: POSTPARTUM CARE, WEEK 1

Key Clinical Information
During the first days postpartum, daily evaluation is performed. The postpartum woman undergoes a multitude of changes as her body returns to the nonpregnant state and she adapts emotionally to the changes in her family. Although the physiologic process is much the same in each individual, every woman responds differently to the birth of a child and has specific and distinct personal needs to be met.

In the first week after the birth, most families begin independent care of their newly born infant. Parents must have clear information regarding the expectations and indications for follow-up care, signs of complications, and when and how to access needed services. Fostering family independence requires ongoing access to support, education, and health care services.

Client History and Chart Review:
Components of the History to Consider
- Age, gravity, and parity
- Pregnancy, labor, and birth history
  - Prenatal course
  - Labor and birth information
    - Length of labor
    - Complicating factors for labor and/or birth
    - Manner of birth
    - Lacerations or episiotomy
  - Infant well-being since birth
    - Feeding
    - Sleeping
    - Activity

- Maternal well-being and adaptation
  - Pain
    - Location
    - Severity
    - Relief measures used and results
  - Adaptation to postpartum status
    - Sleep/rest
    - Appetite
    - Flow
    - Breasts
    - Other symptoms
  - Maternal emotional response to
    - Labor and birth
    - Changes postpartum
    - Changes in family dynamics
  - Observe interaction with infant
    - Feeding
    - Bonding
    - Caretaking
  - Review of systems

Physical Examination:
Components of the Physical Exam to Consider
(Varney et al., 2004)
- Vital signs: blood pressure, temperature, pulse, respirations

- Chest and thorax
  - Heart and lungs
  - Breasts and nipples
    - Cracks or fissures
    - Engorgement
    - Colostrum or milk
  - Costovertebral angle (CVA) tenderness
- Abdomen
  - Fundus: Location, consistency, tenderness
  - Muscle tone: Diastasis, hernia
  - Incision: Dressing, redness, erythema, exudate
  - Bladder: Distension, tenderness
  - Bowel sounds
- Lochia
  - Type, amount, odor
- Perineum and rectum (Davidson, 1974)
  - Evaluate for (see REEDA Scale, Table 5-1)
    - Redness or inflammation
    - Approximation of tissues
    - Bruising and/or hematoma
    - Edema
    - Discharge
  - Hemorrhoids
- Extremities
  - Edema
  - Reflexes

Table 5-1   REEDA Scale

POINTS	REDNESS	EDEMA	ECCHYMOSIS	DISCHARGE	APPROXIMATION
0	None	None	None	None	Closed
1	< 2.5 mm bilateral	< 10 mm bilateral	< 2.5 mm bilateral < 5 mm unilateral	Serum	≤ 3 mm skin separation
2	2.5–5 mm bilateral	10–20 mm	2.5–10 mm bilateral 5–20 mm unilateral	Serosanguinous	Skin and subcutaneous fat separate
3	> 5 mm bilateral	> 20 mm	> 10 mm bilateral > 20 mm unilateral	Bloody, purulent	Skin, subcutaneous fat, and fascia separate

From Davidson, N. (1974). REEDA: evaluating postpartum healing. *Journal of Nurse-Midwifery,* 19, 6–9.

- Homans' sign
- Redness, heat, or pain
- Varicosities

Clinical Impression:
Differential Diagnoses and Code Groups
to Consider
Additional suffix may apply (ICD9data.com, 2007)

- Postpartum care and examination (ICD-9 codes V24)
- Postpartum complications
  - Delayed postpartum hemorrhage (ICD-9 codes 666)
  - Postpartum infection (ICD-9 codes 670)
  - Postpartum venous conditions (ICD-9 codes 671)
  - Postpartum fever (ICD-9 codes 672)
  - Postpartum pulmonary embolism (ICD-9 codes 673)
  - Other and unspecified complications of the postpartum period (ICD-9 codes 674)
  - Other postpartum complications not otherwise specified (ICD-9 codes 669)
- Postpartum follow-up of complications, such as
  - Gestational diabetes (ICD-9 codes 648.8)
  - Postoperative wound infection (ICD-9 codes 670)
  - Preeclampsia (ICD-9 codes 642)
- Postpartum sterilization (CPT codes apply)
  - Tubal ligation
  - Tubal occlusion with device

Diagnostic Testing:
Diagnostic Tests and Procedures to Consider

- Hematocrit and hemoglobin or complete blood count (CBC) first or second postpartum day (Varney et al., 2004)
  - White blood cell count may remain elevated (> 15,000 or more) for 48 hours
  - Hematocrit may take 48 hours to stabilize
- Rh studies
- As indicated for complications of
  - Pregnancy
  - Postpartum
  - Medical condition

Providing Treatment:
Therapeutic Measures to Consider

- Laxatives or stool softeners, such as
  - Colace
  - Senokot
  - Milk of magnesia
- Urinary system
  - Encourage frequent voiding
  - Catheterize as needed for urinary retention
  - Insert Foley catheter if unable to void twice
- Heavy lochia and/or uterine atony
  - Methergine 0.2 mg PO every 4 hours for 6 doses (Varney et al., 2004)
- Pain management (see Immediate Postpartum Assessment)
- Sleep (German & Lee, 2006)
  - Use sleep medications with caution in nursing mothers
  - Nonbenzodiazepines
    - Ambien 5–10 mg at bedtime
    - Lunesta 2–3 mg at bedtime
    - Sonata 10 mg at bedtime
  - Benzodiazepines
    - Dalmane 15–30 mg at bedtime
    - Halcion 0.125–0.25 mg at bedtime
- Immune status (Varney et al., 2004)
  - Rh immune globulin 300 μg IM
  - Rubella vaccine 0.5 mL SC
    - Delay for 3 months in women receiving Rh immune globulin
- Antidepressants for at-risk women (see Care of the Mother: Perinatal Mood Disorders)

Providing Treatment:
Alternative Measures to Consider

- Home visit(s)
- Bowel care
  - Encourage fiber and fluids
    - Whole grains
    - Flax seed meal 1–2 T daily
    - Prune juice
    - Dried fruits

- Perineal care
  - Comfrey compresses (Davis, 1997)
  - Homeopathic arnica montana PO
  - Sitz baths, plain or herbal
- Urinary care
  - Encourage frequent voiding
  - Urinary retention
    - Oil of peppermint drops in toilet
- Sleep
  - Encourage frequent rest periods
  - Lemon Balm tea (Webb, 2006)
  - Chamomile tea

Providing Support:
Education and Support Measures to Consider
- Active listening and queries regarding
  - Birth experience
  - Maternal and family response to infant
  - Infant feeding and care
  - Maternal feelings
- Provide information about
  - Continued care of infant
  - Return to fertility
  - Contraception options, as needed
  - Medication instructions
    - Vitamin and mineral supplements
    - Other medications as indicated
  - When and how to schedule follow-up care
    - Planned postpartum visit(s)
    - Signs and symptoms of postpartum complications
    - When and how to access midwife

Follow-up Care:
Follow-up Measures to Consider
- One- to 2-week recheck
  - New mothers
  - Complicated prenatal or postpartum course
  - Incision check postcesarean or post-tubal
  - Initiate hormonal contraceptives
- Four- to 6-week postpartum examination
  - Involution
  - Lactation
  - Perineum

- Bowel and bladder function
- Sleep patterns
- Family adaptation
- Postpartum depression screening (see Care of the Mother: Perinatal Mood Disorders)
- Concerns and questions
- 8 weeks, as indicated for
  - Intrauterine device (IUD) insertion
  - Diaphragm or cervical cap fitting
- Document all care provided

Collaborative Practice:
Criteria to Consider for Consultation or Referral
- OB/GYN service
  - As needed for signs of maternal complications, such as
    - Endometritis or wound infection
    - Persistent subinvolution of the uterus
    - Thrombophlebitis
    - Pulmonary embolism
- Social services
  - Women, Infant, and Children (WIC)
  - Aid to Families with Dependent Children (AFDC)
  - Support groups
- For diagnosis or treatment outside the midwife's scope of practice

CARE OF THE MOTHER: POSTPARTUM CARE, WEEKS 2–6

Key Clinical Information
Most women adjust rapidly after the birth of their baby. By 4–6 weeks after the birth most women are returning to their usual functioning and are adapting to the changes that the baby has brought into the family's life. Postpartum maternal evaluation is directed toward determining the presence of any complications or concerns and addressing needs for birth control information or supplies. The midwife tailors information about child spacing, pregnancy prevention methods, infant care, and resources to the woman's cultural background, level of understanding, economic resources, and stated needs.

Some women feel isolated or insecure in the initial weeks after the birth of their baby. The empathetic midwife may be able to enhance maternal adaptation by providing care that is culturally acceptable and fosters social support in the mother's home community. Guidance and support during this time of transition may positively impact maternal self-care and the care she provides her infant by providing a nurturing environment where development of a healthy maternal self-image and feelings of competence and confidence as a woman and mother may result.

Women who have difficulty with postpartum adjustment may benefit from referrals to local resources, such as parenting groups or classes, breastfeeding groups, play groups, counseling, and other support services. Feelings of isolation are not uncommon, and many women may need to be given permission or actively directed to participate in activities other than newborn care.

Client History and Chart Review:
Components of the History to Consider
- Review
  - Labor and birth events and outcomes
  - Initial postpartum course
  - Gynecologic history
  - Medical/surgical history
  - Social history
- Physical return to nonpregnant status (Varney et al., 2004)
  - Amount, color, and consistency of lochia
  - Breasts, status of lactation
  - Perineal or abdominal discomfort
  - Bladder and bowel function
  - Physical activity and sleep patterns
  - Resumption of sexual activity
  - Preference for contraception, as indicated
  - Signs or symptoms of delayed involution or medical problems
- Emotional adaptation
  - 🌐 Cultural practices used during the postpartum period
  - Adjustment to parenting

- Satisfaction with parenting, sexuality
- Interactions and support of family/ significant others
- Signs or symptoms of depression or maladaptation
- Infant care
  - Interactions with infant
  - Infant growth and feeding
  - Access to pediatric care
- Review of systems

Physical Examination:
Components of the Physical Exam
to Consider
- Examination components vary based on
  - Timing of visit
  - Indication for visit
  - Client history
- Vital signs, including temperature
- Thyroid
- Thorax
  - Breast examination
    - Lactation
    - Nipple integrity
    - Masses
    - Axilla
  - Heart
  - Lungs
  - Costovertebral angle tenderness
- Abdominal examination
  - Diastasis recti
  - Muscle tone
  - Cesarean section or tubal ligation incision
- Pelvic examination
  - External genitalia for status of perineum/lacerations
  - Speculum examination
    - Appearance of cervix
    - Specimen collection
  - Bimanual examination
    - Uterine involution
    - Vaginal muscle tone
    - Presence of cystocele or rectocele
  - Rectal examination

- Extremities
  - Edema
  - Varicosities
  - Phlebitis
  - Reflexes

Clinical Impression:
Differential Diagnoses and Code Groups
to Consider
Additional suffix may apply (ICD9data.com, 2007)
- Normal postpartum course (ICD-9 codes V24)
- Postpartum complications, such as
  - Endometritis (ICD-9 codes 670)
  - Venous complications (i.e., phlebitis) (ICD-9 codes 671)
  - Postpartum fever (ICD-9 codes 672)
  - Other unspecified complications of postpartum period, such as subinvolution of the uterus (ICD-9 codes 674)
  - Mastitis (ICD-9 codes 675)
  - Breastfeeding difficulties (ICD-9 codes 676)
  - Postpartum depression (ICD-9 codes 648.44)
  - Postpartum adaptation problems (ICD-9 codes V24 and 309)

Diagnostic Testing:
Diagnostic Tests and Procedures to Consider
- Pap smear follow-up as needed
- Sexually transmitted infection testing as indicated by history
- Follow-up of anemia: hematocrit and hemoglobin, CBC
- Fasting blood sugar (gestational diabetics)
- Thyroid testing: thyroid-stimulating hormone (TSH)
- Other laboratory testing as indicated by history

Providing Treatment:
Therapeutic Measures to Consider
- Initiation of birth control, as desired (see Chapter 6)
  - Natural family planning
  - Nonprescription methods
  - Prescription methods

- Postpartum depression screening
- Vitamin and mineral supplementation
  - $FeSO_4$ replacement
  - Calcium
  - Multivitamin

Providing Treatment:
Alternative Measures to Consider
- Nutritional support to promote healing and foster well-being
  - Increased fluid and fiber to stimulate regular bowel function
  - Whole foods: adequate protein, vitamins, and minerals

Providing Support:
Education and Support Measures to Consider
- Encourage social support
  - Assistance and caring from family and friends
  - Resources in the area for specific needs
    - Play or support groups for new mothers
    - Mothers of twins
    - La Leche League
    - Parenting classes
    - Teen parent groups
- Home or office visit for support and education
  - Infant care and feeding
  - Initiation of physical activity
  - Warning signs or symptoms
  - Recommended diet
  - Anticipated weight changes postpartum
  - Potential decrease in libido and natural lubrication
    - Postpartum
    - With breastfeeding
  - Birth control options

Follow-up Care:
Follow-up Measures to Consider
- ⚠ Validate maternal understanding of recommendations
- Document all care provided, including phone triage

- Return visit in 12 months or as indicated by visit
  - Annual gynecologic examination and/or birth control
  - Problem evaluation or follow-up
  - Prenatal care
- Call with questions or concerns

Collaborative Practice:
Consider Consultation or Referral
- Psychotherapist or psychiatrist
  - Significant postpartum depression
  - Poor maternal adaptation
- OB/GYN service
  - For poor wound healing or infection
- Medical service, follow-up of medical problems
  - Diagnosis of diabetes or glucose intolerance
  - Essential hypertension
  - Thyroid disorder
- Social service
  - WIC/AFDC
  - Housing
  - Drug rehabilitation
  - Child welfare
- For diagnosis or treatment outside the midwife's scope of practice

CARE OF THE MOTHER: PERINATAL MOOD DISORDERS

Key Clinical Information
Comprehensive midwifery care includes screening each woman for pregnancy-related mood disorders. Untreated maternal mood disorders have been demonstrated to have adverse effects on the infant's cognitive and language development (Nulman et al., 2002). The risks and benefits of medical treatment during pregnancy and breastfeeding must be weighed against the benefits to both mother and baby. The midwife is responsible for the screening and identification, with appropriate referral for diagnosis and treatment, of women with perinatal mood disorder during and after pregnancy.

Screening every woman for pregnancy-related mood disorders facilitates early identification and treatment of women who require more than simple support to cope with the emotional changes that may occur during pregnancy and after the birth of the infant. Perinatal mood disorders may range from a mild case of "the blues" to significant depression or postpartum psychosis. Postpartum depression may occur up to 12 months after giving birth.

Many women may be reluctant to divulge negative feelings about themselves or their baby. A supportive nonjudgmental environment fosters the trust many women need to talk about their feelings. Postpartum depression affects 10–15% of women who give birth, with as many as 50–80% of women experiencing postpartum blues (National Institutes of Health, 2005). Postpartum depression occurs in 26–32% of adolescent women who give birth and is more common in women with history of mood disorder (Righetti-Velterna et al., 1998)

Client History and Chart Review:
Components of the History to Consider
(Fernandez, 2005; Miller, 1996)
- Age, gravida, para
- Birth and postpartum history
  - Labor and birth experience
  - Perception of postpartum period
  - Infant's age
  - Method of infant feeding
  - Sleep patterns and amounts
  - Hormone use
- Social history
  - Absence of support systems
  - Sexual abuse
  - Familial discord
  - Socioeconomic stressors
- Risk factors for postpartum mood disorder
  - History of depression
  - Depression or anxiety during pregnancy
  - Complications of pregnancy, such as
    - Late onset or erratic prenatal visits
    - Infertility
    - Miscarriage
    - Perinatal loss
    - Multiple gestation
    - Hyperemesis

- Social factors, such as
  - ◆ Adolescents and single women
  - ◆ Social stigma, conflict, or lack of support
  - ◆ Poor socioeconomic status
  - ◆ Major life events unrelated to pregnancy
- Onset and type of symptoms
  - Postpartum blues
    - ◆ Moodiness
    - ◆ Tearfulness
    - ◆ Elation
    - ◆ Heightened reactivity
    - ◆ Onset within 3–5 days after birth
    - ◆ Occurs across all cultures
    - ◆ Transient and self-limiting
    - ◆ Resolves in 7–14 days
    - ◆ ⚠ Twenty percent of women with blues progress to depression
  - Adjustment disorder (present > 2 weeks)
    - ◆ Greater difficulty with adjustment than normal
    - ◆ Decreased coping ability
  - Depression (present > 2 weeks)
    - ◆ Agitation
    - ◆ Anxiety
    - ◆ Sadness
    - ◆ Insomnia
    - ◆ Fatigue
    - ◆ Diminished interest or pleasure
    - ◆ Feelings of worthlessness and guilt
    - ◆ Feelings of detachment from infant
    - ◆ Thoughts of harming infant
    - ◆ Suicidal ideation
    - ◆ Perinatal up to 12 months postpartum
    - ◆ Appetite changes
    - ◆ Irritability/mood changes (Righetti-Velterna et al., 1998)
  - 🕐 Mania
    - ◆ Euphoria
    - ◆ Decreased need for sleep
    - ◆ Racing thoughts
    - ◆ Distractibility
    - ◆ May convert into depression or psychosis

- 🕐 Psychosis
  - ◆ ⚠ Medical emergency
  - ◆ Disorganized thinking, behavior, or speech
  - ◆ Perceptual disturbances (auditory or visual)
  - ◆ Delusions
- Assess
  - Stressors
  - Social and economic resources
  - Sleep–wake patterns
  - Potential for harming self or infant
- Review of systems (ROS)

Physical Examination:
Components of the Physical Exam to Consider
- Vital signs, including temperature
- Signs or symptoms of
  - Postpartum thyroidosis
  - Anemia
  - Infection
- Evaluate for
  - Sleep deprivation
  - Changes in personal appearance
  - Signs of peripartum mood disorder

Clinical Impression:
Differential Diagnoses and Code Groups
to Consider
Additional suffix may apply (ICD9data.com, 2007)
- Perinatal mood disorder, such as (Fernandez, 2005)
  - Postpartum blues (ICD-9 codes 309)
  - Adjustment disorder (ICD-9 codes 309)
  - Depression (ICD-9 codes 296)
  - Mania in the postpartum period (ICD-9 codes 296)
  - Psychosis in the postpartum period (ICD-9 codes 296)
  - Postpartum (ICD-9 codes 674.9) applicable within 4 weeks of delivery
- Preexisting mood disorder exacerbated by birth (ICD-9 codes V24 and 296)

- Severe sleep deprivation (ICD-9 codes V69.4)
- Medical illness, such as
  - Thyroid disorder (ICD-9 codes V24 and 240–246)

Diagnostic Testing:
Diagnostic Tests and Procedures to Consider
(Fernandez, 2005)
- Thyroid profile
- Urinalysis
- CBC with differential
- Comprehensive metabolic panel
- Edinburgh Postnatal Depression Scale

Providing Treatment
Therapeutic Measures to Consider
(Fernandez, 2005; Gjerdingen, 2003)
- 🕐 Referral for diagnosis and treatment may be the best option
- Interpersonal psychotherapy
  - May avoid need for medication
  - Addresses relationships
  - Provides techniques to decrease symptoms
- Antidepressant therapy (Clark & Paine, 1996; Fernandez, 2005)
  - Medication choice based on
    - Symptom type and severity
    - Method of infant feeding (Leopold & Zoschnick, 1997)
  - Selective serotonin reuptake inhibitors (SSRIs)
    - Zoloft or Paxil preferred for breastfeeding mothers
  - Serotonin norepinephrine reuptake inhibitors (SNRIs)
  - Late pregnancy administration for high-risk women
    - Reach therapeutic levels before delivery
    - May result in neonatal behavioral syndrome (Fernandez, 2005)
- Estrogen therapy
  - Use for mild to moderate symptoms with early onset

- Transdermal estradiol 0.1–0.2 mg daily
- Use 3–6 months if improvement noted (Gregoire et al., 1996)
- Combination hormonal contraceptives may improve or exacerbate depression

Providing Treatment:
Alternative Measures to Consider
- Omega-3 polyunsaturated fatty acids (Hendrick, 2003)
- Herbal remedies
  - St. John's wort 300 mg TID (Hendrick, 2003)
    - May decrease effectiveness of hormonal contraceptives
  - Lemon balm tea, 2–3 cups daily
  - Valerian root, 1–3 capsules daily
- Light therapy (Hendrick, 2003)
- Home visits by midwife, doula, or nurse (Gjerdingen, 2003)
- 🌐 Culturally appropriate treatments
- Adequate nutrition
  - Whole foods
  - Adequate fluids
  - Avoid caffeine, alcohol, and cigarettes
- Time scheduled for
  - Sleep
  - Personal care
  - Daily walking or activity
  - Personal time away from infant
  - Favorite activities
  - Intimate time with partner
- ⚠ Alternative therapies should not be a substitute for supervised psychiatric care for the woman who threatens, or appears at risk, to harm herself or her family.

Providing Support:
Education and Support Measures to Consider
(Fernandez, 2005)
- Shared decision-making related to therapies
- Prenatal education
  - Normalcy of feelings associated with postpartum blues

- Signs and symptoms of postpartum mood disorders
- Screening process at postpartum visit
- Local resources
- Self-help or maternal support groups
- Breastfeeding education and support
- Parenting organizations
- Crisis hotline number
- Mental health professionals
- Postpartum education
  - Review resources
  - Mobilize family support
  - Rest with infant
  - Avoid isolation
  - Maintain nutrition
  - Signs and symptoms of postpartum depression
  - How to access help and support
  - Skills training
  - Family interventions

Follow-up Care:
Follow-up Measures to Consider
- Document
  - Screening results
  - Mental health referral
  - Midwife follow-up plan and actions
  - Update plan as condition changes
- Follow-up visits
  - Telephone contact within 24–48 hours
  - Weekly visits (home or office) while acute
  - As needed for titration of medication
- During ongoing care, assess (Fernandez, 2005)
  - Maternal–child interaction and relationship
  - Infant development
  - Partner relationship
  - With delayed recovery explore history for sexual abuse

Collaborative Practice:
Criteria to Consider for Consultation or Referral
- Mental health or psychiatric service
  - Psychotherapy or counseling

- Pharmacologic treatment as indicated by client need and midwife scope of practice
- Clients who do not respond to midwife-initiated therapy within 7–14 days, or as appropriate for medication
- ⚠ Psychiatric emergency
  - Presence of psychosis
  - For any client who is suicidal or homicidal
  - Client or infant is perceived to be at risk for harm
  - Rejection of or physical aggression (threatened or actual) against infant
- Support services
  - Lactation consultant
  - Postpartum doula
- Social services
  - Housing
  - Food
  - Finances
  - Child care
- Medical service
  - Suspected or confirmed medical condition
- For diagnosis or treatment outside the midwife's scope of practice

CARE OF THE MOTHER: POSTPARTUM ENDOMETRITIS

Key Clinical Information

Postpartum endometritis is a polymicrobial disorder where bacteria, such as streptococcus, staphylococcus, *Ureaplasma,* and/or *Escherichia coli,* ascend from the lower genital tract to infect the uterus. Postpartum endometritis may occur after either cesarean delivery (3–10% incidence) or vaginal birth (1–3% incidence) (Simmons & Bammel, 2005). The incidence of postcesarean endometritis is related to the number and types of risk factors present and the use of intraoperative antibiotic prophylaxis (Chandran & Puccio, 2006).

Postpartum endometritis usually presents on the second to seventh postpartum day (Varney et al., 2004). Diagnosis is based primarily on clinical findings as the physiologic elevation of the white blood cell count that occurs during labor typically persists into the postpartum period. Endometritis should be suspected in the presence of postpartum fever, defined as two temperature elevations to 38°C (100.4°F) or greater on any two days more than 24 hours after and within 10 days after delivery (Chandran & Puccio, 2006; Varney et al., 2004).

Client History and Chart Review:
Components of the History to Consider
- Duration of postpartum status
- Presence, onset, duration, and severity of symptoms
  - Fever and chills
  - Malaise
  - Uterine pain
  - Foul odor to lochia
  - Change in amount of lochia flow
- General well-being
  - Appetite
  - Urinary function
  - Respiratory function
  - Other associated symptoms
- Risk factors for postpartum endometritis (Chandran & Puccio, 2006; Simmons & Bammel, 2005)
  - Cesarean delivery
  - Manual removal of the placenta
  - Prolonged rupture of membranes
  - Long labor associated with multiple vaginal examinations
  - Extremes of patient age
  - Prolonged internal fetal monitoring
  - Anemia
  - Poor nutrition
- Medical/surgical history
  - Appendicitis
  - Diverticular disease
  - Immunocompromised condition
- Review of systems

Physical Examination:
Components of the Physical Exam to Consider
- Vital signs: blood pressure, temperature, pulse, respirations
- Cardiopulmonary system
  - Tachycardia
  - Pallor
  - Breath sounds
    - Rales
    - Respiratory effort
- Breast examination
  - Redness
  - Mass
  - Pain
- Abdominopelvic and thoracic examination
  - Uterine size
  - Tenderness with uterine palpation
  - Guarding
  - Rebound tenderness
  - Masses
  - Costovertebral angle tenderness
- Incision or laceration examination
  - Exudate
  - Redness
  - Swelling
  - Masses
- Evaluation of lochia
  - Odor
  - Volume
- Extremities
  - Edema
  - Homans' sign
  - Femoral and pedal pulses

Clinical Impression:
Differential Diagnoses and Code Groups
to Consider
Additional suffix may apply (ICD9data.com, 2007)
- Genital tract
  - Postpartum endometritis (ICD-9 codes 670)
  - Wound infection (ICD-9 codes 674.3)
    - Surgical incision

- ◆ Episiotomy
- ◆ Laceration
- ▪ Pelvic or vaginal hematoma (ICD-9 codes 664.5)
- ▪ Retained placental parts (ICD-9 codes 667.1)
- Breast infection (ICD-9 codes 675)
- Urinary tract
  - ▪ Infection (ICD-9 codes 646.64)
  - ▪ Renal calculi (ICD-9 codes 592)
- Cardiopulmonary system
  - ▪ Respiratory infection (ICD-9 codes 674)
  - ▪ Deep vein thrombosis (ICD-9 codes 674.3)
  - ▪ Pulmonary embolus (ICD-9 codes 673)
- Appendicitis (ICD-9 codes 540)

Diagnostic Testing:
Diagnostic Tests and Procedures to Consider
- CBC w/differential
- Urinalysis
- O_2 saturation
- Cultures as indicated
  - ▪ Urine
  - ▪ Blood
  - ▪ Wound
- Radiology studies as indicated
  - ▪ Chest x-ray
  - ▪ Ultrasound or computed tomography (CT)
    - ◆ Pelvic
      - ➤ Hematoma
      - ➤ Retained placental fragments
    - ◆ Abdominal
      - ➤ Appendix
      - ➤ Kidney, ureter, bladder (KUB)
    - ◆ Extremities

Providing Treatment:
Therapeutic Measures to Consider
- Antimicrobial therapy (Murphy, 2004; Simmons & Bammel, 2005)
  - ▪ IV antibiotic therapy is indicated for serious infection, options include:
  - ▪ Cefotetan 1–2 g IV every 12 hours
  - ▪ Gentamycin 1.5 mg/kg load, then 1 mg/kg every 8 hours, plus Clindamycin 900 mg IV every 6 hours

- ▪ Ampicillin/sulbactam 3 g IV every 4–6 hours
- ▪ Mezlocillin 4 g IV every 4–6 hours
- ▪ Ticarcillin/clavulanate 3.1 g IV every 6 hours
- Hydration
  - ▪ Oral fluids
  - ▪ IV therapy
- Prevention of deep vein thrombosis
  - ▪ Antiembolitic stockings
  - ▪ Isometric exercises

Providing Treatment:
Alternative Measures to Consider
- ⚠ Alternative remedies are not a substitute for prompt medical care
  - ▪ Inadequately treated local infection may become systemic
  - ▪ Systemic infection can rapidly lead to death
- Rescue Remedy to pulse points
- Hot pack to abdomen
- Herbal support
  - ▪ Black walnut tincture
  - ▪ Sage tea
  - ▪ Oregano tea
  - ▪ Echinacea tea or tincture
- Homeopathic arnica montana

Providing Support:
Education and Support Measures to Consider
- Supportive measures
  - ▪ Rest
  - ▪ Adequate nutrition
  - ▪ Provision for infant care
  - ▪ Provide emotional support
  - ▪ Listen
  - ▪ Update information as situation demands
- Discuss with client and family
  - ▪ Working diagnosis
  - ▪ Urgency of condition
  - ▪ Need for diagnostic testing
  - ▪ Potential need for
    - ◆ Medical evaluation
    - ◆ Hospitalization
    - ◆ IV antibiotic treatment
  - ▪ Compatibility of medications with breastfeeding, as needed

Follow-up Care:
Follow-up Measures to Consider

- Anticipate response to medication within 48 hours
- (🕐) If minimal or no response, evaluate for potential complications
  - Pelvic abscess
  - Pelvic hematoma
  - Wound infection
  - Septic pelvic thrombophlebitis
- 🗑 Document
  - Clinical evaluation and working diagnosis
  - Consultation(s) and plan of care
  - Update notes frequently, including
    - Changes in client status
    - Rationale for orders
    - Consultation or transfer of care requests

Collaborative Practice:
Criteria to Consider for Consultation or Referral

- OB/GYN service
  - Evaluation or treatment of postpartum fever or infection
  - Transfer of care from home or birth center for hospitalization
  - Infection that does not respond to treatment within 24–48 hours
- For diagnosis or treatment outside the midwife's scope of practice

CARE OF THE MOTHER: HEMORRHOIDS

Key Clinical Information

Hemorrhoids form as a result of dilatation and engorgement of the arteriovenous plexuses of the anal canal. This condition is often exacerbated during pregnancy, labor, and birth, most likely from direct pressure on the rectal veins (Gurley & Sinert, 2006). Prompt treatment of hemorrhoids postpartum may prevent thrombosis of external hemorrhoids that have become trapped by the anal sphincter. Thrombosed hemorrhoids are exquisitely painful and may require incision and drainage.

Client History and Chart Review:
Components of the History to Consider

- Prior history of hemorrhoids
- Usual diet and bowel function
- Length and positions used during second-stage labor
- Presence of symptoms
  - Itching
  - Aching
  - Severe pain (associated with thrombosis)
- Relief measures used and their effects
- Presence of rectal bleeding

Physical Examination:
Components of the Physical Exam to Consider

- Perineal assessment
  - Approximation of repair, if applicable
  - Edema
- Presence of hemorrhoids
  - May be single or rosette
  - Note
    - Size
    - Location
    - Edema
    - Redness
  - Palpate to evaluate for thrombosis
    - Firm clot felt within vein
    - Exquisitely painful to touch
- Rectal examination
  - Rectal prolapse
  - Anal fissure, lesions or mass
  - Undiagnosed third- or fourth-degree laceration

Clinical Impression:
Differential Diagnoses and Code Groups to Consider
Additional suffix may apply (ICD9data.com, 2007)

- Hemorrhoids
  - Hemorrhoids, not otherwise specified (ICD-9 codes 455.6)
  - Hemorrhoids, thrombosed (ICD-9 codes 455.7)
- Rectovaginal hematoma (ICD-9 codes 665.72)

- Undiagnosed third- or fourth-degree laceration (ICD-9 codes 664)
- Anal abscess or mass (ICD-9 codes 566)
- Anal fissure (ICD-9 codes 565)

Diagnostic Testing:
Diagnostic Tests and Procedures to Consider
- Anoscopy

Providing Treatment:
Therapeutic Measures to Consider
- Topical analgesics for discomfort, with or without hydrocortisone (National Library of Medicine, 2006)
  - Pramoxine (Proctofoam/Proctofoam HC/Anusol ointment)
  - Dibucaine (Nupercainal ointment)
  - Benzocaine (Americaine spray or ointment)
- Steroid hemorrhoid preparations for itching (German & Lee, 2006)
  - Anusol-HC (25 mg hydrocortisone) suppositories
  - Cortifoam (10% hydrocortisone)
  - Proctocort suppositories (30 mg hydrocortisone)
  - ⚠ May decrease resistance to local infection
- Maintain soft formed stool
  - Stool softeners
    - Colace: 50–200 mg daily
    - Surfak: 240 mg PO daily until normal
  - Laxatives
    - Peri-Colace (softener + stimulant)
      - 1–2 capsules at bedtime
    - Perdiem (fiber + stimulant)
      - 1–2 tsp in 8 oz water at bedtime or in the morning
    - Senokot (senna stimulant)
      - 2 tablets at bedtime
  - Fiber supplements
    - Citrucel: 1 Tbs in 8 oz water one to three times daily
    - Metamucil: one packet or 1 tsp in 8 oz water one to three times daily

- Glycerin suppositories
- Enemas
  - Fleet enema
  - Soapsuds enema
- Severe hemorrhoids, no thrombosis
  - Manually reduce hemorrhoids as necessary
  - May require rectal packing
    - Provides counterpressure
    - Lubricate with hemorrhoid cream
    - Remove after 12–24 hours
- Thrombosis
  - May require incision and drainage

Providing Treatment:
Alternative Measures to Consider
- Topical measures to aid soft tissue healing
  - Sitz baths
    - Warm water
    - Herbal infusions
      - Comfrey
      - Plantain
      - Calendula
  - Ice packs
  - Witch hazel compresses
  - Aloe vera gel
  - Comfrey compresses TID
- Knees-to-chest position to drain hemorrhoids
  - Hands and knees
  - Head on pillow
  - Hips elevated
- Homeopathics
  - Arnica 30× 2 tablets QID
  - Hamamelis 30C (Smith, 1984)

Providing Support:
Education and Support Measures to Consider
- Diet adequate in fluids and fiber
  - Dried fruit
  - Psyllium or flax seed
  - Prune juice
  - Rhubarb
  - Blueberries
  - Whole grains
  - Fresh fruit and vegetables

- Discussion of treatment options and instructions
  - Avoidance of
    - Straining
    - Prolonged sitting on toilet
    - Holding stool
  - When to call
    - Bleeding
    - Increasing pain

Follow-up Care:
Follow-up Measures to Consider
- Reevaluate
  - 12–24 hours after treatment
  - Persistent rectal bleeding
- Document
  - Examination findings
  - Recommended treatment plan
  - Response to treatment

Collaborative Practice:
Consider Consultation or Referral
- OB/GYN service
  - Thrombosed hemorrhoids for incision and drainage (I & D)
  - Suspected third- or fourth-degree laceration
  - Rectal
    - Abscess
    - Anal fissure
    - Hematoma
    - Bleeding
- For diagnosis or treatment outside the midwife's scope of practice

CARE OF THE MOTHER: MASTITIS

Key Clinical Information

Mastitis primarily occurs in first 8 weeks postpartum and affects 20–30% of breastfeeding women. Early identification and prompt treatment at the first signs may preclude the need for antibiotic therapy. Untreated mastitis may result in inadequate milk production, abscess formation, recurrent mastitis, or systemic infection (Semba et al., 1999). Educating breastfeeding women about presenting signs and symptoms of mastitis, preventive measures, when and how to contact their midwife for evaluation, and treatment options is an essential part of midwifery practice. This is especially important in breastfeeding women who are infected or at risk for HIV infection, where subclinical mastitis leads to an increase in the viral load carried by breast milk (Nussenblatt et al., 2006).

Client History and Chart Review:
Components of the History to Consider
- Presence of conditions that may affect immune status
  - Chronic illness
  - HIV status and/or risk assessment
- Breastfeeding history
  - Duration of breastfeeding
  - Infant feeding style
  - Recent changes to nursing patterns
  - Usual breast care
- Previous history of breast problems
  - Mastitis
  - Abscess
  - Breast biopsies
  - Breast reduction or implants
- Presence of risk factors for mastitis (Mitchie et al., 2003)
  - Breast trauma
  - Milk stasis
  - Ineffective breast emptying
  - Fatigue
  - Primipara
  - Previous mastitis
  - Inadequate nutrition
  - Immune factors
- Onset, duration, and severity of symptoms (Varney et al., 2004)
  - Breast symptoms
    - Painful breast(s), worse when nursing
    - Redness of breast
    - Swelling or induration of breast
  - Generalized symptoms
    - Fever and/or chills
    - Malaise or flulike symptoms

- ◆ Headache
- ◆ Nausea
- Self-help measures used and effectiveness
- Review of systems

Physical Examination:
Components of the Physical Exam
to Consider
- Vital signs, especially temperature and pulse
- General appearance and well-being
- Breast examination
  - Engorgement
  - Tenderness, redness, swelling
  - Induration
  - Warmth, generalized or local
  - Cracks or fissures in nipples
  - Masses
    - ◆ Firm or soft
    - ◆ Fixed or mobile
    - ◆ Tender or nontender
- Axillary examination
  - Engorgement
  - Lymph nodes
- Additional components as indicated by history and physical

Clinical Impression
Differential Diagnoses and Code Groups
to Consider
Additional suffix may apply (ICD9data.com, 2007)
- Mastitis, acute, postpartum nonpurulent (ICD-9 codes 675.2)
- Mastitis, acute, postpartum purulent (ICD-9 codes 675.1)
- Breast abscess (ICD-9 codes 675.1)
- Breast cancer (ICD-9 codes 174)

Diagnostic Testing:
Diagnostic Tests and Procedures to Consider
- CBC
- Breast ultrasound for mass
  - Abscess suspected
  - Differentiate solid versus cystic

- Culture of breast milk for pathogen
  - Unresponsive to therapy
  - Systemic involvement
- 🕐 Mammograms rarely performed during lactation

Providing Treatment:
Therapeutic Measures to Consider
- Fever and pain reducers
  - Ibuprofen
  - Aspirin
  - Acetaminophen
- Antibiotic therapy for infection, such as
  - Dicloxacillin 250 mg QID for 10 days
  - Keflex 500 mg PO every 6 hours or BID for 10 days
  - Erythromycin for 10 days
    - ◆ ERYC 250 mg PO every 6 hours
    - ◆ Ery-Tab 333 mg every 8 hours or 500 mg every 12 hours
    - ◆ Erythromycin ethylsuccinate 1.6 g/day in two, three, or four evenly divided doses
  - Nafcillin 250–500 mg PO every 4–6 hours for 10 days (or other penicillinase-resistant penicillin) (Murphy, 2004; Varney et al., 2004)

Providing Treatment:
Alternative Measures to Consider
- Adequate rest, hydration, and nutrition
- Rest with infant at breast
- For rest
  - Hops infusion
  - Skullcap tincture (Weed, 1985)
- For fever, infusion of
  - Echinacea
  - Yarrow
  - Peppermint
- To diminish infection
  - Black walnut
  - Sage
  - Oregano
  - Garlic
- Comfrey compresses to affected area

- Homeopathics (Davis, 1997)
  - Arnica 30 C
  - Bryonia 30 C
  - Phytolacca 30 C
  - Belladonna 30 C

Providing Support:
Education and Support Measures
to Consider
- Teach careful hand washing and breast care
  - Warm compresses to affected area
  - Gentle massage toward nipple
  - Frequent nursing and/or pumping
    - Vary infant's suckling positions
      - Cradle
      - Side-lying
      - Football
      - Belly to belly
- Increase fluid intake
- Rest, rest, rest
- Obtain assistance with
  - Housekeeping
  - Child care
  - Promoting rest
- Provide medication instructions
  - Take as directed until medication is gone
  - Infant may get diarrhea or gastrointestinal upset
  - Continue to nurse unless contraindicated by
    - Medication used
    - Significant side effects in infant
    - Serious illness of mother
    - Pumping is an option, but not as effective as nursing
- Instructions for when and how to contact
  - Fever ≥ 100.4°F
  - Chills
  - Worsening symptoms

Follow-up Care:
Follow-up Measures to Consider
- Document findings and recommendations

- Reassess within 24 hours
  - To confirm effectiveness of therapy
  - For evaluation if no improvement
- Consider hospitalization
  - Persistent fever
  - Systemic symptoms
  - IV antibiotic therapy indicated

Collaborative Practice:
Consider Consultation or Referral
- OB/GYN service
  - For mastitis unresponsive to therapy
  - For breast abscess
- Lactation consultant
  - Mastitis prevention instruction
  - Breast care and feeding during illness
  - Infant positioning
  - Massage techniques
  - Recommendations and support
  - Assistance with supplements if needed
- Social service
  - Home help
  - Visiting nurse
  - Other support services
- Pediatric service
  - As indicated by infant response to medication
- For diagnosis or treatment outside the midwife's scope of practice

REFERENCES

American Academy of Family Physicians. (2001). *Circumcision: position paper on neonatal circumcision.* Retrieved January 26, 2008 from http://www.aafp.org/online/en/home/clinical/clinicalrecs/circumcision.html

American Academy of Family Physicians. (2006). *OB coding: using other evaluation and management services in maternity care.* Retrieved January 26, 2008 from http://www.aafp.org/online/en/home/practicemgt/codingresources/codingob/emmaternity.html

American Academy of Pediatrics. (n.d.). *Supporting breastfeeding and lactation: the primary care pediatrician's guide to getting paid.* Retrieved January 26, 2008 from http://www.aapdistrictii.org/BreastCoding.pdf

American Academy of Pediatrics (AAP). (1999). Circumcision policy statement. *Pediatrics, 103,* 686–693.

American Academy of Pediatrics (AAP). (2003). Policy statement: controversies concerning vitamin K and the newborn. *Pediatrics,* 112, 191–192.

American Academy of Pediatrics (AAP) and American Heart Association (AHA). (2006). *Textbook of neonatal resuscitation* (5th ed.). Elk Grove Village, IL: Author.

American College of Obstetricians and Gynecologists. (2001). *Committee opinion #260: Circumcision.* In *2006 Compendium of selected publications.* Washington, DC: Author.

American College of Medical Genetics. (1999). *Evaluation of the newborn with single or multiple congenital anomalies: a clinical guideline.* Bethesda: MD. Author. Retrieved January 26, 2008 from http://www.health.state.ny.us/nysdoh/dpprd/exec.htm

Canadian Pediatric Society and College of Family Physicians of Canada. (2004). Joint position statement: Routine administration of vitamin K to newborns. (Reaffirmed March 2004. Originally published 1997.) *Paediatrics & Child Health* 2, 429–431. Retrieved January 26, 2008 from http://www.cps.ca/ENGLISH/statements/FN/fn97-01.htm

Centers for Disease Control and Prevention. (2005). A comprehensive immunization strategy to eliminate transmission of hepatitis B virus infection in the United States. *Morbidity and Mortality Weekly Report,* 54(RR16), 1–23. Retrieved January 26, 2008 from http://www.cdc.gov/MMWR/preview/mmwrhtml/rr5416a1.htm

Centers for Disease Control and Prevention. (2006a). 2006 STD treatment guidelines. *Morbidity and Mortality Weekly Report,* 55(RR11). Retrieved January 26, 2008 from http://www.cdc.gov/std/treatment/default.htm

Centers for Disease Control and Prevention. (2006b). Recommended immunization schedules for persons aged 0–18 years—United States, 2007. *Morbidity and Mortality Weekly Report,* 55, Q1–Q4. Retrieved January 26, 2008 from http://www.cdc.gov/mmwr/preview/mmwrhtml/mm5551a7.htm?s_cid=mm5551a7_e

Centers for Disease Control and Prevention. (2007). *When should a mother avoid breastfeeding?* Retrieved January 26, 2008 from http://www.cdc.gov/breastfeeding/disease/contraindicators.htm

Chandran, L., & Puccio, J. (2006). *Endometritis.* E-medicine. Retrieved January 26, 2008 from http://www.emedicine.com/ped/topic678.htm

Christakis, D. A., Harvey, E., Zerr, D. M., Feudtner, C., Wright, J. A., & Connell, F. A. (2000). A trade-off analysis of routine newborn circumcision. *Pediatrics,* 105, 246–249.

Circumcision Information and Resource Pages. (2007). *Circumcision: Medical Organization Official Policy Statements in Circumcision Reference Library.* Retrieved January, 26, 2008 from http://www.cirp.org/library/statements/

Clark, C., & Paine, L. L. (1996). Psychopharmacologic management of women with common mental health problems. *Journal of Nurse-Midwifery,* 42, 254–274.

Clark, F. I., & James, E. J. (1995). Twenty-seven years of experience with oral vitamin K1 therapy in neonates. *Journal of Pediatrics,* 127, 301–304.

College of Physicians and Surgeons of British Columbia. (2007). Circumcision (infant male). In *The physician resource manual.* Retrieved January 26, 2008 from http://www.cpsbc.ca/cps/physician_resources/publications/resource_manual/malecircum_pf

Davidson, N. (1974). REEDA: evaluating postpartum healing. *Journal of Nurse-Midwifery,* 19(1), 6–9.

Davis, E. (1997). *Hearts and hands: a midwife's guide to pregnancy & birth.* Berkeley, CA: Celestial Arts.

Davis, P. G., Tan, A., O'Donnell, C. P., & Schulze, A. (2004). Resuscitation of newborn infants with 100% oxygen or air: a systematic review and meta-analysis. *Lancet,* 364, 1329–1333.

Fernandez, R. (2005). *Perinatal mood disorders: psychiatric illnesses during pregnancy and postpartum* (online video). Prepared by the Governor's (NJ) Work Group on Postpartum Depression. Retrieved January 26, 2008 from http://www.vodium.com/MediapodLibrary/index.asp?library=pn100177_fleishman_postpartum&SessionArgs=0U1U0000000100000110

German, D., & Lee, A. (2006). *Nurse practitioner prescribing reference.* New York: Prescribing Reference.

Gjerdingen, D. (2003). The effectiveness of Various Postpartum Depression Treatments and the Impact of Antidepressant Drugs on Nursing Infants. *The Journal of the American Board of Family Practice,* 16, 372–382.

Green, M., & Palfrey, J. S. (Eds.). (2002). *Bright futures: guidelines for health supervision of infants, children, and adolescents* (2nd ed.). Arlington, VA: National Center for Education in Maternal and Child Health.

Gregoire, A. J., Kumar, R., Everitt, B., Henderson, A. F., & Studd, J. W. (1996). Transdermal oestrogen for treatment of severe postnatal depression. *Lancet,* 347, 930–933.

Gurley, D., & Sinert, R. (2006). *Hemorrhoids*. E-medicine. Retrieved January 26, 2008 from http://www.emedicine.com/emerg/topic242.htm

Hendrick, V. (2003). Alternative treatments for postpartum depression. *Psychiatric Times*, 10, 8. Retrieved January 26, 2008 from http://www.psychiatrictimes.com/p030850.html

Laurence, R. (1998–2007). *Herbs and breastfeeding*. Retrieved January 26, 2008 from http://www.breastfeeding.com/reading_room/herbs.html

Leeman, L., Spearman, M., & Rodgers, R. (2003). Repair of obstetric perineal lacerations. *American Family Physician*, 68, 1585–1590.

Leopold, K., & Zoschnick, L. (1997). Postpartum depression. *The Female Patient* (OB/GYN Edition), 22(8), 40–49.

Lowenstein, V. (2004). *Circumcision*. In H. Varney, J. M. Kriebs, & C. L. Gegor (Eds.). *Varney's midwifery* (4th ed., pp. 1313–1326). Sudbury, MA: Jones and Bartlett.

March of Dimes. (2006). *Recommended newborn screening tests: 29 disorders*. Retrieved January 26, 2008 from http://www.marchofdimes.com/professionals/14332_15455.asp

McHugh, M. K. (2004a). *Examination of the newborn*. In H. Varney, J. M. Kriebs, & C. L. Gegor (Eds.). *Varney's midwifery* (4th ed., pp. 999–1010). Sudbury, MA: Jones and Bartlett.

McHugh, M. K. (2004b). *Recognition and immediate care of sick newborns*. In H. Varney, J. M. Kriebs, & C. L. Gegor (Eds.). *Varney's midwifery* (4th ed., pp. 1029–1040). Sudbury, MA: Jones and Bartlett.

Mercer, J., & Skovaard, R. (2002). Neonatal transition physiology: a new paradigm. *Journal of Neonatal and Perinatal Nursing*, 15, 56–75.

Miller, L. (1996, April). Beyond "the blues": postpartum reactivity and the biology of attachment. *Primary Psychiatry*, 4, 35–38.

Mitchie, C., Lockie, F., & Lynn, W. (2003). The challenge of mastitis. *Archives of Disease in Childhood*, 88, 818–821.

Murphy, J. L. (Ed.). (2004). *Nurse practitioner's prescribing reference*. New York: Prescribing Reference.

National Institutes of Health. (2005, Dec.). Understanding postpartum depression. *News in Health*. Retrieved January 26, 2008 from http://newsinhealth.nih.gov/2005/December2005/docs/01features_02.htm

National Library of Medicine (U.S.). (2006). Anesthetics (rectal). *Medline Plus Drug Information. Thomson Healthcare*. Retrieved January 26, 2008 from http://www.nlm.nih.gov/medlineplus/druginfo/medmaster/a682429.html

Nulman, I., Rovet, J., Stewart, D., Wolpin, J., Pace-Asciak, P., Shuhaiber, S., et al. (2002). Child development following exposure to tricyclic antidepressants or fluoxetine throughout fetal life: a randomized controlled study. *American Journal of Psychiatry*, 159, 1889–1895.

Nussenblatt, V., Kumwenda, N., Lema, V., Quinn, T., Neville, M., Broadhead, R., et al. (2006). Effect of antibiotic treatment of subclinical mastitis on human immunodeficiency virus type 1 RNA in human milk. *Journal of Tropical Pediatrics,* 52, 311–315.

Righetti-Velterna, M., Conne-Perreard, P., Bousquet, A., & Manzano, J. (1998). Risk factors and predictive signs of postpartum depression. *Journal of Affective Disorders*, 49, 167–180.

Semba, R., Kumwenda, N., Taha, T., Hoover, D., Lan, Y., Mtimavalye, L., et al. (1999). Mastitis and immunological factors in breast milk of lactating women in Malawi. *Clinical and Diagnostic Laboratory Immunology*, 6, 671–674.

Simmons, G. T., & Bammel, B. M. (2005). *Endometritis*. E-medicine. Retrieved January 26, 2008 from http://www.emedicine.com/MED/topic676.htm

Sinclair, C. (2004). *A midwife's handbook*. St. Louis, MO: W. B. Saunders.

Smith, T. (1984). *A woman's guide to homeopathic medicine*. New York: Thorsons.

Straus, C. (2003). *Herbal and dietary supplements: be aware of dangers*. Retrieved January 26, 2008 from http://www2.bluecrossca.com/pdf/Health_Articles/herbal%20and%20dietary%20supplements.pdf

University of Arizona. (2005). *Pediatric history and physical exam*. Retrieved January 26, 2008 from http://www.peds.arizona.edu/medstudents/PedsHistoryandPhysicalExam.asp

Varney, H., Kriebs, J. M., & Gegor, C. L. (2004). *Varney's midwifery* (4th ed.). Sudbury, MA: Jones and Bartlett.

Walker, M. (2006). *Breastfeeding management for the clinician: using the evidence*. Sudbury, MA: Jones and Bartlett.

Webb, S. (Ed.) (2006). *Nursing herbal medicine handbook* (3rd ed.). Philadelphia: Lippincott Williams & Wilkins.

Weed, S. (1985). *Wise woman herbal for the childbearing year*. Woodstock, NY: Ashtree.

BIBLIOGRAPHY

Bachmann, G. A. (1993). Estrogen-androgen therapy for sexual and emotional well-being. *The Female Patient*, 18, 15–24.

Behrman, R. E., Kleigman, R. M., & Arvin, A. M. (1996). *Nelson textbook of pediatrics* (15th ed.). Philadelphia: W. B. Saunders.

Barger, M. K. (Ed.). (1988). *Protocols for gynecologic and obstetric health care*. Philadelphia: W. B. Saunders.

Briggs, G. G., Freeman, R. K., & Yaffe, S. J. (1998). *Drugs in pregnancy and lactation* (5th ed.). Philadelphia: Lippincott Williams & Wilkins.

Foster, S. (1996). *Herbs for your health*. Loveland, CO: Interweave Press.

Frye, A. (1998). *Holistic midwifery*. Portland, OR: Labrys Press.

Gelbaum, I. (1993). Circumcision: refining a traditional surgical technique. *Journal of Nurse-Midwifery*, 38(Suppl.), 18S–30S.

Graves, B. W. (1992). Newborn resuscitation revisited. *Journal of Nurse-Midwifery*, 37(Suppl.), 36S–42S.

Scott, J. R., DiSaia, P. J., Hammond, C. B., Gordon, J. D., & Spellacy, W. N. (1996). *Danforth's handbook of obstetrics and gynecology*. Philadelphia: Lippincott-Raven.

Sinclair, C. (2004). *A midwife's handbook*. St. Louis, MO: W. B. Saunders.

Smith, T. (1984). *A woman's guide to homeopathic medicine*. New York: Thorsons.

Swartz, M. H. (1994). *Textbook of physical diagnosis* (2nd ed.). Philadelphia: W. B. Saunders.

Walls, D. (2007). *Natural families—healthy homes*. LaVergne, TN: Ingram.

Care of the Well Woman

6

Women are assisted to achieve and maintain optimal wellness throughout their lives when they access midwifery care as an integral part of their health care services.

SECTION ONE:
PREVENTIVE HEALTH CARE FOR WELL WOMEN

Midwives are women's health primary care specialists. By providing women's health care in an environment of support and understanding, midwives cultivate each woman's ability to care for herself. Well women may come to the midwife for care that includes reproductive health screening and assessment, sports-, college- or employment-related evaluations, diagnostic testing, family planning, fertility awareness, and/or general health maintenance. For many women the annual reproductive health examination is their only preventive health visit. This necessitates the midwife be diligent in assessing all body systems, rather than focusing exclusively on reproductive health care.

Many women do not routinely access reproductive health care services or may be unable to navigate the complex health care system in a manner to meet their health care needs. Midwives frequently reach out to women in the communities where they live to bridge this chasm. Community well-woman midwifery practices range from home-based care to neighborhood clinics to complex women's health services within the tertiary care setting. In every environment of care the individual midwife has the potential to make a difference in the lives of women of all ages.

In virtually every culture women have a history of meeting others' needs before attending to their own. Although this trend may be due to social expectations and customs surrounding women's roles, other contributing factors may include limited information or awareness of basic women's reproductive health care recommendations, significant communication or language barriers, transportation issues, and/or a lack of resources with which to pay for services. The process of actively listening to women includes validating each woman's experiences, acknowledging her stated needs, offering nonjudgmental support, and considering how any information disclosed may affect this woman within her family and her community.

Opportunities for promoting midwifery care for well women include grassroots encouragement of women's support networks, such as occur within neighborhoods, cultural enclaves, or ethnic gatherings. Women's health education may be provided as a community service or within the local school system. In areas with limited opportunities for midwives to offer pregnancy and birth care, well-woman, menopausal and/or primary care services for women may be effective in establishing a foothold in the health care community while providing a much needed service. A commitment to women's health and an inquiring mind are all that is necessary to begin the adventure of improving the health and well-being of women across the life span using the midwifery model of care.

COMPREHENSIVE WELL-WOMAN VISIT

Key Clinical Information

The well-woman examination provides women with the opportunity to learn about their bodies while caring for themselves. Each visit offers a chance to develop a partnership within which to address the client's unique concerns. During the initial visit the client history and physical examination may be quite comprehensive, whereas on subsequent visits, particularly when the midwife provides ongoing care, a brief update of the history and a limited physical examination may be all that is required.

Midwives caring for young women may be asked to perform a sports or college entry examination during the annual well-woman visit. Comprehensive health evaluation may be requested for numerous indications such as the preoperative history and physical, age-related periodic health screening, or preemployment screening. Education in the additional components of these examinations is easily obtained through continuing professional education programs.

Client History and Chart Review:
Components of the History to Consider
(Schuiling & Likis, 2006; Varney et al., 2004)
- Reason for visit
- Reproductive history
  - Last menstrual period (LMP)
  - Obstetric history
    - Gravity, para
    - Infertility or losses
    - Problems, concerns
    - Plans for future pregnancies
  - Gynecologic history
    - Menstrual patterns
    - Vaginal or pelvic infections
    - 🌐 Gynecologic health practices
      - ➤ Reproductive health examinations
      - ➤ Genital hygiene practices
      - ➤ Female circumcision
  - Sexual history
    - Sexual orientation
    - New or change in partners
    - Method of birth control, if applicable
    - Concerns
- Medical/surgical history
  - Allergies
  - Medications and remedies
    - Over the counter
    - Prescription
    - Herbal/homeopathic remedies
  - Current immunization status
  - Diseases, conditions, or problems
  - Hospitalizations and/or surgeries
- Current health care
  - Health philosophy
  - Health screening (Office on Women's Health, n.d.)
    - Dental care
    - Eye care
    - Hearing testing
    - Mental health
    - Skin cancer
  - Primary care provider
  - Specialty care providers

- Illnesses or diseases
- Treatments
- Social history
  - Cultural influences on health care
  - Use of alcohol, tobacco, drugs
  - Family and community support systems
  - Intimate partner violence screen
  - Emotional well-being screen
  - Health and personal safety habits
  - Diet and physical activity
  - Occupational stressors or requirements
- Family history
  - Medical conditions
  - Hereditary conditions
- Review of systems (ROS)
  - Client impression of her health
    - Physical
    - Emotional
  - General symptoms
    - Changes in weight or appetite
    - Weakness, fatigue, malaise
    - Fever or chills
    - Change in bowel or bladder function
    - Shortness of breath/palpitations
  - Other symptoms by body system
    - Head, eyes, ears, nose and throat (HEENT)
    - Cardiopulmonary
    - Gastrointestinal
    - Neurologic
    - Reproductive
    - Musculoskeletal
    - Endocrine
    - Integumentary

Physical Examination:
Components of the Physical Exam to Consider
(Schuiling & Likis, 2006; Varney et al., 2004)

- Vital signs
  - Height, weight, body mass index (BMI)
  - Blood pressure, pulse, respirations
- General appearance
  - Hygiene and dress
  - Speech and communication patterns

- Body language and posture
- Affect or emotional state
- Skin
  - Lesions
  - Scars
  - Bruises
  - Cyanosis
- Head, eyes, ears, nose, and throat
  - Eyes
    - Visual acuity
    - Ophthalmic examination
    - Nystagmus
  - Ears
    - Hearing
    - Canals
    - Tympanic membranes
  - Nose
    - Patency of nares
    - Lesions
  - Mouth
    - Lesions
    - Condition of teeth and gums
    - Tonsils
- Neck
  - Range of motion
  - Lymph nodes
  - Thyroid
    - Symmetry
    - Size
    - Masses or nodules
- Back and chest
  - Lesions
  - Configuration, symmetry
  - Costovertebral angle tenderness
  - Scoliosis, kyphosis
- Lungs
  - Rate, rhythm, and depth of respirations
  - Breath sounds
  - Changes with percussion
- Heart
  - Rate and rhythm
  - Murmurs or bruits
  - Extra or unusual sounds

- Breasts
  - Shape and symmetry
  - Presence of masses, dimples, or scars
  - Nipple discharge
  - Axillary nodes
- Abdomen
  - Configuration
  - Masses, pain
  - Diastasis recti
  - Hernia
  - Bowel sounds
  - Palpation of organs
- Extremities
  - Configuration
  - Range of motion
  - Peripheral pulses
  - Reflexes
  - Symmetry
  - Strength
  - Joint stability or mobility
  - Edema
  - Varicosities
- Pelvic examination
  - External genitalia and rectum
    - Configuration
    - Lesions, discharge
    - Bartholin's, urethra, Skene's (BUS)
    - Hemorrhoids
  - Speculum examination
    - Vagina
      - Lesions
      - Discharge
      - Odor
    - Cervix
      - Discharge
      - Lesions
      - Configuration
      - Specimen collection
  - Bimanual examination
    - Uterine position
    - Size and shape
    - Pain on cervical motion
    - Adnexal
      - Masses

  - Pain
  - Mobility
  - Rectal examination
    - Hemorrhoids
    - Masses
    - Bleeding
    - Specimen collection

Clinical Impression:
Differential Diagnoses and Code Groups
to Consider
Additional suffix may apply (ICD9data.com, 2007)
- Well-woman preventive health examination (ICD-9 codes V70)
- Preventive immunizations (ICD-9 codes V02–V06)
- Well-woman examination with additional diagnosis, such as
  - Gynecologic examination (ICD-9 codes V72.31)
  - Health issues related to personal or family history (ICD-9 codes V10–V19)
  - Health screening for sexually transmitted infections (STIs) (ICD-9 codes V74.5)
  - Contraceptive care (ICD-9 codes V25)
  - Diagnosis based on symptoms (ICD-9 codes 780–789)

Diagnostic Testing:
Diagnostic Tests and Procedures to Consider
- Testing performed or collected during visit
  - Dip urinalysis
  - Pregnancy testing
  - Fingerstick hematocrit or hemoglobin
  - Pap smear
  - Chlamydia culture or nucleic acid amplification
  - Gonorrhea culture or nucleic acid amplification
  - Wet prep for
    - Bacterial vaginosis (BV) or
    - Trichomoniasis or
    - Candidiasis
  - Stool for occult blood
  - Mantoux test or purified protein derivative (PPD) for tuberculosis (TB)

- Laboratory testing
  - Complete blood count or hematocrit and hemoglobin
  - Hepatitis profile
  - Human immunodeficiency virus (HIV) testing
  - VDRL or RPR
  - Quantitative or qualitative β-human chorionic gonadotropin (HCG)
  - Sickle cell prep
  - Fasting blood glucose or 2 hour postprandial glucose
  - Urinalysis and/or culture
  - Thyroid screening
  - Cholesterol screening
- Radiology
  - Ultrasound
  - Mammogram
  - Bone density testing
  - Chest x-ray, history of
    - Positive purified protein derivative (PPD)
    - BCG vaccine

Providing Treatment:
Therapeutic Measures to Consider
- Administer immunizations as indicated (Table 6-1) and desired by client (Centers for Disease Control and Prevention [CDC], 2007)
- Treatments are based on diagnosis

Providing Treatment:
Alternative Measures to Consider
- Treatment is based on diagnosis

Providing Support:
Education and Support Measures to Consider
- Address client concerns
- Provide preventive health recommendations
  - Diet and nutrition
  - Physical activity
  - Weight management
  - Safety counseling
  - Smoking cessation
  - Emotional wellness

Table 6-1 Immunization Schedule for Adult Women

VACCINE	AGE RANGES AND INDICATIONS		
	19–49 YEARS	**50–64 YEARS**	**≥ 65 YEARS**
Tetanus, diphtheria, pertussis	1 dose every 10 yr. May substitute Tdap for Td		
Measles, mumps, rubella	1–2 doses Contraindicated in pregnancy	1 dose if risk factor present	
Human papilloma virus	3 doses females aged ≤ 26		
Varicella	2 doses 4–8 wk apart	2 doses 4–8 wk apart	
Influenza	1 dose annually if risk factor present	1 dose annually	
Hepatitis A	2 doses 6–18 mo apart, if risk factors present		
Hepatitis B	3 doses 1–3 mo apart, if risk factors present		
Pneumococcal	1–2 doses if risk factors present		1 dose
Meningococcal	1+ doses if risk factors present		

Adapted from Centers for Disease Control and Prevention. (2007). Recommended adult immunization schedule—United States, October 2007–September 2008. *Morbidity and Mortality Weekly Report, 56*, Q1–Q4. Retrieved January 22, 2008 from http://www.cdc.gov/vaccines/recs/schedules/downloads/adult/06-07/adult-schedule.pdf

- Depression screening
- Screening for drug or alcohol abuse
- Notification process for results
- Recommendations for ongoing care

Follow-up Care:
Follow-up Measures to Consider
- Return for care
  - Reading of Mantoux or PPD
  - Periodic health maintenance
  - Follow-up of illness, disease, or disorder
- Document encounter
- Notify clients of test results
- ⚠ Report adverse reactions to vaccines
  - Vaccine Adverse Event Reporting System
  - http://vaers.hhs.gov/
  - 1-800-822-7967

Collaborative Practice:
Consider Consultation or Referral
- OB/GYN service, indications such as
  - Abnormal Pap smear
  - Abnormal breast examination
  - Other gynecologic problems
- Specialty services, indications such as
  - Screening colonoscopy
  - Thyroid disorder
  - Diabetes
  - Hypertension
  - Heart disease
  - Other medical or surgical problems
- Social service, indications such as
  - Transportation services
  - Mental health services
  - Drug or alcohol rehabilitation services
  - Homeless shelters
  - Abused women's services
- For diagnosis or treatment outside the midwife's scope of practice

SMOKING CESSATION

Key Clinical Information
Approximately 18% of adult American women are cigarette smokers (CDC, 2006). Smoking signifi-cantly increases preventable risks associated with cancer, heart and lung disease, stroke, and early death (Brender, 2006; National Cancer Institute, 2004). Cigarette smoking is addictive both physically and psychologically. Women who succeed at smoking cessation demonstrate deter-mination to quit. Success can be enhanced by offering an effective method of treating the physical symptoms of nicotine withdrawal, support, and cultivation of positive coping skills and habits. The midwife's caring, concern, and counseling can be critical components in a woman's decision to quit smoking.

Client History and Chart Review:
Components of the History
to Consider
- Smoking history
  - When and why started
  - Packs per day
  - Current desire to quit
  - Prior attempts to quit
- Personal and/or family medical history
  - Diabetes
  - Heart disease
    - Coronary artery disease
    - Elevated cholesterol
  - Hypertension
  - Respiratory disorders
    - Asthma
    - Chronic cough
    - Bronchitis
    - Chronic obstructive pulmonary disease
    - Emphysema
  - Seizure disorder
- Mental health disorders
  - Eating disorders
  - Depression
  - Bipolar disease
  - Psychosis
- Medication use
  - Antihypertensive medications
  - Seizure medications

- Estrogen products
  - ◆ Oral contraceptives
  - ◆ Hormone replacement therapy (HRT)
  - Antidepressants
    - ◆ Wellbutrin (same as Zyban)
    - ◆ Monoamine oxidase (MAO) inhibitors
- Social history
  - Partner/family support
  - Coping skills
  - Stress levels
  - Work environment
  - Other smokers in family
- Personal factors (Heatherton et al., 1991)
  - Assessment of nicotine dependence
  - Coping skills
  - Weight gain
- Review of systems (ROS)

Physical Examination:
Components of the Physical Exam to Consider
- Vital signs
- Height, weight, BMI
- Note odor of tobacco smoke
- As indicated by
  - History and review of systems
  - Interval since last examination
- Cardiopulmonary system
  - Blood pressure, carotid pulses
  - Heart rate and rhythm
  - Evaluation of heart sounds
  - Lung fields
- Integumentary system
  - Note tobacco staining on fingers

Clinical Impression:
Differential Diagnoses and Code Groups
to Consider
Additional suffix or CPT codes may apply
(ICD9data.com, 2007)
- Tobacco dependence (ICD-9 codes 305.1)
- Preventive medicine counseling and risk factor reduction intervention services (CPT codes)
- Medical diagnosis codes as appropriate

- Healthcare Common Procedure Coding System (HCPCS; Medicare) codes (American College of Physicians, 2005)
  - Smoking cessation counseling
    - ◆ 3–10 minutes (HCPCS code G0375)
    - ◆ 10 minutes (HCPCS code G0376)

Diagnostic Testing:
Diagnostic Tests and Procedures to Consider
- Lipid profile
- Electrocardiogram (ECG)
- Chest x-ray

Providing Treatment:
Therapeutic Measures to Consider
(Murphy, 2004; Pfizer, 2007)
- Nicotine-containing medications
  - Pregnancy Category D
  - Risk may outweigh benefit in pregnancy
  - Provide informed consent
  - Nicoderm or Habitrol
    - ◆ 7 mg/24 hours, 14 mg/24 hours, or 21 mg/24 hours
    - ◆ Begin with 21- or 14-mg patch
    - ◆ Use 2–6 weeks, then decrease dose
    - ◆ Repeat with decreased dose
  - Nicotrol step-down patch (transdermal)
    - ◆ 5–15 mg/16-hour patch, or
    - ◆ Use during waking hours
  - Nicorette gum
    - ◆ 2 mg, 4 mg strength
    - ◆ Use 2 mg if less than one pack per day smoker
    - ◆ Maximum, 24 pieces a day
  - Nicotrol NS, inhaler
    - ◆ 0.5 mg/spray, 10 mg/cartridge inhaler
    - ◆ One to two doses an hour
- Varenicline (Chantix)
  - Reduces symptoms associated with smoking cessation
  - Decreases urge to smoke
  - Decreases nicotine cravings
  - May cause vivid, disturbing dreams
  - Begin 1 week before "stop smoking" date

- Dosage
  - Days 1–3: 0.5 mg PO daily
  - Days 4–7: 0.5 mg PO BID
  - Day 8 to end of treatment: 1 mg PO BID
- Bupropion HCl (Zyban)
  - 150 mg PO for 3 days
  - 150 BID with 8 hours between doses
  - Stop smoking within 1–2 weeks of initiation
  - May use with nicotine medications
  - Pregnancy Category B
  - Not for use in those with
    - Eating disorders
    - Seizures
    - Wellbutrin or MAOIs
- Nortriptyline (deCosta et al., 2002; Hall et al., 2002)
  - Usual dose 75 mg daily
  - Titrate to serum level 50–150 ng/ml
  - As effective as bupropion
  - Pregnancy Category D

Providing Treatment:
Alternative Measures to Consider
- Herbal support
  - Lobelia
- Engage in learning positive coping skills
  - Avoid situations that increase desire to smoke
  - Keep gum or healthy finger food available for oral satisfaction
  - Increase physical activity

Providing Support:
Education and Support Measures to Consider
- Review smoking cessation benefits
- Provide clear medication instructions
- Nicotine-containing medications
  - Stop smoking before or with onset of use
  - Use lower dose with
    - Cardiac history
    - Pregnancy
    - Body weight < 100 lbs
  - Patches
    - Apply new patch daily
    - Upper torso or arm

- Do not reuse skin sites for at least 1 week
- New patch applied each 24 hours
- Bupropion HCl
  - Take as instructed
  - May decrease appetite
  - May cause medication interactions
- Nortriptyline
  - May treat concomitant depression
  - May cause
    - Dry mouth
    - Sedation
    - Cardiac arrhythmias
- Counsel as determined by history and readiness to change
  - Encourage regular physical exercise
  - Provide nutrition information
- Provide information regarding
  - Local resources for developing healthy coping mechanisms
  - Smoking support groups

Follow-up Care:
Follow-up Measures to Consider
- Document
  - Discussions and education
  - Client plan for smoking cessation
- Revisit 2 weeks after beginning smoking cessation
  - Client support and counseling
  - Evaluation of
    - Current smoking patterns
    - Blood pressure, weight changes
    - Symptoms or side effects of medication
- Register pregnant clients on bupropion HCl with Glaxo: (800) 336-2176

Collaborative Practice:
Consider Consultation or Referral
- Medical service
  - Cardiac history
  - Adverse medication reaction
  - Onset of cardiac symptoms with use of nicotine-containing medications

- Mental health service
  - Exacerbation of depression symptoms
- Social service
  - Smoking cessation support services
  - Other services as necessary to reduce stress
- For diagnosis or treatment outside the midwife's scope of practice

FERTILITY AWARENESS

Key Clinical Information

Every woman can benefit from increased awareness and understanding of her body. Fertility awareness offers women a means to become attuned to the functioning of their reproductive system and its impact on their overall health and well-being throughout the life span.

Awareness of changes throughout the menstrual cycle gives many women a greater sense of control over their lives and can be useful in recognizing ovulation, identifying menstrual dysfunction, and understanding changes during breastfeeding and perimenopause. Cycle charting can be easily incorporated into daily routines.

Teaching fertility awareness to adolescents provides a wonderful outreach opportunity for midwives. The knowledge provided can be incredibly empowering; it may be instrumental in delaying the onset of adolescent sexual activity and may motivate appropriate use of safe sex practices, while building the midwife's prospective client base.

Heterosexual couples interested in the nuances of the female cycle can enhance their relationship while seeking pregnancy prevention *or* conception through the use of fertility awareness. Fertility awareness requires interactive dialogue between partners, acceptance of life cycles, and willingness to compromise. This process fosters development of a respectful and an emotionally intimate relationship and places sex at the periphery rather than at the center of the union (Singer, 2004).

Fertility awareness can also be used for the woman who desires pregnancy in determining the best times to have intercourse. For women who have difficulty achieving pregnancy and for lesbian couples, awareness of fertility can help them decide when to access assisted reproductive technologies to achieve pregnancy.

Client History and Chart Review: Components of the History to Consider

- Social history
  - Goals of learning fertility awareness
  - Partner interest, if applicable
- Menstrual history
  - LMP
  - Frequency of menses
  - Duration of menses
  - Mid-cycle pain, discharge
- Sexual history
  - Age at onset of sexual activity
  - Frequency of sexual activity
  - Type of sexual activity
  - Safe sex practices
    - Abstinence
    - STI testing
    - Condom use
    - Monogamy
  - Sexual relationships
    - Long-term monogamy
    - Serial monogamy
    - Multiple partners
    - Same sex and/or opposite sex partner(s)
  - Current method of birth control, if any
- Obstetric history
- Medical, surgical history
- Review of systems (ROS)

Physical Examination: Components of the Physical Exam to Consider

- Not required for fertility awareness education
- Weight, height, BMI
- Physical examination components as indicated by
  - Age and health status
  - History and client interview
  - Screening recommendations (see Comprehensive Well-Woman Visit, above)

Clinical Impression:
Differential Diagnoses and Code Groups
to Consider
Additional suffix or CPT code may apply
(ICD9data.com, 2007)

- Family planning advice and counseling (ICD-9 codes V25.09)
- Health education (ICD-9 codes V65.49)
- General medical examination (ICD-9 codes V70)

Diagnostic Testing:
Diagnostic Tests and Procedures to Consider

- Pap smear
- STI testing
- Thyroid
- Over-the-counter (OTC) testing options
  - Ovulation predictor tests
  - Luteinizing hormone tests

Providing Treatment:
Therapeutic Measures to Consider

- Prescription methods of birth control
- Hormonal treatment of menstrual irregularities

Providing Treatment:
Alternative Measures to Consider

- Fertility awareness charting (Kass-Annese & Danzer, 2003; Singer, 2004)
  - Appropriate for women
    - From menarche through menopause
    - During breastfeeding
    - With menstrual irregularities
- Nonpharmacologic methods of birth control
  - Natural family planning using fertility awareness
  - Abstinence
    - Periodic abstinence (rhythm method)
      - Avoid intercourse during fertile times
    - Withdrawal
      - May work for some couples
      - There may or may not be sperm in preejaculatory fluid
      - May or may not interrupt sexual satisfaction

- Natural spermicides (see Barrier Methods of Birth Control)
- "Outercourse" (Weinstein, 1994)
  - Hugging and kissing
  - Holding and fondling
  - Oral sex
  - Sexual activity that excludes
    - Penetration
    - Genital to genital contact

Providing Support:
Education and Support Measures to Consider

- Provide fertility awareness education (Singer, 2004)
  - Changes during
    - Menstrual cycle
    - Breastfeeding
    - Perimenopause
  - Primary fertility signals
    - Basal body temperature
    - Cervical fluid
    - Cervical changes
  - Secondary fertility signals
    - Mid-cycle pain
    - Ferning of salivary fluid
    - Spotting
    - Breast tenderness
    - Libido changes
  - Benefits/drawbacks and use of resources
    - Basal body thermometer
    - Cycle beads
    - Cycle charts
    - Ovulation predictors
  - Implementing the method
    - Resources
    - Charts and notations
    - Interpretation of data
    - Application to personal situation
- When using fertility awareness for birth control
  - Engage partner in discussions
  - Discuss best method for couple
  - Optional barrier methods or spermicide at mid-cycle

- Lack of STI protection
- Use of emergency contraception

Follow-up Care:
Follow-up Measures to Consider
- Document
  - Education process and components
  - Recommended resources
  - Discussions
  - Plan to verify client understanding and correct use of method
- Return for care
  - For fertility chart review
  - As recommended by age and sexual activity
  - For Pap smear and STI testing as indicated
  - With pregnancy

Collaborative Practice:
Consider Consultation or Referral
- For diagnosis or treatment outside the midwife's scope of practice

PRECONCEPTION EVALUATION

Key Clinical Information
The planned preconception visit provides an opportunity to address health needs that may affect pregnancy before the pregnancy occurs. This type of client-initiated visit indicates a hunger for information related to preconception health, pregnancy and parenting resources, and labor and birth options. Midwife-initiated screenings and discussions related to preconception care may spark awareness and interest in women not previously motivated to modify health behaviors before pregnancy. The woman may decide to delay attempts at pregnancy until particular health care concerns are addressed and remediated.

Client History and Chart Review:
Components of the History to Consider
(March of Dimes, n.d.; Health Canada, 2000)
- Age
- Obstetric history
  - Gravida, para
  - Outcome of previous pregnancies
    - Term births
    - Preterm births
    - Pregnancy losses
    - Infertility
- Gynecologic history
  - LMP
  - Length of cycle and menses
  - STIs or pelvic infections
  - HIV status

Box 6-1   Fertility Awareness and Natural Family Planning Web Resources

- Taking Charge of Your Fertility: http://www.tcoyf.com
- The Garden of Fertility: http://www.gardenoffertility.com
- Billings Ovulation Method: http://www.billingsmethod.com
- Institute for Reproductive Health: http://irh.org
- Institute for Natural Family Planning: http://www.marquette.edu/nursing/NFP/
- Couple to Couple League International: http://www.ccli.org
- Downloadable Fertility Charts: www.fertilityawareness.net
- Additional sites for fertility monitoring supplies
  - www.fertile-focus.com
  - www.ovulation-predictor.com
  - www.birthcontrol.com

- Abnormal Pap smears, cervical treatment
- Most recent method of birth control
- 🌐 Female genital mutilation (FGM) status
- Medical and surgical history
  - Medical conditions
  - Previous surgery
  - Medications and supplements
  - Mental well-being
- Social history
  - Partner/family support
  - Substance abuse
  - Domestic violence
  - Occupational hazards
    - Chemicals
    - Work hours or conditions
- Family history: client and partner (Scherger, 1993)
  - Birth defects
  - Genetic disorders
  - Multiple births
  - Losses
  - Familial health disorders
- Personal concerns
  - Readiness (self and partner)
  - Financial concerns
  - Spouse and/or family concerns
  - Cultural considerations for childbearing
  - Health habits
    - Physical activity patterns
    - Nutrition, including
      - Eating disorders
      - BMI
      - Pica
- Review of systems (ROS)

Physical Examination:
Components of the Physical Exam to Consider
- Complete physical examination as indicated by
  - History
  - Interval since last physical
- Primary focus on
  - Appropriate weight for height
  - Thyroid

- Breast examination
- Gynecologic examination
- Cardiac evaluation

Clinical Impression:
Differential Diagnoses and Code Groups
to Consider
Additional suffix may apply (ICD9data.com, 2007)
- Preconception counseling (ICD-9 codes V26.4)
- Genetic counseling (ICD-9 codes V26.33)
- Genetic screening (ICD-9 codes V82.71)
- Other related screening (ICD-9 codes V70–V82)
- General medical examination (ICD-9 codes V70.0)

Diagnostic Testing:
Diagnostic Tests and Procedures to Consider
(Heath & Acevedo, 2000–2007)
- Tuberculosis testing
  - Purified protein derivative or Mantoux testing
  - Chest x-ray
- Cervicovaginal screening
  - Pap smear
  - Wet prep for BV or trichomonas
  - Group B streptococcus (GBS)
  - Chlamydia
  - Gonorrhea
- Blood tests
  - Complete blood count
  - Rubella and hepatitis B titers
  - Blood type and Rh
  - Hematocrit and hemoglobin, *or*
  - Complete blood count
  - Thyroid-stimulating hormone (TSH) or thyroid panel
  - Toxoplasmosis screen
  - Varicella
  - HIV testing
  - VDRL or RPR
- Genetic studies
- 🌐 Additional screening of one or both partners
  - African heritage: sickle cell anemia
  - Mediterranean heritage: β-thalassemia
  - Southeast Asian or Chinese: α-thalassemia

PRECONCEPTION SCREENING
AND COUNSELING CHECKLIST

NAME	BIRTHPLACE	AGE

DATE: / /   ARE YOU PLANNING TO GET PREGNANT IN THE NEXT SIX MONTHS? __ Y
__N
IF YOUR ANSWER TO A QUESTION IS YES, PUT A CHECK MARK ON THE LINE IN FRONT OF THE QUESTION. FILL IN OTHER INFORMATION THAT APPLIES TO YOU

DIET & EXERCISE

What do you consider a healthy weight for you? _____
___Do you eat three meals a day?
___Do you follow a special diet (vegetarian, diabetic, other)?
___Which do you drink (__coffee __tea __cola __milk __water __other soda/pop other _____)?
___Do you eat raw or undercooked food (meat, other)?
___Do you take folic acid?
___Do you take other vitamins daily (__multivitamin __vitamin A __other)?
___Do you take dietary supplements (__black cohosh __ pennyroyal __other)?
___Do you have current/past problems with eating disorders?
___Do you exercise? Type/frequency:_____
Notes:

LIFESTYLE

___Do you smoke cigarettes or use other tobacco products?
How many cigarettes/packs a day? _____
___Are you exposed to second-hand smoke?
___Do you drink alcohol?
What kind?_____ How often? _____ How much?_____
___Do you use recreational drugs (cocaine, heroin, ecstasy, meth/ice, other?
List:_____
___Do you see a dentist regularly?
What kind of work do you do?_____
___Do you work or live near possible hazards (chemicals, x-ray or other radiation, lead)? List:_____
___Do you use saunas or hot tubs?
NOTES:

MEDICATION/DRUGS

___ Are you taking prescribed drugs (Accutane, valproic acid, blood thinners)? List them_____
___ Are you taking non-prescribed drugs?
List them:_____
___Are you using birth control pills?
___Do you get injectable contraceptives or shots for birth control?
___Do you use any herbal remedies or alternative medicine?
List:_____
NOTES:

MEDICAL/FAMILY HISTORY

Do you have or have you ever had:
___Epilepsy?
___Diabetes?
___Asthma?
___High blood pressure?
___Heart disease?
___Anemia?
___Kidney or bladder disorders?
___Thyroid disease?
___Chickenpox?
___Hepatitis C?
___Digestive problems?
___Depression or other mental health problem?
___Surgeries?
___Lupus?
___Scleroderma?
___Other conditions?
Have you ever been vaccinated for:
___Measles, mumps, rubella?
___Hepatitis B?
___Chickenpox?
NOTES:

WOMEN'S HEALTH

___Do you have any problems with your menstrual cycle?
___ How many times have you been pregnant?
What was/were the outcomes(s)? _____
___Did you have difficulty getting pregnant last time?
___Have you been treated for infertility?
___Have you had surgery on your uterus, cervix, ovaries or tubes?
___Did you mother take the hormone DES during pregnancy?
___Have you ever had HPV, genital warts or chlamydia?
___Have you ever been treated for a sexually transmitted infection (genital herpes, gonorrhea, syphilis, HIV/AIDS, other)? List:_____
NOTES:

GENETICS

Does your family have a history of	or	your partner's family
___Hemophilia?		
___Other bleeding disorders?		___
___Tay-Sachs disease?		___
___Blood diseases (sickle cell, thalassemia, other)?		___
___Muscular dystrophy?		___
___Down syndrome/Mental retardation?		___
___Cystic fibrosis?		___
___Birth defects (spine/heart/kidney)?		___

Your ethnic background is: _____
Your partner's ethnic background is:_____
NOTES:

HOME ENVIRONMENT

___Do you feel emotionally supported at home?
___Do you have help from relatives or friends if needed?
___Do you feel you have serious money/financial worries?
___ Are you in a stable relationship?
___Do you feel safe at home?
___Does anyone threaten or physically hurt you?
___Do you have pets (cats, rodents, exotic animals)? List:_____
___Do you have any contact with soil, cat litter or sandboxes?
Baby preparation (if planning pregnancy):
___Do you have a place for a baby to sleep?
___Do you need any baby items?
NOTES:

OTHER

IS THERE ANYTHING ELSE YOU'D LIKE ME TO KNOW?

ARE THERE ANY QUESTIONS YOU'D LIKE TO ASK ME?

Figure 6-1 *Preconception Screening and Counseling Checklist*

Source: March of DImes. Retrieved January 27, 2008 from http://www.marchofdimes.com/professionals/19583_4182.asp.

- White: cystic fibrosis screening
- Jewish descent: Tay-Sachs disease, Canavan disease
- Other as indicated by history

Providing Treatment:
Therapeutic Measures to Consider
- Medical conditions
  - Adjust medications according to drug pregnancy category
  - 🕐 Consult for those medications and medical conditions outside the midwife's scope of practice
- Vitamin and mineral supplements
  - Folic acid 0.4 mg/400 μg PO daily
  - Begin one to twelve months before planned conception
  - Continue through at least 13 weeks gestation
  - Consider multivitamin with or without iron
- Update immunization status
  - Hepatitis B
  - Tetanus, diphtheria
  - Avoid pregnancy for 1 month after live virus vaccines (CDC, 2007)
    - Varicella
    - Rubella

Providing Treatment:
Alternative Measures to Consider
- Whole foods diet
- Minerals and folic acid from food sources
- Fertility awareness methods for determining ovulation

Providing Support:
Education and Support Measures to Consider
(Heath & Acevedo, 2000–2007)
- Preconception counseling related to risk factors, such as
  - Diabetes
  - Hypertension
  - Genetic disorders
  - Neural tube defects

- Maternal age
- HIV infection
- Substance abuse (Scherger, 1993)
- Pregnancy health risk awareness
  - Age-related risks
  - Hot tubs
  - Toxoplasmosis
  - Listeria
  - Mercury
  - Domestic violence
- Fertility awareness
  - Menstrual cycle and ovulation
  - Signs of fertility
  - Fertility charting
  - Postcontraception fertility rates
  - Signs of conception
- Health promotion
  - Weight and physical activity
  - Nutrition; vitamins, mineral, and folate
  - Counsel regarding pertinent issues as determined by history
    - Use of medications
  - Encourage dental work before conception
  - Avoidance of cigarettes, alcohol, recreational drugs
  - Moderation in caffeine use (300 mg or less daily)
- Environmental concerns
  - Occupational hazards
  - Toxic chemicals
  - Radiation contamination
- Health concerns
  - Effects of health on developing fetus
  - Recommendations for optimal care
  - Pregnancy information and resources
  - Labor and birth options, locations, and services

Follow-up Care:
Follow-up Measures to Consider
- Document care provided
- Return for
  - Reading of Mantoux test
  - Review of fertility charts

- Onset of amenorrhea for HCG testing
- Follow-up per recommendations
- No pregnancy within 6–12 months
- Questions or concerns

Collaborative Practice:
Consider Consultation or Referral
- OB/GYN service
  - Genetic counseling
  - Infertility evaluation or treatment
  - Based on risk assessment
- Social services
  - Substance abuse centers
  - Physical abuse
  - Psychosocial issues
- Nutritional risk assessment by dietician
- Medical service
  - Management of disease or illness, such as
    - Diabetes
    - Hypertension
- For diagnosis or treatment outside the midwife's scope of practice

EMERGENCY CONTRACEPTION

Key Clinical Information

Emergency contraception (EC) offers women an opportunity to effectively prevent pregnancy from occurring in the event of contraceptive failure, such as a condom that breaks while in use. EC is most effective when initiated as soon as possible after unprotected intercourse. Available options include emergency contraceptive pills (ECPs) and the Copper-T intrauterine device (IUD) (Hatcher et al., 2004).

Emergency contraceptive pills (ECP) are available in two forms: progestin-only pills (POP), such as Plan B®, or combined oral contraceptive pills (OCPs) formulated with both estrogen and progestin (Schuiling & Likis, 2006). *ECPs are now available without a prescription for women and men ages 18 and older* (Duramed Pharmaceuticals, 2006a).

Although research has demonstrated that ECPs are approximately 74% effective when taken as long as 120 hours after unprotected sexual exposure, the manufacturer of Plan B® recommends administration within 24 hours and up to 72 hours after exposure (Duramed Pharmaceuticals, 2006a; Ellerson et al., 2003; Trussell & Raymond, 2006). Side effects of ECPs may include nausea and vomiting, and an antiemetic may be helpful (American College of Obstetricians and Gynecologists [ACOG], 2001b). Clients may access the Emergency Contraceptive Hotline by calling 1-(888) NOT-2-Late (1-888-668-2528). ECP providers may be listed on the hotline by calling the same number.

A Copper-T IUD, such as ParaGard®, may be placed up to 5 days after unprotected intercourse as an emergency contraceptive measure and can provide continued contraception for up to 10 years. Although postcoital IUD insertion reduces the risk of pregnancy by over 99%, IUDs are not readily available or suitable for many women (Trussell & Raymond, 2006).

Client History and Chart Review:
Components of the History to Consider
- OB/GYN history
  - LMP and typical menstrual pattern
  - Gravida, para
  - Sexual history
    - Number of hours since unprotected intercourse
    - Reasons for unprotected sexual exposure
      - Contraceptive failure
      - Lack of contraceptive planning
      - Date rape or sexual assault/abuse
      - Judgment altered by substance abuse
  - Current or recent use of contraception
    - Ability to use ECP as directed
    - Plans for long-term birth control
  - Contraindications to ECP use
    - Pregnancy
    - Undiagnosed genital bleeding

- Contraindications to IUD insertion (see Intrauterine Device and Intrauterine System)
- Most recent examination, Pap smear, and STI testing if applicable
  - History of STIs
  - History of abnormal Pap smears
- Medical history
  - Allergies
  - Medications
  - Medical conditions
- Social history

Physical Examination:
Components of the Physical Exam
to Consider

- Not required for ECP, but may be useful when
  - History is unclear
  - STI testing indicated
  - Other symptoms are present
  - No examination within past 12 months
- Limited reproductive examination
- Complete well-woman examination
- ⚠ Requiring an office visit for ECP may be a barrier to access to ECP for some women. ECP is available over the counter in many areas.

Clinical Impression:
Differential Diagnoses and Code Groups
to Consider
Additional suffix or procedure codes may apply
(ICD9data.com, 2007)

- Counseling related to contraceptive pills (ICD-9 codes V25.01)
- Copper-T IUD insertion (ICD-9 codes V25.1)

Diagnostic Testing:
Diagnostic Tests and Procedures to Consider

- Pregnancy testing
  - If menstrual history is uncertain or unclear
- STI screening
- Other screening tests
  - According to age and health history

Providing Treatment:
Therapeutic Measures to Consider

- Provide antiemetic 1 hour before first ECP dose (ACOG, 2001b; Trussell & Raymond, 2006)
  - Meclizine (OTC) two 25-mg tablets
  - Compazine 5- to 10-mg tablet or 15-mg spansule
  - Phenergan 25-mg tablet or suppository
  - Benadryl 25–50 mg PO
- Emergency contraceptive pills (Table 6-2)
- Copper-T IUD insertion (see Intrauterine Device and Intrauterine System)

Providing Treatment:
Alternative Measures to Consider

- Nausea
  - Seabands®
  - Ginger tea
- Herbs that foster onset of menstruation (Soule, 1996)
  - Blue cohosh
  - Angelica root
  - Dong quai
  - Vitex or chasteberry
  - Black cohosh
  - Evening primrose oil
- Homeopathic remedies that foster onset of menstruation (Smith, 1984)
  - Pulsatilla
  - Sepia
  - Caulophyllum
  - Calcarea carb.
- For additional information about herbal remedies to prevent or avoid pregnancy, see Gardner (1986) or Soule (1996).

Providing Support:
Education and Support Measures to Consider

- Verify client does not want to become pregnant
- Emergency contraceptive pills (Office of Population Research & Association of Reproductive Health Professionals, 2006)
  - Emphasize that ECPs are for emergency use only

Table 6-2 Oral Contraceptives Used for Emergency Contraception in the United States

BRAND	COMPANY	FIRST DOSE	SECOND DOSE (12 HR LATER)	ETHINYL ESTRADIOL PER DOSE (µG)	LEVONORGESTREL PER DOSE (MG)
PROGESTIN-ONLY PILLS					
Plan B, option 1	Barr/Duramed	2 white pills	None	0	1.5
Plan B, option 2	Barr/Duramed	1 white pill	1 white pill	0	1.5
COMBINED PROGESTIN AND ESTROGEN PILLS					
Alesse	Wyeth-Ayerst	5 pink pills	5 pink pills	100	0.50
Aviane	Barr/Duramed	5 orange pills	5 orange pills	100	0.50
Cryselle	Barr/Duramed	4 white pills	4 white pills	120	0.60
Enpresse	Barr/Duramed	4 orange pills	4 orange pills	120	0.50
Jolessa	Barr/Duramed	4 pink pills	4 pink pills	120	0.60
Lessina	Barr/Duramed	5 pink pills	5 pink pills	100	0.50
Levlen	Berlex	4 light-orange pills	4 light-orange pills	120	0.60
Levlite	Berlex	5 pink pills	5 pink pills	100	0.50
Levora	Watson	4 white pills	4 white pills	120	0.60
Lo/Ovral	Wyeth-Ayerst	4 white pills	4 white pills	120	0.60
Low-Ogestrel	Watson	4 white pills	4 white pills	120	0.60
Lutera	Watson	5 white pills	5 white pills	100	0.50
Nordette	Wyeth-Ayerst	4 light-orange pills	4 light-orange pills	120	0.60
Ogestrel	Watson	2 white pills	2 white pills	100	0.50
Ovral	Wyeth-Ayerst	2 white pills	2 white pills	100	0.50
Portia	Barr/Duramed	4 pink pills	4 pink pills	120	0.60
Quasense	Watson	4 white pills	4 white pills	120	0.60
Seasonale	Barr/Duramed	4 pink pills	4 pink pills	120	0.60
Seasonique	Barr/Duramed	4 light-blue-green pills	4 light-blue-green pills	120	0.60
Tri-Levlen	Berlex	4 yellow pills	4 yellow pills	120	0.50
Triphasil	Wyeth-Ayerst	4 yellow pills	4 yellow pills	120	0.50
Trivora	Watson	4 pink pills	4 pink pills	120	0.50

Source: Office of Population Research & Association of Reproductive Health Professionals. (2006). *Types of emergency contraception.* Retrieved January 22, 2008 from http://ec.princeton.edu/questions/dose.html#dose

- ECPs not recommended for regular use as contraception
- Common side effects of ECPs
  - Nausea and vomiting
  - Breast tenderness
  - Menses may be earlier or later than usual
  - Antiemetics may cause drowsiness
- Take ECP dose(s) as instructed
  - Must take within 120 hours of exposure
  - Preventive antiemetic recommended
  - Take exact number of ECPs
  - Repeat dose if vomiting occurs within 1 hour
- Return for care if no menses within 21 days
  - Options counseling
  - ECP nonteratogenic
- ⚠ Call immediately for onset of signs or symptoms, such as
  - Severe leg or abdominal pain
  - Shortness of breath, chest pain
  - Headache, dizziness, weakness, or numbness
  - Difficulty speaking or seeing
  - Onset of jaundice
- IUD (see Intrauterine Device and Intrauterine System)
- Discuss
  - Safe sexual practices
  - Pregnancy and STI prevention
  - Long-term contraceptive options

Follow-up Care:
Follow-up Measures to Consider

- ▽ Document instructions and prescription if provided
- ⚠ Improve access to emergency contraception (Trussell & Raymond, 2006)
  - Educate office staff in OTC and prescription EC options
  - Add discussion of emergency contraception to routine visits
    - Provide ECPs and instruction in advance
    - Provide women aged < 17 years with prescription for EC

- ◆ Provide prescription by phone for known clients
- ◆ Offer prescription without clinical examination
- Follow-up visit for information, counseling, or care
  - Initiation of regular contraception
  - Gynecologic examination and STI screening
  - Amenorrhea > 21 days after ECP
  - Symptoms suggesting complications

Collaborative Practice:
Criteria to Consider for Consultation or Referral

- For diagnosis or treatment outside the mid-wife's scope of practice

BARRIER METHODS OF BIRTH CONTROL

Key Clinical Information

Barrier methods include both mechanical devices and chemical agents that act as barriers to prevent motile sperm from reaching the cervical os. Barriers are an effective and low-cost form of birth control that is particularly well suited for women who do not engage in intercourse on a frequent basis. Some barrier methods provide contraception while simultaneously reducing the risk of contracting sexually transmitted infections (STIs). The primary drawback of barrier methods is that they require using the method correctly and consistently for each and every act of intercourse. The effectiveness of each barrier method is related to the method type, use of spermicide, parity of the woman, and actual method use patterns. Efficacy ranges from 60% to 93%. Multiparous women tend to have higher failure rates than nulliparous women. Barrier methods may be used as an adjunct to other methods, used with other barrier methods, or used alone (Hatcher et al., 2004).

Client History and Chart Review:
Components of the History to Consider
(Hatcher et al., 2004; Johnson, 2004)

- Allergies, including latex allergy
- Medications

- OB/GYN history
  - Contraindications to hormonal contraceptives or IUDs
  - LMP and typical menstrual pattern
  - Reproductive history
    - Gravida, para
    - Recent childbirth or abortion
    - Recent abnormal Pap smear or cervical procedure
    - Last examination, Pap smear, and STI testing, as applicable
    - History of STIs—diagnosis and treatment
- Past and current medical and surgical history
- Social history
  - Drug and/or alcohol use
  - Living situation and resources
  - Sexual partner support for method of birth control
  - Client ability to negotiate for barrier use
- Method-related considerations
  - Frequency of sexual relations
  - Ability to learn and use method reliably
  - Assess impact of unplanned pregnancy
  - Previous reaction to spermicide

Physical Examination:
Components of the Physical Exam to Consider
- Well-woman examination, with focus, as indicated, on
  - Vaginal and cervical anatomy and position
  - Fit of diaphragm or cap
  - Woman's ability to insert/remove device

Clinical Impression:
Differential Diagnoses and Code Groups
to Consider
Additional suffix may apply (ICD9data.com, 2007)
- Contraceptive management (ICD-9 codes V25)
  - General counseling and advice (ICD-9 codes V25.09)
  - Diaphragm or cap fitting (ICD-9 codes V25.02)

- Counseling on initiation of OTC methods (ICD-9 codes V25.02)
- Unspecified contraceptive management (ICD-9 codes V25.9)

Diagnostic Testing:
Diagnostic Tests and Procedures to Consider
- Pap smear
- Urinalysis
- Serum or urine pregnancy test
- STI screening
- Other screening tests according to age and health history

Providing Treatment:
Therapeutic Measures to Consider
(Hatcher et al., 2004; Johnson, 2004)
- Diaphragms and cervical caps
  - May increase risk of urinary tract infections
  - Female superior position may dislodge
  - Spermicide use recommended
  - Prescription needed in United States
- Cervical caps
  - Prentif cavity rim cervical cap
    - No longer available in United States
  - FemCap, nonlatex
    - Three sizes based on parity
      - Small, for women who have never been pregnant
      - Medium, for women who have had an abortion or a cesarean delivery
      - Large, for women who have given birth vaginally
  - Lea's shield, nonlatex
    - One size, no fitting required
  - Oves cap, nonlatex
    - Single use cap
    - Available in Canada
    - Requires fitting
    - Three sizes
- Diaphragms
  - Fifty- to 95-mm sizes
  - Flat spring, for women with firm vaginal tone

- Coil spring, for women with average muscle tone
- Arcing spring, for women with lax muscle tone
- Wide seal, greater surface area for seal
- Reality female condom, nonlatex
  - Allows female control for STI protection and contraception
  - Greater protection than male condom
- Male condom
  - Provides some measure of protection against STIs
  - May contribute to latex allergy
  - Requires male cooperation to use effectively
- Contraceptive sponges
  - 83–91% effective
  - Today sponge
    - ◆ Nonoxyl-9
  - Protectaid
    - ◆ Available in Canada
    - ◆ F5 gel (sodium cholate, nonoxy-9, and benzalkonium chloride)
  - Pharmatex sponge
    - ◆ Available in Canada
    - ◆ Benzalkonium chloride

Providing Treatment:
Alternative Measures to Consider
- Fertility awareness
- Abstinence
- Nonpenetrating sexual relations ("outercourse")
- Withdrawal
- Natural spermicide (Trapani, 1984)
  - For use with cervical cap or diaphragm (use instead of nonoxyl-9)
  - 1 cup water
  - 1 tsp fresh lemon juice
  - 5 tsp table salt
  - 10 tsp cornstarch
  - 10 tsp glycerin
  - Mix solids, add liquids while stirring, cook over low heat until thick. Store refrigerated in sealed container. Discard unused portions after 30 days.

Providing Support:
Education and Support Measures to Consider
(Hatcher et al., 2004; Johnson, 2004)
- Review use and effectiveness of chosen method(s)
- Review other birth control methods and their effectiveness
- Help clients learn to negotiate for safe sex
- Condoms are recommended to protect against STIs
  - Use for every act of penile contact
  - Apply before any penile genital/oral/anal contact
  - Hold rim during withdrawal
  - Use only water-soluble lubricants
- Diaphragm or cervical cap
  - Have client demonstrate device insertion and removal
  - Instruct in proper use, cleaning, and care of reusable devices
    - ◆ Wash hands before insertion or removal
    - ◆ Insertion or removal is easier with one leg bent or in the squatting position
    - ◆ Wear the cap or diaphragm during every act of intercourse
    - ◆ Use with a spermicidal gel or cream
    - ◆ Wear until at least 6 hours after intercourse
    - ◆ Check for correct placement before removing device; if dislodged seek emergency contraception as soon as possible
    - ◆ Use in conjunction with a condom until
      - ➤ Confident device is placed and fits correctly
      - ➤ With concern about the risk of STIs
- Educate regarding signs and symptoms of toxic shock syndrome (Deresiewicz, n.d.)
  - Caused by *Staphylococcus aureus*
  - May occur with use of vaginal barriers
    - ◆ Avoid use during menses
    - ◆ Remove within recommended time frame

- Sudden onset of
  - Fever
  - Sunburnlike rash
  - Hypotension
- ⚠ Seek care immediately

Follow-up Care:
Follow-up Measures to Consider
- Document
  - Discussions
  - Method choice(s)
  - Client teaching
  - Fitting and client demonstration of prescription devices
  - Planned follow-up
- Call or return for care
  - Two-week evaluation of diaphragm or cervical cap use
  - Three- to 4-month repeat Pap smear for cap users
  - Annual well-woman visit
  - Method-related problems
  - Amenorrhea
  - Positive pregnancy test

Collaborative Practice:
Consider Consultation or Referral
- Signs or symptoms of
  - Toxic shock syndrome
  - Latex allergy
- For diagnosis or treatment outside the midwife's scope of practice

INITIATION AND FOLLOW-UP OF HORMONAL CONTRACEPTIVES

Key Clinical Information
Reliable hormonal contraceptives are now available to women in a wide array of delivery methods. Hormonal contraceptives offer women prevention of unplanned pregnancy through suppression of ovulation, mechanisms to inhibit sperm motility and penetration of the cervical canal and ovum, and/or thinning of the endometrium (Hatcher et al., 2004; Organon, 2006).

Oral contraceptive pills (OCPs) offer a well-established woman-controlled method of hormonal birth control. Contraceptive rings and patches provide easily reversible cyclic contraceptive hormones on a continual basis, avoiding the peaks and valleys of OCPs. Contraceptive injections, implants, and hormonal IUDs offer long-acting contraception for women who are not candidates for estrogen-containing contraceptives or prefer continuous protection for extended intervals.

Hormonal contraceptives may reduce ovarian cancer risk, decrease the rate of endometrial cancer, improve dysmenorrhea, decrease menstrual blood loss, and result in a lighter menstrual flow (Adams Hilliard, 2007; Hatcher et al., 2004). Some women report premenstrual syndrome–like symptoms when using progestin-only contraceptives. Contraceptive hormones do pass into breast milk. Although estrogen has been demonstrated to decrease milk production, long-term effects of estrogen and progesterone on the newborn are not well documented (Hatcher et al., 2004; Truitt et al., 2003).

Client History and Chart Review:
Components of the History to Consider
(Hatcher et al., 2004)
- OB/GYN history
  - LMP and typical menstrual pattern, potential for pregnancy
  - Gravida, para, date of most recent birth if postpartum
  - Last examination, Pap smear, and STI testing if applicable
  - Incidence of
    - Dysmenorrhea
    - Menorrhagia
    - Dysfunctional uterine bleeding (DUB)
  - Frequency of intercourse
  - Risk factors for STIs: diagnosis and treatment
  - Abnormal Pap smears: diagnosis and treatment
  - Breast, mammogram abnormalities: diagnosis and treatment

- Past and current health history
    - Allergies
    - Medications and supplements
        - Potential for interaction with hormonal contraceptives, such as (Hatcher et al., 2004)
            - Anticonvulsants (may decrease hormonal contraceptive efficacy and medication therapeutic levels)
            - Anti-HIV protease inhibitors (may alter hormonal contraceptive efficacy)
            - Diazepam and chlordiazepoxide (may increase medication effect)
            - Griseofulvin (antifungal) (may decrease hormonal contraceptive efficacy)
            - Rifamycin and rifabutin (may decrease hormonal contraceptive efficacy)
            - St. John's wort (may decrease hormonal contraceptive efficacy)
            - Theophylline (may increase medication effect)
    - Personal or family history
        - Contraindications to hormonal contraceptive use (ACOG, 2000; Organon, 2006)
            - Pregnancy
            - Liver disease
            - Undiagnosed abnormal genital bleeding
            - Thrombophlebitis or thromboembolitic disease
            - Coronary heart disease or cerebrovascular disease
            - Cancer of the reproductive organs or breast
            - Migraine with aura
        - Relative contraindications (see full prescribing information)
            - Breastfeeding < 6 weeks postpartum
            - Women > 35 years old who smoke
            - Hypertension
            - Depression or mood disorder
            - Gallbladder disease
            - Abnormal glucose metabolism or diabetes
            - Asthma
            - Kidney disease
            - Seizure disorder
            - Lupus
- Assess the woman's ability and motivation to use client-regulated hormonal contraception (Reider & Coupey, 2000)
    - Motivation to prevent pregnancy
    - Ability and motivation to comply with recommended care
        - Daily routine for pill taking
        - Weekly routine for patch
        - Three-week cycle for ring
        - Thirteen-week cycle for injections
    - Ability to cope with side effects while adjusting to hormones
- Social history
    - Cigarette smoking
    - Drug and/or alcohol use
    - Living situation and resources
    - Sexual partner support for method of contraception
- Risk factors for osteoporosis
    - Low Ca^+ diet
    - Sedentary
    - Small frame
    - History of anorexia-related amenorrhea
    - Family history
    - Duration of injectable contraceptive use

Physical Examination:
Components of the Physical Exam
to Consider
- Blood pressure
- Height, weight, BMI
- Comprehensive well-woman examination
    - Focus on reproductive system
        - Thyroid
        - Breasts
        - Pelvic examination
            - Speculum examination
            - Bimanual examination

- Method specific focus
  - Inner aspect of upper arm (implants)
  - Depth of uterine cavity (IUD)

Clinical Impression:
Differential Diagnoses and Code Groups
to Consider
Additional suffix or CPT code may apply
(ICD9data.com, 2007)

- Gynecologic examination (ICD-9 codes V72.31)
- OCPs
  - Counseling and prescription of OCPs (ICD-9 codes V25.01)
  - Repeat prescription of OCPs (ICD-9 codes V25.41)
  - Follow-up care for OCPs (ICD-9 codes V25.41)
- IUD
  - Insertion of IUD (ICD-9 codes V25.1)
  - Follow-up care for IUD (ICD-9 codes V25.42)
- Implants
  - Insertion of subdermal contraceptive implant (ICD-9 codes V25.5)
  - Follow-up care for subdermal contraceptive implant (ICD-9 codes V25.43)
- Other hormonal contraceptive methods
  - Initiation of other contraceptive measures (ICD-9 codes V25.02)
  - Follow-up care for other contraceptive measures (ICD-9 codes V25.40)

Diagnostic Testing:
Diagnostic Tests and Procedures to Consider
(Organon, 2006)

- Pregnancy testing
- Pap smear
- Urinalysis
- STI screening
- Screening tests according to age and health history
  - Lipid profile
    - Family history of coronary artery disease
    - Smoker on oral contraceptives

- Fasting blood sugar
- TSH
- Mammogram
- Bone density testing

Providing Treatment:
Therapeutic Measures to Consider
(Hatcher et al., 2004; Pharmacia, 2005)

- Progestin-only contraceptives
  - Injectable contraceptives
    - Amenorrhea common
    - May delay return to fertility
    - May contribute to osteoporosis
    - May diminish
      - Risk of sickle cell crisis
      - Symptoms of endometriosis
    - Initial injection given
      - Within first 5 days of normal menses
      - Within first 5 days postpartum if not breastfeeding
      - At 4–6 weeks postpartum if breastfeeding
    - Depo-Provera given deep IM
    - Depo SubQ given in anterior thigh or abdomen
  - Hormonal IUD (see Intrauterine Device and Intrauterine System)
    - Insert per manufacturer's recommendations
    - May reduce incidence of
      - Menorrhagia
      - Dysmenorrhea
  - Progestin-only pills (POP)
    - Lower effectiveness than combination OCPs
    - Breakthrough bleeding (BTB) common
    - If pregnancy occurs, greater risk of ectopic implantation
  - Implanon (Organon, 2006)
    - Insert subdermally
      - According to manufacturer's instruction
      - Timing based on current method of contraception

- ➤ Palpate immediately after insertion
- ➤ Rod is palpable when inserted correctly
- Combination contraceptives (estrogen and progestin)
  - May decrease breast milk production
    - ◆ Avoid during breastfeeding, *or*
    - ◆ Delay use until infant taking additional foods
  - OCPs
    - ◆ Use lowest effective dose
    - ◆ Higher doses for specific indications
    - ◆ Very-low-dose birth control pills
      - ➤ Breakthrough bleeding may occur
      - ➤ May have improved side-effect profile over regular-dose OCP
    - ◆ Low-dose birth control pills
      - ➤ Slightly higher dose
      - ➤ Less breakthrough bleeding
      - ➤ May have increased side effects
    - ◆ Ninety-day pills (Seasonale)
      - ➤ Take for 84 days continuously
      - ➤ Initial high rate of breakthrough bleeding
      - ➤ Menses four times a year
    - ◆ 365-day a year pill (Lybrel) (Wyeth, 2008)
      - ➤ Low combined daily dose of the hormones levonorgestrel (LNG) and ethinyl estradiol (EE)—90 mcg and 20 mcg
      - ➤ Effectiveness approximately 98–99%
      - ➤ Amenorrhea in 60% at the end of a year of use
      - ➤ Initial high rate of BTB
  - Transdermal patch: Ortho Evra
    - ◆ Patch lasts 7 days; three patches per prescription cycle carton
    - ◆ Effectiveness approximately 99%
    - ◆ Decreased effectiveness in women weighing more than 198 lbs
  - NuvaRing contraceptive vaginal ring
    - ◆ Lower effective dose of hormones
    - ◆ Effectiveness approximately 98–99%

Providing Treatment:
Alternative Measures to Consider
- Fertility awareness/natural family planning
- Outercourse
- Abstinence
- Withdrawal
- Natural spermicides
- Barrier methods

Providing Support:
Education and Support Measures to Consider
(Hatcher et al., 2004)
- Information and instruction
  - Use of hormonal contraceptives
  - Effectiveness
  - Side effects
  - Warning signs
  - Return schedule
- Smoking cessation information and support (see Smoking Cessation)
- OCPs
  - Start methods
    - ◆ Quick start: Take first pill at office visit
    - ◆ First-day start: Take first pill first day of menses
    - ◆ Sunday start: Take first pill Sunday after onset of menses
  - Barrier or alternate method recommended for first cycle
  - Condoms recommended to protect against STIs
  - Breakthrough bleeding is common in first cycles
  - Take pill daily at the same time, link with other activity
  - Take pills as soon as possible if forgotten
  - Use backup method or ECP if more than two pills are missed
- NuvaRing (Organon, 2005)
  - Insert following manufacturer's instructions
    - ◆ Ring inserted into vagina
    - ◆ Remains in place for 3 weeks
    - ◆ Ring-free for 1 week

- ◆ Side effects same as OCPs
- ◆ May use tampons with ring
- ■ Nuvaring start instructions
  - ◆ No hormonal contraceptive
    - ➤ Start cycle day 1, or
    - ➤ Start cycle day 2–5
      - ▸ Requires nonhormonal contraception first 7 days
  - ◆ Combination OCP or patch
    - ➤ Start within 7 days of last pill or patch
  - ◆ Progestin-only method (pills, injection, or IUD)
    - ➤ Requires nonhormonal contraception first 7 days
    - ➤ Pills: Start any day
    - ➤ Injection: Start when next injection is due
    - ➤ Implant: Start on day of removal
  - ◆ After first-trimester spontaneous or induced abortion
    - ➤ Start days 1–5, or
    - ➤ Start with first menses (see No hormonal contraceptive, above)
      - ▸ Requires nonhormonal contraception first 7 days
- • Ortho Evra (Ortho-McNeil Pharmaceutical, 2007)
  - ■ Patches release 60% more estrogen than 35-μg OCP
  - ■ Side effects similar to OCPs
    - ◆ Greater risk of deep vein thrombosis
    - ◆ Patch users are urged not to smoke
  - ■ First day or Sunday start
  - ■ Replace patch each week for three patches
  - ■ One week patch free (maximum, 7 days)
  - ■ Apply patch to clean dry skin of the
    - ◆ Buttocks
    - ◆ Upper outer arm
    - ◆ Lower abdomen
    - ◆ Upper torso
  - ■ Use additional method or abstinence
    - ◆ During first week of use
    - ◆ If patch falls off or is forgotten

- ■ Replace patch if full or partial detachment occurs
- • Injections (Pharmacia, 2004)
  - ■ Significant bone mineral loss may occur
    - ◆ Limit use to < 2 years unless other methods inadequate
    - ◆ Ensure adequate calcium and vitamin D intake
  - ■ Side effects include
    - ◆ Weight gain and fluid retention
    - ◆ Delayed return to fertility (range, 4–31 months)
    - ◆ Bleeding irregularities
- • Implanon (Organon, 2006)
  - ■ Side effects include
    - ◆ Bleeding irregularities
    - ◆ Mood changes, including depression
    - ◆ Headache
    - ◆ Weight gain
- • All methods: Call or return for care
  - ■ Unexpected amenorrhea or menorrhagia
  - ■ Persistent intermenstrual bleeding
  - ■ Depression
  - ■ Suspected pregnancy
  - ■ Persistent side effects, such as
    - ◆ Nausea
    - ◆ Irregular menses
    - ◆ Mood changes
  - ■ ⚠ Seek emergency care immediately
    - ◆ Abdominal or pelvic pain
    - ◆ Chest pain or shortness of breath
    - ◆ Numbness or tingling of arms or legs
    - ◆ Severe headaches
    - ◆ Visual disturbances
- • Potential health benefits
  - ■ Regulation of menses
  - ■ Decreased cramping and flow
  - ■ Protection against uterine and ovarian cancer
  - ■ Decreased risk of bone loss (except Depo-Provera)
- • 🚫 Potential risks
  - ■ Pregnancy
  - ■ Exacerbation of gallbladder disease

- Stroke or blood clots
- Estrogen dependent cancers
- Osteoporosis (Depo-Provera)
- Uterine perforation (IUD)
- Local infection (injection and implants)

Follow-up Care:
Follow-up Measures to Consider
- Document
  - Pertinent history and physical examination
  - Verification of nonpregnant state
  - Method-related education and counseling
  - Plan for continued care
- Follow-up visit
  - Timing
    - Implant 2–4 weeks to assess healing
    - Injectable contraceptive 11–13 weeks for next injection
    - Combined contraceptives 3 months to assess continued use
    - IUD after first menses to verify placement
  - Blood pressure and weight
  - Laboratory
    - Hemoglobin and hematocrit
    - Triglycerides
    - Glucose
  - Satisfaction with method
  - Questions or concerns
  - ⚠ Review warning signs: ACHES
    - **A**bdominal or pelvic pain
    - **C**hest pain
    - **H**eadache
    - **E**ye problems
    - **S**evere leg pain
- Problem-solving (Hatcher et al., 2004)
  - Amenorrhea
    - Choose increased estrogenic OCP
    - Basal body temperature charting
  - Acne and/or hirsutism
    - Ortho Tri-Cyclen or Estrostep

- Breakthrough bleeding
  - Rule out nonhormonal contraceptive causes
    - Pregnancy
    - Cervical abnormalities
    - Infection
  - Progestin-only contraceptives
    - Offer one or more cycles of combined OCP use if estrogen not contraindicated
    - Counsel that BTB typically diminishes over time
  - Combined hormone contraceptives
    - Change OCP formulation
      - BTB on active pills
        - ★ Increase progestin through cycle, or
        - ★ At end of active pills (triphasic)
      - BTB after withdraw bleed
        - ★ Increase estrogen, or
        - ★ Decrease progestin in early pills
- Breast tenderness
  - Low-dose OCPs
  - Extended-cycle OCPs
  - Continuous dose method (ring or patch)
- ▽ Headaches
  - Monitor blood pressure
  - Determine type of headache
    - Timing, duration, location, severity
    - 🕐 Evaluate potential causes, refer as needed
  - Lower dose of estrogen or progestin
  - Discontinue OCPs
- Mood swings, depression
  - Recommend B vitamin supplement
  - Discontinue injection or implant
  - Continuous-dose method (ring or patch)
  - Low-dose or extended-cycle OCPs
- Nausea
  - Take OCP at bedtime
  - Decrease estrogen dose
  - Take missed pills at 12-hour intervals

◆ Continuous dose method (ring or patch)

◆ Increase fresh fruit, vegetable, and fluid intake

Collaborative Practice:
Criteria to Consider for Consultation or Referral

- OB/GYN service
  - Clients with relative contraindications to hormonal contraceptives who wish to try this method
- Specialty care
  - Development of significant complication(s) related to hormonal contraceptive use
    - ◆ Severe headache, stroke, or neurologic symptoms
    - ◆ Depression or mood disorder
    - ◆ Acute abdomen
    - ◆ Cardiac or vascular symptoms
- For diagnosis or treatment outside the midwife's scope of practice

INTRAUTERINE DEVICE AND INTRAUTERINE SYSTEM

Key Clinical Information

The intrauterine device and/or system (IUD/IUS) offers women a highly effective reversible method of birth control that may be hormonal or nonhormonal. The ParaGard® (Copper-T 380A) IUD is impregnated with copper and is effective for 10 years. The Mirena (LNG-IUS) releases the progestin levonorgestrel into the intrauterine cavity and is effective for 5 years. Like any method of birth control, careful evaluation to determine who is an appropriate candidate for this method is required. Benefits of IUD/IUS use include its effectiveness (> 99%) and ease of use (Hatcher et al., 2004). The common IUD side effect of heavy bleeding has been minimized by the Mirena IUS; the continual release of a low dose of progestin thins the lining of the uterus and may be used to treat menorrhagia and/or dysmenorrhea (ACOG, 2005; Schuiling & Likis, 2006). Risks associated with IUD/IUS use

include uterine perforation, pelvic infection, ectopic pregnancy, and expulsion (Hatcher et al., 2004; Varney et al., 2004).

Client History and Chart Review:
Components of the History to Consider

- Age
- Gravida, para
- Allergies
- Medications
- Medical/surgical history
  - Increased susceptibility to infection, such as (Duramed Pharmaceuticals, 2006b; Bayer HealthCare Pharmaceuticals, 2007)
    - ◆ Leukemia
    - ◆ AIDS
    - ◆ IV drug use
  - IUD/IUS appropriate for women with (ACOG, 2005)
    - ◆ Diabetes
    - ◆ Thromboembolism (copper IUD)
    - ◆ Bleeding disorders or anticoagulant therapy (hormonal IUS)
    - ◆ Menorrhagia/dysmenorrhea (hormonal IUS)
    - ◆ Breastfeeding (copper IUD only before 6 weeks)
    - ◆ Breast cancer (copper IUD)
    - ◆ Liver disease (copper IUD)
- Reproductive history
  - LMP or date of delivery
  - Contraceptive history and current use
  - Pap smear and/or human papillomavirus (HPV) history
  - STI diagnosis and treatment history
  - History of fibroids or unusual configuration of uterus
  - Menstrual history
- The ideal candidate for IUD/IUS use (ACOG, 2006; Varney et al., 2004)
  - Women at low risk for STIs
  - Preference for long-term contraception
  - One or more full-term pregnancies

- Comfortable with the thought of an IUD/IUS in her uterus
- Able to check for the IUD/IUS string
- ⚠ Contraindications to IUD/IUS insertion (ACOG, 2006; Hatcher et al., 2004; Varney et al., 2004)
  - Pregnancy
  - Genital tract infection, current or past 3 months
    - STIs
    - Pelvic inflammatory disease
    - Postpartum endometritis
    - Recent septic abortion
  - Untreated genital tract malignancy
    - Cervix
    - Endometrium
    - Molar pregnancy
  - Distortion of the uterine cavity
  - Copper allergy or Wilson's disease (copper IUD)
  - Decreased immune response
  - Acute liver disease (hormonal IUS)
  - Current deep vein thrombosis (hormonal IUS)
- Before removal determine
  - Indication for removal
  - Birth control method desired, if any

Physical Examination:
Components of the Physical Exam to Consider
- Physical examination as indicated by client history
- Before insertion
  - Consider cervical priming for nulligravid women
    - Insertion of osmotic dilator 1 day before insertion
    - Misoprostol 400 μg 4–12 hours before insertion
  - Obtain Pap smear and STI testing as needed
  - Bimanual examination to determine
    - Uterine size and contour
    - Uterine position
    - Involution if postpartum

- Speculum examination
  - Sound uterus (6–9 cm is recommended)
- Before removal
  - Speculum examination for visualization of strings
  - Based on indication for removal

Clinical Impression:
Differential Diagnoses and Code Groups
to Consider
Additional suffix and procedure codes may apply
(ICD9data.com, 2007)
- Contraceptive counseling, IUD (ICD-9 codes V25.02)
- Emergency contraceptive counseling (ICD-9 codes V25.03)
- IUD insertion (ICD-9 codes V25.1)
- IUD, follow-up postprocedure (ICD-9 codes V45.59)
- IUD in situ, surveillance of (ICD-9 codes V25.42)
- IUD removal and/or reinsertion (ICD-9 codes V25.42)
- Complications of IUD insertion/use
  - Failed IUD insertion (modifier-52)
    - Cervical stenosis (ICD-9 codes 622.4) (Witt, 2006)
  - Discontinued procedure (modifier-53)
    - Vasovagal syncope (ICD-9 codes 780.2)
    - Perforation of the uterus (ICD-9 codes 996.32) (Witt, 2006)
  - Displaced IUD (ICD-9 codes 996.32)
  - Infection secondary to IUD (ICD-9 codes 996.65)
  - Menorrhagia, secondary to IUD in situ (ICD-9 codes 996.76)

Diagnostic Testing:
Diagnostic Tests and Procedures to Consider
- Pregnancy testing
- Pap smear and/or human papillomavirus testing
- Chlamydia and gonorrhea testing
- Hepatitis profile

- HIV testing
- Other laboratory tests as indicated by health status, such as
  - Blood glucose
  - Liver function tests

Providing Treatment:
Therapeutic Measures to Consider
(Hatcher et al., 2004)

- Ibuprofen 600 mg or naproxen sodium 550 mg 1 hour before procedure
- Have atropine sulfate available for treatment of vagal response
  - May give IM when IV route not available
  - 0.4–0.5 mg IM for bradycardia (Varney et al., 2004)
- Antibiotic prophylaxis not indicated (ACOG, 2001a)
- Obtain informed consent (see Informed Consent, Chapter One)
  - Timing of insertion
    - Immediately after abortion or delivery
    - Six to 8 weeks postpartum
    - During menses
    - As emergency contraception (copper IUD only)
    - Any time, as long as pregnancy is ruled out
- To sound uterus before insertion
  - Position tenaculum gently
    - Close *slowly* to decrease cramping
    - Position on anterior lip for anteverted uterus
    - Position on posterior lip for retroverted uterus
    - Avoid vessels at 3 and 9 o'clock positions (Varney et al., 2004)
  - Apply traction to tenaculum
    - Straighten uterine curvature
    - Gently insert sterile sound until slight resistance is felt
      - ⚠ Do not use force
      - Dilate cervix if needed
    - Note depth of sound

- Six to 9 cm recommended (Bayer HealthCare Pharmaceuticals, 2007; Duramed Pharmaceuticals, 2006b)
  - Use sound to prepare IUD/IUS insertion device per manufacturer's instruction
- IUD insertion under sterile technique
  - Swab cervix with antiseptic solution (e.g., Betadine)
  - Load IUD/IUS into insertion device
  - Apply gentle traction to tenaculum
    - Straighten uterine curvature
    - Carefully place IUD/IUS according to manufacturer's instructions
    - Remove insertion device
  - Remove tenaculum
  - Obtain hemostasis
    - Apply pressure to bleeding sites
    - Apply silver nitrate to bleeding sites (may cause cramping)
  - Trim strings to approximately 1.5–2 inches (3–4 cm) in length
  - Vagal response may occur during or after procedure
    - ⊛ Treatment of vagal response (Varney et al., 2004)
      - Stop procedure
      - Trendelenburg position
      - Smelling salts
      - Atropine sulfate 0.4–0.5 mg IM
- IUD removal
  - Swab cervix with antiseptic solution (e.g., Betadine)
  - Grasp strings with ring forceps and pull gently but firmly
  - If strings not visible at os
    - Probe cervical canal with sterile forceps
      - Grasp string or IUD/IUS if felt and pull gently
    - If unable to identify IUD/IUS
      - Evaluate for presence of IUD/IUS with ultrasound
      - Removal under anesthesia may be required
  - Initiate other form of birth control as needed

Providing Treatment:
Alternative Measures to Consider
- Fertility awareness/natural family planning
- Outercourse
- Abstinence
- Withdrawal
- Natural spermicides
- Barrier methods

Providing Support:
Education and Support Measures to Consider
- Review all birth control options appropriate for this woman
- Review history with client and partner as needed
- ▽ Discuss risks, benefits, and effectiveness of IUD/IUS (Bayer HealthCare Pharmaceuticals, 2007; Duramed Pharmaceuticals, 2006b; Hatcher et al., 2004)
  - Risks
    - ◆ Uterine perforation or expulsion
    - ◆ Embedment in uterus
    - ◆ Pelvic inflammatory disease
    - ◆ Ectopic pregnancy
    - ◆ Increased incidence of ovarian cysts (hormonal IUS)
  - Benefits
    - ◆ Effective
      - ➤ Mirena 99.9%
      - ➤ ParaGard® 99.2%
    - ◆ Use unrelated to sexual activity
    - ◆ May decrease menses and dysmenorrhea (hormonal IUS)
- Provide information about
  - Preprocedure preparation
  - IUD/IUS cost
  - Details of insertion procedure
  - Potential side effects/complications
    - ◆ Signs and symptoms
    - ◆ When to call
    - ◆ How to call during off hours
- Teach client to feel strings
  - After insertion

- Before intercourse for first cycle
- After menses or monthly

Follow-up Care:
Follow-up Measures to Consider
- Document insertion and/or removal (see Procedure Note, Chapter One)
- Return for care (Bayer HealthCare Pharmaceuticals, 2007; Duramed Pharmaceuticals, 2006b)
  - Two to 6 weeks postinsertion/after next menses
  - ⚠ With onset of
    - ◆ Fever, abdominal pain, or heavy bleeding
    - ◆ Malodorous vaginal discharge
    - ◆ Signs or symptoms of pregnancy
    - ◆ Inability to locate IUD/IUS strings
    - ◆ Other significant side effects
  - Scheduled well-woman care
  - Exposure to STIs
  - Desired return to fertility
  - Scheduled IUD/IUS replacement
    - ◆ Five years for Mirena
    - ◆ Ten years for ParaGard®
- IUD/IUS troubleshooting (Hatcher et al., 2004)
  - Cramping: nonsteroidal antiinflammatory drugs (NSAIDs)
  - Expulsion
    - ◆ Verify nonpregnant status
    - ◆ Insert new IUD/IUS
  - Perforation with intraabdominal IUD
    - ◆ 📞 Refer for laparoscopy
  - Positive pregnancy test
    - ◆ Confirm location of pregnancy
    - ◆ Remove IUD/IUS promptly
    - ◆ ⚠ Influenza-like illness may signal septic abortion
  - Suspected salpingitis
    - ◆ Treat empirically per current CDC recommendations
    - ◆ May leave IUD/IUS in situ
    - ◆ Male partner examination and treatment indicated

Collaborative Practice:
Criteria to Consider for Consultation or Referral
- OB/GYN service
  - Relative contraindications for IUD/IUS insertion
    - Uterine anomalies
    - History of postpartum endometritis or PID in past 3 months
  - Client desire for paracervical block for insertion
  - For complications of IUD/IUS insertion
    - Difficulty sounding uterus
    - Perforation of uterus
  - Complications of IUD/IUS use
    - IUD string not visible or palpated and removal is desired
    - Septic abortion with IUD in situ
    - PID with IUD in situ
- For diagnosis or treatment outside the midwife's scope of practice

THE UNPLANNED PREGNANCY: OPTIONS FOR WOMEN

Key Clinical Information

Women experience unplanned or unwanted pregnancies due to a multitude of factors, such as birth control failure, issues of access to reproductive services or education, impaired judgment or cognitive ability, poor self-image resulting in limited contraceptive or sexual negotiating skills, and sexual coercion or assault. The role of the midwife is to provide sound unbiased information regarding reproductive choices and supportive nonjudgmental care that allows each woman the opportunity to make an informed personal decision when confronted with this difficult situation (American College of Nurse-Midwives [ACNM], 1997).

Many women will come to terms with their unintended pregnancy and become mothers, adapting their lives to all the changes that this pregnancy brings. A few women will continue their unplanned pregnancies and make plans to relinquish the infant for adoption. Other women opt for early termination of unplanned pregnancies. Each woman's decision to continue or terminate a pregnancy includes short- and long-term emotional, financial, and social consequences.

Adoptions range from traditional "closed-record" adoptions, where the infant is removed from the mother immediately after birth, to "open adoption," where the birth mother has more control of the process. During open adoptions the birth mother may meet the prospective parent(s) to determine if she deems them suitable for her child. The adoptive parents may be present for the birth and may receive the infant directly from the birth mother shortly after the birth. Open adoption allows the mother the potential to have future contact with her child and provides adoptive parents with information such as birth parents' medical and family histories. In all forms of adoption a postadoption waiting period is typical to allow the birth mother an opportunity to review her choice before it becomes legally binding.

Early termination of pregnancy offers women another choice for unplanned pregnancy. Medical abortion using mifepristone is approved by the U.S. Food and Drug Administration (FDA) for women less than 49 days from the LMP (FDA, 2006). It offers women the opportunity to end pregnancy without undergoing a surgical procedure and is 95–98% successful (FDA, 2005). Surgical abortion provides an option for women who desire termination of pregnancy beyond 8 weeks gestation or prefer the speed and efficacy (99–100% effective) of surgical abortion.

Participation in pregnancy termination procedures by the midwife is a highly individual choice often based on the midwife's moral and ethical values and her beliefs regarding women's right to reproductive choice (ACNM, 1997). The process for expanding midwifery practice to include abortion services follows the ACNM Guidelines for the Incorporation of New Procedures into Nurse-Midwifery Practice (ACNM, 2000). In many states abortion services are limited to physician-provided services. State-by-state information regarding abortion and reproductive rights is available at NARAL Pro

Choice America online at http://www.prochoice america.org/index.html (ACNM, 2006).

Client History and Chart Review:
Components of the History to Consider
(Hatcher et al., 2004; Varney et al., 2004)

- Age
- Obstetric history
  - Gravida, para
  - Verify pregnancy
    - LMP, cycle history
    - Date of conception, if known
    - Most recent method of birth control
    - Date of pregnancy test
    - Signs and symptoms of pregnancy
  - Blood type and Rh factor if known
- Gynecologic history
  - STI screening and results
  - Last Pap smear and examination
  - Gynecologic procedures
- Medical/surgical history
  - Allergies
  - Medications, prescription and/or OTC
  - Medical conditions, such as
    - Asthma
    - Inflammatory bowel disease
    - Seizure disorder
    - Cardiac valvular disease
    - Bleeding disorders
  - Prior surgery
- Social issues
  - Feelings about pregnancy
  - Personal support systems
  - Financial concerns regarding pregnancy options
  - Cultural considerations affecting decision
  - Drug, alcohol, and tobacco use
  - Sexual coercion or rape
  - Mental health concerns
  - Tentative plans regarding pregnancy
- Contraindications to medical abortion
  - Allergy to medication
  - Confirmed or potential ectopic pregnancy
  - IUD in situ

- Potential for noncompliance with required follow-up
- Presence of significant medical problems
  - Chronic adrenal failure
  - Bleeding disorders or anticoagulant therapy
  - Long-term corticosteroid therapy
  - Inherited porphyria
- Refusal to follow-up with definitive surgical treatment if medical treatment fails

Physical Examination:
Components of the Physical Exam to Consider

- Vital signs
- Pelvic examination
  - Uterine size and position
  - Estimate of gestational age
- Other evaluations as indicated by history

Clinical Impression:
Differential Diagnoses and Code Groups
to Consider
Additional suffix may apply (ICD9data.com, 2007)

- Pregnancy examination with immediate confirmation (ICD-9 codes V22.0–V22.1)
- Pregnancy examination or test, pregnancy unconfirmed (ICD-9 codes V72.4)
- Late effects of injury purposely inflicted by another person (ICD-9 codes E969)
- Legally induced abortion without complication (ICD-9 codes 635.90–635.92)
- Legally induced abortion with complication (ICD-9 codes 635.00–635.82)

Diagnostic Testing:
Diagnostic Tests and Procedures to Consider
(Hatcher et al., 2004)

- Serum or urine human chorionic gonadotropin (HCG)
- Complete blood count, or hematocrit and hemoglobin
- Screening for genital tract infections
  - Bacterial vaginosis
  - Candidiasis

- Trichomoniasis
- Chlamydia
- Gonorrhea
- Blood type and Rh screen
- Pelvic ultrasound
  - Vaginal or abdominal
  - Rule out ectopic pregnancy
  - Estimate gestational age

Providing Treatment:
Therapeutic Measures to Consider
- Initiate treatment for genital tract infection
- Remove IUD if present
- FDA-approved regimen for medical abortion through 49 days post-LMP (FDA, 2006; Hatcher et al., 2004; Mackenzie & Yeo, 1997; Varney et al., 2004)
  - Verify surgical coverage
    - Client preferences
    - Retained products of conception
  - Obtain informed consent
  - Prophylactic antibiotics not indicated
  - Day 1: mifepristone administration
    - Dose: 600 mg PO in presence of provider
    - Observation for 30 minutes
    - Provide for pain relief
      - Acetaminophen
      - Acetaminophen with codeine
      - Nonsteroidal antiinflammatory drugs
        - Compatible with mifepristone
        - Provide significant pain relief
  - Day 3: misoprostol administration
    - 400 µg misoprostol PO in presence of provider
    - Observe for ± 4 hours (expulsion of products of conception [POC] occurs during this time in 60% of clients)
    - Send tissue to pathology for verification of POC
    - Provide RhIG if indicated
      - One dose (full or mini) postabortion
  - Day 14: posttreatment
    - Client returns to confirm complete termination

- Surgical termination for medical abortion treatment failure
- The safety and effectiveness of other Mifeprex dosing regimens, including use of oral misoprostol tablets intravaginally, has not been established by the FDA (2006).
- Evidence-based regimen for medical abortion through 63 days after LMP (Hatcher et al., 2004)
  - Day 1: mifepristone administration
    - Dose: 200 mg PO in presence of provider
    - Misoprostol 800 µg provided
      - Self-administered vaginally 24–72 hours after mifepristone
  - Post-treatment follow-up day 4–8
  - Advantages
    - Comparable efficacy to FDA regimen
    - Extended window for treatment
    - Shorter time to completion
    - Decreased medication costs
    - Fewer office visits
    - Decreased side effects
  - Disadvantages
    - Potential increased risk of anaerobic infection
- Vacuum aspiration abortion (Hatcher et al., 2004)
  - Ensure presence of emergency medications and equipment
  - Local anesthesia and/or sedation may be used
  - Cervix is dilated with osmotic or mechanical dilators
  - Evacuation cannula is inserted through the cervix
    - Size is equivalent to number of weeks gestation (i.e., 5-mm cannula for 5 weeks gestation)
  - Uterus is evacuated using vacuum pump or syringe
  - Tissue examination to evaluate products of conception

Providing Treatment:
Alternative Measures to Consider

- Herbal remedies to foster interruption of pregnancy (see Emergency Contraception)
- Remedies to support the reproductive system during medical or surgical abortion
  - Herbals (Zeus, 2007; Soule, 1996)
    - Echinacea
    - Red raspberry leaf
    - Dong quai
    - Vitex
    - Lemon balm
    - Alfalfa leaf
    - Nettle leaf
    - Yellow dock
  - Homeopathic support (Smith, 1984)
    - Arnica
    - Sabina
    - Pulsatilla
    - Other remedies as indicated by client symptom presentation
  - Bach flower remedies
    - Rescue Remedy
    - Other remedies as indicated by client emotional presentation

Providing Support:
Education and Support Measures to Consider

- Provide factual unbiased information during options counseling (ACNM, 1997)
- Available options may be based on
  - Age of client
  - Availability of services
  - Cultural factors
  - Gestational age of pregnancy
  - Maternal medical factors
  - Financial considerations
- Clear information should be provided regarding
  - Prenatal care and birth options
    - Adoption outside the family
    - Adoption within the family
    - Keeping and caring for infant
  - Voluntary termination of pregnancy
    - Medical
    - Surgical

- Termination procedure(s)
  - Medical abortion process
    - Provide written information/ instructions detailing
      - Medication dose and administration schedule
      - Anticipated sequence of events
      - Plan for follow-up visits
      - Medication side effects
        - Nausea and vomiting
        - Diarrhea
        - Malaise
      - Warning signs (see below)
      - How to contact practitioner
  - Surgical
    - Provide written information/ instructions detailing
      - Procedure
      - Sedation or anesthesia available
      - Anticipated sequence of events
      - Warning signs (see below)
      - How to contact practitioner
  - Coverage options should surgical services be required or desired

Follow-up Care:
Follow-up Measures to Consider

- After options counseling
  - Schedule prenatal care, or
  - Schedule termination after verification of gestation
- For posttermination examination 4–14 days (Hatcher et al., 2004)
  - Examination to verify complete abortion
  - Postabortion counseling
  - Referral for retained products of conception
- Presence of warning signs after medical abortion (Emma Goldman Clinic, 2007; FDA, 2006)
  - Consider sepsis
  - Obtain complete blood count
  - Initiate immediate antibiotic treatment for anaerobic bacteria such as *Clostridium sordellii*
- Contraceptive management

Box 6-2   Caring for Yourself After an Abortion

- **It is normal to experience the following:**
  - Spotting or bleeding that starts and stops
  - Passage of blood clots
  - Menstrual-like cramping (abdominal or back pain)
  - Slightly elevated temperature (100°F or less)
  - Sadness or emotional upset
  - Disappearance of most pregnancy symptoms within 1–7 days
  - Rapid return to fertility
  - Menses in 4–8 weeks

- **It is *not* normal to experience the following:**
  - Bleeding beyond 3 weeks
  - Heavy bleeding
  - Persistence of pregnancy symptoms
  - Severe cramping or abdominal tenderness
  - Temperature of 100.4°F or more
  - Passage of foul-smelling discharge or tissue
  - No menses within 12 weeks
  - Severe mood changes

- **Things to do:**
  - Use sanitary pads, not tampons
  - Get plenty of rest
  - Drink plenty of fluids
  - Resume nonstrenuous activities
  - Eat iron-rich foods
  - Take your temperature if you feel chilled or hot
  - Come to your follow-up visit
  - If antibiotics were given to you, take as directed until gone
  - Use nonaspirin pain relievers for cramping

- **Things to avoid:**
  - Vaginal penetration with sex until bleeding stops
  - Hot tubs or swimming
  - Douching or vaginal sprays
  - Strenuous exercise for 3–7 days
  - Alcohol and drugs, which may mask complications

- ⚠ **If you experience these warning signs and symptoms after your termination procedure seek medical care immediately!**
  - Saturating sanitary pads every 30 minutes for 2 hours
  - Heavy flow for 24 hours
  - Fever (> 100.4°F) more than 8 hours after misoprostol dose
  - Chills
  - Severe abdominal or back pain

Adapted from Emma Goldman Clinic. (2007). *Post-abortion care.* Iowa City, IA: Author. Retrieved January 22, 2008 from http://www.emmagoldman.com/services/abortion/care.htm; and Hatcher, R. A., Trussell, J., Stewart, F., Nelson, A. L., Cates, W., et al. (2004). *Contraceptive technology.* New York: Ardent Media.

Collaborative Practice:
Criteria to Consider for Consultation or Referral

- OB/GYN or women's health service
  - Midwife cannot provide objective options counseling
  - Midwife does not offer termination services
  - Surgical coverage for clients undergoing medical abortion
- Social service
  - Parenting resources
  - Adoption resources
  - Mental health services
  - Support groups
- For diagnosis or treatment outside the midwife's scope of practice

SECTION TWO:
CARE OF THE AGING WELL WOMAN

Some midwives provide well-woman care from menarche through a woman's mature adulthood. Caring for women as they age requires knowledge and understanding of the many changes that occur during the aging process and the impact those changes may have on each woman's life. The changes as women age cannot be quantified simply by where an individual is on the chart of reproductive life stages, but also how she sees herself and how the challenges of aging affect her.

During the perimenopausal period women may simultaneously have families that include young children, adolescent or adult children, grandchildren, and aging parents. The dream of retirement or financial security may recede with the demands of providing care for aged parents or a diminished ability to work. Health problems may become more prevalent and use up a significant proportion of energy that was previously directed to home, family, or livelihood.

The hormonal changes that occur around the time of menopause influence each woman's response to her life situation. These changes may affect her ability to rest, her emotional well-being, her strength and stamina, and her self-image. Health problems specific to women, such as the vasomotor symptoms of menopause, osteopenia or osteoporosis, and breast cancer, become areas of concern.

Although some women age with grace and dignity, for many others the aging process is beset with challenges. Aging frequently results in or exacerbates physical conditions such as heart disease and hypertension, diabetes, arthritis, and cognitive decline; it may bring financial difficulty through widowhood, divorce, or limited job opportunities. In addition, isolation may occur as a woman's physical condition and mental abilities decline.

Alternative or complementary therapies may relieve symptoms of menopause, maintain bone integrity, and enhance mental acuity and a woman's overall sense of well-being. Activities such as yoga may provide multiple benefits such as maintenance of balance and bone strength, improved blood pressure, decreased stress, emotional balance, social interaction, and spiritual solace. Compassionate midwifery care provides women an opportunity to explore new views of themselves as they age while offering health screening and a gateway to needed health care services.

ASSESSMENT OF WOMEN AT THE TIME OF MENOPAUSE

Key Clinical Information
The woman who stands on the threshold of menopause is entering a new phase of her life. The perimenopausal period is frequently a time of introspection, reappraisal, and personal growth. Each woman responds differently to the precursors of menopause—one may sigh with relief that her time of menstruation is nearly done, whereas another may be dismayed by the passing of her fertility. The onset of menopause may be portrayed using negative terms or, alternately, as a healthy life stage that celebrates the accomplishments and strengths of women (Anderson, 2005).

Although menopause is defined as the day when it has been 12 months since the last menstrual period, the time of transition may last several years during which a woman may experience multiple signs and symptoms (Schuiling & Likis, 2006). Early signs of unintended pregnancy may be erroneously dismissed as irregularity of menses. Visits during the perimenopausal and early postmenopausal period allow the midwife to assess each woman's health beliefs and practices while screening for common health problems and to ensure each woman has access to safe and reliable contraception. Providing information and education related to the change of life may help ease the transition for women, particularly in the early postmenopausal period when women experience the greatest incidence of troublesome symptoms (Schuiling & Likis, 2006).

Client History and Chart Review:
Components of the History to Consider
(Schuiling & Likis, 2006)

- Age, race, and cultural heritage
- Reproductive and sexual history
  - Gravida, para
  - Pap history
  - STIs
  - Presence or absence of cervix, uterus, ovaries
  - Menstrual status
    - Frequency, duration, flow
    - Changes in menses
      - Pattern of bleeding
      - Intermenstrual bleeding
      - Prolonged
      - Excessive or scanty flow
  - Vasomotor symptoms
    - Hot flashes or flushes
    - Night sweats
    - Flushing
  - Urogenital symptoms
    - Vaginal dryness
    - Urinary symptoms
    - Decreased libido
  - Other symptoms
    - Insomnia or sleep pattern changes
    - Emotional changes
      - Emotional lability
      - Depression or anxiety
      - Diminished coping ability
      - Forgetfulness
  - Sexual activity and practices
    - Sexual activity
    - Sexual orientation
    - Changes in
      - Libido
      - Vaginal lubrication
      - Sexual functioning
    - Dyspareunia
- Medical/surgical history
  - Allergies
  - Medications and herbal supplements
  - Complementary and alternative therapies
  - Recent diagnostic testing with other health care practitioner(s)
    - Dental examination
    - Hearing testing
    - Vision examination
    - Medical screening tests
  - Chronic illness or disease
  - Surgeries
- Risk factor assessment
  - Coronary artery disease
  - Osteoporosis
  - Thyroid disorder
  - Diabetes mellitus
  - Malignancy
  - Intimate partner violence
- Family history
  - Age of menopause in close female relatives
  - Osteoporosis
  - Female reproductive cancers
  - Colon or gastrointestinal malignancy
  - Heart disease
  - Diabetes
- Social history
  - Attitudes toward menopause
  - Family support systems
  - Social activities
  - Tobacco, alcohol, or drug use
- Ability to care for self
  - Food, shelter
  - Activities of daily living
  - Ability to seek assistance as needed

- Physical activity
- Nutritional assessment
- Review of systems
  - Integumentary
    - Skin changes
    - Lesions
  - HEENT
    - Hearing loss
    - Visual changes
  - Cardiopulmonary
    - Shortness of breath (SOB)
    - Palpitations
    - Edema
  - Gastrointestinal
    - Bowel changes
    - Rectal bleeding
    - Rectocele
  - Genitourinary
    - Urinary frequency
    - Incontinence
    - Dyspareunia
  - Endocrine
    - Fatigue
    - Intolerance to cold/heat
  - Neurologic
    - Confusion
    - Headaches
  - Musculoskeletal
    - Pain
    - Range of motion
    - Joint enlargement

Physical Examination:
Components of the Physical Exam to Consider
- Vital signs, including blood pressure
  - Height, weight, and BMI
  - Changes in height or weight
- General
  - Evidence of self-care
  - Affect and responsiveness
  - Skin turgor and thickness
  - Presence of bruises, cuts or signs of trauma
- HEENT
  - Hearing
  - Vision

- Thyroid
- Cervical nodes
- Nasal patency
- Teeth and gums
- Back
  - Costovertebral angle tenderness
  - Evaluate for kyphosis, lordosis, low back pain
  - Respiratory examination
    - Ausculate lung fields bilaterally
- Cardiac examination
  - Rate and rhythm
  - Murmurs
  - Pulses
  - Peripheral edema
- Breast examination
  - Masses
  - Discharge
  - Axillary nodes
- Abdomen
  - Bowel sounds
  - Liver margins
- Extremities
  - Edema
  - Varicosities
  - Range of motion
- Genital examination
  - Genital atrophy
  - Vaginal dryness
  - Lesions
  - Speculum examination
  - Bimanual examination
    - Uterus
      - Size
      - Consistency
      - Contour
      - Mobility
    - Adnexa
      - Size
      - Consistency
      - Mobility
    - Presence of cystocele or rectocele
- Rectal examination
  - Hemorrhoids
  - Palpate for lesions/masses

Clinical Impression:
Differential Diagnoses and Code Groups
to Consider
Additional suffix may apply (ICD9data.com, 2007)

- Well-woman examination (ICD-9 codes V72.3)
- Amenorrhea (ICD-9 codes 626)
- Mastalgia (ICD-9 codes 611)
- Premenopausal menorrhagia (ICD-9 codes 627)
- Postmenopausal bleeding (PMB) (ICD-9 codes 627)
- Sleep disturbances (ICD-9 codes 780.50)
- Urinary incontinence (ICD-9 codes 788.3)
- Vasomotor symptoms (ICD-9 codes 627.2)

Diagnostic Testing:
Diagnostic Tests and Procedures to Consider
(ACOG, 1995, 2006; Office on Women's Health,
n.d.; U.S. Preventive Services Task Force, 2006)

- Reproductive testing
  - Endometrial biopsy
  - Mammogram
  - Pap smear
  - STI testing, including
    - Hepatitis testing
    - HIV testing
- General medical testing
  - Fasting blood sugar
  - Hemoglobin
  - Liver function tests
  - Lipid profile or cholesterol
  - Thyroid testing (TSH)
  - Urinalysis
  - Bone density testing
  - Colorectal cancer screening
  - Electrocardiogram
  - Tuberculosis testing

Providing Treatment:
Therapeutic Measures to Consider (ACOG, 2006;
U.S. Preventive Services Task Force, 2006)

- Immunization update (CDC, 2007)
  - Tetanus-diphtheria, pertussis
  - Influenza
  - Pneumococcal
  - Meningococcal
  - Varicella
  - Zoster
- Contraception as indicated
  - Low-dose triphasic OCPs offer
    - Reliable contraception
    - Relief from vasomotor symptoms
- Vitamin and mineral supplements
  - Calcium 1200–1500 mg daily
  - Magnesium 400 mg daily
  - Vitamin E 400 IU BID with meals
- Hormone therapy (see Hormone Replacement Therapy)
  - Estrogen replacement therapy
  - Combination HRT
  - Estrogen/androgen therapy
- Treatment for medical conditions, such as
  - Hypertension
  - Diabetes
  - Hypothyroidism

Providing Treatment:
Alternative Measures to Consider

- Dietary changes
  - Decrease fat, caffeine, sugar, alcohol
  - Increase soy, whole grains, dietary fiber
  - Vitamin E, vitamin D, calcium, and magnesium
- Maintain regular weight-bearing exercise
  - Walking, jogging
  - Weight training
  - Aerobics
- Non–weight-bearing exercise for joint mobility
  - Swimming
  - Biking
- Sleep aids
  - Valerian root
  - Chamomile
  - Melatonin
- Utilize creative outlets
  - Journal writing
  - Dance, meditation, or singing
  - Prayer
- Community involvement, groups
  - Schools, child care
  - Church

- Libraries
- Nature preserves
- Homeless shelters
- Soup kitchens
- Nonprofit organizations
- Sexual comfort
  - Vaginal lubricants
  - Alternative sexual practices

Providing Support:
Education and Support Measures to Consider
- Review signs and symptoms of
  - Perimenopause and postmenopause
  - Thyroid dysfunction
  - Diabetes
- Screening recommendations
  - Benefits and drawbacks to testing
  - Preparation for testing, when indicated
  - Interpretation of test results
- Discuss medical therapies for symptoms
  - Risks
  - Benefits
  - Alternatives
- Discuss alternative therapies for symptoms
  - Risks
  - Benefits
- Maintain mental acuity
  - Puzzles, word games
  - Adult education classes
  - Change daily routines
  - Seek mental challenges and new experiences
  - Avoid isolation
- Physical activity
  - Release endorphins
  - Maintain strength and flexibility
    - Yoga
    - Dance
    - Aerobic activities
- Dietary recommendations
  - Flaxseed
  - Whole grains
  - Dark leafy green vegetables
  - Citrus

- Sea vegetables
- Protein from legumes, nuts, and seeds
- Limited organic animal proteins and fats
- Teach warning signs of female reproductive cancers
  - Bleeding
  - Pain
  - Masses
  - Lesions

Follow-up Care:
Follow-up Measures to Consider
- Document finding
- Return for continued care
  - Annually
  - As indicated by test results
  - With onset of problem or symptoms

Collaborative Practice:
Criteria to Consider for Consultation or Referral
- OB/GYN service
  - For abnormal reproductive findings or test results
- Medical service
  - For continued care of medical problems
- Support services
  - Smoking cessation
  - Drug or alcohol rehabilitation
  - Stress management
  - Housing assistance
- Support groups
  - Diabetes
  - Intimate partner violence
  - Substance abuse
- For diagnosis or treatment outside the midwife's scope of practice

EVALUATION AND TREATMENT OF WOMEN WITH SYMPTOMS RELATED TO MENOPAUSE

Key Clinical Information
Common symptoms such as hot flashes, night sweats, and mood swings occur as a result of the physiologic decline in ovarian function or second-

ary to medical or surgical ablation of the ovaries. Vasomotor symptoms peak after menopause or oophorectomy and frequently affect the quality of a woman's life. At the time of physiologic menopause many women have one-third or more of their life ahead of them. Women seek relief from troublesome symptoms to enhance their quality of life and overall well-being. Symptoms may be particularly troubling for women with a history of breast cancer treated with tamoxifen. Practitioners are encouraged to invite women to actively participate in selection of their preferred treatment approach after consideration of the associated risks, benefits, and costs. Treatment choices include life-style changes, hormone-based therapies, and alternative therapies (ACOG, 2001c; North American Menopause Society, 2004; Schuiling & Likis, 2006).

Client History and Chart Review: Components of the History to Consider

- Age
- Reproductive history
  - Gravida, para
  - LMP or age at menopause
  - Current menstrual status
- Menopausal symptoms and perceived severity
  - Identify
    - Frequency
    - Severity
    - Effect of symptoms on woman's
      - Self-image
      - Emotional well-being
      - Relationships
      - Stamina and physical well-being
    - Previous treatment(s) and results
  - Vasomotor symptoms (North American Menopause Society, 2004)
    - Hot flashes or flushes
    - Night sweats
    - Seven to 8 hot flashes a day or ≥ 60 per week = severe symptoms
    - Contributing factors
      - Elevated ambient temperature
      - Cigarette smoking
      - Elevated BMI
      - Sedentary life-style
      - Low socioeconomic status
      - Alcohol or caffeine
  - Sleep disorders
    - Sleep habits
    - Insomnia
    - Wakefulness
    - Night sweats
    - Daytime sleepiness
  - Urogenital and sexual symptoms
    - Decreased libido
    - Vaginal atrophy and dryness
    - Urinary frequency or urgency
    - Dyspareunia
  - Skin changes
    - Fine wrinkles
    - Increase in facial hair
  - Mood disturbance and mental status changes
    - Mood swings
    - Depression
    - Irritability
    - Confusion
    - Memory loss (Varney et al., 2004)
- Medical/surgical history
  - Allergies
  - Medications
  - Herbs, homeopathics, and nutritional supplements
  - Health conditions, such as
    - Breast disorders
    - Gallbladder disease
    - Heart disease
    - Blood clots
    - Liver disease
    - Chronic illness
    - Depression
- Family history
  - Heart disease
  - Diabetes
  - Cancer
- Social history
  - Alcohol, tobacco, and substance use
  - Coping ability

- Intimate partner violence or abuse
- Support systems
  - Partner
  - Friends
  - Social activities
- Significant life stressors
- Physical activity patterns
- Nutritional assessment
- Review of systems (ROS)

Physical Examination:
Components of the Physical Exam
to Consider

- Vital signs, blood pressure
- Weight, height
- General physical examination with focus on
  - Mood and affect
  - Thyroid
  - Cardiopulmonary status
  - Breast examination
  - Pelvic examination
    - Observe for atrophy of tissues
      - Pale
      - Thin
      - Fragile

Clinical Impression:
Differential Diagnoses and Code Groups
to Consider
Additional suffix may apply (ICD9data.com, 2007)

- Symptoms related to physiologic menopause (ICD-9 codes 627.2)
- Symptoms related to medical or surgical menopause (ICD-9 codes 627.4)
- Medical conditions with similar symptoms, such as
  - Thyroid disorders
  - Mood disorders
  - Sleep disorders
  - Tuberculosis

Diagnostic Testing:
Diagnostic Tests and Procedures to Consider

- TSH
- Mantoux TB testing

- Follicle-stimulating hormone (FSH)/luteinizing hormone (LH)
- Other diagnostic tests as indicated

Providing Treatment:
Therapeutic Measures to Consider

- Antidepressants (North American Menopause Society, 2004)
  - Effective for
    - Hot flashes
    - Mood changes
  - Effexor (venlafaxine) 75 mg/day
  - Paxil (paroxetine) 12.5–25 mg/day
  - Prozac (fluoxetine) 20 mg/day
- Hormonal treatment (see Hormone Replacement Therapy)
  - Oral, vaginal, or transdermal
  - Contraindicated for women with breast cancer
- Other nonhormonal treatments (Schuiling & Likis, 2006)
  - May be beneficial for women in whom hormones are contraindicated and antidepressants are ineffective
  - Neurontin (anticonvulsant)
  - Clonidine (antihypertensive)
  - Megace (breast cancer treatment)
- Sleep aids, short-term therapy (Murphy, 2004)
  - Use caution with
    - Suspected clinical depression
    - Alcohol or substance use
    - Hepatic or renal disease
    - Reevaluate 2–3 weeks
  - Ambien 10 mg PO at bedtime
  - Dalmane 15–30 mg at bedtime
  - Halcion 0.125–0.25 mg at bedtime
  - Sonata 10 mg at bedtime
- Urogenital symptoms
  - Vaginal lubricants
  - Hormone therapy (see Hormone Replacement Therapy)
  - Urinary treatments (see Care of the Woman with Urinary Tract Problems, Chapter 8)

Providing Treatment:
Alternative Measures to Consider

- Bioidentical hormones
  - Hormones chemically identical to endogenous hormones
  - Custom compounding of hormone blends
  - Professional compounding pharmacies
  - Hormone creams, absorbed via skin
- Phytoestrogens
  - Reduce symptoms in some women
  - May stimulate endometrial hyperplasia
  - Contraindicated for women with breast cancer
  - Isoflavones (North American Menopause Society, 2004)
    - Soy derivatives
      - 40–80 mg daily
  - Food sources include (ACOG, 2001c)
    - Peanuts and other legumes
    - Oats, corn
    - Apples and citrus
    - Soy
- Vaginal dryness
  - Lubrication
    - Astroglide
    - Massage oil
    - Replens
  - Evening primrose oil
    - 500 mg PO two to four times daily
    - Apply vaginally
      - Capsule
      - Oil-soaked tampon
  - Slippery elm oral capsules
- Herbal treatments (Alternative Medicine Foundation, n.d.; ACOG, 2001c; North American Menopause Society, 2004)
  - Access to scientific herbal information: www.herbmed.org
  - Black cohosh herb or extract
    - Hot flashes
    - Affective changes
    - Estroven
    - Remifemin
      - 40–80 mg daily
    - Contraindicated in women with history of breast cancer

- Don quai
  - Hot flashes
  - Affective changes
  - Contraindicated in women on warfarin
  - May cause skin sensitivity to sunlight
- Ginkgo biloba
  - Mental acuity and memory
- St. John's wort
  - Affective changes
- Vitex or chasteberry (Chopin, 2003)
  - Hot flashes
  - Affective changes
  - Breast tenderness
- Red clover
- Homeopathic remedies (Smith, 1984)
  - Hot flashes
    - Belladonna
    - Lachesis
  - Vaginal dryness
    - Bryonia
    - Natrum muriaticum

Providing Support:
Education and Support Measures
to Consider

- Provide information about
  - Menopause and common symptoms
  - Treatment recommendations
  - Life-style recommendations
  - Indications to return for evaluation
  - Local resources for women
- 🌐 Suggested practices for symptom relief (North American Menopause Society, 2004)
  - Maintain cool ambient temperatures
    - Fan or air conditioner
    - Cool drinks
    - Dress in layers
  - Maintain optimal BMI
  - Reduce or eliminate cigarette smoking
  - Controlled diaphragmatic breathing at onset of hot flash
  - Active relaxation techniques, such as
    - Yoga
    - Meditation
    - Massage

- Allow time for self-care
  - ◆ Moderate daily exercise
  - ◆ Rest and relaxation
- Limit intake of
  - ◆ Caffeine
  - ◆ Saturated fats
  - ◆ Refined sugar and flour
  - ◆ Cigarettes and alcohol
  - ◆ Phosphorus-containing soft drinks

Follow-up Care:
Follow-up Measures to Consider
- Document
  - Care provided
  - Discussion of options
  - Recommendations and client choices
  - Plan for continued care
- Return for continued care
  - As needed to provide ongoing support
  - Unscheduled vaginal bleeding
  - Breast mass or changes
  - Osteoporosis prevention and evaluation
  - Ineffective coping or mood disorder
  - Worsening symptoms, such as
    - ◆ Mood disorders
    - ◆ Mental status changes
    - ◆ Vasomotor symptoms
  - For evaluation of treatment of side effects
  - For annual evaluation

Collaborative Practice:
Criteria to Consider for Consultation
or Referral
- OB/GYN service
  - Symptoms that do not respond or worsen with
    - ◆ Alternative therapy
    - ◆ Standard HRT regimens
  - Unexplained or persistent vaginal bleeding
  - Breast mass
- Medical service
  - Osteoporosis
  - Abnormal liver or renal function test results

- Symptoms of chronic medical condition, such as
  - ◆ Heart disease
  - ◆ Diabetes
- Mental health or social service
  - Depression
  - Ineffective coping
  - Psychosis
  - Support groups
- Sleep specialist
  - Persistent wakefulness
  - Severe insomnia
- For diagnosis or treatment outside the midwife's scope of practice

SCREENING, DIAGNOSIS, AND TREATMENT OF OSTEOPOROSIS

Key Clinical Information
Women, especially postmenopausal women, run a significant risk of developing osteoporosis as they age. Osteoporosis affects an estimated one in three women over age 50. Osteoporosis is defined as a disorder of bone metabolism characterized by a decrease in the level of bone mass itself, resulting in bones that are more porous (Inverness Medical, n.d.). This process leads to deterioration of the structural integrity of the remaining bone, resulting in fragile bones that are more likely to fracture with minimal trauma.

Diagnosis of osteoporosis or osteopenia (the onset of bone loss but not yet to the degree that equals osteoporosis) is made using bone mineral density (BMD) evaluation. All women with a history of a fracture after age 40 should consider BMD testing (ACOG, 2004; World Health Organization, 2003). Osteoporosis is said to be present when the BMD is more than 2.5 standard deviations below the mean. Prevention measures to maintain bone mass and sustain muscle mass to support the bone include adequate calcium and vitamin D intake, regular physical activity, fall prevention, smoking cessation, and limited or no alcohol use. Medical treatment of osteoporosis is aimed at slowing the loss of bone demineralization and rebuilding bone mass (Schuiling & Likis, 2006).

Client History and Chart Review:
Components of the History to Consider (U.S.
Department of Health and Human Services, 2004)

- Age
- Reproductive history
  - LMP, gravida, para
  - Age at menarche
  - Age at menopause
  - Length of time postmenopause
  - Use of hormonal
    - Contraceptives
    - Replacement therapy
    - Herbs or plant extracts
  - Breastfeeding history
- History of screening
  - Previous BMD or Osteomark screening
  - Oral examinations and x-rays
    - Tooth loss may indicate osteoporosis
- Medical/surgical history
  - Allergies
  - Medications
  - Herbs, homeopathics, and nutritional supplements
  - Health conditions, such as
    - Breast disorders
    - Gallbladder disease
    - Heart disease
- Risk factors for osteoporosis (Labinson et al., 2006; National Osteoporosis Foundation, 2003; Siris & Schussheim, 1998; U.S. Department of Health and Human Services, 2004)
  - Sedentary life-style or immobility
  - Poor lifetime calcium intake
  - Postmenopausal status
  - White or Asian race
  - Small or thin frame or body size
  - Personal or family history of osteoporosis
  - Adulthood fracture after minor trauma
  - Current history of cigarette smoking
  - Alcohol use ($\geq$ 7 oz./wk)
  - Advancing age
  - History of estrogen deficiency
    - Medical or surgical oophorectomy
    - Premature menopause

- Endocrine disorders leading to amenorrhea
- Amenorrhea
  - Long-term breastfeeding
  - Anorexia
  - Extended Depo-Provera use
- Breast cancer treated with
  - Chemotherapy
  - Radiation
  - Secondary causes of osteoporosis
    - High cola intake, especially during bone formation
    - Medications, such as
      - Corticosteroids $\geq$ 10 mg prednisone/day
      - Thyroxine $\geq$ 200 micrograms/day
      - Heparin $\geq$ 12,000–15,000 units/day
      - Anticonvulsants
      - Methotrexate
      - Chemotherapy
    - Medical conditions, such as
      - Cushing's disease
      - Hyperthyroidism
      - Hyperparathyroidism
      - Diabetes
      - Malignancy
      - Cerebral palsy
      - Multiple sclerosis
      - Major depression
- Assess for symptoms of osteoporosis
  - Complaints of back pain
  - Changes in posture/height
  - Fractures after perimenopausal period
  - Ability to perform activities of daily living
- Current prevention measures
  - Mineral supplementation
    - Vitamin D intake/sun exposure
    - Calcium intake
  - Weight-bearing exercise
  - Safety measures to prevent falls
- Health habits
  - Daily physical activity
  - Nutrition
  - Alcohol and tobacco use

Physical Examination:
Components of the Physical Exam to Consider
- Vital signs
- Height and weight
  - Compare to previous
  - Current BMI
- Musculoskeletal system
  - Presence of kyphosis, "dowager's hump"
  - Palpation of vertebrae for pain
  - Muscle strength
  - Posture and gait
- Evidence of increased risk for falls
  - Frailty
  - Balance and coordination
  - Eyesight
- Other examination components as indicated by history

Clinical Impression:
Differential Diagnoses and Code Groups
to Consider
Additional suffix may apply (ICD9data.com, 2007)
- Estrogen deficiency (ICD-9 codes 259.9)
- Kyphosis (ICD-9 codes 737)
- Osteopenia (ICD-9 codes 733.90)
- Osteoporosis, drug induced (ICD-9 codes 733.09)
- Osteoporosis, idiopathic (ICD-9 codes 733.02)
- Osteoporosis, postmenopausal (ICD-9 codes 733.01)

Diagnostic Testing:
Diagnostic Tests and Procedures to Consider
- Osteomark enzyme-linked immunosorbent assay (ELISA) testing (Inverness Medical, n.d.)
  - Urine or serum
  - Screens for bone collagen breakdown
  - (800-99OSTEX) or www.ostex.com
- BMD testing
  - Dual x-ray absorptiometry (DXA)
    - Low radiation dose
    - T-score
      - Bone mass in relation to young adult reference population
        - T-score − 1 = 1 standard deviation decrease in bone mass
        - 1 standard deviation = twofold risk in fracture
        - T-score − 2 = fourfold risk of fracture (ACOG, 2004; World Health Organization, 2003)

Providing Treatment:
Therapeutic Measures to Consider
(National Osteoporosis Foundation, 2003)
- Therapy is initiated for women with
  - Hip DXA T-score < −2.0 (no risk factors)
  - Hip DXA T-score < −1.5 (one or more risk factors)
  - Present or prior vertebral or hip fracture
- For women with no contraindications to hormone therapy
  - Single or combination hormone therapy (see Hormone Replacement Therapy)
  - Short-term therapy (< 5 years)
  - Weigh risks versus benefits
  - Consider nonhormonal treatments
- Nonhormonal treatment (Eli Lilly & Co., 2007; Merck & Co, Inc., 2007; Murphy, 2004; Procter & Gamble, 2006; Roche Laboratories, 2006; Schuling & Likis, 2006)
  - Bisphosphonates
    - Alendronate (Fosamax)
      - Dosing
        - Osteopenia: 5 mg PO every day, or 35 mg/wk
        - Osteoporosis: 10 mg PO every day, or 70 mg/wk
        - Fosamax plus D contains 2800 or 5600 IU vitamin D
    - Ibandronate sodium (Boniva)
      - 2.5 mg PO daily, or 150 mg PO monthly
      - Requires 60-minute upright posture and fast after administration
    - Risedronate (Actonel)
      - 5 mg PO daily, or 35 mg/wk
      - Actonel with Ca^+ for weekly dosing includes
        - Actonel 35 mg, one tablet
        - Calcium carbonate 1250 mg, 6 tablets

- May cause irritation of upper gastrointestinal mucosa
- Contraindications
  - Esophageal abnormalities that delay esophageal emptying (e.g., stricture or achalasia)
  - Inability to stand or sit upright for 30–60 minutes
  - Hypo- or hypercalcemia
  - Creatinine clearance < 30–35 ml/min
- Instructions
  - Take upon arising after 6- to 8-hour fast
  - Swallow whole with 6–8 oz. plain water
  - Remain upright and fasting for 30–60 minutes
  - Medications or dietary supplements may be taken after 60 minutes
  - Avoid simultaneous use with aspirin or NSAIDs
  - Take adequate calcium and vitamin D
  - Report
    - Gastrointestinal symptoms
    - Bone, joint, or muscle pain
- Selective estrogen receptor modulator
  - Raloxifene (Evista)
    - 60 mg PO daily
  - Contraindications
    - History of deep vein thrombosis
    - Liver disease
    - Cholestyramine use
  - Side effects
    - May cause hot flashes and blood clots
    - Lowers risk of breast cancer in high risk women
    - Less risk of endometrial cancer than estrogen
  - Instructions
    - Discontinue use at least 72 hours before surgery
- Calcitonin-salmon (Miacalcin, Calcimar, Fortical)
  - 200 units intranasally daily, or
  - 50–100 IU IM or SC every other day
  - For women > 5 years postmenopause

- Parathyroid hormone (teriparatide)
  - 20 micrograms SC daily
    - Supplied in 28-dose delivery system
  - Do not use in women with
    - Inability to perform self-injection
    - Primary or secondary malignancy of bone
    - Prior radiation therapy of bone
    - Hypercalcemia
    - Paget's disease of bone
      - May increase risk of osteosarcoma
  - Side effects
    - Orthostatic hypotension
    - Muscle spasms
    - Nausea and vomiting
  - Instructions
    - Administer per manufacturer's instructions
    - Refrigerate medication
    - Sit or recline if orthostatic hypotension develops
    - Treatment period < 2 years

Providing Treatment:
Alternative Measures to Consider
(National Osteoporosis Foundation, 2003)
- Nutritional support
  - Calcium foods (see Appendices B-4 and B-5)
  - Vitamin and mineral supplements
    - Vitamin D 400–800 IU daily
    - Calcium 1000–1500 mg daily (ACOG, 2004)
- Sunlight exposure for vitamin D synthesis
  - Hands and face
  - Minimum 10 minutes daily
- Physical activity for
  - Fall prevention
  - Weight-bearing exercise
  - Muscle strengthening
  - Improve or maintain balance
  - Options, such as
    - Yoga, dance
    - Strength training
    - Swimming, tennis
    - Housework, gardening
    - Balance or rocker board

Providing Support:
Education and Support Measures to Consider

- Provide information regarding
  - Calcium sources and intake (see Appendices B-4 and B-5)
  - Physical activity
  - Medication use
    - ◆ Side effects
    - ◆ Benefits
    - ◆ Risks (Ferris et al., 1998)
- Recognition of limitations
  - Ask for and accept help
  - Use mechanical devices as needed, such as
    - ◆ Cane or walker for balance
    - ◆ Reaching tools
    - ◆ Shower chair
- Identify modifiable risks
  - Life-style factors
  - Fall risks, such as
    - ◆ Throw rugs
    - ◆ Uneven or slippery surfaces
    - ◆ Lack of grab bars
    - ◆ Balance issues
- Formulate prevention plan
  - Risk reduction actions
  - Access to help in case of fall
  - Screening or treatment
  - Follow-up plan
- Community preventive health programs
  - Smoking cessation
  - Alcoholics Anonymous
  - Exercise programs and opportunities
- Avoid or limit use of
  - Tobacco
  - Alcohol
  - Caffeine
  - Phosphorus-containing soft drinks (i.e., colas)

Follow-up Care:
Follow-up Measures to Consider

- Document
  - Care provided
  - Screening results
  - Recommendations

- Reevaluate for modifiable factors
  - Medication use
  - Smoking
  - Alcohol use
  - Physical activity patterns
- Review risk status during well-woman examination
- BMD testing at 1- to 2-year intervals

Collaborative Practice:
Criteria to Consider for Consultation or Referral

- OB/GYN, medical, orthopedic or endocrine service
  - Treatment for osteoporosis
- Physical therapy
  - Assess for risk of falls
    - ◆ Strengthening program
    - ◆ Improve balance
  - Ability to maintain activities of daily living
- Social service
  - Smoking cessation
  - Alcohol treatment program
- Nutritionist
  - Evaluation of diet
- For diagnosis or treatment outside the midwife's scope of practice

EVALUATION OF POSTMENOPAUSAL BLEEDING

Key Clinical Information

Peri- and postmenopausal bleeding (PMB) require a thorough directed history and evaluation of the genital tract for cervical, vaginal, and/or endometrial lesions. Causes of PMB include hormone use, polyps, fibroids, trauma, and malignant or premalignant genital tract lesions (Albers & Hull, 2004). Hormone imbalance is a common cause of PMB, as is the presence of uterine fibroids or polyps (Miller, 2005). Use of natural estrogen-containing products for the treatment of menopausal symptoms can result in PMB. Women should be advised to report any unexpected or unusual bleeding. Cyclic use of a progestin diminishes the growth of the endometrium in women with intact uteri using estrogen or an estrogen-like product (Albers & Hull, 2004). Use of combination HRT, when indicated, decreases risk of endometrial cancer when compared with both nonhormone users and those women with a uterus who take only estrogen. Endometrial cancer is present in approximately 10% of women with PMB and typically goes undetected until abnormal bleeding occurs (Miller, 2005). When found early, cancer of the endometrium is highly treatable.

Client History and Chart Review:
Components of the History to Consider

- Age
- Obstetric/gynecologic history
  - Gravida, para
  - LMP or age at menopause
  - Presenting symptoms
    - Onset, duration, and severity of bleeding
    - Bleeding intervals
      - Random
      - Cyclic
      - Postcoital
    - Amount, consistency, and color of bleeding
    - Other accompanying symptoms
      - Pain and cramping
      - Diarrhea
      - Backache
      - Respiratory symptoms
- Medical history
  - Diabetes
  - Clotting dysfunction
    - Coagulopathy
    - Liver disorder
  - Endocrine disorders
    - Thyroid
    - Polycystic ovary syndrome (PCOS)
  - Heart disease
- Medication and supplement use
  - Tamoxifen therapy
  - Estrogen replacement therapy
  - Hormone replacement therapy

- Aspirin or anticoagulant use
- Estrogen precursors
- Contributing factors to PMB (American Cancer Society, 2007; Albers & Hull, 2004)
  - Early menarche
  - Late menopause
  - Nulliparous
  - Infertility
  - Polycystic ovary syndrome
  - Estrogen-producing tumors
  - Dietary estrogen precursors
  - Diabetes
  - Thyroid disorders
  - Previous or current breast cancer
  - Family history
    - Northern European
    - North American
- Review of systems (ROS)
  - Jaundice
  - Easy bruising
  - Abdominal enlargement
  - Persistent cough

Physical Examination:
Components of the Physical Exam to Consider

- Vital signs, including blood pressure, BMI
- Speculum examination
  - Blood in vaginal vault
  - Appearance of cervix
  - Presence of lesions or masses
- Bimanual examination
  - Uterine size and contour
  - Cervical contour
  - Adnexal masses
  - Presence of pain
  - Firmness and mobility of reproductive organs
- Inguinal lymph nodes
- Rectal examination
  - Confirm pelvic examination
  - Evaluate posterior pelvis
  - Masses
  - Mobility of tissues

Clinical Impression:
Differential Diagnoses and Code Groups
to Consider
Additional suffix may apply (ICD9data.com, 2007)

- Perimenopausal vaginal bleeding (ICD-9 codes 627.0)
- Postmenopausal vaginal bleeding (ICD-9 codes 627.1)
- Endometrial hyperplasia (ICD-9 codes 621.3)
- Endometrial hyperplasia, with atypia (ICD-9 codes 621.33)
- Uterine fibroid, location unspecified (ICD-9 codes 218.9)
- Uterine polyp (ICD-9 codes 621.0)

Diagnostic Testing:
Diagnostic Tests and Procedures to Consider
(Albers & Hull, 2004; Miller, 2005)

- Complete blood count
- Clotting studies
- Pap smear
- Pelvic ultrasound
    - Routes
        - Transvaginal
        - Transuterine (sonohysterography)
        - Abdominal
    - Evaluation of endometrial stripe
        - A visible stripe less than 5 mm is considered within normal limits
- Histology
    - Endometrial biopsy
    - Endometrial curettage (D&C)
    - Sonohysterography with biopsy
    - Hysteroscopy with biopsy

Providing Treatment:
Therapeutic Measures to Consider

- Consult or refer for treatment
- Malignancy
- Surgical treatment of endometrial cancer (ACS, 2006)
    - Hysterectomy
    - Oophorectomy
    - Pelvic lymph nodes for staging

- Additional surgery may be required
- Radiation therapy
- Chemotherapy

Providing Treatment:
Alternative Measures to Consider

⚠ Alternative therapies should not delay evaluation and treatment.

- Nutritional support for healing
    - Healthy balanced low-fat diet
        - Maintain healthy BMI
        - Increase dietary intake of
            - Whole grains
            - Legumes, including soy
            - Vitamins C and E
            - Antioxidant foods, such as
                - Blueberries
                - Green tea
            - Omega-3 fatty acids
            - Live culture yogurt
        - Avoid hormone-containing
            - Meats and poultry
            - Dairy products
    - Herbal support (Sallamander Concepts, 1998–2007)
        - Alfalfa
        - Astragalus root
        - Chamomile
        - Garlic
- Herbs to avoid 7–14 days before surgery (Murphy, 1999; Sallamander Concepts, 1998–2007)
    - May decrease clotting ability
        - Astragalus
        - Feverfew
        - Garlic
        - Ginseng
        - Ginkgo
- Acupuncture
- Emotional immune support
    - Laughter
    - Visualization
    - Meditation
    - Prayer

Providing Support:
Education and Support Measures to Consider
- Discussion regarding
  - Potential significance of symptoms
  - Need for diagnostic workup
  - Results of
    - Physical examination
    - Diagnostic testing
  - Referral and ongoing care
  - Options for support services
- Active listening
  - Client fears and concerns
  - Questions
  - Preferences for care

Follow-up Care:
Follow-up Measures to Consider
- Document
  - Clinical findings
  - Discussions and teaching
  - Client preferences
  - Plan for ongoing care
  - Referrals
- Offer continued support, as appropriate
- Assess for
  - Depression
  - Altered self-image
  - Barriers to healing
- Encourage
  - Positive attitude
  - Use of healing modalities
- Return visits based on
  - Diagnosis and treatment needs
  - Client need for support
  - Scope of practice

Collaborative Practice:
Criteria to Consider for Consultation or Referral
- OB/GYN service
  - Evaluation of postmenopausal bleeding
  - Diagnosis of
    - Endometrial atypia
    - Endometrial hyperplasia
    - Endometrial cancer

- Support services, such as
  - Social services
  - Nutritionist
  - Support groups
- For diagnosis or treatment outside the midwife's scope of practice

HORMONE REPLACEMENT THERAPY
Key Clinical Information

Hormone replacement therapy (HRT) offers significant benefits to a carefully selected group of women. For other women HRT poses considerable risk. Women who use long-term HRT have an increased risk of heart disease and breast cancer over women who decline HRT. For women with severe symptoms who are planning short-term HRT use (< 5 years) the risk is considered low in the absence of significant risk factors for breast cancer or heart disease.

For women with severe effects of hormone depletion shortly after menopause or during the perimenopausal period, HRT provides highly effective symptom relief. Estrogen therapy is not recommended for women with an intact uterus because of the substantially elevated risk of endometrial cancer when compared with women who use combination HRT or women who decline HRT. Breast cancer incidence is reduced in women who use estrogen therapy for less than 7 years; however, these women have a higher incidence of abnormal mammogram results and undergo more breast biopsies than women who decline estrogen therapy (National Institutes of Health, 2007a). For women with an intact uterus using estrogen or estrogen-like substances it is recommended that the estrogenic effects be balanced with progestin (combination therapy).

Discussion of the risks, benefits, and alternatives to HRT, as well as each woman's personal indications and preferences, is an integral part of providing hormone therapy. Providing women with the most current information allows each woman the opportunity to make the best personal decision while being an active participant in the process. Other treatment modalities exist for the treatment of vasomotor symptoms, osteoporosis, and the physiologic changes associated with post-menopausal status.

Client History and Chart Review: Components of the History to Consider

- Age
- Reproductive history
  - Menstrual history
    - Current menstrual status
    - Age at menopause, or
    - Hysterectomy
  - 🔘 Presence of vasomotor symptoms
    - Hot flashes
    - Night sweats
  - 🔘 Symptoms related to estrogen decline
    - Sleep changes
    - Mood changes
    - Urinary changes
    - Skin changes
      - Development of fine lines
      - Increase in facial hair
      - Vaginal atrophy and dryness
    - Sexual changes
      - Diminished libido
      - Decreased lubrication
      - Dyspareunia
  - Reproductive cancers and disorders (e.g., leiomyomata)
- Review most recent
  - Physical examination
  - Pap smear
  - Mammogram
  - BMD testing
- Medical/surgical history
  - Allergies
  - Medications
  - Heart disease
    - Coronary artery disease
    - Hypertension
    - Prior thromboembolus or thrombosis
  - Risk factors for osteoporosis (see Screening, Diagnosis, and Treatment of Osteoporosis)
  - Mood disorder
- Gallbladder disease
- Liver disease
- Family history
  - Osteoporosis
  - Heart disease
  - Alzheimer's disease
  - Colon cancer
  - Breast cancer
- Social history
  - Tobacco and alcohol use
  - Physical activity patterns
  - Nutritional status
  - Intimate partner violence or abuse
- Contraindications for HRT
  - History of estrogen-sensitive tumors
  - Breast cancer
  - Endometrial hyperplasia
  - Endometrial cancer
  - Undiagnosed PMB
  - Impaired liver function
  - History of thromboembolus or thrombosis
  - Heart disease
- Review of systems (ROS)

Physical Examination: Components of the Physical Exam to Consider

- Vital signs, blood pressure
- Height, weight
  - BMI
  - Height, compare with previous
- Thyroid
- Breast examination
  - Presence of masses
  - Documentation of contour
- Cardiopulmonary evaluation
- Pelvic examination
  - Genital atrophy, pallor
  - Uterine size, and contour
  - Presence of masses
- Bony integrity
  - Range of motion
  - Arthritis
  - Kyphosis
- Rectal examination

Clinical Impression:
Differential Diagnoses and Code Groups
to Consider
Additional suffix may apply (ICD9data.com, 2007)

- HRT (ICD-9 codes V07.4)

Diagnostic Testing:
Diagnostic Tests and Procedures
to Consider

- Serum or salivary hormone levels
- Pap smear
- Blood lipid evaluation
- Electrocardiogram
- BMD testing
- Mammogram
- Pelvic ultrasound
- Postmenopausal women
  - Before initiation of HRT consider
    - Endometrial biopsy
    - Progestin challenge
      - Provera 5–10 mg daily for 10 days
      - Anticipate withdrawal bleed within 10 days of completion of medication
      - If little or no bleed consider continuous HRT
      - If vigorous bleed consider cyclic HRT

Providing Treatment:
Therapeutic Measures to Consider

- Indications for HRT
  - Severe vasomotor symptoms
  - Osteoporosis (consider nonhormonal therapies first)
  - ASC-US Pap smear (local therapy preferred)
  - Mood disturbance related to hormone changes (consider other medications first)
- Perimenopausal woman with moderate to severe vasomotor symptoms
  - Low-dose triphasic oral contraceptives
  - Combination hormonal contraceptives
    - ⚠ Do not use in smokers 35 years or older

- Progestogen
  - Depo-medroxyprogesterone acetate (DMPA)
    - 150 mg IM monthly
    - Oral 20 mg/day
  - Transdermal estrogen
- Abnormal Pap smear (ASC-US)
  - Estrogen vaginal cream
- Transdermal estrogen
  - Estraderm 0.5 or 1.0 mg
  - Progestin not required with regular monthly menses
  - Add progestin when menses irregular
    - Provera 5–10 mg for 5–10 days
    - Prometrium 200 mg at bedtime for 12 days (Murphy, 2005)
- Postmenopausal woman
  - Continuous HRT
  - Use for as brief a period as possible
  - Combination therapy
- CombiPatch (estradiol/norethindrone acetate transdermal system)
  - Apply patch at twice weekly interval
  - For more info: (877) 266-2448 or www.combipatch.com
- Prempro (oral conjugated estrogens/progestin)
  - Use lowest effective dose
  - 0.3 mg/1.5 mg once PO daily
  - 0.45 mg/1.5 mg once PO daily
  - 0.625 mg/2.5 mg once PO daily
  - 0.625/5 once PO daily
- Estrogen: daily
  - Conjugated estrogen 0.3–0.625 mg
  - Estropipate 0.625 mg
  - Esterified estrogen 0.3–0.625 mg
  - Micronized estradiol 0.5–1 mg
  - Transdermal estrogen 0.05 mg
- Progestin: daily
  - Provera 2.5 mg
- Cyclic HRT
  - Estrogen: days 1–25 of month
  - Dose range 0.3–1.25 mg daily, varies with brand and indication

- 0.625 mg is lowest dose recommended to treat osteoporosis
- 🌐 Plant-based estrogens
  - Estrace
  - Cenestin
  - Gynodiol
  - Estratab
  - Ogen
- Progestin use with cyclic estrogen
  - Provera 5–10 mg for 5–10 days
  - Prometrium 200 mg at bedtime for 12 days
  - Use progestin days 11–25 to 16–25 of cycle month
- Estrogen–androgen therapy (Bachmann, 1993; Simon et al., 1999)
  - For decreased libido
  - Given cyclically (e.g., 3–4 weeks on, 1 week off)
  - Short-term therapy
  - Virilization may occur
  - Must use progestin in client with intact uterus
  - Products available
    - Esterified estrogen 0.625 mg/ methyltestosterone 1.25 mg
    - Esterified estrogen 1.25 mg/ methyltestosterone 2.5 mg
    - Conjugated estrogen 0.625 mg/ methyltestosterone 5 mg
    - Conjugated estrogen 1.25 mg/ methyltestosterone 10 mg

Providing Treatment:
Alternative Measures to Consider
- Use of bioidentical hormones
- See indication for HRT, such as
  - Vasomotor symptoms
  - Osteoporosis
- Vitamin and mineral supplements
  - Calcium and magnesium supplementation
  - Vitamin E supplements 400 IU BID with meals

Providing Support:
Education and Support Measures to Consider
- Provide information for informed choice
- HRT recommendations
  - Perimenopause to early postmenopause
  - Short-term use
  - Indications for HRT
    - Osteoporosis
    - Significant vasomotor symptoms
- Limitations and risks of HRT (National Institutes of Health, 2007b)
  - Increased risk of
    - Stroke
    - Breast cancer
    - Coronary artery disease
    - Thromboemboli
    - Risks, benefits, and alternatives to HRT
- Methods of HRT, dose, timing, side effects
- Osteoporosis prevention and evaluation
- Provide medications instructions
  - Dose
  - Timing and method of use
  - Anticipated results
  - Warning signs and symptoms
- Reinforce need to return for evaluation for
  - Unscheduled vaginal bleeding
  - Symptoms of complications related to HRT
- Dietary recommendations
  - Limit caffeine, fat, white sugar, flour, and alcohol
  - Whole grains, dark leafy green vegetables, sea vegetables
  - Protein from legumes, nuts, and seeds
- 🌐 Recommended life-style changes
  - Smoking cessation
  - Regular exercise, rest, and relaxation
  - Support acceptance of life changes

Follow-up Care:
Follow-up Measures to Consider
- Document
  - Indication for HRT
  - Discussions with client
  - Treatment plan

- Return for evaluation
  - Three months after initiating HRT and/or estrogen replacement therapy
    - Weight, blood pressure
    - Reduction in symptoms
    - Bleeding patterns
    - Satisfaction with treatment
    - Concerns or unexpected side effects
- Annually for well-woman examination
- Unanticipated or unscheduled vaginal bleeding
- Breast changes

Collaborative Practice:
Criteria to Consider for Consultation or Referral

- OB/GYN service
  - Symptoms that do not respond to standard HRT regimens
  - Unexplained or persistent vaginal bleeding
  - Gynecologic complications of HRT
- Medical service
  - Diagnosis of osteoporosis (see Screening, Diagnosis, and Treatment of Osteoporosis)
  - Signs or symptoms of heart disease
  - Medical complications of HRT
- Breast specialist
  - Breast mass or abnormal mammogram
- For diagnosis or treatment outside the midwife's scope of practice

REFERENCES

Adams Hilliard, P. J. (2007). *Injectable contraceptives* (online slide presentation). Houston, TX: Baylor College. Retrieved July 16, 2007 from http://www.contraceptiononline.org/slides/talk_cme_activity.cfm?tk=34&&cmepage=presentations

Albers, J. R., & Hull, S. K. (2004). Abnormal uterine bleeding. *American Family Physician, 69,* 1915–1926. Retrieved January 27, 2008 from http://www.aafp.org/afp/20040415/1915.html

Alternative Medicine Foundation, Inc. (n.d.). *HerbMed database.* Retrieved January 27, 2008 from http://www.herbmed.org

American Cancer Society. (2007). Detailed Guide: Endometrial cancer. Retrieved January 27, 2008 from http://www.cancer.org/docroot/CRI/CRI_2_3x.asp?rnav=cridg&dt=11

American College of Nurse-Midwives (ACNM). (1997). *ACNM position statement: Reproductive choices.* Silver Spring, MD: Author. Retrieved January 27, 2008 from http://www.midwife.org/siteFiles/position/Reproductive_Choices_05.pdf

American College of Nurse-Midwives (ACNM). (2000). *Medical abortion: a tip sheet for ACNM state legislative contacts.* Number 36, March 2000. Silver Spring, MD: Author. Retrieved January 27, 2008 from http://www.midwife.org/display.cfm?id=533

American College of Nurse-Midwives (ACNM). (2006). *QuickInfo: midwives and abortion services.* Silver Spring, MD: Author. Retrieved January 27, 2008 from http://www.midwife.org/siteFiles/education/Abortion_Services_12.06.pdf

American College of Obstetricians and Gynecologists (ACOG). (1995). Health maintenance for perimenopausal women. In *2002 compendium of selected publications* (technical bulletin no. 210). Washington, DC: Author.

American College of Obstetricians and Gynecologists (ACOG). (2000). Use of hormonal contraception in women with co-existing medical conditions. In *2005 compendium of selected publications* (practice bulletin no. 18). Washington, DC: Author.

American College of Obstetricians and Gynecologists (ACOG). (2001a). Antibiotic prophylaxis for gyn procedures. In *2005 compendium of selected publications* (practice bulletin no. 23). Washington, DC: Author.

American College of Obstetricians and Gynecologists (ACOG). (2001b). Emergency oral contraception. In *2005 compendium of selected publications* (practice bulletin no. 25). Washington, DC: Author.

American College of Obstetricians and Gynecologists (ACOG). (2001c). Use of botanicals for management of menopausal symptoms. In *2005 compendium of selected publications.* Washington, DC: Author.

American College of Obstetricians and Gynecologists (ACOG). (2004). Osteoporosis. In *2005 compendium of selected publications* (practice bulletin no. 50). Washington, DC: Author.

American College of Obstetricians and Gynecologists (ACOG). (2005). Intrauterine device. In *2006 compendium of selected publications* (practice bulletin no. 59). Washington, DC: Author.

American College of Obstetricians and Gynecologists (ACOG). (2006). Primary and preventive care: periodic assessments (committee opinion no. 357). *Obstetrics & Gynecology, 108,* 1615.

American College of Physicians. (2005). Medicare ushers in new smoking cessation coverage. *ACP Observer,* May

2005. Retrieved January 27, 2008 from http://www.acponline.org/journals/news/may05/smoking.htm

Anderson, B. A. (2005). *Reproductive health: women's and men's shared responsibility*. Sudbury, MA: Jones and Bartlett.

Bachmann, G. A. (1993). Estrogen-androgen therapy for sexual and emotional well-being. *The Female Patient*, 18, 15–24.

Bayer HealthCare Pharmaceuticals (2007). Mirena package insert. Wayne, NJ: Author. Retrieved January 27, 2008 from http://berlex.bayerhealthcare.com/html/products/pi/Mirena_PI.pdf

Brender, E. (2006). Smoking cessation. *Journal of the American Medical Association*, 296, 130. Retrieved January 27, 2008 from http://jama.ama-assn.org/cgi/content/full/296/1/130

Centers for Disease Control and Prevention. (2007). Recommended adult immunization schedule—United States, October 2007–September 2008. *Morbidity and Mortality Weekly Report*, 56, Q1–Q4. Retrieved January 22, 2008 from http://www.cdc.gov/vaccines/recs/schedules/downloads/adult/06-07/adult-schedule.pdf

Centers for Disease Control and Prevention (CDC). (2006). *Women and tobacco fact sheet*. Retrieved January 27, 2008 from http://www.cdc.gov/tobacco/data_statistics/Factsheets/women_tobacco.htm

Chopin, L. B. (2003). Vitex agnus castus essential oil and menopausal balance: a research update. *Complementary Therapies in Nursing and Midwifery*, 8, 148–154.

deCosta, C. L., Younes, R. N., & Lorneco, M. T. (2002). Stopping smoking: a randomized double-blind study comparing nortriptyline to placebo. *Chest*, 122, 403–408.

Deresiewicz, R. (n.d.). *Toxic shock syndrome: a health professional's guide*. Retrieved January 27, 2008 from http://www.toxicshock.com/

Duramed Pharmaceuticals. (2006a). *Plan B® prescribing information*. Retrieved January 27, 2008 from http://www.go2planb.com/PDF/PlanBPI.pdf

Duramed Pharmaceuticals. (2006b). *ParaGard® T380A intrauterine copper contraceptive prescribing information*. Pomona, NY: Barr Pharmaceuticals. Retrieved January 27, 2008 from http://www.paragard.com/hcp/custom_images/ParaGard_HCP_PI.pdf

Eli Lilly & Co. (2007). *Forteo prescribing information*. Indianapolis, IN: Author.

Ellertson, C., Evans, M., Ferden, S., Leadbetter, C., Spears, A., Johnstone, K., et al (2003). Extending the time limit for starting Yuzpe regimen of emergency contraception to 120 hours. *Obstetrics and Gynecology*, 101, 1168–1171.

Emma Goldman Clinic. (2007). *Post-abortion care*. Iowa City, IA: Author. Retrieved January 27, 2008 from http://www.emmagoldman.com/services/abortion/care.htm

Ferris, D., Brotzman, G., & Mayeaux, E. J. (1998). Improving compliance with estrogen therapy for osteoporosis. *The Female Patient*, 23(4), 29–45.

Gardner, J. (1986). *A difficult decision: a compassionate book about abortion*. Berkeley, CA: Crossing Press.

Hall, S. M., Humfleet, G. L., Rhus, V. I., Munoz, R. F., Hartz, D. T., & Maude-Griffin, R. (2002). Psychological intervention and antidepressant treatment in smoking cessation. *Archives General Psychiatry*, 59, 930–936.

Hatcher, R. A., Trussell, J., Stewart, F., Nelson, A. L., Cates, W., et al. (2004). *Contraceptive technology*. New York: Ardent Media.

Health Canada. (2000). *Family-centred maternity and newborn care: national guidelines*. Ottawa: Minister of Public Works and Government Services. Retrieved January 27, 2008 from http://www.phac-aspc.gc.ca/dca-dea/publications/pdf/fcmc00_e.pdf

Heath, C., & Acevedo, R. (2000–2007). Preconception screening and counseling. *The Female Patient*. Retrieved January 27, 2008 from http://www.femalepatient.com/html/arc/sig/screening/articles/029_10_052.asp

Heatherton, T. F., Kozlowski, L. T., Frecker, R. C., & Fagerstrom, K. O. (1991). The Fagerstrom test for nicotine dependence: a revision of the Fagerstrom tolerance questionnaire. *British Journal of Addiction*, 86, 1119–1127.

Inverness Medical. (n.d.). *Osteomark NTx*. Princeton, NJ: Author. Retrieved January 27, 2008 from http://www.ostex.com

Johnson, J. (2004). *Diaphragms, caps and shields*. Planned Parenthood. Retrieved January 27, 2008 from http://www.plannedparenthood.org/birth-control-pregnancy/birth-control/diaphragms-caps-andshields.htm

Kass-Annese, B., & Danzer, H. (2003). *Natural birth control made simple*. Alameda, CA: Hunter House.

Labinson, P., Taxel, P., Gagel, R. F., & Hoff, A. O. (2006). Implications of breast and prostate cancer on bone health. In *Osteoporosis clinical updates*. Washington, DC: National Osteoporosis Foundation. Retrieved January 27, 2008 from http://www.nof.org/cmeexam/Issue10ImplicationsBreastProstate/BreastProstateCancerIssue-forweb.pdf

March of Dimes. (n.d.). Preconception screening and counseling checklist. Author. Retrieved January 27, 2008 from: http://www.marchofdimes.com/professionals/19583_4182.asp

Mackenzie, S. J., & Yeo, S. (1997). Pregnancy interruption using mifepristone (RU-487): a new choice for women in the USA. *Journal of Nurse-Midwifery*, 42, 86–98.

Merck & Co., Inc. (2007). *Fosamax D prescribing information*. Whitehouse Station, NJ: Author.

Miller, J. C. (2005). *Ultrasound in the evaluation of abnormal vaginal bleeding*. Radiology Rounds. Massachusetts General Hospital. Retrieved January 27, 2008 from http://www.mghradrounds.org/index.php?src=gendocs&link=2005_april

Murphy, J. L. (Ed.). (2004). *Nurse practitioner's prescribing reference*. New York: Prescribing Reference.

National Cancer Institute. (2004). *Cigarette smoking and cancer: questions and answers*. Retrieved January 27, 2008 from http://www.cancer.gov/cancertopics/factsheet/Tobacco/cancer

National Osteoporosis Foundation. (2003). *Physicians guide to the prevention and treatment of osteoporosis*. Washington, DC: Author. Retrieved September 16, 2007 from http://www.nof.org/professionals/index.htm

North American Menopause Society. (2004). Position statement: Treatment of menopause-associated vasomotor symptoms. *Menopause* 11, 11–33.

Office of Population Research & Association of Reproductive Health Professionals. (2006). *Types of emergency contraception*. Retrieved January 27, 2008 from http://ec.princeton.edu/questions/dose.html#dose

Office on Women's Health. (n.d.). *Preventive screening tests and immunizations: screening tests and immunizations guidelines for women*. U.S. Department of Health and Human Services. Retrieved January 27, 2008 from http://www.womenshealth.gov/screeningcharts/general/

Organon. (2005). *NuvaRing provider insert*. Roseland, NJ: Author. Retrieved January 27, 2008 from http://www.nuvaring.com/Authfiles/Images/309_76063.pdf

Organon. (2006). *Implanon provider insert*. Roseland, NJ: Author. Retrieved January 27, 2008 from http://www.implanon-usa.com/HCP/prescribingImplanon/index.asp

Ortho-McNeil Pharmaceutical. (2007). *Ortho Evra: updated label*. Retrieved January 27, 2008 from http://www.orthoevra.com/

Pfizer Labs. (2007). *Chantix product information*. Retrieved January 27, 2008 from http://www.pfizer.com/files/products/uspi_chantix.pdf

Pharmacia. (2004). *Depo-Provera contraceptive injection prescribing information*. New York: Pfizer Inc. Retrieved January 27, 2008 from http://www.pfizer.com/pfizer/download/uspi_depo_provera_contraceptive.pdf

Pharmacia. (2005). *Physician information: Depo sub-Q Provera 104*. New York: Pfizer Inc. Retrieved January 27, 2008 from http://www.pfizer.com/pfizer/download/uspi_depo_provera_contraceptive.pdf

Procter & Gamble. (2006). *Actonel prescribing information*. Cincinnati, OH: Author.

Roche Laboratories. (2006). *Prescribing information for Boniva tablets*. Nutley, NJ: Author.

Sallamander Concepts. (1998–2007). *Herbal encyclopedia*. Retrieved January 27, 2008 from http://www.ageless.co.za/herbal-encyclopedia.htm

Scherger, J. E. (1993). Preconception care: a neglected element of prenatal services. *The Female Patient*, 18, 78–83.

Schuiling, K., & Likis, F. (2006). *Women's gynecologic health*. Sudbury, MA: Jones and Bartlett.

Simon, J., Klaiber, E., Wiita, B., Bowen, A., & Yang, H. M. (1999). Differential effects of estrogen-androgen and estrogen-only therapy on vasomotor symptoms, gonadotropin secretion, and endogenous androgen bioavailability in postmenopausal women. *Menopause*, 6, 138–146.

Singer, K. (2004). *The garden of fertility*. New York: Avery.

Siris, E. S., & Schussheim, D. H. (1998). Osteoporosis: assessing your patient's risk. *Women's Health in Primary Care*, 1, 99–106.

Smith, T. (1984). *A woman's guide to homeopathic medicine*. New York: Thorsons.

Soule, D. (1996). *The roots of healing*. Secaucus, NJ: Citadel Press.

Trapani, F. J. (1984). *Contraception naturally*. Coopersburg, PA: CJ Frompovich.

Truitt, S. T., Fraser, A., Gallo, M. F., Lopez, L. M., Grimes, D. A., & Schulz, K. F. (2003). Combined hormonal versus nonhormonal versus progestin-only contraception in lactation. *Cochrane Database of Systematic Reviews*, Issue 2, Art. No. CD003988.

Trussell, J., & Raymond, E. (2006). *Emergency contraception: a cost-effective approach to preventing unintended pregnancy*. Princeton NJ: Office of Population Research. Retrieved January 27, 2008 from http://ec.princeton.edu/questions/ec-review.pdf

U.S. Department of Health and Human Services. (2004). *Bone health and osteoporosis: a report of the Surgeon General*. Rockville, MD: U.S. Department of Health and Human Services, Office of the Surgeon General.

U.S. Food and Drug Administration (FDA). (2005). *Mifeprex (mifepristone)*. Retrieved January 27, 2008 from http://www.fda.gov/cder/drug/infopage/mifepristone/default.htm

U.S. Food and Drug Administration (FDA). (2006). *FDA public health advisory: sepsis and medical abortion update.* March 17, 2006. Retrieved January 27, 2008 from http://www.fda.gov/cder/drug/advisory/mifeprex200603.htm

U.S. Preventive Services Task Force. (2006). *The guide to clinical preventive services 2006: recommendations of the U.S. Preventive Services Task Force.* Washington, DC: U.S. Department of Health and Human Services, Agency for Healthcare Research and Quality.

Varney, H., Kriebs, J. M., & Gegor, C. L. (2004). *Varney's midwifery* (4th ed.). Sudbury, MA: Jones and Bartlett.

Weinstein, M. (1994). *Your fertility signals.* St. Louis, MO: Smooth Stone Press.

Witt, M. (2006). If IUD insertion fails and payer balks try the manufacturer. *Journal of Family Practice.* Retrieved January 27, 2008 from http://www.jfponline.com/Pages.asp?AID=4031

World Health Organization. (2003). *Prevention and management of osteoporosis* (WHO technical report no. 921). Geneva: Author.

Wyeth (2008). *Lybrel: Inhibition of Menses.* Retrieved on January 27, 2008 from http://www.wyeth.com/hcp/lybrel/efficacy/inhibitionofmenses

Zeus, S. (2007). *Taking care after abortion, miscarriage or herbally induced abortion.* Retrieved January 27, 2008 from http://www.sisterzeus.com/post_ca.htm

BIBLIOGRAPHY

Advocates for Youth. (n.d.). *Intrauterine device.* Retrieved January 27, 2008 from http://www.advocatesforyouth.org/youth/health/contraceptives/iud.htm

Barger, M. K. (Ed.). (1988). *Protocols for gynecologic and obstetric health care.* Philadelphia: W. B. Saunders.

Foster, S. (1996). *Herbs for your health.* Loveland, CO: Interweave Press.

Frye, A. (1998). *Holistic midwifery.* Portland, OR: Labrys Press.

Office on Women's Health. (n.d.). Program for Appropriate Technology in Health. (1997). *Emergency contraception: a resource manual for providers.* Seattle, WA: Author.

Ringel, M. (1998). HRT: is it for you? *The Female Patient,* 11(Suppl.), 13–17.

Starr, D. S. (2000). The legal advisor: missing a smoking gun. *The Clinical Advisor,* March 25, pp. 105–106.

Sweet, B. R. (Ed.). (1999). *Mayes' midwifery* (12th ed.). London: Bailliere Tindall.

U.S. Preventive Services Task Force. *Recommendations.* Retrieved January 27, 2008 from http://www.ahrq.gov/clinic/uspstfix.htm#Recommendations

Walls, D. (2007). *Natural families—healthy homes.* LaVergne, TN: Ingram.

Weed, S. (1985). *Wise woman herbal for the childbearing year.* Woodstock, NY: Ashtree.

7

Care of the Woman with Reproductive Health Problems

When faced with reproductive health problems, women who use midwifery services beyond childbearing look to midwives for continued care and appropriate referrals.

Many women routinely rely on midwives for reproductive health care unrelated to pregnancy. Professional midwifery practice often includes providing care to women with reproductive health problems and variations from normal. The scope of care provided to women with reproductive health issues is based not only on the midwife's education and training but also on additional factors such as the location and type of practice, clinical site expectations, and the needs of the population of women served.

The expert midwife develops the ability to differentiate those conditions or findings that represent the wide spectrum of "normal" from those that are subtle presentations of abnormal conditions. Skill as a diagnostician is vital to midwifery practice and is an integral component of providing comprehensive care to women.

A problem-oriented directed history is essential to accurate diagnosis and validation of the woman's concerns. Physical examination centers on pertinent body systems and the organs that influence them. The resulting clinical impression, or list of potential differential diagnoses, guides the midwife's decisions regarding appropriate diagnostic studies and when consultation or referral is indicated. The optimal midwifery plan of care clearly delineates anticipatory thinking and addresses planned follow-up both with and without resolution of symptoms.

Maintaining competency in women's reproductive health care requires ongoing professional education to keep up with changes in diagnostic techniques and terminology and with current treatment methods. There is a wide range of resources available to develop, maintain, and improve competence in the diagnosis and treatment of commonly encountered women's health problems.

ABNORMAL MAMMOGRAM INTERPRETATION AND TRIAGE

Key Clinical Information

Abnormalities found on mammography represent breast lesions that may be benign or malignant. An abnormal mammogram indicates the need for further evaluation to determine whether treatment is indicated. Most women with abnormal results are understandably anxious and may not accurately take in information presented by the clinician. Many practitioners prefer to give abnormal results in person, offering women an opportunity to ask questions and take written information home to discuss with loved ones.

Mammography frequently identifies women with premalignant lesions or early signs of breast cancer before a palpable mass is present. Prompt evaluation and treatment of women with early breast malignancy provides the best chance for long-term survival. Women with negative axillary lymph nodes at time of breast biopsy have a 70% chance for 5-year survival without recurrence (Simpson et al., 2000). Many communities now have breast centers where women with breast abnormalities can obtain specialty care.

Client History and Chart Review:
Components of the History to Consider
(Aliotta & Schaeffer, 2006)
- OB/GYN history
  - Current menstrual status
  - Pregnancy history
    - Gravida, para status
    - Age at first birth
    - Breastfeeding history
      - Number of children breastfed
      - Duration of breast-feeding
  - Contraceptive history
  - Breast history
    - Mastitis
    - Prior breast masses
    - Prior breast surgery
    - Prior treatment for breast disease
- Current symptoms, such as
  - Pain (mastalgia)
  - Skin changes
  - Presence of mass
  - Spontaneous nipple discharge
    - Sexual history
      - Breast stimulation

- Symptom history
  - Location
  - Onset
  - Duration
  - Severity
- Family history
  - Breast cancer
  - Ovarian cancer
  - Benign breast disease
  - Ethnic heritage
- Breast cancer risk assessment (National Institutes of Health, 2007; American College of Obstetricians and Gynecologists [ACOG], 2003)
  - Most breast cancer occurs randomly
  - Contributing factors include
    - Older age
    - Early menarche
    - Alcohol use
    - Postmenopausal hormone therapy
    - Eastern European Jewish heritage
    - Nulliparous women
    - Never having breast fed
    - Significant family history
    - Personal history of breast cancer
    - Exposure to radiation

Physical Examination:
Components of the Physical Exam to Consider
(Aliotta & Schaeffer, 2006)
- Complete breast examination
  - Positioning
    - Seated, arms at sides
    - Seated, arms raised
    - Seated, leaning forward
    - Supine
  - Evaluate for
    - Mass
    - Dimpling
    - "Orange peel" sign
    - Nipple retraction
    - Nipple discharge
    - Redness
    - Induration

- ◆ Axillary lymphadenopathy
- ◆ Breast or axillary tenderness
- ■ Note characteristics of mass
  - ◆ Size and contour
  - ◆ Mobility
  - ◆ Definition of borders
  - ◆ Firmness
  - ◆ Associated
    - ➤ Pain or tenderness
    - ➤ Skin changes
    - ➤ Distortion of breast contour
- ■ Note characteristics of nipple discharge
  - ◆ Presence in one or both breasts
  - ◆ Color and consistency
  - ◆ Spontaneous emission

Clinical Impression:
Differential Diagnoses and Code Groups to Consider
Additional suffix may apply (ICD9data.com, 2007)

- Abnormal mammogram, unspecified (ICD-9 codes 793.80)
- Abnormal mammogram, microcalcifications (ICD-9 codes 793.81)
- Other abnormal findings on radiologic examination of breast (ICD-9 codes 793.89)
- Benign breast conditions (ICD-9 codes 611)
- Breast malignancy (ICD-9 codes 174)
- Axillary lymphadenopathy (ICD-9 codes 785.6)

Diagnostic Testing:
Diagnostic Tests and Procedures to Consider

- Ultrasound (ACOG, 2003)
  - ■ Benign process suspected
  - ■ Differentiates solid from cystic mass
- Follow-up mammogram
  - ■ Based on radiologist recommendations
    - ◆ Magnification views
    - ◆ Three- to 6-month follow-up
- Biopsy
  - ■ Based on
    - ◆ Clinical findings
    - ◆ Radiologist recommendations
    - ◆ Client preference

- ■ Biopsy methods
  - ◆ Fine-needle aspiration
  - ◆ Core-needle biopsy
  - ◆ Stereotactic biopsy
  - ◆ Excisional biopsy
- Genetic testing
  - ■ *BRCA1*
  - ■ *BRCA2*
- Magnetic resonance imaging (MRI)

Providing Treatment:
Therapeutic Measures to Consider

- Excisional biopsy
  - ■ Definitive treatment for benign masses
  - ■ Treatment for small malignancies, combined with
    - ◆ Chemotherapy
    - ◆ Radiation treatment
- Cancer treatments
  - ■ Surgery
    - ◆ Lumpectomy
    - ◆ Mastectomy
      - ➤ Partial
      - ➤ Simple
      - ➤ Modified radical
      - ➤ Radical
    - ◆ Axillary node evaluation
      - ➤ Sentinel node(s)
      - ➤ Axillary node dissection
- Medical therapy
  - ■ Radiation treatment
  - ■ Chemotherapy
  - ■ Chemoprevention
    - ◆ Tamoxifen
    - ◆ Evista
- Prophylactic mastectomy for women at high risk for breast cancer

Providing Treatment:
Alternative Measures to Consider

- Alternative therapies should not delay diagnostic measures or substitute for medical or surgical treatment

- Healthy whole foods diet
  - Avoid foods with
    - Hormones (meat, milk)
    - Hormone-like activity
    - Pesticides or herbicides
    - Preservatives
  - Limit
    - Animal fats
    - Alcohol
    - Refined sugar and flour
    - Processed foods
- ⚠ Herbal and homeopathic remedies may interact with medications
- Immune support
  - Echinacea—use with caution (Foster, 1996; Soule, 1995)
  - Love and laughter boost immune response
    - Rent comedy videos
    - Enjoy time with friends
- Emotional support
  - Bach flower essences, such as
    - Rescue remedy
  - St. John's wort
  - Lemon balm tea (Foster, 1996)
  - Cultivate a positive attitude
    - Meditation or prayer
    - Enjoy each day as a gift
    - Seek healing and optimal health

Providing Support:
Education and Support Measures to Consider
- Advise client of abnormal screening test results
- Provide information
  - Abnormal mammogram is not indicative of cancer
  - Options for diagnostic testing
  - Tissue sample (biopsy) is diagnostic test
  - Written information helpful
- Allow time for client to express concerns
  - Validate concerns
  - Address fears
- Develop management plan
  - Referral for biopsy
  - Plan for follow-up

- With cancer diagnosis, provide information on
  - Community resources, such as
    - Reach to Recovery
    - American Cancer Society (ACS)
    - Cancer support groups

Follow-up Care:
Follow-up Measures to Consider
- Document
  - Characteristics of clinical findings
  - Discussions with client
  - Referral indication and plan
- Provide client with referral information
  - Appointment time and date
  - Directions
  - Anticipated sequence of events
- Return for care
  - To review findings
  - Provide client education
  - For support and counseling
  - For well-woman care

Collaborative Practice:
Criteria to Consider for Consultation or Referral
- Surgery or breast care service
  - Suspicious mammogram result
  - Evaluation of lesion
  - Second opinion
- Community resources
  - Social service
  - Transportation
  - Counseling
  - Support groups
- For diagnosis or treatment outside the midwife's scope of practice

ABNORMAL PAP SMEAR INTERPRETATION AND TRIAGE

Key Clinical Information

Triage of women with a Pap smear other than *"Satisfactory for evaluation. Negative for intraepithelial lesion or malignancy,"* is confusing for many clinicians. First, the specimen must be adequate for interpretation. Adequacy is determined by the presence of cells representing the transformation zone, including endocervical cells, except in women who have undergone total hysterectomy. Continued cytologic screening is indicated in women after hysterectomy who have had a supracervical hysterectomy, a hysterectomy for cervical cancer, women with HIV disease or other immune system disorders, multiple sexual partners, are diagnosed with sexually transmitted diseases, and DES daughters.

Interpretation may be hampered by partially obscuring blood or inflammatory exudate, particularly when the specimen is collected on a slide rather than in a liquid-based medium (Davey et al., 2002). Pap smear slides remain the most effective and cost-efficient means of screening a large population of women. However, liquid-based cytology offers the opportunity to perform "reflex" human papilloma virus (HPV) testing if an atypical result is returned and increases specimen adequacy (Davey et al., 2002). HPV testing is useful for determining which clients with abnormal squamous cells of unknown significance (ASC-US) or low-grade squamous intraepithelial lesions (LSIL) require a diagnostic workup (Wright et al., 2007a). Atypical glandular cells (AGC), high-grade squamous intraepithelial lesions (HSIL), or cancer findings (carcinoma in situ [CIS] or adenocarcinoma in situ [AIS]) require prompt evaluation by a skilled colposcopist. When in doubt about the interpretation of any Pap smear result, discussion with the cytology laboratory is recommended.

Client History and Chart Review:
Components of the History to Consider
- Last menstrual period (LMP), gravida, para
- Special circumstances
  - Pregnant client
  - Adolescent client
  - Postmenopausal client
- History of prior
  - Abnormal Pap smears
  - Diagnostic testing
  - Treatment
- Sexual history
  - Age at onset of sexual activity
  - Number of sexual partners
  - Condom use

- History of STIs
  - HPV
  - HIV
- Medical history
- Surgical history
  - Hysterectomy
    - Complete or partial
    - Indication
- Social history
  - Smoking
  - Drug and alcohol use
- Family history
  - Cervical disease
  - DES exposure in utero
- Risk factors for abnormal Pap smear
  - More than three sexual partners
  - History of STIs, especially HPV and HIV
  - Prior abnormal Pap smears
  - Lack of self-care, noncompliance
  - Cigarette smoking
  - Presence of cervical intraepithelial neoplasia (CIN) grades 2 and 3
- Symptoms consistent with cervical cancer
  - Persistent watery discharge
  - Intermenstrual bleeding

Physical Examination:
Components of the Physical Exam to Consider
- Examination of the external genitalia for HPV lesions (Saslow et al., 2003)
  - Visible HPV is considered low risk for CIN
  - External HPV may contribute to
    - Vulvar intraepithelial neoplasia (VIN)
    - Vaginal intraepithelial neoplasia (VaIN)
- Visualization of the cervix and vaginal vault
  - Presence of gross lesions
  - Signs of genital atrophy
  - Cervical cuff in women with hysterectomy
- Colposcopic examination, if indicated
  - Squamocolumnar junction
  - Presence of acetowhite lesions
    - Punctation
    - Mosaicism
    - Abnormal vessels
  - Lesion borders
  - Abnormal Lugol's uptake

Clinical Impression:
Differential Diagnoses and Code Groups
to Consider
Additional suffix may apply (ICD9data.com, 2007)

- Cervicitis (ICD-9 codes 616.0)
- Vaginitis, non-specific (ICD-9 codes 616.10)
- Atypical glandular cells of unknown significance (AGC-US) (ICD-9 codes 795.00)
- ASC-US (ICD-9 codes 795.01)
- Atypical squamous cells, cannot exclude high grade (ASC-H) (ICD-9 codes 795.02)
- LSIL (ICD-9 codes 795.03)
- HSIL (ICD-9 codes 795.04)
- Positive test results for high-risk HPV DNA (ICD-9 codes 795.05)
- Pap smear suspicious for cervical cancer (ICD-9 codes 795.06)

Diagnostic Testing:
Diagnostic Tests and Procedures to Consider
(Davey et al., 2002; Wright et al., 2007a)

- Based on Pap smear results
- Negative Pap smear with obscuring
  - Repeat in 6 months in women with
    - Previous abnormal Pap smear within 2 years
    - Previous Pap smear with AGC
    - High-risk HPV diagnosed within 12 months
    - Inability to sample endocervix
    - Immunosuppression
    - Similar obscuring on previous Pap smear
    - Irregular infrequent screening
- Specimen unsatisfactory
  - Treat any underlying infection
  - Repeat Pap smear in 2–4 months
  - ⚠ Persistent unsatisfactory results
    - Associated with progressive lesions
    - Colposcopy
    - Biopsy
- ASC-US
  - "Reflex" high-risk HPV DNA testing, *or*
  - Repeat Pap smear every 6 months for 2 years, *or*
  - Colposcopic evaluation

- Follow-up testing/evaluation within normal limits
  - Repeat Pap smear in 12 months
  - Liquid cytology preferred
- Evaluation abnormal
  - Colposcopy indicated
- Adolescent women (up to age 20)
  - Repeat Pap smear in 12 months
    - Less than HSIL
      - Repeat Pap smear in 12 months
        - Negative → routine screening
        - ASC or greater → colposcopy
    - HSIL → colposcopy
- ASC-H
  - Colposcopy
- LSIL
  - Colposcopic evaluation
    - Identification of lesions
    - Directed biopsy
    - Endocervical curettage
  - Adolescents
    - See ASC-US, above
    - ⚠ High-risk HPV testing unacceptable
  - Pregnancy
    - Colposcopy, *or*
    - Defer colposcopy until postpartum
    - Endocervical curettage not acceptable
  - Postmenopausal women
    - Triage with high-risk HPV testing, *or*
    - Repeat cytology in 6 and 12 months, *or*
    - Colposcopy
    - Negative testing/evaluation
      - Repeat cytology in 12 months
    - ASC or greater, or positive HPV
      - Colposcopy
- HSIL
  - Colposcopic evaluation
    - Identification of lesion
    - Directed punch biopsy
    - Endocervical curettage
  - Loop electrical excision procedure (LEEP) biopsy
    - ⚠ Unacceptable for
      - Pregnant women
      - Adolescent women

- AGC *or* adenocarcinoma in situ
  - Colposcopic evaluation
  - Biopsy of lesions
  - Endocervical sampling
  - Endometrial sampling
    - Age > 35 with
      - Unexplained vaginal bleeding
      - Diagnosed chronic anovulation
  - High-risk HPV DNA testing
- Atypical endometrial cells
  - Endocervical sampling
  - Endometrial sampling
  - Normal results → colposcopy

Providing Treatment:
Therapeutic Measures to Consider
- Menopausal clients with ASC or LSIL
  - Vaginal estrogen for 3 months
  - Repeat cytology as indicated
- Ⓥ Ablation therapies
  - Cryotherapy
  - Laser
- Ⓥ Excisional therapies
  - LEEP procedure
  - Cold knife cone

Providing Treatment:
Alternative Measures to Consider
- ⚠ Alternative therapies are not a substitute for prompt evaluation and treatment
- Dietary support (Soule, 1995)
  - Beta-carotene—50,000 IU BID with meals
  - Vitamin C—1000–2000 mg TID
  - Vitamin E—400 IU daily
  - Folic acid—2 mg daily for 3 months, then 0.4 mg daily
  - Selenium—200 mg daily
  - Zinc—30 mg daily
- Herbs to support the immune and reproductive systems
  - Echinacea (Foster, 1996)
  - Red raspberry leaf (Soule, 1995)
  - Vitex (Foster, 1996; Soule, 1995)
- Visualization of healing

Providing Support:
Education and Support Measures to Consider
- Provide information regarding cervical disease
  - Written information preferred
  - Meaning of abnormal Pap smear result
  - Information about diagnostic testing options
  - Potential treatment measures
- Importance of, and schedule for, follow-up
- Smoking cessation, as needed
- Recommended vitamin and mineral supplements
- Safe sexual practices

Follow-up Care:
Follow-up Measures to Consider
- Document
  - Cytology result
  - Discussion with client
  - Plan for continued care
  - Consultations and referrals
- Triage as recommended by American Society for Colposcopy and Cervical Pathology (see Figures 7-1 to 7-10)
- Treat and follow-up according results

Collaborative Practice:
Criteria to Consider for Consultation or Referral
- OB/GYN service
  - Unusual cervical configuration or appearance
    - Visually
    - By palpation
    - By colposcopy
  - Colposcopy for HSIL lesions
  - Evaluation of AGC-US lesions
    - Treatment
      - CIN lesions
      - Malignancy
- For diagnosis or treatment outside the midwife's scope of practice

CARE OF THE WOMAN WITH AMENORRHEA

Key Clinical Information
Primary amenorrhea is an uncommon condition that is defined as an absence of menarche in a young woman who by age 14 has not begun developing

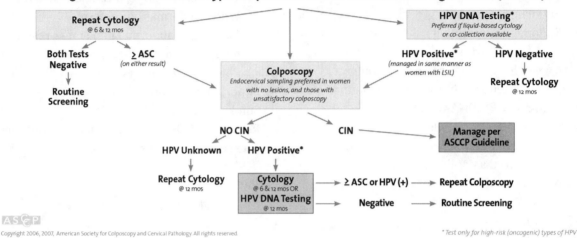

Figure 7-1   *Management of Women with Atypical Squamous Cells of Undetermined Significance (ASC-US)*

Copyright 2006, 2007. American Society for Colposcopy and Cervical Pathology. All rights reserved.

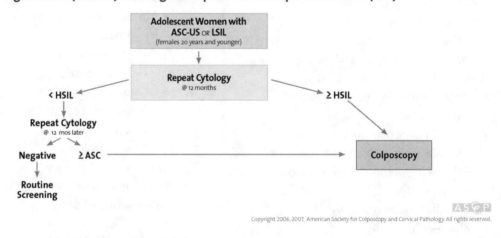

Figure 7-2   *Management of Adolescent Women with Either Atypical Squamous Cells of Undetermined Significance (ASC-US) or Low-grade Squamous Intraepithelial Lesion (LSIL)*

Copyright 2006, 2007. American Society for Colposcopy and Cervical Pathology. All rights reserved.

Management of Women with Atypical Squamous Cells: Cannot Exclude High-grade SIL (ASC - H)

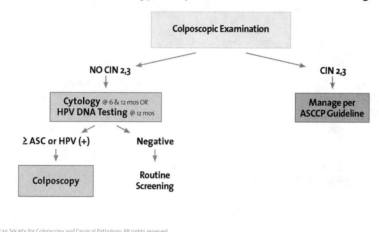

Copyright 2006, 2007. American Society for Colposcopy and Cervical Pathology. All rights reserved.

Figure 7-3 *Management of Women with Atypical Squamous Cells: Cannot Exclude High-grade SIL (ASC-H)*

Copyright 2006, 2007. American Society for Colposcopy and Cervical Pathology. All rights reserved.

Management of Women with Low-grade Squamous Intraepithelial Lesion (LSIL) *

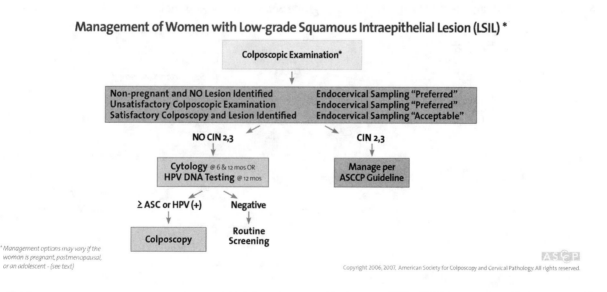

Copyright 2006, 2007. American Society for Colposcopy and Cervical Pathology. All rights reserved.

Figure 7-4 *Management of Women with Low-grade Squamous Intraepithelial Lesion (LSIL)*

Copyright 2006, 2007. American Society for Colposcopy and Cervical Pathology. All rights reserved.

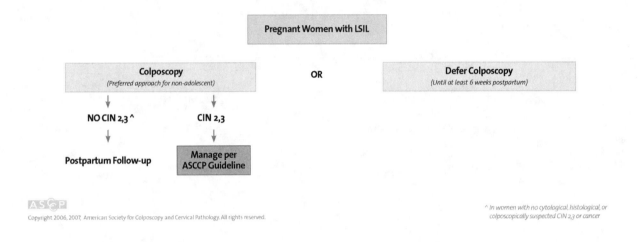

Figure 7-5   *Management of Pregnant Women with Low-grade Squamous Intraepithelial Lesion (LSIL)*
Copyright 2006, 2007. American Society for Colposcopy and Cervical Pathology. All rights reserved.

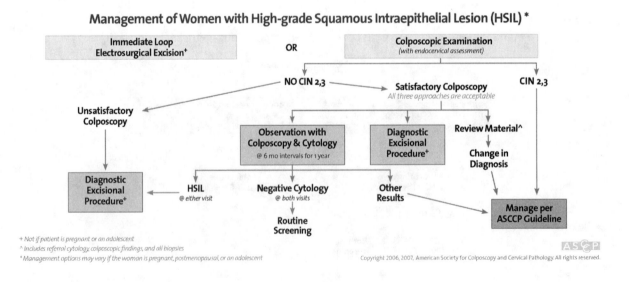

Figure 7-6   *Management of Women with High-grade Squamous Intraepithelial Lesion (HSIL)*
Copyright 2006, 2007. American Society for Colposcopy and Cervical Pathology. All rights reserved.

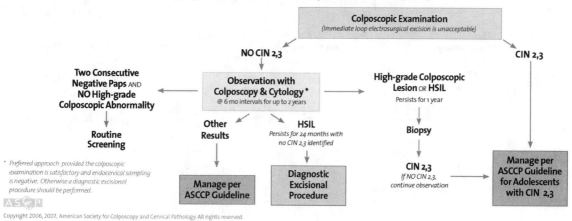

Figure 7-7 *Management of Adolescent Women (20 Years and Younger) with High-grade Squamous Intraepithelial Lesion (HSIL)*

Copyright 2006, 2007. American Society for Colposcopy and Cervical Pathology. All rights reserved.

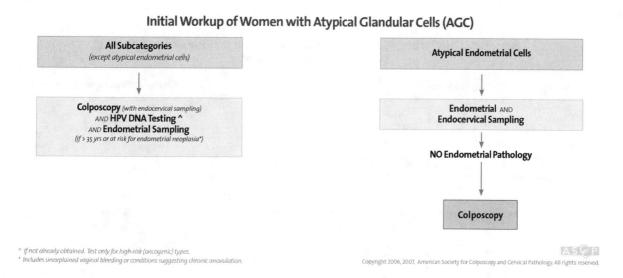

Figure 7-8 *Initial Workup of Women with Atypical Glandular Cells (AGC)*

Copyright 2006, 2007. American Society for Colposcopy and Cervical Pathology. All rights reserved.

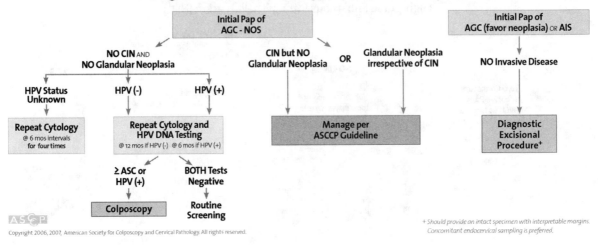

Figure 7-9   *Management of Women with Atypical Glandular Cells (AGC)*

Copyright 2006, 2007. American Society for Colposcopy and Cervical Pathology. All rights reserved.

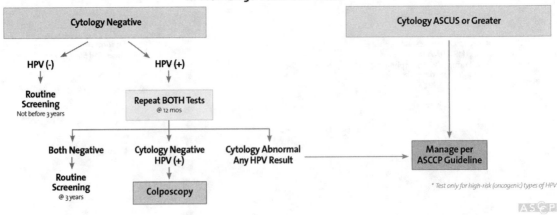

Figure 7-10   *Use of HPV DNA Testing* as an Adjunct to Cytology for Cervical Cancer Screening in Women 30 Years and Older*

Copyright 2006, 2007. American Society for Colposcopy and Cervical Pathology. All rights reserved.

secondary sex characteristics or who by age 16 or older has developed secondary sex characteristics but not started menstruation (Varney et al., 2004). Primary amenorrhea may result from genetic and congenital disorders or from medical conditions such as malnutrition or hyperthyroidism. Up to 10% of young women with primary amenorrhea have a constitutional delay of menarche, with onset of menarche as late as age 18.

Secondary amenorrhea is defined as the absence of menses for 3–6 months in a woman who has previously menstruated and is not pregnant, breast-feeding, or menopausal, frequently secondary to anovulation (Faucher & Schuiling, 2006; Varney et al., 2004). Secondary amenorrhea occurs in approximately 4% of women (MedlinePlus, 2006). There is crossover between potential causes of primary and secondary amenorrhea, and all differential diagnoses should be considered when evaluating the woman with amenorrhea (Faucher & Schuiling, 2006).

Client History and Chart Review:
Components of the History to Consider (Faucher & Schuiling, 2006; MedlinePlus, 2006)

- Age
- Menstrual history
  - Age at menarche
  - Previous menstrual pattern
  - Onset and duration of amenorrhea
  - Presence of associated symptoms
    - Galactorrhea
    - Hirsutism
    - Headache
    - Vaginal dryness
    - Visual changes
- Gynecologic history
  - Presence of secondary sex characteristics
  - Gynecologic surgery, such as
    - Cervical cryosurgery
    - Dilatation and curettage (D&C)
    - Dilatation and evacuation (D&E)
    - Endometrial ablation
  - Sexual history
    - Sexual activity
    - Sexual abuse

- Contraceptive history
  - Depo-Provera
  - Mirena
  - Continuous oral contraceptives
  - Implanon or Norplant
- Pregnancy and breast-feeding history
  - Pregnancy terminations
  - Length of breast-feeding
- Medical and surgical history
  - Thyroid disorders
  - Weight changes
    - Loss/gain
    - Distribution
  - Systemic illness
- Medications that may contribute to amenorrhea (MedlinePlus, 2006)
  - Busulfan
  - Chlorambucil
  - Cyclophosphamide
  - Phenothiazines
  - Oral contraceptives
  - Non–oral contraceptives such as
    - Depo-Provera
    - Mirena intrauterine device (IUD)
- Psychosocial assessment
  - Stressors
  - Nutrition patterns
    - Adequacy of diet
    - Eating disorders
  - Physical activity level
    - Competitive sports
  - Effects of amenorrhea on self-image
- Review of systems (ROS)

Physical Examination:
Components of the Physical Exam to Consider (Faucher & Schuiling, 2006)

- Vital signs
- Height/weight
  - Body mass index (BMI)
  - Weight changes
  - Weight distribution
  - Ratio of muscle to adipose tissue

- Thyroid examination
  - Enlargement
  - Nodularity
  - Physical findings consistent with thyroid disorders
- Tanner staging (Moses, 2007a)
  - Age appropriate height increases
  - Pubic hair development
    - ◆ Texture
      - ➤ Fine villus hair
      - ➤ Minimal coarse pigmented hair
      - ➤ Dark curly coarse hair
    - ◆ Distribution
      - ➤ Labia
      - ➤ Mons
      - ➤ Axilla
      - ➤ Medial thigh
  - Breast development
    - ◆ Breast buds
    - ◆ Areolar enlargement
    - ◆ Breast mound develops
    - ◆ Areola forms secondary mound
    - ◆ Adult contour
  - Acne vulgaris develops
- Pelvic examination
  - Examination for physical cause of amenorrhea
    - ◆ Outflow tract disorders
      - ➤ Imperforate hymen
      - ➤ Labial fusion
      - ➤ Cervical stenosis
    - ◆ Absence of vagina, cervix, or uterus
    - ◆ Ambiguous genitalia
  - Signs of endocrine/central nervous system disorders
    - ◆ Vaginal atrophy
    - ◆ Clitoral hypertrophy
- Ⓥ Visual field examination
  - Pituitary tumor

Clinical Impression:
Differential Diagnoses and Code Groups
to Consider
Additional suffix may apply (ICD9data.com, 2007)

- Amenorrhea, primary or secondary (ICD-9 codes 626.0)

- Amenorrhea, due to
  - Asherman's syndrome (ICD-9 codes 621.5)
  - Ovarian dysfunction (ICD-9 codes 256.8)
  - Pregnancy (ICD-9 codes V22.2)
  - Hormonal contraception use (ICD-9 codes V25.40)
  - Premature menopause (ICD-9 codes 256.31)
  - Hypothalamic dysfunction secondary to (ICD-9 codes 253.4)
    - ◆ Low body fat
    - ◆ Stress
  - Endocrine disorders
    - ◆ Premature ovarian failure (ICD-9 codes 256.39)
    - ◆ Polycystic ovary syndrome (ICD-9 codes 256.4)
    - ◆ Androgen-producing tumors (ICD-9 codes 183)
    - ◆ Hyperprolactinemia (ICD-9 codes 253.1)
    - ◆ Hypothyroidism (ICD-9 codes 244.8)
    - ◆ Pituitary disease (ICD-9 codes 253)
  - Genetic factors
    - ◆ Constitutional rate of maturation (ICD-9 codes 259.0)
    - ◆ Congenital anomalies
      - ➤ Congenital anomalies of genital tract (ICD-9 codes 752)
      - ➤ Congenital adrenogenital disorders (ICD-9 codes 255.2)
- Galactorrhea (ICD-9 codes 611.6)

Diagnostic Testing:
Diagnostic Tests and Procedures to Consider
(Varney et al., 2004)

- Secondary amenorrhea
  - Serum β-human chorionic gonadotropin (β-HCG)
  - If β-HCG negative
    - ◆ Thyroid-stimulating hormone (TSH) (elevated TSH = hypothyroidism)
    - ◆ Prolactin level (< 100 ng/ml normal)
  - Consider progesterone trial

- Primary amenorrhea
  - Normal secondary sex characteristics
    - Pelvic sonography
  - Uterus present
    - Serum HCG
    - Serum T$_4$, TSH
    - Prolactin level
      - Elevated prolactin level
        - MRI of head/pituitary, or
        - Computed tomography (CT) of sella turcica
      - Normal prolactin level
        - Evaluate for
          - Imperforate hymen
          - Vaginal and cervical patency
  - Uterus absent
    - Evaluate testosterone level, and/or
    - Karyotype
- No secondary sex characteristics
  - Follicle-stimulating hormone (FSH)/ luteinizing hormone (LH) levels
  - FSH 5–30 IU/l
  - LH 5–20 IU/l
    - Elevated FSH/LH → karyotype
    - Normal or low FSH/LH
      - Refer for trial of gonadotropin-releasing hormone

Providing Treatment:
Therapeutic Measures to Consider
- Progesterone trial
  - Medication options
    - Provera 10 mg for 10 days *or*
    - Prometrium 400 mg at bedtime for 10 days *or*
    - Crinone 4%, progesterone gel 45 mg vaginally QID for six doses
  - Expect withdrawal bleeding within 10 days after medication
- Refer for treatment based on working diagnosis
  - Gynecologic
  - Endocrine
  - Congenital

Providing Treatment:
Alternative Measures to Consider
- Herbal remedies that support menstruation (Soule, 1995)
  - Red raspberry leaf tea
  - Vitex tea, tincture or capsules
  - Dong quai tea (not to be used while nursing)
  - Wild yam root tea or tincture
  - Blue cohosh root tea or tincture
  - Use for 3 months, even after cycle resumes
- Acupuncture

Providing Support:
Education and Support Measures to Consider
- Provide age-appropriate information
  - Menstrual cycle and function
  - Potential causes
    - Breast-feeding
    - Exercise and low body fat
    - Endocrine disorders
    - Chromosomal abnormalities
    - Congenital anomalies
- Plan for testing and results
- Expectation for treatment
- Potential for associated
  - Infertility
  - Endometrial hyperplasia
  - Osteopenia and osteoporosis (Sinclair, 2004)

Follow-up Care:
Follow-up Measures to Consider (Faucher & Schuiling, 2006)
- Document
  - Working diagnosis
  - Plan for continued care
- Office follow-up
  - As indicated by results and diagnosis
    - Results of progestin challenge
      - Withdrawal bleed with normal prolactin and TSH = anovulation
      - Negative withdrawal bleed requires further workup
  - For support during gynecologic workup
  - As indicated for routine care

Collaborative Practice:
Criteria to Consider for Consultation or Referral

- OB/GYN or gynecologic endocrinologist
  - Primary amenorrhea
    - Presence of anomalies
    - Abnormal laboratory results
    - Reproductive
    - Endocrine
    - Genetic
  - Secondary amenorrhea
    - Primary evaluation
    - After progestin challenge
      - If no withdrawal bleed
- Mental health service
  - Presence of eating disorder
- Social service
  - Evidence of malnutrition
- For diagnosis or treatment outside the midwife's scope of practice

CARE OF THE WOMAN WITH BACTERIAL VAGINOSIS

Key Clinical Information

Bacterial vaginosis (BV) is one of the most commonly occurring forms of vaginitis, characterized by the classic "fishy" odor and accounting for up to 50% of vaginitis diagnoses. Although not an STI, a higher incidence of BV is found in women with new or multiple partners. Untreated BV may contribute to endometritis and reproductive postoperative wound infections and may increase susceptibility to STIs, including HIV (Fogel, 2006a). Although controversy exists as to whether BV contributes to the onset of preterm labor, persistent recurrent BV has been linked to background mycoplasma infection. Many women consider all vaginal infections as "yeast infections" and self-treat before being seen for evaluation.

Client History and Chart Review:
Components of the History to Consider
(Fogel, 2006a)

- Onset and duration of symptoms
  - Vulvovaginal irritation or burning

- Presence of discharge
  - Copious
  - Homogenous
  - Thin
  - Grayish white
- Odor
  - Described as foul or "fishy"
  - Stronger after menses and intercourse
- Treatments used and results
- OB/GYN history
  - LMP
  - Birth control method
  - Previous BV infection
    - Testing
    - Treatment
  - BV associated with
    - Early pregnancy losses
    - Preterm labor (ACOG, 2001)
    - Endometritis/pelvic inflammatory disease (PID)
    - STIs
    - Postoperative wound infection
- Sexual practices that may contribute to BV (Centers for Disease Control and Prevention [CDC], 2006a; Fogel, 2006a)
  - Oral–genital contact
  - Vaginal contact after anal penetration
  - Multiple partners (woman or partner)
    - Inquire regarding discharge or symptoms in partner(s)
  - Female partner(s)
  - Douching
- Medical history
  - Allergies
  - Medications
    - Antibiotics
    - Hormones
  - Systemic illness
    - Diabetes

Physical Examination:
Components of the Physical Exam to Consider

- Vital signs
- Pelvic examination

- External examination
  - Redness
  - Erythema
  - Lesions
  - Discharge
  - Odor
- Speculum examination
  - Discharge
  - Lesions
  - Retained tampon or foreign body
- Bimanual examination
  - Cervical motion tenderness
  - Adnexal masses

Clinical Impression:
Differential Diagnoses and Code Groups
to Consider
Additional suffix may apply (ICD9data.com, 2007)

- Bacterial vaginosis (BV) (ICD-9 codes 616.10)
- Candida vaginitis (ICD-9 codes 112.1)
- Cervicitis (ICD-9 codes 616.0)
- Foreign body (ICD-9 codes 939.2)
- Chlamydia (ICD-9 codes 099.53)
- Gonorrhea (ICD-9 codes 098)
- Mycoplasma (ICD-9 codes 616.10)
- Trichomoniasis (ICD-9 codes 131.01)
- Vaginitis complicating pregnancy (ICD-9 codes 646.6)

Diagnostic Testing:
Diagnostic Tests and Procedures to Consider
(CDC, 2006a)

- Wet preparation (provider performed microscopy)
  - Vaginal pH > 4.5
  - KOH preparation
    - Positive KOH whiff test
    - Negative mycelia or branching hyphae
  - Saline preparation
    - Positive clue cells
    - Rare lactobacilli
    - Occasional white blood cells
- Gram stain
- DNA probe, such as BD Affirm VPIII

- Point-of-service rapid tests
  - QuickVue Advance
  - Osom BV test
- ⚠ Note: The vaginal discharge and visual inspection of the discharge is nonspecific and cannot be used alone for diagnosis. Multiple pathogens may be present. Perform additional testing as required for accurate diagnosis.

Providing Treatment:
Therapeutic Measures to Consider (CDC, 2006a)

- Metronidazole
  - Pregnancy Category B
  - Use in second or third trimester preferred
  - Pregnancy dosing
    - 500 mg PO BID for 7 days, *or*
    - 250 mg orally TID for 7 days
  - Nonpregnancy dosing
    - 500 mg PO BID for 7 days, *or*
    - 750 mg extended release 1 PO for 7 days
    - MetroGel-Vaginal
      - One applicator per vagina
      - At bedtime for 5 days
- Cleocin (clindamycin)
  - Pregnancy Category B
  - Avoid pregnancy use from 20 weeks to term (CDC, 2006a)
  - Pregnancy dosing
    - Clindamycin 300 mg PO BID for 7 days
    - Vaginal cream
      - 5 g intravaginally at bedtime for 7 days
  - Nonpregnancy dosing
    - Vaginal cream
      - 5 g intravaginally at bedtime for 7 days
    - Clindamycin 300 mg PO BID for 7 days
    - Clindamycin ovules 100 mg intravaginally at bedtime for 3 days

Providing Treatment:
Alternative Measures to Consider

- Infection of imbalance
  - Provide immune support
  - "Tincture of time" to allow spontaneous resolution

- Black walnut tincture
- Boric acid capsules (Soule, 1996)
    - Boric acid powder
    - Slippery elm powder
    - One per vagina at bedtime five nights
    - Follow with
        - *Lactobacillus* capsules
        - One per vagina at bedtime five nights, *or*
        - Yogurt douche
            - ➤ 1 cup live culture yogurt
            - ➤ 1 quart warm water
- Garlic vaginal suppository
    - One clove garlic, peeled
    - Attach 6-inch length of dental floss
    - Use nightly for five nights
- Herbal douche
    - Tincture of
        - Calendula—2 parts
        - Echinacea root—2 parts
        - Myrrh—2 parts
        - Place 50 gtts in 1 cup warm calendula tea
        - Douche for 6 nights
- Homeopathic remedies (Smith, 1984)
    - Graphites—discharge is thin and watery and causes burning
    - Sepia—discharge is offensive and may be yellowish

Providing Support:
Education and Support Measures to Consider
- Review genital hygiene
    - Limit alkaline soaps (Soule, 1996)
    - Wipe front to back
    - Urinate after sexual relations
    - Cotton panties or liners
    - Avoid close-fitting clothing
- Provide information about BV
- Treatment instructions
    - Avoid sexual relations during treatment
    - Return for care for persistent symptoms
    - Additional testing may be needed
    - Partner may need treatment

- Diagnosis during pregnancy
    - Risk and benefits of treatment
    - Warning signs of preterm labor

Follow-up Care:
Follow-up Measures to Consider
- Document
    - Clinical findings
    - Wet prep and pH results
- If symptoms recur or persist
    - Consider testing for
        - Chlamydia
        - Mycoplasma
        - Trichomoniasis
    - Treat partner and retreat patient
- Diagnosis during pregnancy
    - Reevaluate in 1 month (CDC, 2006a)
    - Assess for signs of
        - Preterm labor
        - Postpartum endometritis
        - Postoperative wound infection

Collaborative Practice:
Criteria to Consider for Consultation or Referral
- OB/GYN service
    - For persistent or unresponsive vaginitis
    - For preterm labor
- For diagnosis or treatment outside the midwife's scope of practice

CARE OF THE WOMAN WITH BREAST MASS

Key Clinical Information
Every breast mass must be considered suspicious for breast cancer until shown to be otherwise. Breast cancer is second only to lung cancer as a cause of cancer mortality in women, with death rates 37% higher in African-American women than in white women (ACS, 2007a). Up to 80% of women who develop breast cancer have no risk factors for breast cancer. Pregnancy does not exclude breast cancer from the differential diagnosis; 2% of all breast cancers are diagnosed during pregnancy (Simpson et al., 2000; Varney et al., 2004).

Client History and Chart Review:
Components of the History to Consider
(Klein, 2005)

- Age
- Gravida, para
- Diet history
  - Caffeine intake
  - Fat intake
  - Alcohol consumption
  - Overcooked or charred meat
  - Unwashed fruits and vegetables (pesticides)
- Medications
  - Oral contraceptives
  - Hormone replacement therapy
- LMP and menstrual status
- Location and onset of symptoms
  - When first noted
  - Relation to menstrual cycle
  - Characteristics of mass
    - Location
    - Consistency
    - Mobility
    - Pain
- Associated breast changes
  - Nipple discharge
  - Dimpling
  - "Orange peel" sign
  - Skin changes
- Axillary masses
- Previous mammography
- Presence of risk factors for breast cancer
  (ACS, 2007a; ACOG, 2003)
  - Female gender
  - Age
  - Presence of *BRCA1* or *BRCA2*
  - Positive family history
  - Previous history of breast cancer
  - Atypical hyperplasia on biopsy
  - Exposure to high-dose radiation
  - High postmenopausal bone density
  - Early menarche/late menopause
  - Nulliparous, or first child born after age 30
  - Long-term hormone replacement therapy

- Obesity, diabetes, high-fat diet
- Tall women
- Jewish heritage
- Alcohol consumption
- Previous or current breast conditions
  - Lactation
  - Benign disorders, such as
    - Fibrocystic breasts
    - Mastitis
    - Breast abscess
  - Biopsies
- Self-breast examination habits and techniques
- Review of systems (ROS)

Physical Examination:
Components of the Physical Exam to Consider
(ACS, 2007a; Klein, 2005)

- Height/weight/BMI
- Complete breast examination, sitting and supine
- Visual findings
  - Scarring
  - Dimpling and retraction
  - Skin changes
    - "Orange peel" sign
    - Paget's
  - Asymmetry
  - Nipple retraction
  - Redness
- Palpation of superficial, intermediate and
  deep tissue
- Palpable findings of mass(es)
  - Single or multiple
  - Location(s)
    - Upper outer quadrant most common
      for cancer
    - Diffuse distribution more common with
      cystic breasts
  - Contour
    - Smooth
    - Stellate
  - Size
    - Describe in centimeters
  - Round, oval, or irregular

- Mobility
  - ◆ Mobile
  - ◆ Fixed
- Consistency
  - ◆ Firm
  - ◆ Hard
  - ◆ Soft
- Heat
- Nipples
  - Palpate for masses
  - Spontaneous nipple discharge
  - Expression of discharge
- Palpation for lymph nodes
  - Axilla
  - Supraclavicular
  - Neck

Clinical Impression:
Differential Diagnoses and Code Groups
to Consider
Additional suffix may apply (ICD9data.com, 2007)
- Breast mass(es) (ICD-9 codes 611.72)
- Breast abscess, postpartum (ICD-9 codes 675.14)
- Breast abscess (ICD-9 codes 611.0)
- Breast cyst, solitary (ICD-9 codes 610.0)
- Fibrocystic breasts (ICD-9 codes 610.1)
- Fibroadenosis of breast (ICD-9 codes 610.2)
- Traumatic hematoma of breast (ICD-9 codes 611.8)
- Mastitis, postpartum (ICD-9 codes 675.2)
- Mastitis (ICD-9 codes 611)
- Nipple discharge (ICD-9 codes 611.79)
- Enlarged lymph node(s) (ICD-9 codes 785.6)
- Malignancy of breast (ICD-9 codes 174)

Diagnostic Testing:
Diagnostic Tests and Procedures to Consider
(Klein, 2005)
- Ultrasound
  - Young women with dense breast tissue
  - Cyst or abscess suspected
  - May support or oppose physical findings

- Shows fluid-filled soft-tissue changes best
- Differentiates palpable solid masses
- Mammogram
  - Difficult to interpret with
    - ◆ Young women
    - ◆ During lactation
    - ◆ Dense breast tissue
  - Diagnostic mammogram
    - ◆ Indications (Madigan Army Medical Center, 2006)
      - ➤ Persistent breast mass
      - ➤ Spontaneous unilateral nipple discharge
      - ➤ Nipple or skin retraction
    - ◆ Lesion marked with radiopaque marker
      - ➤ Spot compression
      - ➤ Magnified views
  - Digital
    - ◆ Allows for enhancement
  - MRI
    - ◆ Women with silicone breast implants
    - ◆ Difficult to interpret mammogram or ultrasound
      - ➤ Dense or scarred breast tissue
      - ➤ Breast cancer follow-up
      - ➤ Axillary metastasis with unknown primary
- Biopsy
  - Definitive diagnosis with tissue specimen
  - Each technique has limitations
    - ◆ Fine- or core-needle aspiration biopsy
    - ◆ Stereotactic biopsy
    - ◆ Excisional biopsy
- Genetic screening
  - *BRCA1* and *BRCA2*
  - Family history
    - ◆ Breast cancer
    - ◆ Ovarian cancer
  - Ashkenazi Jewish heritage
  - Negative screen does not exclude risk (ACOG, 2003)

Providing Treatment:
Therapeutic Measures to Consider
(Klein, 2005)

- Red clover tea
- Cystic mass
  - Observation for one cycle
  - Aspiration
  - Excision
- Abscess
  - Treat with oral antibiotics (see Care of the Mother: Mastitis, Chapter 5)
  - May require incision and drainage
- Solid mass with
  - Sharp margins by ultrasound
  - Uniform shape
  - No characteristics of malignancy
    - Reevaluation within 1–3 months
    - Needle or stereotactic biopsy
    - Excision of mass
  - Characteristics of malignant or premalignant lesions
    - Needle or stereotactic biopsy
    - Excisional biopsy
- Breast cancer treatments (ACS, 2007a)
  - Surgery
  - Radiation
  - Biologic therapy
  - Chemotherapy
  - Hormone therapy

Providing Treatment:
Alternative Measures to Consider

- ⚠ Alternative measures are not a substitute for prompt evaluation and treatment
- Improve diet
  - Decrease or eliminate
    - Caffeine
    - Chocolate
    - Alcohol
    - Carbonated beverages
  - Products from hormone-fed animals
    - Meat
    - Poultry
    - Milk
    - Cheese
  - Grains, fruits, and vegetables grown with
    - Pesticides
    - Herbicides
  - Limit fat intake
  - Increase vitamin intake
    - Vitamin C
    - Beta-carotene
    - Vitamin E
    - Vitamin B complex
- Increase intake of
  - Deep green vegetables
  - Grains
  - Legumes
  - Sea vegetables
  - Fruit
- Homeopathic treatment for fibrocystic breast discomfort (Smith, 1984)
  - ⚠ Use only after malignancy has been ruled out
  - Belladonna for tenderness and sensitivity
  - Conium for premenstrual tenderness
  - Lapis albis for a painful nodule with burning
- Homeopathic remedies for cysts
  - Calcarea for single cyst without tenderness or pain
  - Conium for right-sided, hard, mobile cyst
- Breast cancer
  - Healthy diet to promote healing
  - Homeopathic arnica to promote healing
  - Rescue Remedy for emotional distress

Providing Support:
Education and Support Measures to Consider

- Teach self-breast examination techniques
  - Daily versus monthly
  - No reminder needed monthly
  - Familiarity with breast changes through cycle
  - Do in bath or shower
  - Soap hands to allow deeper palpation

- Provide information related to
  - Working diagnosis
  - Informed choice
  - Evaluation modalities
  - Testing recommendations
  - Treatments
  - Support services and options
- Prevention measures (ACS, 2007a)
  - Maintain optimal BMI
  - Regular physical activity
  - Reduce alcohol consumption to less than two drinks a day
  - Hormone replacement therapy
    - Avoid, or
    - Use as short a time as possible
    - Use lowest dose
    - High risk women (*BRAC* positive)
      - Tamoxifen therapy
      - Prophylactic mastectomy
      - Prophylactic oophorectomy

Follow-up Care:
Follow-up Measures to Consider

- Document
  - Findings
  - Discussion
  - Plan for continued care
    - Follow-up
    - Referral
- Screening recommendations (ACS, 2007a)
  - Age 40+
    - Mammogram annually for women in good health
    - Clinical breast examination annually
    - Regular self-breast examination
  - Ages 20–39, low risk
    - Clinical breast examination annually
    - Regular self-breast examination
  - Ages 20–39, mother or sister with breast cancer (Madigan Army Medical Center, 2006)
    - Screening mammography 10 years before age at onset for mother or sister
- Assess
  - Emotional state
  - Understanding of information

- Ability to proceed with recommendations
- Need for counseling/support
- Return for care
  - Cystic mass
    - One to three cycles
    - After menses
    - Immediately if enlargement occurs
  - Solid masses, not referred for biopsy
    - Must appear benign by
      - Clinical findings, and
      - Mammogram and/or ultrasound
    - One-month rechecks
      - After menses (if cycling)
      - No growth or regression
      - ⚠ Benign mass may mask malignancy
  - Women postbiopsy for benign lesion
    - Unilateral mammogram in 6 months to establish new baseline

Collaborative Practice:
Criteria to Consider for Consultation or Referral

- Breast center or surgery service
  - Breast mass that is suspicious for cancer
  - Diagnostic evaluation
    - Abnormal mammogram
    - Abnormal ultrasound
    - Persistent mass
  - For excision if cyst recurs after aspiration
  - Client preference for definitive therapy (e.g., excisional biopsy)
- For diagnosis or treatment outside the midwife's scope of practice

CARE OF THE WOMAN WITH CHLAMYDIA

Key Clinical Information

Chlamydia remains the most common STI in the United States. Women with chlamydial infection may present with symptoms that range from mucoid discharge to fulminant PID. Chlamydial infection contributes to decreased tubal patency that may result in infertility and ectopic pregnancy. Chlamydial infection is also associated with persistent pelvic pain, preterm labor or rupture of membranes, and neonatal conjunctivitis and/or trachoma. Chlamydia frequently coexists with gonorrhea or other STIs and may be asymptomatic. Routine annual chlamydia screening is recommended for women under 25 and for women over 25 with a new sexual partner or multiple partners. Screening is a cost-effective means of reducing the incidence of chlamydia (CDC, 2006a).

Client History and Chart Review:
Components of the History to Consider
(Ross et al., 2007)
- Gravida, para
- LMP
  - Onset, duration
  - Abnormal bleeding
    - Intermenstrual
    - Postcoital
  - Potential for pregnancy
    - Current method of birth control
    - Ectopic pregnancy may mimic chlamydia
    - Gestational age if pregnant
- Onset, duration, and type of symptoms
  - Pain
    - Location
      - Urethral
      - Adnexal
      - Suprapubic
    - Severity
    - Precipitating factors
  - Discharge
    - Amount
    - Color
    - Consistency
- Sexual history
  - New sexual partner for self or partner
  - Multiple sexual partners
  - Previous diagnosis of STIs
  - Presence of IUD
  - Condom use
- Medical/surgical history
  - Allergies
  - Medications
  - Chronic health problems
- Social history
  - Alcohol or drug use
- Review of systems (ROS)

Physical Examination:
Components of the Physical Exam to Consider
(Ross et al., 2007)
- Vital signs, including temperature
- Abdominal palpation for
  - Rebound tenderness
  - Guarding
- Pelvic examination
  - External genitalia
  - Speculum examination
    - Vaginal discharge
    - Appearance of cervix
      - Presence of mucopurulent cervical discharge
      - Edema, erythema of cervix
  - Bimanual examination
    - Cervical motion tenderness
    - Uterine enlargement or tenderness
    - Adnexal mass
    - Adnexal pain

Clinical Impression:
Differential Diagnoses and Code Groups
to Consider
Additional suffix may apply (ICD9data.com, 2007)
- Chlamydia (ICD-9 codes 099.50)
- Gonorrhea (ICD-9 codes 098)
- PID (ICD-9 codes 614–616)
- Endometriosis (ICD-9 codes 617)
- Ectopic pregnancy (ICD-9 codes 633)
- Ovarian cyst (ICD-9 codes 620)
- Cervicitis (ICD-9 codes 616.0)
- Cervical cancer (ICD-9 codes 180)
- Irritable bowel (ICD-9 codes 564.1)
- Appendicitis (ICD-9 codes 540–543)

Diagnostic Testing:
Diagnostic Tests and Procedures to Consider
(CDC, 2006a)
- Chlamydia testing
  - Urine
  - Cervical swab
- Gonorrhea testing
- Vaginal wet preparation
- Serum/urine pregnancy testing

- Serum testing for
  - HIV
  - Hepatitis B
  - Syphilis
- ⚠ Note: The vaginal discharge and visual inspection of the discharge is nonspecific and cannot be used alone for diagnosis. Multiple pathogens may be present. Perform additional testing as required for accurate diagnosis.

Providing Treatment:
Therapeutic Measures to Consider (CDC, 2006a; Ross et al., 2007)
- Intrauterine device
  - Treat before insertion
  - Remove if present at time of diagnosis
  - Provide alternate method of birth control
- Analgesia for pain relief
- Recommended treatments
  - Single-dose treatment under observation is ideal
  - Azithromycin 1 g PO single dose
    - First-line therapy
    - Acceptable for use in pregnancy
    - Pregnancy Category B
  - Doxycycline 100 mg PO BID for 7 days
    - First-line therapy for nonpregnant women
    - ⚠ Do not use in pregnancy
    - Pregnancy Category D
  - Amoxicillin 500 mg TID for 7 days
    - First-line therapy for pregnant women
    - Pregnancy Category B
- Alternate treatments
  - Erythromycin base 500 mg PO QID for 7 days—Pregnancy Category B
  - Erythromycin ethylsuccinate 800 mg PO QID for 7 days—Pregnancy Category B
  - Ofloxacin 300 mg PO BID for 7 days—Pregnancy Category C
  - Levofloxacin 500 mg PO QID for 7 days

Providing Treatment:
Alternative Measures to Consider
- ⚠ Alternative measures are not a substitute for antibiotic therapy

- Promote well-being
  - Rest
  - Balanced diet
- Herbal/homeopathic remedies to boost immune response
  - Echinacea
  - Homeopathic Mercurius solubilis
- Acidophilus to offset effects of antibiotics on gut
  - Capsules
  - Yogurt
  - Probiotics

Providing Support:
Education and Support Measures to Consider
- Provide age-appropriate information regarding
  - Infection cause and transmission
  - Effects on reproductive organs and future fertility
  - Reportable infection
  - Treatment plan and follow-up
    - Need to evaluate and/or treat partner(s)
    - Medication instructions
  - Avoid intercourse until
    - Partner has been tested and treated, and
    - 7 days after medication is begun (CDC, 2006a)
  - Prevention measures
    - Risk behaviors
    - Safe sexual practices

Follow-up Care:
Follow-up Measures to Consider
- Document
  - Results
  - Treatment
  - Reporting
  - Client discussion and education
  - Plan for follow-up
- Further STI testing
- Return to office or clinic
  - Three to 4 weeks after treatment for test of cure
    - Pregnancy
    - Noncompliant client
    - High-risk behaviors (CDC, 2006a)

- For continued symptoms
- For persistent pain
- New partner for self or partner
- Client preference for testing
- Rescreen within 3–12 months
- With new diagnosis of pregnancy
  - Test all clients
  - Early ultrasound after PID to rule out ectopic pregnancy
- Assess postpartum and newborn clients
  - Endometritis
  - Salpingitis
  - Newborn ophthalmic infection
  - Newborn respiratory infection (CDC, 2006a)

Collaborative Practice:
Criteria to Consider for Consultation or Referral
- OB/GYN service
  - For complicated infection, such as with
    - Persistent symptoms
    - Pelvic infection
    - Unresponsive infection
    - Positive HIV or hepatitis B status
    - Persistent pelvic pain
    - Ectopic pregnancy
- Pediatric service
  - Imminent delivery with
    - Chlamydia infection or symptoms
    - Preterm labor
    - Newborn with signs of
      - Chlamydia
      - Ophthalmia neonatorum
      - Pneumonia
- For diagnosis or treatment outside the midwife's scope of practice

CARE OF THE WOMAN UNDERGOING COLPOSCOPY

Key Clinical Information
Colposcopy remains the gold standard for the evaluation of abnormal Pap smear results and genital tract lesions. Colposcopy allows a directed examination of the genital area for areas of abnormality, including the cervix, vagina, and vaginal opening (vulva), using a special binocular microscope (colposcope) to illuminate and magnify the area of examination by 10 to

40 times. During the procedure one or more solutions are applied to the tissues and colored filters may be used to help delineate or highlight abnormal lesions and allow detailed examination. Directed biopsies are then taken from the most abnormal area(s). Neither cytology nor histology reliably predicts the biologic potential of a lesion to progress to invasive cancer (Wright et al., 2007b). A wonderful resource for additional information or education is the American Society for Colposcopy and Cervical Pathology (800-787-7227 or www.asccp.org).

Client History and Chart Review:
Components of the History to Consider
- Age
- Indications for colposcopy (Wright et al., 2007b)
  - ASC-US
    - Recurrent ASC-US
    - High-risk HPV positive
  - ASC-H
  - LSIL
  - Adolescent women younger than age 20 with
    - Persistent ASC-US
    - HSIL
  - HSIL
  - AGC
  - Vulvar or vaginal lesions
- Presence of symptoms
  - Vaginal discharge
  - Postcoital bleeding
  - Postmenopausal bleeding
  - Pelvic pain
- Reproductive history
  - Gravida, para
  - LMP, pregnancy status
  - Method of birth control
  - History of STIs
  - Prior abnormal Pap smears
    - HPV test results
    - Diagnostic procedures
    - Treatment
  - Intermenstrual or postcoital bleeding
- Medical history
  - HIV infection
  - Decreased immune response

- Social history
  - Smoking
  - Diet
  - Support
- Factors that contribute to risk (ACS, 2006a)
  - High-risk HPV infection
  - Multiple sexual partners (self or partner)
  - Unprotected sex
  - Chlamydia
  - Smoking
  - Diet low in fruits and vegetables
  - Low socioeconomic status
  - Grand multipara
  - Immune deficiency
  - Long-term oral contraceptive use
  - Family history
  - Diethylstilbestrol (DES) exposure in utero
- Verify client preparation for procedure
  - Premedication (see below)
  - Informed consent
  - Questions and concerns

Physical Examination:
Components of the Physical Exam to Consider
(Moses, 2007b; Wright & Lickrish, 1989)
- Vulvar examination
  - Apply 5% acetic acid-soaked 4 × 4 pads
    - White vinegar
  - Examine for evidence of potential vulvar intraepithelial lesion (VIN)
    - Pigmented or acetowhite lesions
    - Visible warts
    - Discharge
- Vaginal examination
  - Apply 5% acetic acid wash
  - Examine for evidence of vaginal intra-epithelial lesion (VaIN)
    - Acetowhite lesions
    - Warts or other signs of HPV
    - Punctation and/or mosaicism
  - Visible lesion present
    - Gentle biopsy, or
    - Refer for biopsy
    - Vagina is very thin

- Cervical examination
  - Obtain specimens only if indicated
    - May cause tissue disruption and limit examination
    - Pap smear
    - HPV testing
  - Apply 5% acetic acid wash
    - Examine without magnification
    - Examine colposcopically
      - No filter
      - Green filter
    - Satisfactory examination includes visualization of the
      - Squamocolumnar junction
      - Transformation zone
    - Evaluate lesion(s)
      - Size
      - Location
      - Clarity of margins
      - Thickness of edge
      - Brightness of acetowhite tissue
      - Presence of punctation and/or mosaicism
        - Intercapillary distance
        - Fine versus coarse changes
        - Abnormal vessels
    - Apply Lugol's solution if needed to clarify presence of lesion or borders
    - Obtain biopsies as indicated
      - After biopsies of lesion(s)
      - Ensure hemostasis
        - Pressure
        - Monsel's paste
          - ★ Ferric subsulfate solution
          - ★ Leave open to thicken to paste
        - Silver nitrite application
          - ★ Insert one to three sticks into biopsy wound
          - ★ Apply gentle steady pressure
          - ★ Release pressure
          - ★ Do not pull on sticks
          - ★ Tap gently until sticks spontaneously release
      - Allow patient to rest supine for several minutes

Clinical Impression:
Differential Diagnoses and Code Groups to Consider
Additional suffix or procedure codes may apply (ICD9data.com, 2007)

- Abnormal Pap smear (ICD-9 codes 795)
- HPV (ICD-9 codes 079.4)
  - High risk, DNA test positive (ICD-9 codes 795.05)
  - Low risk, DNA test positive (ICD-9 codes 795.09)
- Condyloma acuminatum (ICD-9 codes 078.11)
- Postcoital bleeding (ICD-9 codes 626.7)
- Postmenopausal bleeding (ICD-9 codes 627.1)
- Leukoplakia of cervix (ICD-9 codes 622.2)
- Vaginal discharge, noninfectious (ICD-9 codes 623.5)
- Cervical dysplasia (ICD-9 codes 622.1)
- Carcinoma in situ of cervix (ICD-9 codes 233.1)
- Procedures (CPT codes apply)
  - Colposcopy, no biopsy
  - Colposcopy, with biopsy
  - Cervical biopsy
  - Endocervical biopsy

Diagnostic Testing:
Diagnostic Tests and Procedures to Consider (Wright et al., 2007b)

- Pap smear—rarely indicated
  - Obtaining may obscure lesion
  - Benefit with HSIL, for correlation of results
- HPV DNA testing
- STI testing per client history
- Biopsies as indicated by colposcopic examination
  - Directed biopsies of lesion(s)
  - Endocervical curettage
    - If unsatisfactory examination or
    - All clients

Providing Treatment:
Therapeutic Measures to Consider

- Treatment options
  - Cryotherapy (ablative therapy)
  - LEEP procedure (excisional therapy)
  - Laser (ablative therapy)
  - Cold knife cone (excisional therapy)
- Treatment triage (Wright et al., 2007b)
  - Client with consistent results
    - No high-risk HPV, no lesion, ASC-US Pap smear
      - No treatment indicated
      - Observation with close follow-up for 2 years
    - ASC-US, ASC-H, LSIL Pap smear
      - Pap, lesion, and biopsy consistent with CIN grade 1
      - Conservative management: close follow-up
      - Ablative treatment acceptable
        - Persistent CIN grade 1 lesion
        - Satisfactory examination
        - Negative endocervical sampling
      - Excisional treatment indicated for
        - Persistent CIN grade 1 lesion
        - Unsatisfactory examination
        - Positive endocervical sampling
        - Previous treatment
    - HSIL or AGC—not otherwise specified (NOS) Pap smear
      - Pap smear, lesion, and biopsy consistent with CIN grade 1
      - Conservative management: close follow-up for 1 year
        - Satisfactory examination, and
        - Negative endocervical sampling
        - Follow-up
          - ★ Pap smear every 6–12 months, *or*
          - ★ HPV test every 12 months
        - Negative follow-up return to routine screening

- ▸ HSIL on follow-up progress to
  - ★ Colposcopy
  - ★ Excisional biopsy
- ➤ Excisional treatment
- ◆ Adolescents with CIN grade 1
  - ➤ Repeat cytology in 12 months
    - ▸ Less than HSIL → 12 months Pap smear
      - ★ Normal Pap smear → routine screening
      - ★ ASC or greater → colposcopy
    - ▸ HSIL → colposcopy
- ◆ Pregnant women with CIN grade 1
  - ➤ Follow without treatment until after delivery
- ◆ CIN grades 2 and 3
  - ➤ Satisfactory colposcopy
    - ▸ Ablative treatment
    - ▸ Excisional treatment
  - ➤ Unsatisfactory colposcopy
    - ▸ Diagnostic excision
  - ➤ Two follow-up options
    - ▸ Cytology every 6 months twice
      - ★ Routine screening after two negative results
      - ★ Colposcopy and endocervical curettage for ASC or greater
    - ▸ HPV DNA testing every 6 months twice
      - ★ Routine screening after two negative results
      - ★ Colposcopy and endocervical curettage for high-risk HPV
  - ➤ Adolescents with CIN grades 2 and 3
    - ▸ Observation or treatment acceptable
    - ▸ Cytology and colposcopy every 6 months
    - ▸ Repeat biopsy for persistent or worsening lesion
    - ▸ Treat for
      - ★ CIN grade 3, *or*
      - ★ CIN grades 2 and 3 that persist ≥ 24 months

Providing Treatment:
Alternative Measures to Consider
- Supplements or food sources for
  - ▪ Folic acid
  - ▪ Vitamins C and E
  - ▪ Selenium
- Whole foods diet, especially
  - ▪ Dark yellow and orange vegetables
    - ◆ Winter squash
    - ◆ Carrots
    - ◆ Rutabaga
  - ▪ Tomatoes
- Support immune system (short-term therapy)
  - ▪ Echinacea
  - ▪ Goldenseal
  - ▪ Yarrow
- Visualization of healing

Providing Support:
Education and Support Measures
to Consider
- Provide information
  - ▪ Indication for colposcopy
  - ▪ Colposcopic procedure
  - ▪ In stirrups with speculum
  - ▪ Takes 5–20 minutes
  - ▪ May cause cramping
  - ▪ Occasional vagal response (syncope)
- Decrease stress during procedure (Galaal, 2007)
  - ▪ Play music during procedure
  - ▪ Use video colposcopy if available
  - ▪ Premedicate with nonsteroidal antiinflam-matory drug (NSAID)
- Postcolposcopy instructions
  - ▪ Brownish discharge common
  - ▪ Vaginal rest for 7 days
  - ▪ Call with bright bleeding
- Postcolposcopy information
  - ▪ Working diagnosis
  - ▪ Anticipated treatment and/or follow-up
  - ▪ Provide written information
    - ◆ Abnormal Pap smears
    - ◆ HPV

- Decrease risk of progression
  - Smoking cessation
  - Healthy diet
  - Safe sex practices

Follow-up Care:
Follow-up Measures to Consider
- Document
  - Indication for colposcopy
  - Findings: pictorial and descriptive
  - Anticipated biopsy result(s)
  - Actual biopsy result(s)
  - Correlate results to formulate plan
    - Pap smear
    - HPV test
    - Clinical picture
    - Biopsy results
- Close follow-up per American Society for Colposcopy and Cervical Pathology recommendations (see Figures 7-11 to 7-16)

Collaborative Practice:
Criteria to Consider for Consultation or Referral
- OB/GYN or colposcopy service
  - Colposcopy not within midwife's scope of practice
  - High-grade lesions
  - Confirmed CIN grades 2 and 3 or greater for treatment
  - Clients with demonstrated progression
  - Noncompliant clients for treatment
  - For management plan for woman in whom results are not consistent
- For diagnosis or treatment outside the midwife's scope of practice

CARE OF THE WOMAN WITH DYSFUNCTIONAL UTERINE BLEEDING

Key Clinical Information
Dysfunctional uterine bleeding (DUB) occurs in approximately 10% of American women at some point in their lives. Anovulation, and the associated unopposed estrogen that results, accounts for nearly 90% of noncyclic bleeding, which occurs primarily in adolescent and perimenopausal women (Dodds & Sinert, 2006). In women with regular ovulatory cycles, the DUB typically occurs secondary to hormone imbalance or in conditions such as thyroid disease, uterine fibroids, or pelvic infection (ACOG, 2000a; Dodds & Sinert, 2006). Investigation into the etiology of heavy, irregular, or intermenstrual bleeding is integral to development of a management plan that is both acceptable to the woman and appropriate for the diagnosis.

Client History and Chart Review:
Components of the History to Consider
(Dodds & Sinert, 2006)
- Age
- Reproductive history
  - Gravida, para
  - Date of LMP, delivery, or abortion
  - Current method of contraception
    - IUDs
    - Hormonal methods
  - History of and risk for STIs
  - Results of prior Pap smears
  - Date of last Pap smear and examination
  - Menstrual history
    - Onset of menarche or menopausal symptoms
    - Usual flow patterns
    - Changes in menses/bleeding
      - Onset, frequency, and duration of bleeding
      - Number of pads/tampons per day
      - Incidence of
        - Clots
        - Heavy blood flow
      - Association of bleeding with
        - Menstrual cycle
        - Intercourse
        - Pain
  - Other associated signs and symptoms
    - Tachycardia
    - Pallor

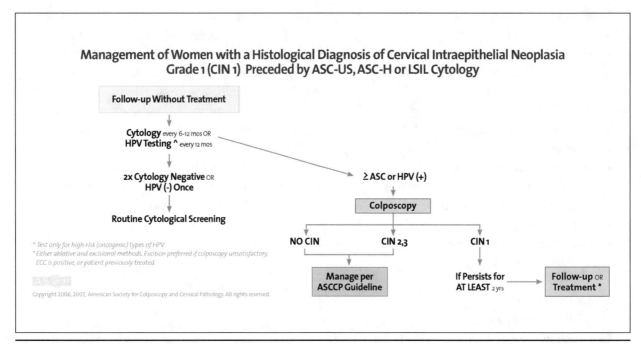

Figure 7-11   *Management of Women with a Histological Diagnosis of Cervical Intraepithelial Neoplasia Grade 1 (CIN 1) Preceded by ASC-US, ASC-H or LSIL Cytology*

Copyright 2006, 2007. American Society for Colposcopy and Cervical Pathology. All rights reserved.

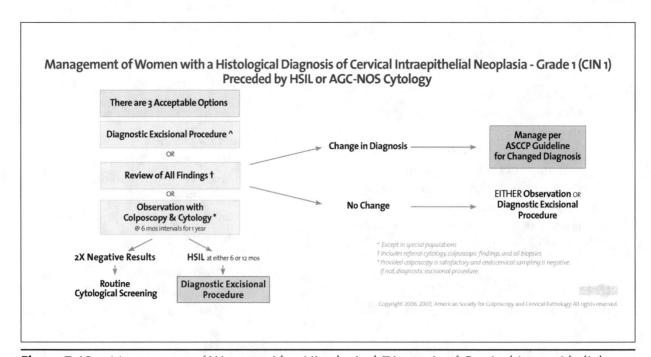

Figure 7-12   *Management of Women with a Histological Diagnosis of Cervical Intraepithelial Neoplasia—Grade 1 (CIN 1) Preceded by HSIL or AGC-NOS Cytology*

Copyright 2006, 2007. American Society for Colposcopy and Cervical Pathology. All rights reserved.

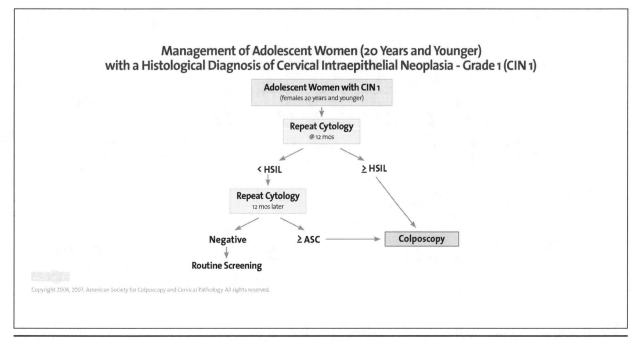

Figure 7-13 *Management of Adolescent Women (20 Years and Younger) with a Histological Diagnosis of Cervical Intraepithelial Neoplasia—Grade 1 (CIN 1)*

Copyright 2006, 2007. American Society for Colposcopy and Cervical Pathology. All rights reserved.

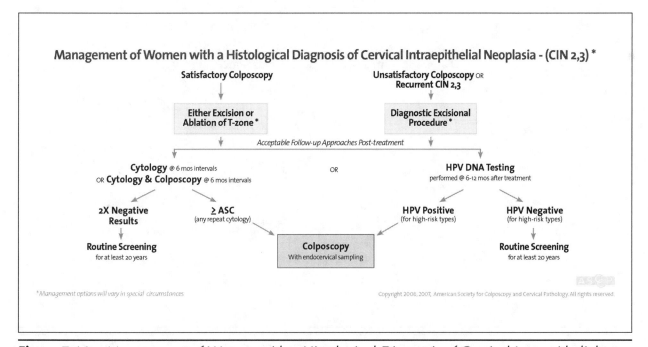

Figure 7-14 *Management of Women with a Histological Diagnosis of Cervical Intraepithelial Neoplasia—(CIN 2,3)*

Copyright 2006, 2007. American Society for Colposcopy and Cervical Pathology. All rights reserved.

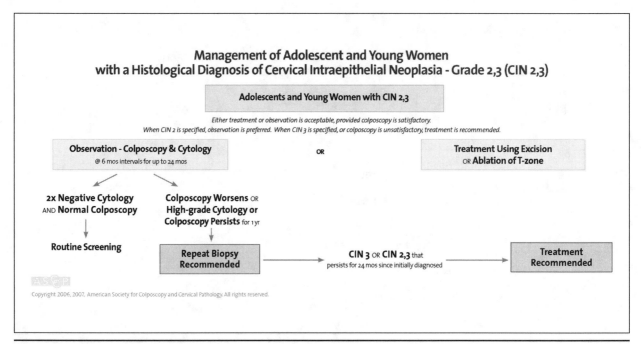

Figure 7-15 *Management of Adolescent and Young Women with a Histological Diagnosis of Cervical Intraepithelial Neoplasia—Grade 2,3 (CIN 2,3)*

Copyright 2006, 2007. American Society for Colposcopy and Cervical Pathology. All rights reserved.

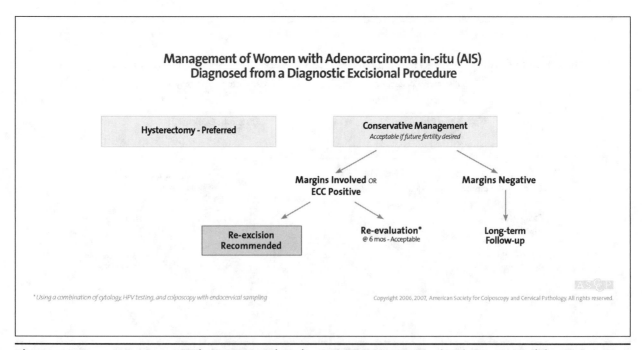

Figure 7-16 *Management of Women with Adenocarcinoma in-situ (AIS) Diagnosed from a Diagnostic Excisional Procedure*

Copyright 2006, 2007. American Society for Colposcopy and Cervical Pathology. All rights reserved.

- ◆ Fatigue, breathlessness
- ◆ Weight changes
- ◆ Change in hair texture or distribution
- ◆ Pain with intercourse
- ◆ Urinary frequency
- ◆ Abdominal bloating
- Medical history
  - ▪ Allergies
  - ▪ Medications
  - ▪ Herbal or over-the-counter remedies
  - ▪ Medical conditions
- Social history
  - ▪ Potential for hypothalamic suppression
    - ◆ Stress
    - ◆ Anorexia
    - ◆ High level of physical activity
- Directed history to potential causes of DUB (Albers et al., 2004; ACOG, 2000a)
  - ▪ Pregnancy related conditions
    - ◆ Spontaneous abortion
    - ◆ Ectopic pregnancy
    - ◆ Placenta previa or abruption
  - ▪ Gynecologic conditions
    - ◆ Infection
    - ◆ Benign lesions, such as fibroids
    - ◆ Trauma
    - ◆ Malignant or premalignant lesions
    - ◆ Polycystic ovary syndrome
  - ▪ Systemic conditions
    - ◆ Thyroid disease
    - ◆ Hypothalamic suppression
    - ◆ Diabetes
    - ◆ Hypertension
    - ◆ Adrenal disorders
    - ◆ Blood dyscrasias and coagulopathies, such as
      - ➤ Von Willebrand's disease
    - ◆ Liver disease
    - ◆ Pituitary adenoma
    - ◆ Kidney disease
  - ▪ Prescription medications
    - ◆ Hormones
    - ◆ Tamoxifen
        - ◆ Selective serotonin reuptake inhibitors
        - ◆ Anticoagulants
        - ◆ Antipsychotics
        - ◆ Corticosteroids
  - ▪ Herbal or over-the-counter remedies
    - ◆ Aspirin
    - ◆ Blue or black cohosh
    - ◆ Ginkgo biloba
    - ◆ Ginseng
    - ◆ Soy
- Review of systems (ROS)

Physical Examination: Components of the Physical Exam to Consider (Albers et al., 2004; Dodds & Sinert, 2006)

- Assess vital signs for
  - ▪ Hypotension
  - ▪ Tachycardia or bradycardia
  - ▪ Subnormal temperature
- Weight: note changes
- Body habitus
- Skin and mucous membranes
  - ▪ Pallor
  - ▪ Dry coarse texture
  - ▪ Diaphoresis
  - ▪ Petechiae
  - ▪ Hirsutism
- Thyroid
  - ▪ Size
  - ▪ Symmetry
  - ▪ Nodules
- Breasts
  - ▪ Presence of galactorrhea
- Speculum examination
  - ▪ Origin of bleeding
  - ▪ Cervix and vagina
    - ◆ Erosion
    - ◆ Lesions
    - ◆ Friability
    - ◆ Presence of IUD strings
  - ▪ Presence of polyps
  - ▪ Evidence of trauma or foreign body

- Bimanual examination
  - Uterine, cervical, and adnexal
    - Position
    - Size
    - Contour
    - Consistency
  - Masses
  - Pain
  - Cervical motion tenderness

Clinical Impression:
Differential Diagnoses and Code Groups
to Consider
Additional suffix may apply (ICD9data.com, 2007)
- Functional DUB (ovarian dysfunction) (ICD-9 codes 256.9)
- Cervicitis (ICD-9 codes 616.0)
- Cervical polyps (ICD-9 codes 622.7)
- Endometrial hyperplasia (ICD-9 codes 621.3)
- Uterine fibroids (ICD-9 codes 218)
- Menorrhagia, primary (ICD-9 codes 626.2)
- Menorrhagia, adolescent (ICD-9 codes 626.3)
- Menorrhagia, perimenopausal (ICD-9 codes 627.0)
- Menorrhagia, postmenopausal (ICD-9 codes 627.1)
- Premature ovarian failure (ICD-9 code 256.31)
- Polycystic ovary syndrome (ICD-9 codes 256.4)
- Thyroid dysfunction (ICD-9 codes 240–246)

Diagnostic Testing:
Diagnostic Tests and Procedures to Consider
(Dodds & Sinert, 2006; Varney et al., 2004)
- Office testing
  - Pregnancy testing
  - Pap smear
  - Chlamydia and/or gonorrhea testing
  - Endometrial biopsy
    - Older than age 35
    - Elevated BMI
    - Polycystic ovarian syndrome (PCOS)
- Endocrine testing
  - Thyroid testing: TSH, thyroid antibodies, T_3, T_4
  - Hormonal evaluation
    - FSH and LH
    - Prolactin (ACOG, 2000a)

- Estradiol
- Testosterone
- Hematology
  - Complete blood count (CBC) with differential
  - Hematocrit and hemoglobin
  - Bleeding time, prothrombin time (PT), partial thromboplastin time (PPT)
- Pelvic imaging
  - Abdominal or vaginal ultrasound
    - Placenta previa
    - Uterine fibroids
    - Thickness of endometrial stripe
    - Intrauterine polyps
    - Ovarian or adnexal masses
  - CT: abdomen and pelvis
- Surgical biopsy methods
  - Saline-infusion sonohysterography
  - Hysteroscopy
  - Dilation and curettage

Providing Treatment:
Therapeutic Measures to Consider (Albers et al., 2004; Dodds & Sinert, 2006)
- Functional DUB (primary ovarian dysfunction)
  - Hyperplasia without atypia on endometrial biopsy
  - NSAIDs
    - Begin 24 hours before menses
    - Continue through menses
      - Naproxen 500 mg PO BID
      - Ponstel 500 mg PO TID
      - Ibuprofen 200–400 mg PO every 4–6 hours
  - Combination hormonal contraceptives
    - 35 microgram oral contraceptive pill
    - One PO two to four times a day for 5–7 days and bleeding controlled
    - Taper to one pill daily
    - Complete 28-day pill pack
    - Continue oral contraceptive pill for 3–6 months
  - Cyclical progestins
    - Begin 14 days before next anticipated menses
    - Provera 5–10 mg/day for 5–10 days/mo

- ◆ Aygestin 2.5–10 mg/day for 5–10 days/mo
- ◆ Prometrium 200 mg for 10–12 days/mo
- ■ Mirena IUD
- ■ Iron replacement therapy
- ⚠ Acute bleeding with DUB
  - ■ 🕑 Refer to emergency services
  - ■ 🕑 IV estrogen to control bleeding
  - ■ 🕑 Surgical treatment measures
    - ◆ Dilation and curettage
    - ◆ Endometrial ablation
    - ◆ Hysterectomy
- 🕑 Additional treatment as indicated by differential diagnosis

Providing Treatment:
Alternative Measures to Consider
- Balanced nutrition
  - ■ Iron foods to treat anemia (see Appendix B-3)
  - ■ Vitamins C and E
  - ■ Bioflavonoids
  - ■ Phytoestrogens
- Moderate physical activity
- Stress management
  - ■ Planned time for
    - ◆ Regular physical activity
    - ◆ Rest and recreation
    - ◆ Personal time
  - ■ Counseling for emotional issues
- Herbal remedies (Davidson, 2006; Soule, 1995)
  - ■ Milk thistle
  - ■ Red raspberry
  - ■ Blue cohosh
  - ■ Shepherd's purse
  - ■ Vitex
- Acupuncture

Providing Support:
Education and Support Measures to Consider
- Client education
  - ■ Normal menstrual functioning
  - ■ Workup related to working diagnosis
- Maintain menstrual calendar

- Results and diagnosis
  - ■ Informed choice regarding treatment options
  - ■ Follow-up plan
  - ■ Treatment instructions
  - ■ When/how to contact for problems
  - ■ Consultation and/or referral criteria

Follow-up Care:
Follow-up Measures to Consider
- Document
  - ■ Working diagnoses
  - ■ Evaluation plan
  - ■ Discussions with client
  - ■ 🔖 Referral criteria
- Return for continued care
  - ■ Hyperplasia (no atypia)
    - ◆ Follow-up endometrial biopsy 6–12 months
  - ■ For persistent or worsening symptoms
  - ■ For support during evaluation and/or treatment
  - ■ For well-woman care after treatment

Collaborative Practice:
Criteria to Consider for Consultation or Referral
(Dodds & Sinert, 2006)
- OB/GYN service
  - ■ Diagnostic testing, such as
    - ◆ Sonohysteroscopy
  - ■ Women with acute bleeding
    - ◆ Hemodynamic stabilization
    - ◆ Parenteral estrogen therapy
    - ◆ Surgical treatment
  - ■ Presence of
    - ◆ Uterine fibroids
    - ◆ Reproductive cancer or precancerous condition
    - ◆ Ectopic pregnancy
    - ◆ Placenta previa
  - ■ DUB
    - ◆ Persistent and progressive bleeding
    - ◆ Unresponsive to herbal or hormone therapy
    - ◆ Unknown cause
  - ■ Client preference

- Medical or endocrinology service
  - Bleeding secondary to
    - Systemic condition
    - Endocrine dysfunction
- For diagnosis or treatment outside the midwife's scope of practice

CARE OF THE WOMAN WITH DYSMENORRHEA

Key Clinical Information

Painful periods may be related to functional uterine contractions or may be caused by endometriosis, infection, hormonal dysfunction, or enlarging uterine fibroids. When dysmenorrhea does not respond to treatment, evaluation for endometriosis should be considered. The pain of endometriosis frequently begins before the onset of menses, unlike physiologic pain, which is caused by uterine contractions expelling the menstrual flow (ACOG, 1999a). Pain with menstruation is often accompanied by heavy flow, headache, diarrhea, or other symptoms and may cause women lost days from work or limit their ability to care for themselves or their family. Careful investigation into this common problem may provide options for relief or a decrease in symptoms.

Client History:
Components of the History to Consider

- Age
  - Common in women aged < 20 years (Varney et al., 2004)
- OB/GYN history
  - Gravida, para, LMP
    - Common in nulliparous women
  - Menstrual history
    - Age of menarche
    - Usual menstrual patterns
    - Age at onset of dysmenorrhea
    - Characteristics of discomfort
      - Location
      - Duration
      - Severity
      - Timing in cycle at onset
      - Association with other body functions
      - Bowel and bladder changes with pain
      - Other associated symptoms
    - Relief measures used and results
    - Impact on life-style and daily functioning
  - Current method of birth control
    - Hormonal contraceptive use
    - IUD use, type
  - PID/STIs
  - Endometriosis
    - Symptoms
    - Diagnosis
  - Previous pelvic surgery
  - Congenital pelvic anomaly
- Medical/surgical history
  - Medications
  - Allergies
  - Health conditions
- Family history
  - Dysmenorrhea
  - Endometriosis
- Social history
  - 🌐 Cultural attitudes regarding menstruation
- Review of systems (ROS)

Physical Examination:
Components of the Physical Exam to Consider

- Vital signs
- Body Mass Index (BMI)
- Abdominal palpation
  - Lower abdominal tenderness
  - Costovertebral angle tenderness
- Pelvic examination
  - Speculum examination
    - Appearance of cervix
    - Appearance of vagina
    - Specimen collection as needed
  - Bimanual examination
    - Uterine size, position, and contour
    - Uterine or cervical motion tenderness
    - Uterine and adnexal mobility
    - Adnexal tenderness
    - Pelvic masses
    - Cystocele or rectocele
- Rectal examination

Clinical Impression:
Differential Diagnoses and Code Groups to Consider
Additional suffix may apply (ICD9data.com, 2007)

- Functional dysmenorrhea (ICD-9 codes 625.3)
- Endometriosis (ICD-9 codes 617)
- PID (ICD-9 codes 614)
- Pelvic anomaly (ICD-9 codes 752)
- Uterine fibroids (ICD-9 codes 218)
- Pelvic organ prolapse (ICD-9 codes 618)
- Premenstrual syndrome (ICD-9 codes 625.4)
- Urinary tract infection (ICD-9 codes 595)
- Bowel disorder or disease (ICD-9 codes 555–569)

Diagnostic Testing:
Diagnostic Tests and Procedures to Consider

- Pap smear
- Chlamydia/gonorrhea testing
- Urinalysis
- Stool for occult blood after rectal examination
- Pelvic ultrasound based on pelvic examination findings

Providing Treatment:
Therapeutic Measures to Consider

- Functional dysmenorrhea
  - Ibuprofen 300–600 mg TID
  - Naproxen 275–500 mg BID
  - Begin 24 hours before menses expected
- Hormonal control
  - Combination hormonal birth control
    - Extended cycling doses
  - Mirena IUD
  - Depoprovesa
- Suspected endometriosis
  - Low-dose birth control pills
    - Regulate menses
    - Diminish symptoms
  - Consider definitive diagnosis and treatment
  - Laparoscopy is used for evaluation and treatment
- Other diagnoses, evaluate and treat as appropriate

Providing Treatment:
Alternative Measures to Consider

- Heat to abdomen
- Balanced diet
  - Vitamin E
  - Decrease salt intake
  - Natural diuretics
    - Tea, coffee
    - Asparagus
  - Plenty of fiber
- Vigorous exercise for endorphin release
- Herbal remedies
  - Vitex tea, tincture or capsules
  - Dandelion root tea or tincture (Soule, 1996, p. 78)
    - Three to five times daily 5 days/wk
    - Continue 1–6 months
    - Safe for use in pregnant and nursing women
  - Evening primrose oil, three to six capsules a day (WholehealthMD.com, 2000)
  - Dong quai tea (not to be used while pregnant or nursing or if menses are excessive)
  - Crampbark tea or tincture, may combine with valerian root

Providing Support:
Education and Support Measures to Consider

- Provide age-appropriate information
  - Reproductive anatomy and physiology
    - Symptoms may improve after pregnancy
    - Teach fertility awareness
      - Foster awareness of cycle
      - NSAID use before onset of menses
  - Working diagnosis
    - Evaluation options
    - Testing and treatment recommendations
    - Self-help measures
    - When to return for care
  - Indications for consult or referral
- Validate client concerns

Follow-up Care:
Follow-up Measures to Consider
- Document
- Return for care
  - After treatment to evaluate effectiveness
  - As indicated by test results
  - For worsening symptoms

Collaborative Practice:
Criteria to Consider for Consultation or Referral
- OB/GYN service
  - For evaluation and treatment of suspected endometriosis
  - For symptoms that do not improve with treatment
  - For abnormal ultrasound, prolapse, or occult bleeding
- For diagnosis or treatment outside the midwife's scope of practice

CARE OF THE WOMAN UNDERGOING ENDOMETRIAL BIOPSY

Key Clinical Information
Endometrial cancer is the most common invasive cancer affecting women (American College of Nurse-Midwives [ACNM], 2001). Diagnosis is made by histology, that is, the microscopic evaluation of an endometrial tissue sample. Evaluation of a woman's uterine endometrium can be easily and safely accomplished in the office setting with endometrial biopsy. This form of tissue sampling is commonly used to evaluate for endometrial hyperplasia, atypia or malignancy. The woman who presents with persistent DUB may also be evaluated using endometrial biopsy (ACOG, 1999a). Evaluation of Pap smear results with endometrial cells or atypical glandular cells (AGC-US) requires endometrial biopsy; however, in these instances endometrial biopsy is best performed in conjunction with colposcopy performed by an expert colposcopist because of the possibility of highly aggressive disease (Wright et al., 2007a). Gentle technique minimizes discomfort during the procedure and aids in preventing complications.

Client History and Chart Review:
Components of the History to Consider
(ACNM, 2001; Grube & McCool, 2004)
- Age
- Gravida, para
- History of cervical trauma
  - May contribute to cervical stenosis
  - Abnormal Pap smear treatment
  - Abortion
  - Dilation and curettage
- Indications for endometrial biopsy
  - DUB
  - Rule out endometrial cancer or premalignant lesions
    - Abnormal uterine bleeding
    - Postmenopausal bleeding
    - Endometrial stripe > 5 mm
  - Infertility investigation
  - Pap smear results with (Wright et al., 2007a)
    - Atypical glandular cells
    - Adenocarcinoma in situ
    - Endometrial cells
- Contraindications for endometrial biopsy
  - Positive HCG or suspected pregnancy
  - Genital tract infection
  - Cervical cancer
- Risk factors for endometrial cancer (ACS, 2006b; ACNM, 2001)
  - Age over 50 years
  - Polycystic ovary syndrome
  - Elevated BMI
  - Prolonged exposure to estrogen
    - Nullipara
    - Unopposed estrogen therapy
    - Delayed menopause (age 52 or older)
  - Diabetes mellitus
  - Tamoxifen
- LMP or menstrual status
  - Luteal phase for infertility investigation
    - Confirmation of ovulation days 22–23
  - Potential for pregnancy
  - Method of birth control if applicable
- Last Pap smear and results

- Medical history
  - Allergies
  - Medications, such as
    - Hormone replacement
    - Hormonal contraception
    - Tamoxifen
    - Aspirin
  - Medical conditions, such as
    - Current undiagnosed fever
    - Bleeding or clotting disorders
    - Heart valve replacement
    - Coronary artery disease
- Verify client preparation
  - Questions or concerns
  - Informed consent obtained
  - Premedication, as needed
  - Nutritional intake
  - Support person available

Physical Examination:
Components of the Physical Exam to Consider
(ACNM, 2001)
- Vital signs pre- and postprocedure
- Bimanual examination
  - Verify size and position of uterus
  - Cervical motion tenderness
- Speculum examination
  - Vaginal or cervical discharge
  - Cervical scarring
- Presence of reproductive tract infection
  - If present treat and reschedule

Clinical Impression:
Differential Diagnoses and Code Groups
to Consider
Additional suffix or procedure codes may apply
(ICD9data.com, 2007)
- Endometrial biopsy, procedure (CPT codes apply)
- Indications
  - Postmenopausal bleeding (ICD-9 codes 627.1)
  - Postmenopausal hormone replacement therapy (ICD-9 codes V07.4)
  - Endometrial hyperplasia (ICD-9 codes 621.3)
  - Persistent DUB (ICD-9 codes 626)
  - Luteal phase defect (ICD-9 codes 256.8)
  - Atypical glandular cells (ICD-9 codes 795.00)

Diagnostic Testing:
Diagnostic Tests and Procedures to Consider
(ACNM, 2001; Grube & McCool, 2004)
- Urine or serum HCG
- Vaginal wet preparation slide
- STI testing
- Pelvic ultrasound
  - Transvaginal
  - Abdominal
- Sonohysteroscopy
- Hysteroscopy with directed biopsy
- Endometrial biopsy procedure
  - Cleanse cervix with prep solution
  - Use careful aseptic technique
  - Apply tenaculum to straighten uterus
    - Apply 20% benzocaine gel to application site if desired
    - Slow application decreases cramping
    - Upper lip of cervix for anteverted/anteflexed uterus
    - Posterior lip of cervix for retroverted/retroflexed uterus
    - Avoid 3 and 9 o'clock positions
  - Apply gentle steady traction to tenaculum
  - Sound uterus
    - Helps to dilate cervix
    - Determines depth of
      - Endometrial cavity
      - Biopsy collection device insertion
    - Gently insert sound or device in direction of uterine curvature
    - Apply gentle pressure at os to relax os
    - When resistance releases
      - Gently advance sound to fundus
      - Do not force sound
      - If perforation occurs, remove sound and do not proceed
      - Remove sound
      - Note centimeter marking on sound

- Insert endometrial biopsy collection device to fundus
  - Determine depth by sound measurement
  - Apply suction according to manufacturer's instructions
  - Rotate 360 degrees while gently moving along length of uterus several times
  - Suction lost when tip removed from uterus
- Deposit specimen into formalin
  - Label formalin container
  - Cut off end of collection device (into formalin)
  - Expel remainder of specimen into formalin
- Remove tenaculum
  - Hemostasis of puncture sites
    - Pressure
    - Silver nitrate
- Assess for
  - Bleeding
  - Vasovagal response
- Allow client to rest supine
- Obtain postprocedure vital signs

Providing Treatment:
Therapeutic Measures to Consider
(Varney et al., 2004)
- Preprocedure medication
  - Ibuprofen 600–800 mg PO
  - One to 2 hours before procedure
- ⚠ Vasovagal syncope
  - Atropine sulfate indicated for heart rate under 40
    - Preferred route is IV but may be given IM
    - Dose: 0.4 mg
  - Be prepared for cardiopulmonary resuscitation
  - 🕐 Call for additional help
- Uterine perforation (Patel, 2005)
  - Rate 1–2/1000 procedures
  - Expectant management
    - Stable, no hemorrhage
    - Empiric antibiotics

- Surgical intervention
  - Unstable, hemorrhage
  - Bowel visible

Providing Treatment:
Alternative Measures to Consider
- ⚠ Alternative measures are not a substitute for evaluation of abnormal uterine bleeding
- Herbal support
  - Red raspberry leaf
  - Yarrow
  - Dong quai (Foster, 1996)
  - Black cohosh
- Homeopathic support
  - Lachesis
  - Natrum muriaticum
  - Sepia

Providing Support:
Education and Support Measures to Consider
- Provide information
  - Potential side effects
    - Cramping
    - Light bleeding
    - Vasovagal syncope
  - Potential complications
    - Cervical stenosis preventing adequate biopsy
    - Uterine perforation
    - Postprocedure infection
- Plan for continued care
  - Obtaining results
  - Warning signs of complications
  - Indications for consultation or referral
  - When to return for care

Follow-up Care:
Follow-up Measures to Consider
- Document procedure, see Procedure Note— Chapter 1
  - Note depth of uterus
  - Client response
  - Adequacy of sample

- Return for continued care
  - As indicated by biopsy results
  - Treatment based on diagnosis
  - With bleeding, pain, or fever
  - Recurrent or unresolved symptoms
- Interpretation of results
  - Negative findings
    - Atrophic endometrium
    - Proliferative endometrium
    - Secretory endometrium
  - Positive findings
    - Luteal phase defect
    - Simple or complex hyperplasia (no atypia)
    - Simple or complex hyperplasia with atypia
    - Endometrial adenocarcinoma

Collaborative Practice:
Criteria to Consider for Consultation
or Referral

- OB/GYN service
  - Cervical stenosis
  - Uterine perforation
  - Treatment recommendations
  - Diagnostic testing
    - Sonohysteroscopy
    - Hysteroscopy with directed biopsy
  - Postprocedure infection
  - Pathology result diagnostic of
    - Endometrial hyperplasia
    - Endometrial atypia
    - Endometrial cancer
- Medical service
  - Clearance for clients with
    - Valve replacement
      - Antibiotic prophylaxis recommendations
    - Coronary artery disease
  - Follow-up of clients with coronary artery disease or significant vagal response
- For diagnosis or treatment outside the midwife's scope of practice

CARE OF THE WOMAN WITH ENDOMETRIOSIS

Key Clinical Information

Endometriosis is a combination endocrine and immune disorder (Ballweg, 2005) characterized by implants of endometrial tissue outside the uterus that form in response to multiple genetic, hormonal, environmental, and immune factors (Brinton, 2005). Endometriosis implants may affect the reproductive organs, the bowel, the bladder, and the pelvic side-walls (ACOG, 1999a) and are linked to higher than expected rates of reproductive cancer (Brinton, 2005). Endometriosis is found in 5–20% of women of reproductive age during pelvic laparoscopy. As many as one-third of these women have endometriosis-related infertility, second only to tubal causes of infertility (Brinton, 2005). Moderate to severe pain is the primary presenting complaint in women with endometriosis. Pelvic laparoscopy is used to diagnose and treat endometriosis in an effort to reduce symptoms and improve fertility (Ballweg, 2005).

Client History and Chart Review:
Components of the History to Consider

- Age
- OB/GYN history
  - Gravida, para
  - Menstrual history
    - Age at menarche
    - LMP
    - Usual menstrual patterns
  - Sexual activity
    - Contraception
      - Hormonal contraceptives
      - IUD
    - STIs
- Onset, duration, and frequency of symptoms
  - Age at onset of symptoms
  - Presence of symptoms related to endometriosis (ACOG, 1999a; Ballweg, 2005)
    - Significant cyclic pre- and peri-menstrual pain
      - Onset in adolescence common
      - Limits ability to perform daily activities

- ◆ Dyspareunia
- ◆ DUB
- ◆ Infertility
- ◆ Effect on bowel and bladder function
  - ➤ Diarrhea or gastrointestinal upset with menses
  - ➤ Urinary urgency or frequency
- ◆ Other symptoms
  - ➤ Fatigue, exhaustion
  - ➤ Associated with increased allergic responses
  - ■ Relief measures used and their effect
- • Medical/surgical history
  - ■ Allergies
    - ◆ Environment
    - ◆ Food
    - ◆ Atopic
  - ■ Medications
  - ■ Cystitis
  - ■ Pelvic surgery
  - ■ Diverticular disease
  - ■ Appendicitis
- • Family history
  - ■ Prenatal exposure
    - ◆ Diethylstilbestrol exposure
    - ◆ Dioxin
  - ■ Dysmenorrhea
  - ■ Infertility
  - ■ Endometriosis
  - ■ Diabetes
  - ■ Bowel disorders
- • Social history
  - ■ Risk factors for
    - ◆ PID
    - ◆ Ectopic
- • Review of systems (ROS)

Physical Examination:
Components of the Physical Exam to Consider
- • Vital signs
- • Weight/BMI
- • Body habitus
- • Thyroid

- • Abdominal examination
  - ■ Tenderness
  - ■ Rebound
  - ■ Guarding
  - ■ Masses
- • Speculum examination
  - ■ Cervical discharge
- • Bimanual examination
  - ■ Uterine position, size, and consistency
  - ■ Cervical motion tenderness
  - ■ Adnexal size, location, and tenderness
    - ◆ Mobility
    - ◆ Masses
- • Findings suggestive of endometriosis
  - ■ Fixed, retroverted uterus
  - ■ Adnexal thickening, nodularity, or irregularity
  - ■ Limited mobility of
    - ◆ Uterus
    - ◆ Adnexa

Clinical Impression:
Differential Diagnoses and Code Groups
to Consider
Additional suffix may apply (ICD9data.com, 2007)
- • Pelvic pain (ICD-9 codes 625.9) secondary to
  - ■ Endometriosis (ICD-9 codes 617)
  - ■ Fibroid uterus (ICD-9 codes 218)
  - ■ Salpingitis (ICD-9 codes 614)
  - ■ Ectopic pregnancy (ICD-9 codes 633)
  - ■ Interstitial cystitis (ICD-9 codes 595.1)
  - ■ Appendicitis (ICD-9 codes 540–543)
  - ■ Abdominal adhesions (ICD-9 codes 568) related to
    - ◆ PID
    - ◆ Pelvic surgery
    - ◆ Peritonitis
    - ◆ Diverticular disease

Diagnostic Testing:
Diagnostic Tests and Procedures to Consider
(Metzger, 2005)
- • STI testing
- • Hepatitis C

- HIV
- Mycoplasma
- Epstein-Barr virus
- CBC
- TSH, thyroid antibodies, T_3, free T_4
- Fasting blood sugar
- Pelvic ultrasound
  - May be suggestive of endometriosis
  - May demonstrate endometrioma
  - Used to rule out other differential diagnoses
- Laparoscopy to confirm diagnosis (ACOG, 1999a)
  - Visualization of pelvis
  - Tissue sample for histology

Providing Treatment:
Therapeutic Measures to Consider
- Symptomatic treatment while awaiting diagnosis
  - Anti-inflammatory medication
    - Naproxen sodium
    - Ponstel
- Ovulation suppression (ACOG, 1999a)
  - Oral/hormonal contraceptives
  - Progestins, including Mirena IUD
  - Danazol
  - Gonadotropin-releasing hormone (GnRH) analogues
- Laparoscopy for diagnosis and preliminary treatment
  - Ablation of endometrial implants
- Persistent symptoms (ACOG, 1999a)
  - Continue medications
  - Surgical treatment
    - Retreat with ablative therapy
    - Hysterectomy with oophorectomy

Providing Treatment:
Alternative Measures to Consider
- Dietary (Metzger, 2005)
  - Shiitake mushroom
  - Low-glycemic diet

- Essential fatty acids
  - Fish oil
  - Primrose oil
  - Borage oil
- Vitamin/mineral supplements
  - Vitamins C and E
  - Vitamin B complex
  - Magnesium
- Live culture yogurt or probiotics
- Digestive enzymes
- Limit dairy and meat
- Avoid food allergens
- Symptomatic treatment (see Care of the Woman with Dysmenorrhea)
  - Local heat
  - Castor oil packs
  - Heating pad
  - Massage
  - Acupuncture
- Stress reduction
  - Yoga
  - Meditation

Providing Support:
Education and Support Measures
to Consider
- Encourage participation in evaluation and treatment process
  - Active listening
  - Women may opt to live with symptoms
- Provide information
  - Endometriosis
  - Endometriosis Association (800-992-3636 or http://www.endometriosisassn.org)
  - Fertility awareness
  - Evaluation process
  - Potential modes of treatment
- Indications for surgery (Nezhat, 2005)
  - Diagnosis
    - Severe endometriosis
    - Infertility
    - Failed medical management

- Surgical options
    - ◆ Conservative surgery
        - ➤ Ablation or excision of implants
            - ▸ Laser
            - ▸ Cautery
            - ▸ Scalpel
        - ➤ Lysis of adhesions
        - ➤ Resection of endometriomas
        - ➤ Pregnancy rates after surgery 5–50%
        - ➤ Recurrence rates 10–44%
    - Definitive treatment
        - ◆ Hysterectomy with bilateral salpingo-oophorectomy

Follow-up Care:
Follow-up Measures to Consider
- Document
    - Criteria used for diagnosis
    - Discussions with client
    - Treatment plan
- Return for care
    - As needed during diagnosis and/or treatment
    - For well-woman care
    - With pregnancy

Collaborative Practice:
Criteria to Consider for Consultation or Referral
- OB/GYN service
    - Suspected endometriosis
    - Persistent pelvic pain
    - Pain accompanied by bowel or bladder involvement
    - Pain accompanied by fever or elevated white blood cells
- For diagnosis or treatment outside the midwife's scope of practice

CARE OF THE WOMAN WITH UTERINE FIBROIDS

Key Clinical Information
Fibroids are a common benign tumor of the uterus affecting over 30% of women (Indman, 2006). Fibroids may enlarge continuously in the premenopausal woman and typically regress during menopause. Fibroids occur as a result of the effects of growth factors and hormonal influences in women with a genetic predisposition or mutation that stimulates the overgrowth of uterine muscle cells (Wallach & Vlahos, 2004). Fibroids are classified by location and may occur in multiple locations in the uterus: the fundus, the wall of the uterus, inside the uterus, or the cervix. Current uterine-sparing treatments are based primarily on relieving symptoms: pain, bleeding, abdominal enlargement, and infertility (ACOG, 1999b; Indman, 2006). Although fibroids are most often benign, there is a small risk of malignancy developing, and women with uterine fibroids have an associated higher incidence of uterine malignancy (Brinton et al., 2005).

Client History and Chart Review:
Components of the History to Consider
- Age, gravida, para
- OB/GYN history
    - LMP and menstrual status
    - Menstrual history
        - ◆ Duration, frequency, and length
        - ◆ Amount of flow
        - ◆ Dysmenorrhea
        - ◆ Intermenstrual bleeding
    - Previous clinical findings
        - ◆ Uterine size and contour
        - ◆ Previous pelvic ultrasounds
    - Reproductive problems
        - ◆ DUB
        - ◆ Infertility
    - Hormone use
        - ◆ Contraception
        - ◆ Hormone replacement
- Current symptoms
    - Onset, duration, severity
- Symptoms of uterine fibroids
    - Pelvic pressure or pain
        - ◆ Suprapubic pain
        - ◆ Lower back pain
    - Abdominal enlargement
        - ◆ Rapid enlargement suggests malignancy
        - ◆ Pressure may result in lower limb
            - ➤ Varicosities
            - ➤ Edema

- Changes in bowel or bladder function
  - Urinary frequency
  - Constipation
  - Menorrhagia with anemia
  - Pregnancy losses
- Risk factors for uterine myoma (Faerstein et al., 2001)
  - African-American ethnicity
  - Late reproductive and perimenopausal women
  - Early menarche
  - Elevated BMI
  - Family history of uterine myoma
- Medical history
- Review of systems (ROS)

Physical Examination:
Components of the Physical Exam to Consider

- Vital signs, including blood pressure and weight
- Abdominal examination
  - Fundal height
  - Abdominal girth
- Pelvic examination
  - Cervical or vaginal discharge
  - Uterine
    - Size and position
    - Contour
    - Consistency
  - Cervical motion tenderness
  - Presence of adnexal
    - Masses or fullness
    - Pain
- Rectal or rectovaginal examination
  - Rectal lesions
  - Palpate posterior uterus
  - Stool for occult blood

Clinical Impression:
Differential Diagnoses and Code Groups to Consider
Additional suffix may apply (ICD9data.com, 2007)

- Enlarged uterus (ICD-9 codes 621.2)
- Uterine fibroids (ICD-9 codes 218)

- Pregnancy (ICD-9 codes V22)
- Menorrhagia, premenopausal (ICD-9 codes 627.0)
- Postmenopausal bleeding (ICD-9 codes 627.1)
- Gastrointestinal bleeding (ICD-9 codes 578.1)
- Anemia, iron deficiency (ICD-9 codes 280)

Diagnostic Testing:
Diagnostic Tests and Procedures to Consider (Indman, 2006)

- Pelvic ultrasound
  - Vaginal
  - Abdominal
- CBC
- Hemoglobin and hematocrit
- Hemoccult
- Hysteroscopy or sonohysteroscopy
- Endometrial biopsy
- Lesion biopsy

Providing Treatment:
Therapeutic Measures to Consider

- Hormonal regulation of menses
  - May inhibit development of myoma
- Iron supplementation as indicated (Murphy, 2004)
  - Ferro-Sequels 1–2 PO daily
  - Niferex 150 1–2 PO daily
  - Ferrous gluconate 1–2 PO daily
- Fertility-sparing treatments (Parker, 2007)
  - Watchful waiting
  - Myomectomy (ACOG, 1999b)
    - Excision of fibroid(s)
    - Retains fertility
    - Uterine scarring may require cesarean
    - Approaches
      - Hysteroscopic
      - Laparoscopic
      - Abdominal
- Medical therapy
  - Lupron Depot (Murphy, 2004; National Institutes of Health, 2005)
    - Short-term treatment
    - Indicated to decrease myoma before surgery

- Dosing
  - 3.75 mg IM monthly for 3 months, *or*
  - 11.25 mg IM for 1 month (lasts 3 months)
  - ⚠ Contraindicated for women with
    - Undiagnosed uterine bleeding
    - Pregnancy
  - May cause vasomotor symptoms
- Endometrial ablation
- Uterine artery embolization or occlusion (National Institutes of Health, 2005)
- Hysterectomy
  - Indications
    - Grossly enlarged uterus
    - Degenerative fibroids
    - Potential or suspected malignancy
    - Severe menorrhagia
    - Client preference
  - Methods
    - Abdominal
    - Vaginal
    - Laparoscopic

Providing Treatment:
Alternative Measures to Consider
- Vitex tea, tincture or capsules
- Dietary sources of iron replacement (see Appendix B-3)
  - Floradix iron supplement
- Avoid phytoestrogens
- Homeopathic remedies (Smith, 1984)
  - Aurum muriaticum natronatum
  - Belladonna
  - Calcarea iodata
  - Tarentula hispana

Providing Support:
Education and Support Measures to Consider
- Discussion regarding
  - Clinical findings
  - Recommended testing

- Planned follow-up
- Medications recommended
  - Indications
  - Side effects
  - Anticipated results
- Warning signs
  - Excessive bleeding
  - Pain
  - Change in bowel or bladder function
- Active listening to elicit
  - Concerns
  - Family/personal support
  - Coping mechanisms
- Provide information and support if surgery indicated
  - Preoperative testing
  - Anticipated hospital stay
  - Self-care after discharge
  - Allow grieving
    - Loss of fertility/body part
    - Body image changes with surgery
    - Potential perceived loss of femininity

Follow-up Care:
Follow-up Measures to Consider
- Document
  - Findings
  - Diagnostic test results
  - Discussions with client
  - Management plan
- Return for care
  - Reevaluation of uterine size
    - Annual or semiannual
    - Serial ultrasound sizing
    - Change in bleeding pattern
    - Progression of symptoms
  - Assess for uterine malignancy
    - Women with documented myoma and intact uterus
  - Preoperative history and physical, as needed
  - Informed consent as indicated for
    - Lupron Depot
    - Operative procedures

Collaborative Practice:
Criteria to Consider for Consultation
or Referral

- OB/GYN service
  - Grossly enlarged uterus
  - Severe or progressive symptoms
  - Evidence or suspicion of malignancy
  - Client preference
- Social service support, as needed
- For diagnosis or treatment outside the midwife's scope of practice

CARE OF THE WOMAN WITH GENITAL CANDIDIASIS

Key Clinical Information

Genital candidiasis is so common that many women assume that every form of vaginitis is a "yeast infection." *Candida* yeasts are part of the normal vaginal flora. Changes to the balance of the vaginal environment that affect the acidity or hormonal balance often result in overgrowth of *Candida* (CDC, 2005). Candidal vulvovaginitis has many different appearances, from curdy white vaginal discharge to the excoriated skin creases common in diabetic women with chronically elevated blood glucose levels. Careful attention to the microscopic evaluation of the wet preparation is necessary to determine the presence of yeast and to confirm the absence of additional causes of vaginitis.

Client History and Chart Review:
Components of the History to Consider

- Age
- Reproductive health history
  - Gravida, para, LMP
    - Current method of birth control, or
    - Gestation
  - Sexual practices
    - Change in sexual partners/habits
    - Anal/vaginal intercourse
    - Sex toys, use and care of
  - Douching/genital hygiene

- Problem history
  - Exacerbating factors
    - Menses
    - Intercourse
  - Symptoms
    - Onset, location, and duration
    - Common description (CDC, 2005)
      - Intense itching
      - Curdy discharge
      - Moist raw skin
      - Other associated symptoms
        - Burning with urination
        - Pain with intercourse
  - Treatments tried and efficacy
  - Associated with (CDC, 2005)
    - Pregnancy
    - Diabetes
    - Antibiotic therapy
- Medical/surgical history
  - Allergies
  - Medications
    - Antibiotic use
    - Steroid use
  - Chronic illness
    - Diabetes or gestational diabetes
    - Immunocompromised condition
      - HIV/acquired immunodeficiency syndrome (AIDS)
      - Cancer
- Social history
  - Use of tight or damp clothing
  - Stress

Physical Examination:
Components of the Physical Exam
to Consider

- Pelvic examination
  - Presence of red excoriated external genitalia
  - White, adherent, curdy discharge within vagina
  - Collect vaginal discharge specimen for provider performed microscopy

- Assess for signs of monilia
  - On skin folds
  - Cutaneous infection
  - Oral cavity
- Observe for signs or symptoms of STIs

Clinical Impression:
Differential Diagnoses and Code Groups
to Consider

Additional suffix may apply (ICD9data.com, 2007)

- Vulvovaginal candidiasis (ICD-9 codes 112.1)
- Oral candidiasis (thrush) (ICD-9 codes 112.0)
- Intertriginous candidiasis (ICD-9 codes 112.3)
- Vulvovaginitis, unspecified (ICD-9 codes 616.10)
- Bacterial vaginosis (ICD-9 codes 616.10)
- Trichomoniasis (ICD-9 codes 131)
- Vulvar vestibulitis or vulvodynia (ICD-9 codes 625)
- Chlamydia (ICD-9 codes 099.5)
- Gonorrhea (ICD-9 codes 098)
- Chronic cervicitis (ICD-9 codes 616.0)
- Foreign body, vaginal (ICD-9 codes 939.2)
- Impetigo (ICD-9 codes 684)

Diagnostic Testing:
Diagnostic Tests and Procedures to Consider

- Wet preparation; provider performed microscopy (American College of Physicians, 1998; Varney et al., 2004)
  - Saline
    - Mycelia
    - Branching hyphae
    - White blood cells
    - 10× and 40× magnification
  - KOH slide
    - Negative whiff test
    - Budding yeast
    - 10× magnification
- Vaginal pH testing
  - pH 3.8–4.5
  - pH > 4.5
    - Bacterial vaginosis (BV)
    - Trichomoniasis

- Severe or recurrent infection
  - Fasting blood sugar
  - HIV testing (CDC, 2004c)
  - Culture of skin exudate
- Other STI testing as indicated by history

Providing Treatment:
Therapeutic Measures to Consider

- Diflucan
  - 150 mg PO for one or two doses
  - Pregnancy Category C
- Terconazole
  - Three- or 7-day therapy
  - Pregnancy Category C
- Nystatin vaginal tablets
  - One tablet per vagina for 14 days
  - Pregnancy Category A
- Monistat Derm for cutaneous symptoms (Murphy, 2004)
- Over-the-counter antifungals
  - Tioconazole (Vagistat vaginal)
  - Miconazole (Monistat)
  - Clotrimazole (Gyne-Lotrimin, Mycelex)
  - Butoconazole (Femstat)

Providing Treatment:
Alternative Measures to Consider

- Dietary support
  - Cranberries or cranberry juice
  - Yogurt or acidophilus capsules
  - Probiotics 4–8 billion units/day
- Tub bath with 1 cup vinegar in water
- Vaginal treatments
  - Acidophilus capsules 1 per vagina at bedtime for 5–7 days
  - Boric acid capsules 1 per vagina at bedtime for 5–7 days; ⚠ poisonous if taken orally!
  - Herbal douche two times a week (use acidophilus capsules other nights)
    - 1 T tea tree oil
    - 2 T cider vinegar
    - 2 cups warm water
  - Black walnut tincture

- Sage
- Oregano
- Olive leaf

Providing Support:
Education and Support Measures to Consider
- Medication instructions
  - Take complete course of medication
  - Avoid intercourse while using medication
- General hygiene
  - Wipe front to back after toileting
  - Promptly change out of damp clothing or swimsuits
  - Wear loose well-ventilated clothing
- After bathing
  - Dry genital region thoroughly before dressing (use blow dryer on cool setting)
  - Wear cotton panties, loose clothing (boxer shorts are good)
- Avoid
  - Excessive sugar or alcohol in diet
  - Douching
  - Products containing perfume or deodorant, such as
    - Bubble bath
    - Feminine hygiene sprays
    - Tampons or sanitary pads
    - Toilet paper

Follow-up Care:
Follow-up Measures to Consider
- Document
  - Wet preparation and pH findings
- Return for care
  - Symptoms not improved within 5–7 days
  - For additional testing
    - Consider vaginal culture
  - As indicated by other test results

Collaborative Practice:
Criteria to Consider for Consultation or Referral
- OB/GYN service
  - Recurrent or unresponsive infection

- Medical service
  - For fasting glucose over 126 g/dl (diagnostic of diabetes)
  - Positive HIV titer
  - Evidence of immunocompromise
- For diagnosis or treatment outside the midwife's scope of practice

CARE OF THE WOMAN WITH GONORRHEA

Key Clinical Information
Gonorrhea is often accompanied by chlamydia or trichomoniasis and may infect eyes, mouth, and joints as well as the reproductive tract. Significant effects of gonococcal infections include infertility, premature rupture of membranes, preterm labor, and infection of the newborn's eyes resulting in blindness if left untreated. Gonorrhea, like other STIs, may increase the transmission risk of those exposed to HIV infection. Fluoroquinolone-resistant gonorrhea is now widespread throughout the United States, prompting the CDC to change its recommendations for use of this class of antimicrobials for the treatment of gonorrhea (CDC, 2007a). The CDC STI treatment guidelines may be downloaded to a hand-held device from the CDC Web site (www.cdc.gov).

Client History:
Components of the History to Consider
- Age
- Reproductive history
  - Gravida, para, LMP
    - Potential for pregnancy
    - Birth control method
  - Review previous history
    - Pap smear
    - STI testing
    - STI treatments
  - Sexual history
    - Sexual practices
      - Long-term mutually monogamous relationship
      - Multiple partners for self or partner(s)

- ➤ Vaginal, oral, anal intercourse
- ➤ Condom use
    - ▸ Male condom
    - ▸ Female condom
- Problem-focused history
    - Onset, duration, and severity of symptoms
    - Last unprotected intercourse
    - Symptom profile for gonorrhea
        - ◆ May be asymptomatic
        - ◆ Urinary frequency and dysuria
        - ◆ Urethritis
        - ◆ Vaginal or anal discharge
        - ◆ Sore throat
        - ◆ Pelvic inflammation (PID)
            - ➤ Pain with intercourse
            - ➤ Genital pain and discharge
            - ➤ Fever
            - ➤ Lower abdominal pain
            - ➤ Intermenstrual bleeding
            - ➤ Painful bowel movements
- Medical/surgical history
    - Allergies
    - Medications
    - Chronic health conditions
- Social history
    - Behavioral risk factors
    - Alcohol/drug use
    - Exposure to more than five sexual partners
    - Male partner who is bisexual
    - Social support
    - Access to health care
- Review of systems (ROS)

Physical Examination:
Components of the Physical Exam to Consider
- Vital signs, including temperature
    - Temperature > 38°C suspicious for PID
- Pelvic examination (Varney et al., 2004)
    - Bartholin's gland, urethra, and Skene's gland (BUS) for evidence of
        - ◆ Discharge
        - ◆ Inflammation
    - Vaginal, cervical, or anal discharge
        - ◆ Yellow or mucopurulent

- ▪ Evidence of PID
    - ◆ Pain on cervical motion
    - ◆ Adnexal or uterine tenderness
    - ◆ Lower abdominal pain
    - ◆ Presence of inflammatory mass on pelvic examination

Clinical Impression:
Differential Diagnoses and Code Groups
to Consider
Additional suffix may apply (ICD9data.com, 2007)
- Gonorrhea (ICD-9 codes 098)
- Chlamydia (ICD-9 codes 099.50)
- PID (ICD-9 codes 614–616)
- Endometriosis (ICD-9 codes 617)
- Ectopic pregnancy (ICD-9 codes 633)
- Ovarian cyst (ICD-9 codes 620)
- Cervicitis (ICD-9 codes 616.0)
- Cervical cancer (ICD-9 codes 180)
- Irritable bowel (ICD-9 codes 564.1)
- Appendicitis (ICD-9 codes 540–543)

Diagnostic Testing:
Diagnostic Tests and Procedures
to Consider
- Gonorrhea testing (Payne, 2003)
    - Gram stain
    - Positive gram stain
        - ◆ Gram-negative intracellular diplococci
        - ◆ 10 white blood cells per high-power field
    - Culture
        - ◆ DNA probe
        - ◆ Enzyme-linked immunosorbent assay (antigen specific)
        - ◆ Nucleic acid amplification tests
- Chlamydia testing
- Wet preparation
- Pelvic ultrasound
    - Presence of inflammatory mass
- CBC with sedimentation rate
    - Sedimentation rate > 15 mm/hr suspicious
- HIV counseling and testing
- ⚠ Note: The vaginal discharge and visual inspection of the discharge is nonspecific and

cannot be used alone for diagnosis. Multiple pathogens may be present. Perform additional testing as required for accurate diagnosis.

Providing Treatment:
Therapeutic Measures to Consider
- Begin treatment based on symptoms
- CDC recommendations for uncomplicated gonorrhea (CDC, 2007a)
  - One-time dosing
    - Provided on site
    - Compliance assured by direct observation
  - Cefixime 400 mg PO (Pregnancy Category B), or
  - Ceftriaxone 125 mg IM (Pregnancy Category B)
    - 1% lidocaine as diluent to reduce injection pain
  - *Plus*, treatment for chlamydia if it has not been ruled out
- Alternate regimens
  - Ceftizoxime 500 mg IM, *or*
  - Cefoxitin 2 g IM, administered with probenecid 1 g orally, *or*
  - Cefotaxime 500 mg IM
  - *Plus*, treatment for chlamydia if it has not been ruled out
- If chlamydia has not been ruled out, add
  - Azithromycin 1 g PO (Pregnancy Category B), *or*
  - Doxycycline 100 mg PO (Pregnancy Category D) BID for 7 days
- Pharyngeal infection
  - Ceftriaxone 125 mg IM (Pregnancy Category B)
  - 1% lidocaine used as diluent to reduce injection pain
  - *Plus,* treat for chlamydia if it has not been ruled out

Providing Treatment:
Alternative Measures to Consider
- ⚠ Alternative therapies are not a substitute for medical treatment

- Supportive measures to promote healing
  - Adequate rest
  - Sitz baths with comfrey leaf tea or Epsom salts
  - Nutritional support
    - Balanced diet
      - ➤ Live culture yogurt
      - ➤ Blue-green algae
      - ➤ Vitamins C and E
- Herbal support formulas (Soule, 1995)
  - Adjunct to medical therapy
  - Use two to three times daily
  - Prepare as tea or tincture
    - Red clover—2 parts
    - Calendula—2 parts
    - Yarrow—1 part
    - Dandelion root—1 part
- Homeopathic remedies
  - Adjunct to medical therapy
  - Use 30× grains three times daily
    - Arnica montana (promotes soft tissue healing)
    - Mercurius solubilis (to offset side effects of antibiotic treatment)
- Acidophilus capsules per vagina to prevent yeast overgrowth

Providing Support:
Education and Support Measures
to Consider
- Diagnosis
  - Potential sequelae
  - Treatment recommendations
  - Partner notification
  - State reporting requirements
  - Symptoms of acute PID
- Treatment instructions
  - Avoid sexual relations
    - Until treatment is completed
    - Symptoms have resolved
    - Partner treatment completed
- When and how to access care
- STI transmission and prevention

Follow-up Care:
Follow-up Measures to Consider

- Document
  - Confirmation of diagnosis
  - Medication administration
  - Epidemiologic reporting
- Indications to return for care (CDC, 2006a)
  - Symptoms of acute PID
  - Persistent symptoms
    - Reinfection
    - Drug-resistant organism
    - Noninfectious process
- Repeat testing
  - Persistent symptoms
  - New partner for self or partner
- Offer HIV and other STI counseling and testing

Collaborative Practice:
Criteria to Consider for Consultation or Referral

- OB/GYN service or STI clinic
  - Signs and symptoms of PID
  - Client requiring hospitalization
  - Gonorrhea infection with
    - Symptoms of meningitis
    - Disseminated infection
- Social services
- For diagnosis or treatment outside the midwife's scope of practice

CARE OF THE WOMAN WITH HUMAN IMMUNODEFICIENCY VIRUS

Key Clinical Information

Human immunodeficiency virus (HIV) infection of women in the United States continues to rise (National Institute of Allergy and Infectious Diseases [NIAID], 2006). Although HIV affects women of all ages, races, and backgrounds, HIV/AIDS affects a greater percentage of African-American and Hispanic women (CDC, 2007b). HIV is transmitted to women during insertion intercourse, oral/genital, or digital/genital contact with an infected sexual partner and through HIV-contaminated needles during IV drug use. Most women contract HIV infection through heterosexual contact, whether consensual or involuntary (CDC, 2007b; NIAID, 2006). Transmission is enhanced when the HIV-exposed woman is menstruating or has breaks in the skin or mucous membrane, such as occurs with ulcerative STIs or trauma. A lack of access to early diagnosis and adequate treatment, including during pregnancy, further contributes to increases in HIV progression among women and infection in newborns (NIAID, 2006). Prompt treatment improves survival rates considerably, stimulating the CDC to recommend routine HIV screening of adult adolescents and pregnant women (CDC, 2006d).

Not all exposed women contract HIV; genetic and/or immunologic factors may protect against HIV infection (Hessol et al., 2005). Promising new research is directed toward the effectiveness of vaginal topical microbicides, which disrupt attachment of the virus to the vaginal wall (NIAID, 2006). Effective topical microbicides provide women with a means to protect themselves from exposure by offering an HIV protection measure that does not rely on partner participation, knowledge, or acceptance. Multiple HIV prevention vaccines (for use in HIV-negative clients) and therapeutic HIV vaccines (to improve the immune system of HIV-positive individuals) are currently undergoing clinical trials (Johnson & Fauci, 2007).

Client History and Chart Review:
Components of the History to Consider (CDC, 2006d, 2007b; Varney et al., 2004)

- Age
- Obstetric/gynecologic and sexual history
  - LMP and contraception method
    - Pregnancy status
  - Previous diagnosis and/or treatment
    - STIs
    - Abnormal cervical cytology
  - HIV risk assessment
    - HIV knowledge and perception of risk
    - Current HIV prevention behaviors
    - Previous HIV screening

- Risk factors for HIV infection (CDC, 2007b)
  - Younger age (15–39)
  - Black or Hispanic ethnicity
  - Lack of awareness of partner's risk factors
  - Substance abuse/IV drug abuse
  - Sexual inequality resulting in
    - Nonconsensual sex
    - Lack of condom use
  - Sex with incarcerated male(s)
  - Risk factors for HIV-1 infection
    - Client or partner with more than five partners
    - Diagnosis or symptoms of any STI
    - IV drug use, self or partner
    - Exposure to blood or body fluids
  - Risk factors for HIV-2 infection
    - Travel or residence in HIV-2 endemic areas
      - West Africa
      - Angola
      - France
      - Mozambique
      - Portugal
    - Clinical evidence of HIV infection with negative HIV-1 test
- Medical/surgical history
  - Allergies
  - Medications
  - Chronic diseases or disorders
  - HIV-associated illnesses
    - Herpes zoster
    - Oral hairy leukoplakia
    - Candidiasis
      - Oral
      - Persistent vaginal
    - Idiopathic thrombocytopenic puerpera
    - Listeriosis
    - Tuberculosis
- Social history (Varney et al., 2004)
  - Support systems
    - Living situation
    - Economic factors
    - Access to services

- Substance abuse
- Mental health issues
- Signs and symptoms of acute retroviral syndrome (CDC, 2006a; Niu et al., 1993)
  - Fever
  - Lymphadenopathy
  - Pharyngitis
  - Rash
  - Maculopapular lesions
  - Mucocutaneous ulceration
  - Myalgia or arthralgia
- Signs and symptoms of active HIV infection
  - Abnormal cytology: CIN grades 2 or 3
  - PID
  - Constitutional symptoms > 1 month
    - Fever
    - Weight loss
    - Diarrhea
    - Peripheral neuropathy
- Review of systems (ROS)

Physical Examination:
Components of the Physical Exam
to Consider
- Vital signs, including temperature
  - Weight—compare with previous
- Skin
  - Rash
  - Erythematous maculopapular rash
  - Mucocutaneous ulceration
  - Lesions
  - Herpes zoster
- Head, eyes, ears, nose and throat (HEENT)
  - Cervical lymph nodes
  - Oral candidiasis or ulcerative lesions
  - Pharyngeal erythema
- Chest
  - Cardiac assessment
  - Lung sounds
  - Presence of cough
- Abdomen
  - Enlargement of liver or spleen
  - Bowel sounds

- Extremities
  - Range of motion
  - Joint tenderness or swelling
  - Femoral lymph nodes
- Pelvic examination
  - Lesions
  - Mucocutaneous ulceration of genitals
  - Discharge
    - Mucopurulent cervicitis
    - Bacterial vaginosis (BV)
  - Cervical lesions
    - Cervicitis
    - Friability
    - Masses
  - Uterine motion tenderness
  - Adnexal mass or pain
- Neurologic examination (Niu et al., 1993)
  - Peripheral neuropathy
  - Facial palsy
  - Mental status
  - Cognitive impairment

Clinical Impression:
Differential Diagnoses and Code Groups
to Consider
Additional suffix may apply (ICD9data.com, 2007)
- HIV infection, asymptomatic (ICD-9 codes V08)
- IV drug abuse/addiction (ICD-9 codes 304–305)
- Acute retroviral syndrome (ICD-9 codes 042)
- AIDS (ICD-9 codes 042)
- Opportunistic infection (ICD-9 codes 136.9)
- Kaposi's sarcoma (ICD-9 codes 176)
- Candidiasis (ICD-9 codes 112)
- Tuberculosis (ICD-9 codes 010–018)
- Cervical cancer (ICD-9 codes 180)
- Viral hepatitis (ICD-9 codes 070)

Diagnostic Testing:
Diagnostic Tests and Procedures to Consider
- HIV screening (CDC, 2006d)
  - Screen women aged 13–64
  - Screen all pregnant women
  - Screen high-risk women annually

- "Opt-out" testing is recommended
    - Client advised testing is routine
    - Testing done unless client declines
  - Antibody screen is positive > 2–14 weeks postinfection
- HIV-1 antibody testing
  - Rapid HIV-1 testing (AIDS Education & Training Centers [AETC], 2007b; CDC, 2004c; Greenwald et al., 2006)
    - Oral, blood, or plasma
    - False-positive result may occur
    - Test may occur at point of care, such as
      - STI clinic
      - Labor and delivery
    - Reactive test results requires confirmatory testing
      - Western blot, *or*
      - Immunofluorescent assay, *and*
      - Retest with blood specimen in 4 weeks
  - Indications for Rapid HIV testing in labor and delivery
    - Unknown HIV status
    - Little or no prenatal care
  - Enzyme immunoassay
    - Venous sample (tiger-top tube)
    - False-positive result may occur
    - Positive test results requires confirmatory testing
- Other laboratory testing
  - Gonorrhea and chlamydia testing
  - Pap smear
  - Wet preparation
  - Hepatitis A, B, and C serology
  - Syphilis serology
- HIV infection strongly suspected
  - CBC
  - Chemistry profile
  - Blood urea nitrogen and creatinine
  - Toxoplasmosis antibody test
  - Tuberculosis testing
    - Mantoux skin test
    - Chest x-ray
  - CD4 cell count

Providing Treatment:
Therapeutic Measures to Consider

- Antiretroviral therapy (ART)
  - May delay onset of HIV-related complications
  - Current treatment guidelines http://aidsinfo.nih.gov/guidelines
  - Administer based on rapid test while awaiting confirmation (AETC, 2007b)
    - Labor and delivery
    - Neonates
    - Acute retroviral syndrome
- Problem-specific treatments as indicated

Providing Treatment:
Alternative Measures to Consider

- ⚠ Drug–herb interactions
  - Avoid with ART (Dharmananda, 2005)
    - St. John's wort
    - Grapefruit
    - Garlic
  - Avoid echinacea and other immunostimulants
- HIV immune support
  - Adequate rest
  - Stress reduction
  - Balanced diet
    - Fresh fruits and vegetables
    - Limit nonorganic meat and dairy
    - Antioxidant foods
    - Fish oil (omega-3)
  - Herbs (Sahelian, n.d.)
    - Red bush tea
    - Hyssop
    - Calendula
    - Olive leaf extract
    - Licorice

Providing Support:
Education and Support Measures
to Consider

- HIV-1 antibody testing
  - Antibody screen is positive > 2–14 weeks postinfection

- Pretest counseling
  - Opt out
  - Routes of transmission
  - Prevention measures
- Information regarding testing
  - Specimen collection technique
  - Confidentiality
  - Test interpretation
  - Timing of results
  - Partner notification
- HIV risk-reduction practices
  - Abstaining from intercourse
  - Selecting low-risk partners
  - Negotiating partner monogamy
  - Condom use
- Client resources
  - CDC Division of HIV/AIDS Prevention: www.cdc.gov/hiv/dhap.htm
  - American Medical Association HIV/AIDS Patient Info: www.ama-assn.org
  - HIV/AIDS Treatment Information Center: www.aidsinfo.nih.gov
  - National AIDS Hotline
    - English (800) 342-AIDS
    - Spanish (800) 344-7432
- Encourage creative and supportive measures, such as
  - Meditation or spiritual practices
  - Art therapy
  - Dance
  - Support groups
  - Religious involvement
  - Community involvement
  - Participation in HIV prevention programs

Follow-up Care:
Follow-up Measures to Consider

- Document
  - Results
  - Posttest counseling
  - Plan for continued care
- HIV-negative client (Baeten et al., 2005)
  - Provide HIV prevention education
  - Perform HIV risk assessment at return visits

- HIV-positive client
  - 🕐 Arrange case management
- Provide ongoing reproductive health care as appropriate
- Labor care for women with HIV (AECT, 2007b)
  - Vaginal birth appropriate for women with
    - ART, *and*
    - Viral HIV-RNA load < 1000 copies/ml
    - Avoid fetal exposure to maternal blood and body fluids
      - ➤ Prolonged rupture of membranes
        - ▸ Active management of labor
      - ➤ External fetal evaluation
      - ➤ No invasive intrauterine monitoring
      - ➤ Maintain intact perineum
  - Cesarean at 38 weeks gestation indicated in women with
    - No current ART
    - Viral HIV-RNA load > 1000 copies/ml
    - Client preference

Collaborative Practice:
Criteria to Consider for Consultation or Referral
- Women with previously diagnosed HIV
  - Medical evaluation
  - Treatment plan
  - Coordination of case management
- Women with new HIV diagnosis
  - Case management and medical care
    - Reproductive health counseling
    - Medical evaluation and treatment
      - ➤ Detailed medical history
      - ➤ Physical examination including pelvic
      - ➤ Comprehensive laboratory work
      - ➤ Tuberculosis testing
      - ➤ Chest x-ray
      - ➤ Monitoring of medical status
- Psychosocial services
  - Psychosocial evaluation
  - Mental health
  - Crisis counseling
  - Substance abuse services
  - Housing and financial support services

- Behavioral health services
  - Risk reduction for women with
    - HIV-negative status with HIV behavioral risk factors
    - HIV-positive status behavioral risk factors affecting
      - ➤ Potential for
        - ▸ Coinfection with other STIs
        - ▸ Spread of infection
      - ➤ ART and/or medical treatment compliance
      - ➤ Perinatal HIV transmission
  - Support services as indicated
- For diagnosis or treatment outside the midwife's scope of practice

CARE OF THE WOMAN WITH HEPATITIS

Key Clinical Information

Hepatitis is defined as inflammation of the liver (Mercksource.com, 2002). It includes a number of liver diseases that may be broken down based on viral characteristics into the categories of hepatitis A, hepatitis B, hepatitis C, hepatitis D, and hepatitis E. Hepatitis B and C are the forms most frequently seen in women's health practice. Hepatitis B is 100 times more infectious than HIV, with both hepatitis B and C occurring concurrently with HIV infection in some women and complicating management of these disorders (Khalili, 2006). Approximately 10% of infected adults develop chronic hepatitis B infection, which may lead to permanent liver damage, liver failure, or liver cancer (AETC, 2007a). Noninfectious hepatitis may be caused by autoimmune dysfunction, alcohol abuse, and/or drug-related liver injury, particularly combined alcohol and acetaminophen use.

Client History and Chart Review:
Components of the History to Consider
(CDC, 2006a)
- Age
- Medical/surgical history
  - Allergies

- Medications
  - ◆ Acetaminophen-based products
- Chronic illnesses
  - ◆ Organ transplant
  - ◆ Anemia
  - ◆ HIV/AIDS
- Social history
  - Drug and/or alcohol use
  - 🌐 Emigration, travel, or adoption from endemic areas
    - ◆ Asia
    - ◆ Africa
    - ◆ Pacific Islands (including Hawaii)
    - ◆ South or Central America and Mexico
- Presence, onset, duration, and severity of symptoms
  - May be asymptomatic
  - Malaise and lethargy
  - Fever and chills
  - Right upper quadrant pain
  - Jaundice
  - Nausea and vomiting
  - Dark urine
  - Pale-colored stools (Mercksource, 2003)
- Risk factors for hepatitis exposure
  - IV drug use, shared needles
  - Sexual contacts
  - Presence of tattoos, body piercings
  - Health care workers
  - Ingestion of raw shellfish
  - Children born to women with viral hepatitis
  - Partner with tattoos, body piercing
  - Hemodialysis patients
  - Blood or organ recipient before 1992
- Indications for hepatitis A vaccine (CDC, 2006b)
  - Children at ages 12–23 months
  - People going to any area of the world for longer than 12 months except the United States, Canada, Western Europe, Japan, New Zealand, and Australia
  - Illegal drug users, both oral and injecting
  - People who have blood clotting disorders

- People who work with hepatitis A-infected primates or hepatitis A in a research laboratory setting
- Any person who wishes to be immune to hepatitis A
- Indications for hepatitis B vaccine (CDC, 2006c)
  - Universal immunization of
    - ◆ Infants
    - ◆ Adolescents
    - ◆ Adults
  - Immunization of those at risk
    - ◆ Adolescents before sexual activity
    - ◆ Diagnosis of STI, including HIV
    - ◆ Travel to hepatitis B endemic areas
    - ◆ Occupational risk
    - ◆ Multiple sexual partners
    - ◆ IV drug use
  - Client preference
- Contraindications to hepatitis B vaccine
  - Allergy to yeast
- Review of systems (ROS)

Physical Examination:
Components of the Physical Exam to Consider (AETC, 2007b)
- Vital signs, including weight
  - Watch for hypertension
- Skin
  - Examine for evidence of jaundice
    - ◆ Mucous membranes
    - ◆ Sclera
  - Petechiae
  - Bruising
- Chest
  - Cardiac rate and rhythm
  - Lung fields
- Abdomen
  - Right upper quadrant pain
  - Liver margins
  - Splenomegaly
  - Abdominal ascites
  - Abdominal girth

- Extremities
  - Edema
- Neurologic system
  - Mental status
  - Coordination

Clinical Impression:
Differential Diagnoses and Code Groups
to Consider
Additional suffix may apply (ICD9data.com, 2007)

- Hepatitis B immunization (ICD-9 codes V04.89)
- Jaundice (ICD-9 codes 782.4)
- Nausea and vomiting (ICD-9 codes 787.01)
- Hepatitis, nonviral (ICD-9 codes 573.3)
- Viral hepatitis (ICD-9 codes 070)
- Biliary disease (ICD-9 codes 575–576)
- Cholelithiasis (ICD-9 codes 574)
- Other liver disorders (ICD-9 codes 753)

Diagnostic Testing:
Diagnostic Tests and Procedures to Consider
(Guidelines and Protocols Advisory
Committee, 2005)

- Hepatitis workup
  - Anti-HAV-IgM (IgM class antibody to the hepatitis A virus)
  - HBsAg (hepatitis B surface antigen)
  - Anti-HBs (total antibody to hepatitis B surface antigen)
  - Anti-HCV (antibody to hepatitis C virus antigens)
  - Alanine aminotransferase (ALT) elevated with liver inflammation
- Jaundice present
  - International Normalized Ratio (INR); prothrombin time
    - ⚠ 🕑 Elevated levels indicate fulminant infection
- Hepatitis A
  - Anti-HAV-IgM
    - Negative—infection is ruled out
    - Positive—acute infection

- Hepatitis B
  - HBsAg (hepatitis B surface antigen)
    - Detected 1–12 weeks postinfection
    - Positive result indicates infection with hepatitis B
    - Negative result indicates susceptibility to hepatitis B
  - HBsAb or anti-HBs (hepatitis B surface antibody)
    - Positive result indicates immunity
    - Negative result indicates infection
  - HBcAb or anti-HBc (hepatitis core antibody)
    - Indicates past or present infection
    - May be present in those chronically infected
      - False positive is possible
      - With positive HBsAb indicates recovery
      - With positive HBsAg indicates chronic infection
- Hepatitis C
  - Anti-HCV (antibody to hepatitis C virus antigens)
    - Test reliable 5–6 weeks postinfection
    - Negative—infection unlikely
      - Repeat in 1–2 months if no other etiology for symptoms
      - Immunocompromised client consider HCV-RNA testing
    - Positive—acute or chronic infection
      - Consider HCV-RNA testing
- Liver function tests (LFTs)
  - Aspartate aminotransferase (AST)
  - Alanine aminotransferase (ALT)
  - Lactate dehydrogenase (LDH)
  - Bilirubin
    - During acute phase
    - 🕑 Elevated levels indicate need for specialist care
- HIV testing
- Ultrasound, right upper quadrant
  - Gallbladder

Providing Treatment:
Therapeutic Measures to Consider (CDC, 2006a)

- Hepatitis A vaccine
  - Inactivated virus vaccine
  - Two doses, 6 months apart
- Hepatitis B vaccines
  - Recombinant vaccines
    - Age-related doses by manufacturer
    - Series of immunizations (three doses)
    - Given with hepatitis B immune globulin (HBIG) immediately after exposure
- Hepatitis B immune globulin
  - Given as soon as possible after exposure (up to 7 days)
    - One or two doses

Providing Treatment:
Alternative Measures to Consider

- Supportive care
  - Whole foods diet with minimum of toxins
  - Adequate rest
- Herbal support
  - Milk thistle tea (Soule, 1996)
  - Silymarin 140–560 mg TID for 6 weeks (Ferenci et al., 1989; Hepatitis C Technical Advisory Group, 2005)
  - Licorice root tincture

Providing Support:
Education and Support Measures to Consider

- Provide information about hepatitis
  - Types
  - Route(s) of transmission
    - Fecal–oral, contaminated food or water (hepatitis A)
    - Blood or body fluids (hepatitis B)
    - Blood (hepatitis C)
  - Prevention measures (Mercksource.com, 2003)
    - Avoid contact with blood or body fluids
    - Wash hands before eating and after toileting
    - Safe sexual practices

- Avoid undercooked food in endemic areas
- Avoid shared needles or razors
- Acetaminophen use
  - Abstain from alcohol when taking
  - Do not exceed recommended dose
  - Over-the-counter medications may contain acetaminophen, avoid double closing
- Discussion regarding
  - Hepatitis A and B immunizations
  - Options for treatment and supportive care, as needed
  - Potential effects of illness
  - Medications
  - Criteria for referral

ONLINE RESOURCES

Hepatitis Foundation International:
http://www.hepfi.org/

The Hepatitis Information Network:
http://www.hepnet.com/

CDC Viral Hepatitis:
http://www.cdc.gov/ncidod/diseases/hepatitis/

Hepatitis B Foundation:
http://www.hepb.org

Hepatitis C Information Center:
http://hepatitis-central.com/

Follow-up Care:
Follow-up Measures to Consider

- Document
  - Symptoms
  - Risk factors
  - Test results
  - Discussions with client
  - Follow-up plan
- Retest (CDC, 2006a)
  - Postimmunization
  - After illness or exposure
    - Incubation lasts 1–4 months
    - It may take up to 6 months to
      - Determine whether a client has recovered, or
      - Remains chronically infected (hepatitis B)

- Return for care
  - Weekly during acute phase of infection
  - Periodic liver function tests
  - STI testing, as needed

Collaborative Practice:
Criteria to Consider for Consultation or Referral

- Medical service
  - Diagnosis of hepatitis for detailed evaluation and treatment
  - Evidence of
    - Liver failure
    - Ascites
    - Acetaminophen overdose
- Social services
  - Addiction treatment
  - Clean needle programs
- For diagnosis or treatment outside the midwife's scope of practice

CARE OF THE WOMAN WITH HERPES SIMPLEX VIRUS

Key Clinical Information

Herpes simplex virus (HSV) is a chronic lifelong infection caused by HSV-1 and HSV-2. These common viruses may be sexually transmitted and frequently cause significant discomfort to those with active genital lesions. The goal of therapy is to encourage the virus to become dormant and to support the immune system so that it stays dormant and the client remains asymptomatic. Herpes infection in the HIV-positive client increases the likelihood of transmission of HIV (CDC, 2004b). Unfortunately, it is possible to spread herpes infection without a noticeable lesion. Infants who are exposed to HSV may acquire systemic infection resulting in serious illness or death. For this reason cesarean birth may be offered to pregnant women with a history of recurrent HSV outbreaks during pregnancy. Cesarean birth is recommended for pregnant women with an active HSV lesion during late pregnancy. See Care of the Pregnant Woman with Herpes Simplex Virus, Chapter 3.

Client History and Chart Review:
Components of the History to Consider
(CDC, 2004b)

- Age
- Reproductive history
  - LMP
  - Current method of birth control
  - Sexual orientation
  - Sexual practices
    - Oral–genital sex
    - Anal sex
    - Safe sex practices
  - Last examination and testing results
    - HSV and other STI testing
    - HIV status
    - Pap smear results
- Problem-oriented history (CDC, 2006a)
  - Previous history of genital or oral lesions
  - Partner with oral or genital HSV
  - Present symptoms
    - Onset, duration, and severity
    - Presence and location of lesions
      - Vesicular lesions
      - Ulcerative lesions
    - Pain, tingling, dysuria
    - Other associated symptoms
    - Precipitating factors
      - Stress
      - Fever or infection
      - Menses
      - Sun exposure
- Review of systems (ROS)
- Medical/surgical history
  - Allergies
  - Medications
  - Chronic illnesses
  - Immunosuppression
    - HIV/AIDS
    - Cancer
    - Burns
    - Organ transplant
    - Steroid use

- Psychosocial assessment
  - Impact of symptoms
  - Ability to pay for medication
- Primary HSV infection associated with (CDC, 2006a)
  - Fever
  - Headache
  - Malaise
  - Local lesions at site of infection
  - Lymphadenopathy
  - ⚠ Herpes meningitis
  - ⚠ Increased risk of perinatal transmission at term
- Risk factors for HSV infection
  - 🌐 African-Americans more likely to test positive for HSV
  - Whites more likely to have active symptoms
  - White teens are fastest growing HSV-positive population (CDC, 2000)
  - Compromised immune system

Physical Examination:
Components of the Physical Exam
to Consider
- Vital signs, including temperature
- Palpate inguinal lymph nodes
- External genital examination
  - Examine for characteristic lesions
    - Vesicles
    - Shallow ulcers
  - Lesions may occur on
    - Vulva
    - Urethra
    - Vagina
    - Cervix
    - Thighs
    - Anus
    - Buttocks
- Speculum examination
  - Vaginal or cervical discharge
- Bimanual examination
  - Cervical or uterine motion tenderness

- Neurologic examination
  - Neck tenderness
  - Light sensitivity

Clinical Impression:
Differential Diagnoses and Code Groups
to Consider
Additional suffix may apply (ICD9data.com, 2007)
- Genital herpes (ICD-9 codes 054.10)
- Herpetic vulvovaginitis (ICD-9 codes 054.11)
- Herpes gestationis (ICD-9 codes 646.8)
- Herpetic meningoencephalitis (ICD-9 codes 054.3)
- Contact dermatitis (ICD-9 codes 692.9)
- Chancre (ICD-9 codes 091.0)

Diagnostic Testing:
Diagnostic Tests and Procedures to Consider
(CDC, 2006a)
- Culture lesions using viral media for
  - HSV
- Serum testing for HSV-1 or -2 antibody titer
  - Documents primary infection
  - Important in early pregnancy
  - Repeat 7–10 days
  - Fourfold increase indicates primary infection
- Additional STI testing as indicated

Providing Treatment:
Therapeutic Measures to Consider (CDC, 2006a)
- Zovirax (Acyclovir)
  - Pregnancy Category C
  - Pregnancy registry: (800) 722-9292, ext. 58465
  - Topical ointment 5% apply TID for 7 days
  - Initial outbreak
    - 200 mg PO five times a day, *or*
    - 400 mg TID for 10 days
  - Recurrent outbreak
    - 200 mg PO five times a day, *or*
    - 400 mg TID or 800 mg BID for 5 days
  - Suppression, severe recurrent outbreaks
    - 400 mg PO BID for 12 months

- Famvir (famciclovir)
  - Pregnancy Category B
  - Initial outbreak: 250 mg TID for 7–10 days
  - Recurrent outbreak: 125 mg BID for 5 days
  - Begin medication within 6 hours of first symptom
- Valtrex (valacyclovir hydrochloride)
  - Pregnancy Category B
    - Pregnancy registry: (800) 722-9292, ext. 39437
  - Initial outbreak: 1000 mg PO BID for 7–10 days
  - Recurrent outbreak: 500 mg PO BID for 3–5 days, *or*
  - 1000 mg BID for 5 days
  - Begin medication within 24 hours of first symptom
- Acetaminophen or ibuprofen for pain relief

Providing Treatment:
Alternative Measures to Consider
- Nutritional supplements
  - L-lysine
    - 500 to 1000 mg QID for prevention
    - 2000 mg BID or QID for outbreak (Soule, 1995)
  - Vitamin C 250–500 mg
    - BID with outbreak
    - Combine with acidophilus
      - 1 cap with meals
  - Zinc 30 mg daily (Sinclair, 2004)
  - Vitamin A
    - 200,000 IU PO for 3 days, *or*
    - 50,000 IU daily
    - Decreases length and severity of symptoms
    - Not for use during pregnancy or with liver disorders
- Selenium 0.25 mg (250 µg) daily
- Herbal support
  - Lemon balm, tea or topical application
  - Tea tree oil topical application

- Echinacea tea, tincture, tablets, or capsules TID for 2 weeks
- Aloe vera ointment
- Sitz bath or salve made with
  - Lemon balm (Foster, 1996)
  - Calendula
  - Comfrey
- Homeopathics (University of Maryland Medical Center, n.d.)
  - Graphites
    - Large itchy lesions
    - Client with elevated BMI
  - Natrum muriaticum
    - Outbreaks caused by emotional stress
    - Symptoms that are worse in daytime
  - Petroleum
    - Lesions on anus and thighs
    - Symptoms worse in winter
  - Sepia
    - Stubborn outbreaks
    - Client with lack of energy and cold intolerant

Providing Support:
Education and Support Measures
to Consider
- Diet
  - Avoid foods high in arginine: chocolate, cola, peanuts, cashews, pecans, almonds, sunflower and sesame seeds, peas, corn, coconut, and gelatin
  - Include foods high in lysine: margarine, yogurt, cheese, milk, brewer's yeast, potatoes, fish, chicken, eggs (Soule, 1996)
- Rest and comfort measures
- Discuss and provide written information about
  - Nutritional support
  - Herpes management (CDC, 2006a)
    - Medications
      - Episodic
      - Suppressive therapy
    - Abstinence during outbreaks

- ◆ Potential for transmission with no lesions
  - ➤ Partner notification
  - ➤ Condom use
  - ◆ Wash hands after lesion contact
  - ◆ Avoid handling infants during active lesion
- ■ Effects on
  - ◆ Sexuality
  - ◆ HIV susceptibility
  - ◆ Childbearing
  - ◆ Self-image
- ■ Review warning signs and symptoms
  - ◆ Meningitis
  - ◆ Secondary infection
  - ◆ Depression
- • Client resources
  - ■ The American Social Health Association: www.ashastd.org
  - ■ National Women's Health Network: www.womenshealthnetwork.org
  - ■ Centers for Disease Control and Prevention: (800) 311-3435 www.cdc.gov

Follow-up Care:
Follow-up Measures to Consider
- • Document
  - ■ Location, size, and appearance of lesions
- • Return for care
  - ■ Symptoms persist > 10 days
  - ■ Worsening symptoms
    - ◆ Stiff neck
    - ◆ Unremitting fever
    - ◆ Inability to urinate
  - ■ Ineffective coping
- • Pregnancy (CDC, 2006a)
  - ■ ⚠ Initial outbreak in third trimester
    - ◆ 🕐 Infectious diseases specialist consultation
  - ■ HSV-negative woman HSV-positive partner
    - ◆ Avoid intercourse in last trimester
    - ◆ Avoid oral/genital contact

- ■ Onset of labor
  - ◆ Inquire regarding prodromal symptoms
  - ◆ Examine for lesions
  - ◆ Plan vaginal delivery
    - ➤ No prodrome or lesions
  - ◆ Cesarean delivery
    - ➤ Prodrome or lesions
    - ➤ Initial outbreak at term (per specialist)

Collaborative Practice:
Criteria to Consider for Consultation or Referral
- • OB/GYN service
  - ■ Symptoms of
    - ◆ Herpes meningitis
    - ◆ Systemic infection
    - ◆ Ocular herpes
  - ■ Pregnancy
    - ◆ Initial outbreak during pregnancy
    - ◆ Cesarean birth during active genital outbreak
- • For diagnosis or treatment outside the midwife's scope of practice

CARE OF THE WOMAN WITH HUMAN PAPILLOMA VIRUS

Key Clinical Information
Over 40 types of human papilloma virus (HPV) affect the genital tract. Only a few types are considered high risk. Types 16, 18, 31, 33, and 35 are associated with cervical dysplasia and may contribute to the development of anal, cervical, penile, and vulvar cancers. Other types may cause visible genital warts. Women may be infected with more than one type of HPV. With an intact immune system and healthy immune response, over 90% of HPV infections resolve within 2 years (ACS, 2007b). The HPV vaccine Gardasil provides protection against virus types 6, 11, 16, and 18 and is currently recommended for girls before the onset of sexual activity. Screening tests indicate the presence or absence of one or more high-risk types of HPV and are used to guide clinical management of women infected with HPV (CDC, 2006a; Saslow et al., 2003).

Client History and Chart Review:
Components of the History to Consider
(ACS, 2007b)
- Age
- Reproductive history
  - LMP
  - Current method of birth control
  - Previous
    - HPV testing
    - Abnormal cervical cytology
- Sexual practices
  - Condom use
  - Number of sexual partners
  - Anal sex with penetration
- Onset, duration, and severity of current symptoms
  - Location of lesions
  - Other associated symptoms
- Medical/surgical history
  - Allergies
  - Medications
  - Chronic illnesses
- Social history
  - Tobacco use (increases risk of progression)
  - Drug and/or alcohol use (associated with risk behaviors)
- Risk factors for HPV infection
  - Previous or current STIs
  - Diminished immune response
  - Unprotected sexual activity
  - Over five lifetime sexual partners for self or partner(s)
- Review of systems (ROS)

Physical Examination:
Components of the Physical Exam
to Consider
- External genitalia
  - Genital warts
  - Friable lesions
- Speculum examination
  - Cervical or vaginal lesions

- Bimanual examination
  - Palpate for abnormality of cervix or vagina
    - Contour
    - Consistency
    - Mass
- Consider colposcopy of
  - External genitalia
  - Vagina
  - Cervix
- Consider application of
  - 5% acetic acid (white vinegar)
    - HPV lesions turn acetowhite
  - Lugol's solution (strong iodine)
    - Normal squamous cells stain mahogany brown
    - HPV lesions and columnar cells remain unstained

Clinical Impression:
Differential Diagnoses and Code Groups
to Consider
Additional suffix may apply (ICD9data.com, 2007)
- Genital warts (ICD-9 codes 078.19)
- Condyloma acuminatum (ICD-9 codes 078.11)
- Syphilitic condyloma latum (ICD-9 codes 091.3)
- Musculosum contagiosum (ICD-9 codes 078.0)
- Dysplasia
  - Vulvar (ICD-9 codes 624.01–02)
  - Vaginal (ICD-9 codes 623.0)

Diagnostic Testing:
Diagnostic Tests and Procedures to Consider
- HPV testing
  - Cervicovaginal
  - Anal
- Other STI testing as indicated, such as
  - Gonorrhea/chlamydia nucleic acid amplification tests
  - Rapid plasma regain (RPR)
  - HIV counseling and testing

- Cytology
  - Specimen source
    - Cervicovaginal
    - Anal
  - Specimen collection
    - Slide (most cost-effective for screening)
    - Liquid-based cytology
      - Allows for reflex HPV testing
- HCG as indicated, before treatment
- Stool for occult blood

Providing Treatment:
Therapeutic Measures to Consider (CDC, 2006a)
- Gardasil vaccine
  - Recommended age of vaccination 11–12 years
  - Range: 9–26 years
  - Dose 0.5 ml IM at 0, 2, and 6 months
- Vitamin therapy
  - Vitamin E 400 IU daily
  - Vitamin C 500–1000 mg daily
- Client-applied therapy for visible warts
  - Imiquimod cream 5%
    - Apply every night three times a week until clear
    - Wash off after 6–10 hours
    - Not for use in pregnancy
    - More info: (800) 428-6397 or www.3M.com/ALDARA
  - Podofilox 0.5% solution or gel
    - Apply BID for 3 days
    - No treatment for 4 days
    - Repeat up to four cycles
    - Not for use in pregnancy
- Provider applied therapy for visible warts
  - Cryotherapy
  - Podophyllin resin
    - Apply weekly to lesions
    - Wash off in 6–8 hours
    - Not for use in pregnancy
  - Trichloroacetic acid or bichloracetic acid
    - Apply weekly to lesions
    - Protect normal tissue with petrolatum
  - Surgical removal

- Alternate treatment
  - Intralesional interferon injection
  - Laser ablation

Providing Treatment:
Alternative Measures to Consider
- Balanced whole foods diet
- Antioxidant foods
  - Blueberries
  - Red peppers
  - Plums
  - Pumpkin
  - Tomatoes
- Herbal remedies
  - Tea tree oil
  - Echinacea tea or tincture daily to boost immune response
- Stress management
- Visualization of area healed and whole

Providing Support:
Education and Support Measures
to Consider
- 🌐 Age and culturally appropriate information
  - Male and female condoms provide limited protection
    - Uncovered areas not protected
  - Wart virus is not curable but may become dormant
    - Regression most likely in adolescents
    - May spread virus with no visible warts
  - Oral, pharyngeal, or anal warts may occur with exposure
  - Partner evaluation/treatment as needed
- Treatment recommendations
  - Medication/remedy use
  - Anticipated response to treatment
  - Signs or symptoms indicating need to return for care
- Risk of cervical dysplasia
  - Increased risk for abnormal Pap smear results
  - Emphasize need for annual Pap smears

- - Smoking increases risk of progression
  - Immune response affects regression or progression
- Encourage smoking cessation
- For more information
  - American Social Health Association: www.ashastd.org
  - Centers for Disease Control and Prevention: www.cdc.gov

Follow-up Care:
Follow-up Measures to Consider

- Document
  - Location, number, and size of lesions
  - Treatment method
  - Anticipated follow-up
- Return for care
  - As necessary for treatment chosen
  - HPV screening results and interpretation
  - As indicated by
    - Clinical response to treatment
    - Cytology results (see Abnormal Pap Smear Interpretation and Triage)
    - HPV test results (see Abnormal Pap Smear Interpretation and Triage)

Collaborative Practice:
Criteria to Consider for Consultation or Referral

- OB/GYN service
  - Ablative therapy
    - Cryotherapy
    - Laser
  - Interferon injection of lesions
  - Extensive lesions
  - Anal lesions
- Behavior risk modification
  - Safe sex practices
  - Drug and alcohol rehabilitation
  - Smoking cessation
- For diagnosis or treatment outside the midwife's scope of practice

CARE OF THE WOMAN WITH NIPPLE DISCHARGE

Key Clinical Information

Nipple discharge in the absence of pregnancy and lactation occurs in 10–15% of women with benign breast conditions. It may represent a physiologic variation of normal or may be the presenting symptom of a pathologic process. Regular and frequent stimulation of the nipples and breasts, such as nursing a baby with a Lactaid device or engaging in frequent sexual foreplay, may result in milk production. Bilateral galactorrhea is associated with hypothyroidism, with amenorrheic syndromes such as occur with pituitary adenoma, or with pharmacologic causes (Breast Expert Workgroup, 2005). Fortunately, many pituitary tumors are benign and grow exceedingly slowly. However, without treatment enlarging tumors may cause pressure on optic nerves, resulting in permanent visual loss or blindness.

Unilateral spontaneous nipple discharge that is clear, serous, or bloody requires prompt evaluation for underlying malignancy. Spontaneous discharge is suspected when a woman notes staining on her clothing or bedding. Spontaneous discharge from a single duct or that associated with a proximate underlying mass is of particular concern (Breast Expert Workgroup, 2005).

Client History and Chart Review:
Components of the History to Consider

- Age
- Reproductive history
  - Gravida, para, LMP
  - Usual menstrual patterns
  - Current method of birth control
  - Infertility
- Breast history
  - Lactation, duration, and most recent dates
  - Self-breast examination practices
  - Breast disorders
    - Mastitis
    - Breast abscess

- ◆ Fibrocystic breast disorder
- ◆ Breast cancer
- ■ Breast stimulation or trauma
- Onset and duration of symptoms
  - ■ Nature of discharge
    - ◆ Bloody, serous, greenish, or milky
    - ◆ Unilateral or bilateral
    - ◆ Spontaneous or expressed
    - ◆ Recent breast changes
  - ■ Associated symptoms
    - ◆ Breast pain, tenderness, masses
    - ◆ Fever
    - ◆ ⚠ Headache
    - ◆ ⚠ Visual changes
    - ◆ Presence of menstrual dysfunction
      - ➤ Amenorrhea
      - ➤ Irregular or scanty menses
    - ◆ Change in libido
- Causes of nipple discharge (Thompson, 2004)
  - ■ Pregnancy and lactation
  - ■ Breast manipulation
  - ■ Medications
  - ■ Endocrine disorders
  - ■ Malignancy
- Medical/surgical history
  - ■ Medications that may cause nipple discharge (Thompson, 2004)
    - ◆ Phenothiazine
    - ◆ Cimetidine
    - ◆ Methyldopa
    - ◆ Metoclopramide
    - ◆ Oral contraceptives
    - ◆ Reserpine
    - ◆ Tricyclic antidepressants
    - ◆ Verapamil
  - ■ Health conditions
    - ◆ Hypothyroidism
    - ◆ Family history
      - ➤ Breast disease
      - ➤ Endocrine disorder
- Review of systems (ROS)

Physical Examination:
Components of the Physical Exam
to Consider
- Breast examination (Breast Expert Workgroup, 2004)
  - ■ Sitting and supine
  - ■ Presence of spontaneous nipple discharge
    - ◆ Crusting of discharge on nipple
  - ■ Breast asymmetry or retraction
  - ■ Venous patterns
  - ■ Masses
    - ◆ Size
    - ◆ Proximity to nipple
    - ◆ Characteristics
  - ■ Breast skin changes
    - ◆ Thickening or coarseness
    - ◆ Edema
    - ◆ Scaling
    - ◆ Redness and/or heat
    - ◆ "Orange peel" sign
  - ■ Lymph nodes
    - ◆ Axillary
    - ◆ Clavicular
- Hirsutism
- Thyroid palpation

Clinical Impression:
Differential Diagnoses and Code Groups
to Consider
Additional suffix may apply (ICD9data.com, 2007)
- Nipple discharge (ICD-9 codes 611.79)
- Galactorrhea (ICD-9 codes 611.6)
- Hyperprolactinemia (ICD-9 codes 253.1)
- Hypothyroidism, acquired (ICD-9 codes 244)

Diagnostic Testing:
Diagnostic Tests and Procedures to Consider
(Leung & Pacaud, 2004)
- Pregnancy testing
- Purulent discharge
  - ■ Culture of discharge
  - ■ Ultrasound for fluctuant mass

- ⚠ Spontaneous bloody, serous, or clear discharge (Breast Expert Workgroup, 2005)
  - Mammogram
  - 🔇 Breast biopsy
- Milky discharge
  - Thyroid testing, TSH
  - Prolactin level
    - ◆ Nonpregnant < 0–20 ng/ml
    - ◆ Pregnant 10–300 ng/ml
    - ◆ Prolactinoma > 200 ng/ml
  - Head CT for prolactinoma
  - MRI for abnormalities of prolactin or sella turcica

Providing Treatment:
Therapeutic Measures to Consider (Leung & Pacaud, 2004)
- Treatment based on cause of discharge
- Idiopathic galactorrhea, normal prolactin levels
  - Eliminate cause, if determined
  - No treatment required
- Pharmacologic cause
  - Alter medication if appropriate
  - No treatment required
- Pituitary tumor or elevated prolactin levels
  - 🔇 Refer for evaluation and treatment
    - ◆ Bromocriptine used to
      - ➤ Normalize prolactin levels
      - ➤ Shrink pituitary tumor
    - ◆ Large or bromocriptine-resistant tumors
      - ➤ Surgical removal
- Hypothyroidism
  - 🔇 Thyroid replacement therapy
- Breast infection (see Care of the Mother: Mastitis, Chapter 5)
- Ductal ectasia
  - Observation
  - Surgical repair of duct
- Intraductal papilloma
  - Observation
  - Surgical removal
- Malignancy
  - Surgical treatment

Providing Treatment:
Alternative Measures to Consider
- Provide emotional support
- Comfort measures
  - Warm castor oil packs
  - Bach flower remedies to balance emotional state
- Immune support formulas

Providing Support:
Education and Support Measures to Consider
- Provide information related to
  - Diagnosis
  - Recommendations for evaluation
  - Treatment options
- Teach or review self-breast examination
- Offer active listening
- Address client fears and concerns

Follow-up Care:
Follow-up Measures to Consider
- Document
  - Characteristics of discharge
  - Presence or absence of mass
  - Diagnostic testing and results
  - Discussions with client
  - Plan for continued care
  - Referrals
- Pregnancy: options counseling as indicated
- Galactorrhea, negative diagnostic imaging
  - Pharmacologic or physiologic cause
    - ◆ Observation
    - ◆ Periodic prolactin levels to assess stability
    - ◆ Persistent galactorrhea refer to endocrinologist
    - ◆ Assess for recurrence after treatment
- Galactorrhea, pathologic
  - Return for care after evaluation and medical or surgical treatment
    - ◆ Response evaluated with
      - ➤ Serum prolactin levels
      - ➤ MRI of any tumor

- ◆ Assess for
  - ➤ Symptom recurrence
  - ➤ Prolactinoma tumor regrowth
  - ➤ Contralateral breast disease
- Spontaneous unilateral nipple discharge (Breast Expert Workgroup, 2005)
  - ▪ Negative testing
    - ◆ Reevaluate in 3 months
    - ◆ Persistent discharge refer to breast specialist
- Routine well-woman care

Collaborative Practice:
Criteria to Consider for Consultation or Referral
- Breast care specialist
  - ▪ Ductal ectasia
  - ▪ Intraductal papilloma
  - ▪ Breast cancer
- Endocrinology service
  - ▪ Pituitary adenoma
  - ▪ Hypothyroidism
  - ▪ Persistent galactorrhea
- For diagnosis or treatment outside the midwife's scope of practice

CARE OF THE WOMAN WITH PARASITIC INFESTATION

Key Clinical Information
Lice and scabies are two common parasites that can be particularly challenging in midwifery practice. An infestation of lice can be hard to eradicate, and because they are mobile, lice may affect the office environment and housekeeping practices after a client has been diagnosed. Lice and scabies live on human blood and may contribute to the spread of impetigo. Head lice prefer the nape of the neck, whereas body lice inhabit seams of clothing or bedding and move onto the host to feed. Pubic or crab lice live in the genital region but may be found on any hairy aspect of the body. The scabies mite burrows under the skin. Persistent itching may result from reinfestation, allergic dermatitis, or secondary skin infection (CDC, 2006a). More information on additional parasites that

affect women can be found at the CDC Division of Parasitic Disease (http://www.cdc.gov/ncidod/dpd/index.htm).

Client History and Chart Review:
Components of the History to Consider
- LMP, pregnancy status
- Symptoms
  - ▪ Onset, duration, location
    - ◆ Itching
    - ◆ Presence of nits (lice)
    - ◆ Presence of skin tracks (scabies)
  - ▪ Other associated symptoms
    - ◆ Joint aches
    - ◆ Rash or skin changes
    - ◆ Headache
    - ◆ Fever
- Medical/surgical history
  - ▪ Allergies
  - ▪ Medications
  - ▪ Health conditions
    - ◆ Asthma
- Social history
  - ▪ Exposure to lice, nits, or scabies
    - ◆ Environmental exposure
      - ➤ Shared personal items
      - ➤ Infested clothes or bedding
    - ◆ Interpersonal exposure
      - ➤ Intimate contacts
      - ➤ Household contacts
      - ➤ Public contacts
        - ▸ School or day care
        - ▸ International travel
  - ▪ Sexual partner or family member symptoms
  - ▪ General hygiene and housekeeping habits
- Review of systems (ROS)

Physical Examination:
Components of the Physical Exam to Consider
- Observe for signs of parasites (Emmons et al., 1997)
  - ▪ Anogenital region
  - ▪ Extremities
  - ▪ Nape of neck

- Presence of
  - Lice (1-mm crablike organism)
  - Nits (small white tear drop shaped orb attached to hair shaft)
  - Skin tracks from scabies burrows
  - Tick or other insect(s) or bites
- Secondary signs
  - Redness and erythema
  - Rash
  - Blisters
  - Scabbing
- Pelvic examination as indicated
  - STI symptoms
- Lymph nodes for enlargement

Clinical Impression:
Differential Diagnoses and Code Groups to Consider
Additional suffix may apply (ICD9data.com, 2007)
- Pediculosis (ICD-9 codes 132)
- Scabies (ICD-9 codes 133.0)
- Allergic dermatitis (ICD-9 codes 692.9)
- Impetigo (ICD-9 codes 684)
- Viral exanthem, unspecified (ICD-9 codes 057.9)

Diagnostic Testing:
Diagnostic Tests and Procedures to Consider
- Microscopic examination of parasites
- Culture of skin lesions
- Vaginal wet preparation
- STI testing
- Additional testing as needed
  - Lyme titer
  - Viral tests

Providing Treatment:
Therapeutic Measures to Consider
(CDC, 2006a; Food and Drug Administration, 2003)
- Pediculosis
  - Permethrin 1% cream rinse
    - Pregnancy Category B
  - Pyrethrin with piperonyl butoxide
    - Pregnancy Category C

- Instructions
  - Apply to affected area(s)
  - Wash off after 10 minutes
  - Avoid pyrethrin or permethrin with
    - Asthma
    - Ragweed allergy
- Alternate options
  - Malathion 0.5% lotion
    - Apply to affected area(s)
    - Wash off after 8–12 hours
    - Pregnancy Category B
  - Ivermectin 250 μg/kg PO, repeat in 2 weeks
    - Pregnancy Category C
    - Avoid in pregnancy or lactation
- Avoid lindane due to toxicity
- Scabies treatment
  - Permethrin cream (5%)
    - Apply to all areas of the body from the neck down
    - Wash off after 8–14 hours
  - Ivermectin 200 μg/kg PO, repeat in 2 weeks
  - Alternate regimen
    - Lindane (1%) 1 oz. of lotion or 30 g of cream
      - Apply in a thin layer to body from the neck down
      - Thoroughly wash off after 8 hours
      - ⚠ May cause severe neurotoxic reaction
      - Do not use
        - Immediately after a bath or shower
        - Persons with extensive dermatitis
        - Women who are pregnant or lactating
        - Children aged < 2 years
- Impetigo (superficial staphylococcus or streptococcus infection)
  - Antibacterial soap or cleanser
  - Topical antibiotic such as Bactroban
  - Oral antibiotic therapy

Providing Treatment:
Alternative Measures to Consider
- Lice R Gone Shampoo
  - Safe Solutions, Inc.
    - (888) 443-8738
    - www.safesolutionsinc.com
- Head or pubic lice
  - Coat affected area in olive oil
  - Comb with fine-toothed comb
  - Wash with soap or shampoo
  - Apply cream rinse
  - Comb again
  - Apply vinegar rinse
  - Use caution as may cause burning of
    - Eyes
    - Genitals
- Salt scrub to affected area
  - Mix coarse salt with oil
  - Follow with soap wash
- Wash of herbal painted daisy infusion
  - Source of pyrethrins
  - Use wash to affected area TID
- Shave affected area

Providing Support:
Education and Support Measures
to Consider
- Provide written medication instructions
- Recommend treatment for all contacts
- Avoid sexual contact until treatment complete
- Review transmission mechanisms
- Cleanse bedding and clothing
  - Hot water wash with bleach
  - Hot dryer
- Vacuum living quarters
- Wash throw rugs

Follow-up Care:
Follow-up Measures to Consider
- Document
  - Presence of parasite
  - Medication recommendations and instructions

- Return for care
  - One week if symptoms not eliminated
  - Reinfestation
  - Secondary infection
  - Medication side effects

Collaborative Practice:
Criteria to Consider for Consultation or Referral
- Infection control department
  - Evidence or risk of epidemic
- Laboratory
  - Identification of unusual parasite
- Emergency department or medical service
  - Symptoms of neurotoxicity with lindane
- For diagnosis or treatment outside the mid-wife's scope of practice

CARE OF THE WOMAN WITH ACUTE PELVIC PAIN

Key Clinical Information
Pelvic pain has many potential causes, both reproductive and nonreproductive related. Acute pelvic pain is defined as moderate to severe pain of less than 7 days duration. (Sauerland et al., 2006). Acute pelvic pain requires timely evaluation and accurate diagnosis to institute appropriate corrective action. On occasion the ability to differentiate between acute and nonacute pain can be challenging. A careful workup is essential to determine whether prompt referral for emergency care is indicated.

Client History and Chart Review:
Components of the History to Consider
- Age
- Reproductive history
  - LMP, gravida, para
    - Potential for pregnancy
    - Method of birth control
  - Last examination, Pap smear, and STI testing
  - History of
    - STIs/PID
    - Endometriosis
    - Ectopic pregnancy
  - Change in sexual partner for self or partner

- Pain profile
  - Location: local or radiating
  - Onset: sudden, gradual, or cyclic
  - Duration of pain
  - Severity of symptoms
  - Precipitating or exacerbating factors
  - Associated symptoms
    - Fever and chills
    - Shoulder pain
    - Nausea and vomiting
    - Diarrhea, constipation, or obstipation
    - Cervicovaginal discharge
      - Bloody
      - Mucopurulent
    - Painful urination
- Potential causes of acute pelvic pain (Kripke, 2007; Sauerland et al., 2006)
  - Reproductive system
    - Mucopurulent cervicitis
    - PID or endometritis
    - Ectopic pregnancy
    - Septic abortion
    - Spontaneous abortion or miscarriage
    - Ovarian cyst
    - Torsion of ovary
    - Endometriosis
    - Degenerating fibroids
  - Urinary system
    - Renal calculi
    - Acute cystitis
  - Gastrointestinal system
    - Acute appendicitis
    - Diverticulitis
    - Ulcerative colitis
    - Bowel obstruction
    - Incarcerated inguinal hernia
  - Lower abdominal trauma
- Medical/surgical history
  - Medications
  - Allergies
  - Health conditions
    - Diverticular disease
    - Appendicitis
    - Previous abdominal surgery

- Psychosocial history and status
  - Physical or sexual violence
  - Drug/alcohol use
  - Living situation
  - Mental health status
- Client affect and presentation
- Review of systems (ROS)

Physical Examination:
Components of the Physical Exam
to Consider
- Vital signs, including temperature
  - Orthostatic hypotension
- Abdominal examination
  - Distention
  - Mass
  - Rebound tenderness
  - Guarding
  - Presence or absence of bowel sounds
- Costovertebral angle tenderness
- Pelvic examination
  - Speculum examination
    - Presence of cervical discharge
    - Chadwick's sign
- Bimanual examination
  - Cervical motion tenderness
  - Uterine enlargement or tenderness
  - Palpation of
    - Adnexa
    - Fornices
- Rectal examination
  - Pain
  - Masses

Clinical Impression:
Differential Diagnoses and Code Groups
to Consider
Additional suffix may apply (ICD9data.com, 2007)
- Abdominal tenderness, lower left quadrant (ICD-9 codes 789.64)
- Abdominal tenderness, lower right quadrant (ICD-9 codes 789.63)
- Abdominal tenderness, periumbilical (ICD-9 codes 789.65)

- Abdominal tenderness, generalized (ICD-9 codes 789.67)
- Abdominal pain, lower left quadrant (ICD-9 codes 789.04)
- Abdominal pain, lower right quadrant (ICD-9 codes 789.03)
- Abdominal pain, periumbilical (ICD-9 codes 789.05)
- Abdominal pain, unspecified (ICD-9 codes 789.00)
- Abdominal rigidity, generalized (ICD-9 codes 789.47)

Diagnostic Testing:
Diagnostic Tests and Procedures to Consider
- Urinalysis
- Serum or urine HCG
- CBC with differential
- Erythrocyte sedimentation rate
- STI testing
- Pelvic ultrasound or CT (American Roentgen Ray Society, 2006)
- Diagnostic laparoscopy

Providing Treatment:
Therapeutic Measures to Consider
- ⚠ Prompt medical care is indicated for acute abdominal or pelvic pain
  - Adequate analgesia during diagnostic studies (Kripke, 2007)
    - NSAIDs
    - Opioids
  - Nothing by mouth until definitive diagnosis
- Treatment is based on definitive diagnosis

Providing Treatment:
Alternative Measures to Consider
- Symptomatic treatment while test results pending
  - Rest
  - Local heat
  - Positioning
- Active listening of client concerns

Providing Support:
Education and Support Measures to Consider
- Information and discussion regarding
  - Working diagnosis
  - Plan for evaluation
  - Access to care if condition worsens
  - Indications for consultation and/or referral
- Acute pain with referral
  - Anticipate hospital admission
  - Nothing by mouth
  - Medical or surgical treatment

Follow-up Care:
Follow-up Measures to Consider
- Document
  - Criteria used for diagnosis
  - Indications for consultation
  - Client instructions
  - Consultation and/or referral
  - Plan for continued care
- Nonacute presentation
  - Reevaluate within 24–48 hours
  - Phone or face to face
- Return for care
  - Worsening symptoms
  - Persistent symptoms
  - As indicated by testing

Collaborative Practice:
Criteria to Consider for Consultation or Referral
- OB/GYN service
  - Suspected or confirmed obstetric/gynecologic cause, such as
    - Pelvic abscess
    - Ectopic pregnancy
    - Septic abortion
  - Uncertain diagnosis
  - Clients with no improvement in 24–48 hours with treatment

- Medical/surgical or emergency service
  - Non-gynecologic surgical emergency
  - Uncertain diagnosis
  - Temperature $\geq$ 102°F with rebound tenderness or guarding
- For diagnosis or treatment outside the midwife's scope of practice

CARE OF THE WOMAN WITH CHRONIC PELVIC PAIN

Key Clinical Information

Chronic pelvic pain is a common finding in women's health and may be related to reproductive functioning, the bladder or bowel, or residual effects of abdominal infection or surgery. Many women with chronic pelvic pain are ultimately diagnosed with endometriosis. Low-grade pelvic pain may occur in women who have been subject to sexual assault or molestation, whereas ovarian cancer typically presents with vague pelvic symptoms. Client involvement and support during investigation of chronic pelvic pain is essential. Validation of the client's discomfort and concerns are as essential to evaluation and treatment of this challenging problem as a skillfully obtained history, review of systems, and thorough physical examination. The evaluation of chronic pelvic pain often takes place over many visits. Client acceptance of the chronic nature of the symptoms and development of positive coping behaviors reduces anxiety during this process.

Client History and Chart Review: Components of the History to Consider (Moses, 2007c)

- Age
- Reproductive history
  - Gravida, para, menstrual status
    - Menstrual patterns
    - Potential for pregnancy
    - Current method of contraception
    - Vaginal birth and/or cesarean delivery
  - Most recent examination, Pap smear, and STI testing

- Current sexual practices
  - Number of lifetime sexual partners
  - New sexual partner for self or partner
- History of
  - Premenstrual dysphoric disorder
  - STI/PID
  - Endometriosis
  - Ectopic pregnancy
- Pain profile
  - Onset, duration, severity
  - Location: radiating or fixed
  - Timing
    - Intermittent or constant
    - Correlation with
      - Menstrual cycle
      - Pelvic infection
      - Sexual violence
      - Abortion
  - Precipitating factors
    - Menses
    - Intercourse
    - Bowel or bladder function
  - Character of symptoms, such as
    - Cramping
    - Aching
    - Knifelike
  - Presence of associated symptoms
    - Fever and chills
    - Nausea and vomiting
    - Vaginal discharge
    - Change in bowel or bladder function
    - Weight loss
    - Dyspareunia
  - Relief measures used and client response
- Potential causes of chronic pelvic pain (Swanton et al., 2006)
  - Physiologic causes
    - Mid-cycle pain
    - Pelvic relaxation
  - Infections
    - Chlamydia
    - Gonorrhea
    - Low-grade PID
    - Urinary tract infection

- Reproductive pelvic disorders, such as
  - Endometriosis
  - Pelvic congestion
  - Uterine fibroids
  - Chronic pelvic pain post-PID
  - Ovarian mass or cancer
  - Ectopic pregnancy
- Non-gynecologic pelvic disorders, such as
  - Peritoneal adhesions
  - Hernia
  - Gastrointestinal cause
  - Interstitial cystitis
- Psychogenic pain
- Medical/surgical history
  - Medications
  - Allergies
  - Health conditions
    - Diverticular disease
    - Renal calculi
    - Abdominal surgery
- Family history
  - Endometriosis
  - Dysmenorrhea
  - Ovarian cancer
  - Diverticular disease
  - Colon cancer
- Psychosocial history and status
  - Physical or sexual violence
  - Drug/alcohol use
  - Living situation
  - Client interpretation of pain
- Mental health status
  - Affect and presentation
  - Coping ability
- Review of systems (ROS)

Physical Examination:
Components of the Physical Exam to Consider
(Moses, 2007c)
- Vital signs
- Abdominal examination
  - Palpate for masses and/or pain
  - Note guarding or rebound tenderness
  - Auscultate bowel sounds

- Pelvic examination
  - Speculum examination
    - Vaginal discharge
    - Bleeding
    - Cervical discharge or lesions
  - Bimanual examination
    - Urethra
    - Cervical motion tenderness
      - Mild
        - Endometriosis
        - Adhesions
      - Moderate
        - PID
    - Uterus: contour, position, or pain
      - Retroverted uterus associated with
        - Endometriosis
        - Adhesions
        - Dyspareunia
    - Adnexa: size, mass, or pain
    - Fornices and posterior pelvis: mass or pain
  - Rectovaginal examination
    - Vague pelvic ache with pressure associated with
      - Cystocele
      - Rectocele
      - Enterocele
      - Uterine prolapse
  - Rectal examination
    - Pain
    - Masses

Clinical Impression:
Differential Diagnoses and Code Groups
to Consider
Additional suffix may apply (ICD9data.com, 2007)
- Abdominal tenderness, lower left quadrant (ICD-9 codes 789.64)
- Abdominal tenderness, lower right quadrant (ICD-9 codes 789.63)
- Abdominal tenderness, periumbilical (ICD-9 codes 789.65)
- Abdominal tenderness, generalized (ICD-9 codes 789.68)

- Abdominal pain, lower left quadrant (ICD-9 codes 789.04)
- Abdominal pain, lower right quadrant (ICD-9 codes 789.03)
- Abdominal pain, periumbilical (ICD-9 codes 789.05)
- Abdominal pain, unspecified (ICD-9 codes 789.00)

Diagnostic Testing:
Diagnostic Tests and Procedures to Consider (Moses, 2007c)

- Pregnancy testing
- Pap smear
- STI testing
- Urinalysis
- Urine culture and sensitivity
- Stool for occult blood
- CBC, with differential
- Cancer antigen (CA-125) (postmenopausal clients)
  - Nonspecific, elevated in ovarian cancer
  - 35 μ/ml suspicious
  - May be falsely elevated in premenopausal women
- Carcinoembryonic antigen (CEA)
  - Elevated in the presence of some cancers
- Pelvic ultrasound
  - Transvaginal
  - Abdominal
- Diagnostic laparoscopy
- Colonoscopy

Providing Treatment:
Therapeutic Measures to Consider

- Symptom relief
  - NSAIDs
    - Ibuprofen 600 mg TID for 5–7 days
    - Naproxen sodium 500 mg BID for 7–10 days
- Other treatments based on confirmed diagnosis

Providing Treatment:
Alternative Measures to Consider

- Local symptomatic relief measures
  - Heat
  - Positioning

- Physical activity
- Rest
- Dietary support
  - Well-balanced diet
  - Maintain optimal bowel and bladder function
    - Limit fatty foods, caffeine, and alcohol
    - Adequate fiber and fluid intake
- Stress management
  - Acupuncture
  - Expressive therapy
    - Visualization
    - Acceptance
  - Coping skills for living with chronic pain

Providing Support:
Education and Support Measures to Consider

- Encourage client participation in evaluation process
  - Pain mapping: symptom diary and menstrual record (Swanton et al., 2006)
  - Provide reassurance, comfort, active listening
  - Teach coping skills for living with chronic pain
  - Review danger signs (e.g., fever, acute pain, syncope)
- Information and discussion
  - Differential diagnosis
  - Recommendations for evaluation
  - Treatment options
  - Community resources
  - Support groups

Follow-up Care:
Follow-up Measures to Consider

- Document
  - Symptom profile
  - Clinical findings
  - Criteria used for diagnosis
  - Criteria for consultation or referral
- Return for continued care
  - At frequent intervals until pathology ruled in/out
  - For continued support
- Consider laparoscopic evaluation for diagnosis

Collaborative Practice:
Criteria to Consider for Consultation or Referral

- OB/GYN service
  - Suspected endometriosis
  - Pain of suspected or documented patho-logic origin
  - Persistent low-grade pelvic pain unrespon-sive to therapy
  - Signs of pelvic prolapse
- Mental health service
  - Pain with apparent psychogenic basis
  - Ineffective coping ability
  - Diagnosis of chronic disorder
- Pain management clinic
- For diagnosis or treatment outside the mid-wife's scope of practice

CARE OF THE WOMAN WITH PELVIC INFLAMMATORY DISEASE

Key Clinical Information

Pelvic inflammatory disease (PID) is one of the most common and serious complications of STIs. PID is caused by bacteria ascending from the vagina into the upper genital tract, most often occurring during menses (Fogel, 2006). The most common causative bacteria are *Neisseria gonorrhoeae* and *Chlamydia*; however, the normal flora of the gas-trointestinal and genital tracts may also cause PID. Diagnosis of PID is based on clinical presentation, which may be vague. It is essential that the sexual partner(s) of women with suspected PID be treated before resumption of sexual activity. PID may cause significant scarring in the fallopian tubes as well as in the pelvis. Scarring may contribute to infertility, chronic pelvic pain, and other related disorders. Women with HIV are more likely to require hospi-talization with PID (CDC, 2006a).

Client History and Chart Review:
Components of the History to Consider
(CDC, 2006a; Fogel, 2006b)

- Age
  - Most common in adolescents

- Reproductive history
  - LMP, gravida, para
    - Menstrual/pregnancy status
    - Current method of contraception
  - Most recent Pap smear and STI testing
  - Sexual orientation and practices
  - New sexual partner for self or partner
  - Recent procedure, delivery, or termination of pregnancy
- Risk factors for PID
  - Active infection with chlamydia or gonorrhea
  - Previous infection with STI
  - Sexually active adolescent
  - IUD insertion
  - Multiple sexual partners
  - Douching
- Symptom profile
  - Location, onset, duration, severity of symptoms
  - Triad of symptoms for empiric treatment (CDC, 2006a)
    - Lower abdominal pain
    - No other apparent cause of illness, *and*
      - Cervical motion tenderness, *or*
      - Uterine tenderness, *or*
      - Adnexal tenderness
    - Additional diagnostic criteria
      - Fever > 101°F (> 38.3°C)
      - Mucopurulent vaginal or cervical discharge
      - Many white blood cells on saline wet preparation
      - Elevated erythrocyte sedimentation rate
      - Elevated C-reactive protein
      - Positive CT or GC results
  - Other associated symptoms
    - Dyspareunia
    - Referred pain
    - Menstrual irregularities
    - Malaise
- Medical/surgical history
  - Allergies
  - Medications

- Chronic illnesses
- Previous surgery
- Social history
  - Drug or alcohol use
  - Living situation
- Review of systems (ROS)

Physical Examination:
Components of the Physical Exam to Consider
- Vital signs, including temperature
- Abdominal examination
  - Lower abdominal tenderness
    - Guarding
    - Distention
    - Rebound tenderness
  - Presence or absence of bowel sounds
- Pelvic examination
  - Speculum examination
    - Mucopurulent cervical discharge
    - Collection of cervical cultures
  - Bimanual examination
    - Cervical motion tenderness
    - Uterine enlargement or tenderness
    - Adnexal mass or tenderness

Clinical Impression:
Differential Diagnoses and Code Groups
to Consider
Additional suffix may apply (ICD9data.com, 2007)
- Pelvic inflammatory disease (PID) (ICD-9 codes 614)
- Ectopic pregnancy (ICD-9 codes 633)
- Ovarian cyst (ICD-9 codes 620)
- Septic abortion (ICD-9 codes 639)
- Endometritis (ICD-9 codes 615)
- Endometriosis (ICD-9 codes 617)
- Cystitis (ICD-9 codes 595)
- Appendicitis (ICD-9 codes 540–543)

Diagnostic Testing:
Diagnostic Tests and Procedures to Consider
(CDC, 2006a)
- Urinalysis
- Serum or urine HCG

- STI testing, including HIV
- CBC with differential
- Erythrocyte sedimentation rate
- C-reactive protein
- Gram stain and culture of cervical discharge
  - Presence of gram-negative intracellular diplococci
  - 10 white blood cells per high-power field
- Pelvic ultrasound or MRI
  - Thickened fluid-filled tubes
  - Free fluid in pelvis
  - Tuboovarian abscess
- Diagnostic laparoscopy

Providing Treatment:
Therapeutic Measures to Consider (CDC, 2007a;
CDC, 2006a)
- Choice and location of treatment varies with
  - Severity of illness
  - Anticipated client compliance
- Outpatient treatment for PID
  - Option one
    - Ceftriaxone 250 mg IM in a single dose, *plus*
    - Doxycycline 100 mg PO twice a day for 14 days, *or*
  - Option two
    - Cefoxitin 2 g IM in a single dose, *with*
    - Probenecid 1 g PO in a single dose, *plus*
    - Doxycycline 100 mg PO twice a day for 14 days, *or*
  - Other parenteral third-generation cephalosporins, such as
    - Ceftizoxime or cefotaxime, *plus*
    - Doxycycline 100 mg orally twice a day for 14 days
  - Alternate regimens for PID with
    - Low community prevalence of gonorrhea
    - Low individual risk of gonorrhea
    - Fluoroquinolones
      - Levofloxacin 500 mg orally once daily, *or*
      - Ofloxacin 400 mg twice daily for 14 days

- Outpatient regimen may be given *with* or *without*
  - Metronidazole 500 mg orally twice a day for 14 days
- Hospital-based treatment
  - 🩺 Criteria for considering hospital-based treatment
    - Acute abdominal cause such as appendicitis cannot be excluded
    - Pregnant women
    - Oral antimicrobial therapy ineffective or inappropriate
    - PID accompanied by
      - Nausea and vomiting, *or*
      - High fever, *and*
      - Tuboovarian abscess
  - Transition to oral treatment 24–48 hours after clinical improvement
  - Oral antibiotics are given to provide 14 total days of coverage
  - Parenteral regimen A
    - Cefotetan 2 g IV every 12 hours, *or*
    - Cefoxitin 2 g IV every 6 hours, *plus*
    - Doxycycline 100 mg PO or IV every 12 hours
  - Parenteral regimen B
    - Clindamycin 900 mg IV every 8 hours, *plus*
    - Gentamicin
      - Loading dose IV or IM (2 mg/kg of body weight)
      - Maintenance dose (1.5 mg/kg) every 8 hours
      - Single daily dosing may be substituted
  - Alternate parenteral regimen
    - Ampicillin/Sulbactam 3 g IV every 6 hours, *plus*
    - Doxycycline 100 mg PO or IV every 12 hours

Providing Treatment:
Alternative Measures to Consider
- ⚠️ Alternative therapies are not a substitute for prompt medical care

- Comfort measures
  - Warm heat to abdomen
  - Adequate rest
- Remedies for healing and immune support
  - Balanced nutrition
  - Echinacea
  - Rescue Remedy
  - Visualization

Providing Support:
Education and Support Measures to Consider
- Provide information related to
  - Diagnosis
  - Need to evaluate and/or treat partner(s)
  - Treatment recommendations
    - Complete all medication
    - Avoid intercourse until
      - Medications completed + 7 days
      - Partner treated + 7 days
  - Mandatory STI reporting
  - Test of cure as indicated
  - Potential complications
    - Pelvic abscess
    - Infertility
    - Ectopic pregnancy
    - Chronic pelvic pain
- Provide written materials
  - Medication instructions
  - Transmission of infection
  - Warning signs
  - When to return for care
- Prevention of recurrence
  - Abstinence
  - Condom use
  - Mutual monogamy
  - Regular STI screening

Follow-up Care:
Follow-up Measures to Consider
- Document
  - Criteria used for diagnosis
  - Treatment regimen
  - Medication administration
  - Client education

- Mandatory reporting
- Plan for continued care
- Criteria for consultation or referral
- Outpatient therapy
  - Client contact within 24–48 hours
  - Hospitalization if limited improvement by 72 hours (CDC, 2006a)
- Test of cure 4–6 weeks with diagnosis of
  - Chlamydia
  - Gonorrhea
- HIV testing if not done with initial workup

Collaborative Practice:
Criteria to Consider for Consultation or Referral
- OB/GYN service
  - Acutely ill women requiring hospitalization
  - Pregnant women with PID
  - Clients who do not improve within 24–72 hours of treatment
- Emergency care
  - Other nonreproductive-related acute abdomen
- For diagnosis or treatment outside the midwife's scope of practice

CARE OF THE WOMAN WITH CYCLIC MENSTRUAL SYMPTOMS

Key Clinical Information
Women experience symptoms of varying severity related to the menstrual cycle. In some women recurring symptoms are significant enough to interfere with normal daily functioning. Menstrual symptom disorders are classified as cyclic perimenstrual pain and discomfort or premenstrual syndrome (PMS). Both conditions include primary dysmenorrhea, whereas PMS also includes premenstrual dysphoric disorder (PMDD), a severe form of PMS with a preponderance of affective symptoms (Taylor et al., 2006). Women who suffer from PMS frequently feel they are not in control of their moods or actions. Treatment is aimed at finding relief measures that are acceptable to the individual woman and supporting her within the

context of her life. Attention to life-style, diet, home life, and other life choices is an integral part of the assessment and treatment for cyclic perimenstrual pain and discomfort and PMS.

Client History and Chart Review:
Components of the History to Consider
(Taylor et al., 2006)
- Age
  - Ages 30–45 may have most severe symptoms
- Reproductive history
  - LMP, gravida, para
  - Method of contraception
  - Current stage of reproductive life
- Menstrual history
  - Age at menarche
  - Years of menstruation
  - Normal cyclic pattern
- ▽ Symptom profile
  - Timing of symptoms in cycle
  - Age at onset of symptoms
  - Onset, duration, and severity of symptoms
  - Emotional symptoms
    - Turmoil
      - Hostility
      - Aggression
      - Mood swings
      - Anxiety
    - Depression
      - Sadness
      - Guilt
      - Tearfulness
      - Desire to be alone
    - ⚠ Potential for harm to self or others
  - Behavioral symptoms
    - May be related to decreased serotonin activity
    - Irritability, anger, panic attacks
    - Alcohol abuse, sweet cravings, binge eating
  - Physical symptoms
    - Weight gain and bloating
    - Fluid retention

- ◆ Pelvic pain
- ◆ Breast tenderness
- ◆ Migraine
- ◆ Constipation
- ◆ Joint and muscle pain
- ◆ Lack of energy
- ◆ Forgetfulness
- ◆ Confusion
- Effect of symptoms on daily living
  - ▪ Self-image
  - ▪ Relationships
  - ▪ Employment
- Ability to effectively self-treat symptoms
  - ▪ 🔘 Relief measures used and rate of success
- Medical/surgical history
  - ▪ Allergies
  - ▪ Medications
  - ▪ Health conditions
    - ◆ Endocrine disorders
    - ◆ Heart disease, hypertension
  - ▪ Other medical conditions
- Psychosocial history and status
  - ▪ Potential contributing factors
    - ◆ Life stressors
    - ◆ Ineffective stress response
    - ◆ Sexual abuse
    - ◆ Cultural expression of symptoms
  - ▪ Drug/alcohol, tobacco use
  - ▪ Usual physical activity
  - ▪ Diet review
  - ▪ Social and family support
  - ▪ Stressors
- Review of systems (ROS)

Physical Examination:
Components of the Physical Exam
to Consider

- Age-appropriate physical examination
  - ▪ If none within previous 6–12 months
  - ▪ With new onset of symptoms
  - ▪ To update pertinent systems

Clinical Impression:
Differential Diagnoses and Code Groups
to Consider
Additional suffix may apply (ICD9data.com, 2007)

- PMS (ICD-9 codes 625.4)
- Premenstrual dysphoric disorder (ICD-9 codes 625.4)
- Perimenopausal changes (ICD-9 codes 627.2)
- Mood disorder (ICD-9 codes 296)
- Endocrine disorder (ICD-9 codes 240–259)

Diagnostic Testing:
Diagnostic Tests and Procedures to Consider

- Premenstrual symptoms screening tool (American Psychiatric Association, 1995)
- Premenstrual dysphoric disorder diagnosis
  - ▪ Symptoms only present during luteal phase
  - ▪ Symptoms occur most cycles
  - ▪ Confirmation of symptoms for at least two consecutive cycles
  - ▪ 🔻 Five or more symptoms
    - ◆ At least one must be from the first four listed
      - ➤ Symptoms
        - ▹ Depressed mood
        - ▹ Tension
        - ▹ Mood swings
        - ▹ Irritability
        - ▹ Decreased interest in usual activities
        - ▹ Lack of energy
        - ▹ Insomnia or hypersomnia
        - ▹ Physical symptoms such as bloating and breast tenderness
        - ▹ Difficulty concentrating
        - ▹ Marked change in appetite
        - ▹ Feeling overwhelmed
- Laboratory testing is based on age and findings on history and physical examination
  - ▪ Thyroid panel
  - ▪ TSH
  - ▪ LH/FSH
  - ▪ Renal function testing
  - ▪ Hepatic function testing

Providing Treatment:
Therapeutic Measures to Consider
(ACOG, 2000b; Murphy, 2004; Taylor
et al., 2006)

- Hormonal treatment, such as
  - Oral contraceptive pills
    - Yaz
    - Seasonale
  - Progesterone
    - Perimenopausal women
    - Days 12–28 of cycle
      - Micronized progesterone
        - 300 mg qhs
      - Provera
        - 10 mg qhs
- Selective serotonin reuptake inhibitors (SSRI)
  - Fluoxetine (Sarafem)
    - 20 mg daily
    - Pregnancy Category C
  - Sertraline (Zoloft)
    - 50 mg daily
    - Pregnancy Category C
- Anxiolytic medications
  - ⚠ Short-term use only
  - May exacerbate symptoms
  - Alprazolam
  - Diazepam
  - Lorazepam
  - Buspirone
- Diuretic
  - Aldactone 25–100 mg
  - Use daily during luteal phase
- NSAIDs
  - Prostaglandin inhibitors
  - Use during luteal phase
  - Mefenamic acid (Ponstel)
  - Naproxen sodium (Anaprox or Aleve)
- Vitamin and mineral supplementation
  - Calcium 400 mg QID
  - Magnesium 200–400 mg/day
  - Vitamin E 400 IU/day
  - Vitamin B_6, taken in B complex

Providing Treatment:
Alternative Measures to Consider (ACOG,
2000b; Holden, n.d.; Taylor et al., 2006)

- Regular aerobic exercise
- Tryptophan-containing foods
  - Chocolate
  - Cheddar cheese
  - Salmon
  - Oats
  - Chick peas
  - Sunflower and pumpkin seeds
  - Bananas, mangos, and dates
  - Peanut and sesame butter
  - Red meats and turkey
- Evening primrose oil
- Herbal balancing formula (for additional formulas, see Soule, 1996, pp. 124–134)
  - Mix equal parts
    - Chamomile
    - Red raspberry leaf
    - Chasteberry (Vitex)
    - Prepare as tea or tincture
    - Use daily
- Diuretic formula for premenstrual phase of cycle
  - Dandelion leaf or root—2 parts
  - Stinging nettle—2 parts
  - Peppermint—1 part
  - Black cohosh—1 part
  - Mix and prepare as tincture (preferable) or tea
  - Use 10–30 gtts tincture TID or tea morning and night
- Premenstrual depression
  - St. John's wort
  - May alter effectiveness of hormonal birth control
- Homeopathic remedies
  - 30× tabs QID for acute symptoms
  - 100× pellets daily as constitutional remedy
  - Calcarea phosphorica—general sense of weakness and fatigue accompanied by breast tenderness, genital sweating, and itching

- Pulsatilla—for tears and anxiety, nausea, tension; menses are unpredictable
- Sepia—symptoms of exhaustion, irritability, low back pain, decreased sex drive, anger, and intolerance

Providing Support:
Education and Support Measures to Consider
- Review menstrual cycle and function
  - Menstrual charting
  - Symptom charting
    - Onset
    - Duration
    - Relation to cycle
- Reinforce benefits of
  - Excellent and balanced nutrition
  - Regular daily exercise
  - Personal time
- Discuss potential life-style changes
  - Stress reduction techniques, such as
    - Music or art therapy
    - Dance
    - Yoga
    - Prayer/meditation
  - Foster self-image and autonomy
  - Encourage family and friends to help
  - Allow for personal time
  - Shared responsibility
- Explore fertility/sexuality/relationship issues

Follow-up Care:
Follow-up Measures to Consider
- Document
  - Symptom profile
  - Criteria used for diagnosis
  - Treatment plan
    - Behavioral
    - Pharmacologic
    - Nutritional supplements
- Differentiate between premenstrual dysphoric disorder and depression
  - Client to keep symptom diary for three or more cycles

- Review symptoms
- Plot on menstrual calendar
- Return for continued care
  - For symptom diary review
  - For persistent or worsening symptoms
  - For medication follow-up
  - For well-woman care

Collaborative Practice:
Criteria to Consider for Consultation or Referral
- OB/GYN or medical service
  - For underlying medical or gynecologic problem
- Mental health service
  - For mental health issues unrelated to PMS
  - Severe premenstrual dysphoric disorder
  - Client who is a danger to self or others
- Support groups/community resources
  - Women's groups
  - PMS support group
- For diagnosis or treatment outside the midwife's scope of practice

CARE OF THE WOMAN WITH SYPHILIS

Key Clinical Information

Syphilis is a complex systemic sexually transmitted disease that is infectious only when mucocutaneous lesions are present, although testing and treatment are recommended for any exposure (CDC, 2006a). Syphilis infection includes the following possible stages: primary infection (ulcer or chancre at infection site), secondary infection (rash, mucocutaneous lesions, and lymphadenopathy), and latent stage (asymptomatic) and tertiary infection (cardiac, neurologic, ophthalmic, auditory, or gummatous lesions). Early latent syphilis is defined as infection acquired within 1 year, whereas late latent syphilis is infection acquired more than 1 year previously yet still in the latent stage. Treatment is most successful when the disease is diagnosed in the primary or secondary stages. Perinatal transmission commonly results in development of congenital syphilis in the newborn (CDC, 2006a).

Client History and Chart Review:
Components of the History to Consider
(CDC, 2006a)

- Age
- Reproductive history
  - LMP, gravida, para
    - Perinatal losses
    - Current method of contraception
  - Last examination, Pap smear, and STI screen
  - Previous diagnosis or treatment of STIs
  - Sexual activity
    - Number of lifetime partners
    - New partner for self or partner
- Duration, onset, and severity of symptoms
- Signs and symptoms of syphilis
  - Primary syphilis
    - Chancre at site of infection
    - Develops 10–90 days postexposure
    - Single painless sore
    - Raised edges
    - Lasts 1–5 weeks
    - Infection persists after chancre heals
  - Secondary syphilis
    - Symptoms develop 2–28 weeks postexposure
    - Symmetric, macular, papular, nonitchy rash
    - Condylomata lata
    - Mucous membrane lesions
    - Alopecia
    - Symptoms of systemic illness
      - Generalized malaise
      - Fever
  - Latent phase
    - No clinical manifestations
    - Lasts 2–30 years after infection
    - Testing is essential for diagnosis
- Tertiary syphilis
  - Gumma development
  - Neurologic symptoms
    - Headache
    - Symptoms of central nervous system involvement

- Auditory or visual symptoms
- Paralysis
- Mental illness
- Cardiopulmonary symptoms
  - Shortness of breath
  - Hypertension
- Medical/surgical history
  - Allergies
  - Medications
  - Chronic or acute health conditions
  - HIV status, if known
- Review of systems (ROS)

Physical Examination:
Components of the Physical Exam
to Consider

- Vital signs, including blood pressure and temperature
- Observe skin and soft tissue for signs of primary infection (Varney et al., 2004)
  - Alopecia
  - Generalized adenopathy
  - Rash
    - Palms and soles
    - Neck and head
    - Torso
  - Mucous membrane ulcers
- Cardiopulmonary assessment
  - Presence of murmur
  - Lung sounds
- Neurologic assessment
  - Cranial nerve abnormalities
  - Diminished reflexes
  - Change in personality
- Pelvic examination
  - Primary chancre
    - Characteristic painless firm ulcer
  - Condylomata lata
  - Evaluation for signs of other STIs
  - Collection of specimens for testing

Clinical Impression:
Differential Diagnoses and Code Groups
to Consider
Additional suffix may apply (ICD9data.com, 2007)
- Syphilis
  - Primary (ICD-9 codes 091.0–091.2)
  - Secondary (ICD-9 codes 091.3–091.9)
  - Latent (early or late) (ICD-9 codes 092 or 096)
  - Tertiary (ICD-9 codes 093–095)
- Acute bacterial infection (ICD-9 codes 030–041)
- Viral infections (ICD-9 codes 050–079)
- Mononucleosis (ICD-9 codes 075)
- Hansen's disease (ICD-9 codes 030)
- HPV-related condyloma (ICD-9 codes 078.1)

Diagnostic Testing:
Diagnostic Tests and Procedures to Consider
(CDC, 2006a)
- Rapid plasma reagin (RPR) or venereal disease Research Laboratory (VDRL) titers
  - Signs or symptoms
  - Exposure
  - Diagnosis of any STI
  - Pregnancy
    - Initial prenatal visit
    - Stillborn > 20 weeks gestation
    - Repeat for high-risk population at
      - 28–32 weeks gestation
      - On admission for delivery
  - Positive VDRL or RPR 1–4 weeks after chancre
    - False positive may occur with
      - Acute infection
      - Autoimmune disorders
      - Malignancy
      - Pregnancy
      - After immunization
    - FTA-ABS or MHA-TP to confirm
      - FTA-ABS = fluorescent treponemal antibody absorbed
      - MHA-TP = microhemagglutination assay for antibody to *T. pallidum*

- Wet preparation
- Chlamydia and gonorrhea testing
- HCG testing
- Hepatitis screen
- HIV counseling and testing

Providing Treatment:
Therapeutic Measures to Consider (CDC, 2006a)
- Parenteral penicillin G is treatment of choice
- Primary and secondary syphilis and early latent syphilis
  - Benzathine penicillin G
    - 2.4 million units IM as one-time dose
    - In pregnancy may repeat dose in 7 days for
      - Primary
      - Secondary
      - Early latent
- 🔖 Penicillin allergy, primary or secondary
  - Desensitization to penicillin recommended
  - Doxycycline 100 mg PO BID for 14 days
    - Pregnancy Category D
  - Tetracycline 500 mg PO QID for 14 days
    - Pregnancy Category D
- Indications for 3-week series
  - Late latent syphilis
  - Syphilis of unknown duration
  - Treatment failure in absence of tertiary disease
  - Benzathine penicillin G 7.2 million units *total dose*
    - Give IM weekly for three doses
    - 2.4 million units

Providing Treatment:
Alternative Measures to Consider
(Herbs2000.com, 2002)
- ⚠️ Alternative measures are not a substitute for prompt antibiotic treatment
- General measures to promote healing
  - Probiotic supplement
  - Avoid tryptophan-containing foods or supplements

- Herbal support
  - Astragalus—capsules or tincture
  - Butcher's broom—capsules
  - Rooibos tea

Providing Support:
Education and Support Measures to Consider (American Social Health Association, 2005; CDC, 2006a)
- Reinforce need for sex partners to be tested
  - Partner exposed within 90 days may be infected yet seronegative
  - Partner exposed > 90 days should be treated presumptively while awaiting serology
- Time periods before treatment used for identifying at-risk partners
  - More than 3 months duration of symptoms for primary syphilis
  - More than 6 months duration of symptoms for secondary syphilis
  - Twelve months for early latent syphilis
- Provide written information
  - Prevention education materials
  - Medication information and instructions
  - STI reporting and contact follow-up
  - Return visit and follow-up testing
- Active listening
- Discussion of strategies for
  - Informing partner(s)
  - Behavioral change

Follow-up Care:
Follow-up Measures to Consider (American Social Health Association, 2005; CDC, 2006a)
- Document
  - Method of infection confirmation
  - Changes in titers
  - Treatment plan
  - Follow-up protocol
  - Required case reporting
    - Disease diagnosis and treatment
    - Sexual contacts

- Return for continued care
  - As indicated during pregnancy
  - Reevaluate and retest
    - Primary or secondary syphilis: 6 and 12 months
    - Latent syphilis: 6, 12, and 24 months
    - HIV-positive client: every 3 months for 2 years
  - Retreat for
    - Persistent symptoms
    - Failure to have fourfold decline in non-treponemal test titers
  - HIV testing for treatment failures
  - Observe for Jarisch-Herxheimer reaction
    - May occur within 24 hours after therapy for syphilis
    - Acute febrile reaction
    - Headache, myalgia, and other symptoms
    - Most common with early syphilis
    - May cause fetal distress or preterm labor

Collaborative Practice:
Criteria to Consider for Consultation or Referral
- OB/GYN service
  - For acute illness with primary infection
  - Pregnancy complicated by syphilis
  - Jarisch-Herxheimer reaction
  - Treatment failures
- Medical service
  - For tertiary or neurosyphilis
- Pediatric service
  - Infants at risk for congenital syphilis
- For diagnosis or treatment outside the midwife's scope of practice

CARE OF THE WOMAN WITH TRICHOMONIASIS

Key Clinical Information
Trichomoniasis is the term for the infection caused by the parasitic protozoan *Trichomonas vaginalis*. It is a highly contagious STI that affects both men and women, with approximately 120 million women affected worldwide each year (Forna & Gulmezogly,

2003). Trichomoniasis is characterized by malodorous, frothy, yellow-green vaginal discharge and petechiae on the cervix. These objective signs may be accompanied by vaginal pruritus and irritation, dyspareunia, and/or dysuria. The effects of *Trichomonas* infection range from simple discomfort in the woman to increased morbidity and mortality for her fetus secondary to preterm labor, rupture of membranes or delivery, and/or low birth weight infants (Okun et al., 2005). Because infection with *T. vaginalis* infection can increase the likelihood of HIV transmission, all women with trichomonal infections as well as their sex partners should be promptly treated (Okun et al., 2005). However, recent findings suggest that treatment of asymptomatic trichomoniasis infections with metronidazole during pregnancy may actually increase the risk of preterm labor, raising questions and concerns regarding current treatment guidelines for trichomoniasis treatment in pregnancy. The CDC continues to recommend treating *T. vaginalis* infections in pregnancy (CDC, 2006a).

Client History and Chart Review:
Components of the History to Consider
(CDC, 2006a)

- Age
- Reproductive history
  - LMP gravida, para
    - Onset, duration
    - Method of birth control
    - Symptoms of pregnancy
    - Gestational age if pregnant
  - Obstetric history
    - Preterm labor and birth
    - Premature rupture of membranes
    - Low birth weight infants
  - Sexual history and practices
    - Use of condoms
    - Previous diagnosis of STI
    - Risk factors for PID
    - New sexual partner for self or partner
    - Multiple partners for self or partner
    - Heterosexual relationship
    - Same sex relationship
    - Use of sex toys
- Symptom history
  - Pain
    - Location
    - Severity
    - Precipitating factors
  - Vulvovaginal symptoms
    - Itching
    - Irritation
    - Burning
    - Dyspareunia
    - Dysuria
  - Presence of discharge
    - Frothy
    - Yellow-green
    - Malodorous, described as foul or fishy
  - Treatments used and results
  - Aggravating and alleviating factors
  - Signs or symptoms of PID
- Medical/surgical history
  - Allergies
  - Medications
  - Chronic health problems
- Social history
- Alcohol or drug use
- Sexual, physical, or emotional abuse

Physical Examination:
Components of the Physical Exam to Consider
(CDC, 2006a)

- Vital signs
- Abdominal palpation for signs of PID
  - Rebound tenderness
  - Guarding
- Pelvic examination
  - External genitalia
    - Frothy discharge at introitus
    - Vulvar irritation
  - Speculum examination
    - Vaginal discharge
    - Vaginal walls may appear erythematous

♦ "Strawberry spots" (tiny petechiae) on cervix and/or vaginal wall

♦ Friable cervix

▪ Bimanual examination

♦ Cervical motion tenderness

♦ Uterine enlargement or tenderness

♦ Painful adnexal mass

- ⚠ Note: The vaginal discharge and visual inspection of the discharge is nonspecific and cannot be used alone for diagnosis. Multiple pathogens may be present. Perform additional testing as required for a complete diagnosis.

Clinical Impression:
Differential Diagnoses and Code Groups to Consider

Additional suffix may apply (ICD9data.com, 2007)

- Trichomoniasis (ICD-9 codes 131)
- BV (ICD-9 codes 616.10)
- Candida vulvovaginitis (ICD-9 codes 112.1)
- Chlamydia (ICD-9 codes 099.5)
- Gonorrhea (ICD-9 codes 098)
- PID (ICD-9 codes 614)
- Ectopic pregnancy (ICD-9 codes 633)
- Round ligament pain (ICD-9 codes 625.9)
- Appendicitis (ICD-9 codes 540–543)

Diagnostic Testing:
Diagnostic Tests and Procedures to Consider (CDC, 2006a)

- Wet preparation for motile trichomonads
  - ▪ Sensitivity 60–70%
- Rapid point-of-service tests
  - ▪ OSOM Trichomonas Rapid Test
  - ▪ Affirm VP III
  - ▪ Sensitivity up to 83%
- Liquid-based Pap smear (Aslan et al., 2005)
  - ▪ Sensitivity up to 98%
- Culture of discharge—gold standard
  - ▪ Standard culture
  - ▪ InPouch TV culture system

Providing Treatment
Therapeutic Measures to Consider (CDC, 2006a)

- Nonpregnant client
  - ▪ Metronidazole 2 g PO one time, *or*
  - ▪ Tinidazole 2 g PO one time, *or*
  - ▪ Metronidazole 500 mg PO BID for 7 days
- ⚠ Therapeutic considerations
  - ▪ Metronidazole gel is not effective in treating *trichomonas* because therapeutic levels of the medication do not reach infected perivaginal glands or urethra.
  - ▪ Nursing mothers
    - ♦ Refrain from breast-feeding and discard milk
      - ➤ Metronidazole: onset of treatment— 24 hours after last dose
      - ➤ Tinidazole: onset of treatment— 3 days after last dose
- Pregnant client
  - ▪ Metronidazole 2 g PO in a single dose
  - ▪ Pregnancy Category B
  - ▪ May delay treatment to > 37 weeks (Hynes, 2007)
    - ♦ Asymptomatic client

Providing Treatment:
Alternative Measures to Consider

- ⚠ Alternative measures are not a substitute for antibiotic therapy
- Nutritional support to offset effects of antibiotics on gut
  - ▪ Yogurt
  - ▪ Applesauce
  - ▪ Acidophilus or probiotics
- Remedies to boost immune response
  - ▪ Echinacea
  - ▪ Homeopathic mercurius solubilis

Providing Support:
Education and Support Measures to Consider

- Provide information regarding
  - ▪ Infection cause and transmission
  - ▪ Effects on reproductive organs and future fertility

- Potential effect on pregnancy
  - Premature rupture of membranes
  - Preterm labor
  - Preterm birth
  - Low birth weight
- Need for partner notification and treatment
- Treatment plan
- Medication instructions
  - Reinforce importance of taking medication as prescribed
  - Avoid alcohol during treatment
    - Metronidazole: 24 hours after last dose
    - Tinidazole: 72 hours after last dose
  - Abstinence until
    - Treatment complete
    - Symptoms resolve in both partners
- Prevention measures
  - Safe sexual practices
  - Reduce risk behaviors
  - Condom use for prevention of STI
  - Return for care if potential for STI

Follow-up Care:
Follow-up Measures to Consider
- Document
  - Criteria for diagnosis
  - Treatment regimen
  - Discussion and instructions
  - Plan for continued care
- Follow-up testing not indicated with
  - Client asymptomatic at diagnosis
  - Symptom resolution with treatment
- Return to office with persistent symptoms (CDC, 2006a)
  - HIV testing
  - Treatment failure with Metronidazole 2 g
    - Reinfection excluded
    - Tinidazole 2 g PO one time, *or*
    - Metronidazole 500 mg PO BID for 7 days
  - Persistent treatment failure
    - Metronidazole 2 g PO for 5 days, *or*
    - Tinidazole 2 g PO for 5 days

- Continued treatment failure
  - CDC consultation, *and*
  - *T. vaginalis* susceptibility testing
  - (770) 488-4115; http://www.cdc.gov/std

Collaborative Practice:
Criteria to Consider for Consultation or Referral
- OB/GYN service
  - Persistent symptoms
  - Antibiotic-resistant trichomoniasis
  - Pelvic infection (PID)
  - Positive HIV or hepatitis B status
  - Persistent pelvic pain
  - Ectopic pregnancy
- Pediatric service
  - Delivery of infant to infected mother
  - Infant shows signs of fever and/or abnormal vaginal discharge
- For diagnosis or treatment outside the midwife's scope of practice

REFERENCES

AIDS Education & Training Centers (AETC). (2007a). *Hepatitis B infection.* Retrieved January 29, 2008 from http://www.aidsetc.org/aidsetc?page=cm-511_hepb

AIDS Education & Training Centers (AETC). (2007b). *Clinical manual for management of the HIV-infected adult.* Retrieved January 29, 2008 from http://www.aidsetc.org/aidsetc?page=cm-00-00

Albers, J. R., Hull, S. K., & Wesley, M. S. (2004). Abnormal uterine bleeding. *American Family Physician.* Retrieved January 30, 2008 from http://www.aafp.org/afp/20040415/1915.html

Aliotta, H. M., & Schaeffer, N. J. (2006). Breast conditions. In K. D. Schuiling & F. E. Likis (Eds.). *Women's gynecological health.* Sudbury, MA: Jones and Bartlett.

American Cancer Society (ACS). (2006a). *What are the risk factors for cervical cancer?* Retrieved January 30, 2008 from http://www.cancer.org/docroot/CRI/CRI_2_3x.asp?rnav=cridg&dt=8

American Cancer Society (ACS). (2006b). *Detailed guide: endometrial cancer: what are the risk factors for endometrial cancer?* Retrieved January 30, 2008 from http://www.cancer.org/docroot/CRI/CRI_2_3x.asp?dt=11

American Cancer Society (ACS). (2007a) *Breast cancer facts and figures 2007–2008.* Atlanta: American Cancer Society. Retrieved January 30, 2008 from http://www.cancer.org/docroot/stt/stt_0.asp

American Cancer Society (ACS). (2007b). *ACS recommendations for HPV vaccine use to prevent cervical cancer and pre-cancers.* Retrieved January 31, 2008 from http://www.cancer.org/docroot/CRI/content/CRI_2_6X_ACS_Recommendations_for_HPV_Vaccine_Use_to_Prevent_Cervical_Cancer_and_PreCancers_8.asp?sitearea=&level=

American College of Nurse-Midwives (ACNM). (2001). *Endometrial biopsy.* Clinical bulletin no. 5. Silver Spring, MD: Author.

American College of Obstetricians and Gynecologists (ACOG). (1999a). Medical management of endometriosis. Practice bulletin #11. In *2005 Compendium of selected publications.* Washington, DC: Author.

American College of Obstetricians and Gynecologists (ACOG). (1999b). Surgical alternatives to hysterectomy in the management of leiomyomas. Practice bulletin #16. In *2005 Compendium of selected publications.* Washington, DC: Author.

American College of Obstetricians and Gynecologists (ACOG). (2000a). Management of anovulatory bleeding. Practice bulletin #14. In *2002 Compendium of selected publications.* Washington, DC: Author.

American College of Obstetricians and Gynecologists (ACOG). (2000b). Premenstrual syndrome. Practice bulletin #15. In *2006 Compendium of selected publications.* Washington, DC: Author.

American College of Obstetricians and Gynecologists (ACOG). (2001). Assessment of risk factors for preterm birth. Practice bulletin #31. In *2002 Compendium of selected publications.* Washington, DC: Author.

American College of Obstetricians and Gynecologists (ACOG). (2003). Breast cancer screening. Practice bulletin #42. In *2005 Compendium of selected publications.* Washington, DC: Author.

American College of Physicians. (1998). *Wet mount examinations.* Retrieved January 31, 2008 from http://www.acponline.org/mle/wm_exams.htm

American Psychiatric Association. (1995). *Diagnostic and statistical manual of mental disorders* (4th ed.). Washington, DC: Author.

American Roentgen Ray Society. (2006). CT and ultrasound are equally valuable in diagnosing pelvic pain in women. *Women's Health Law Weekly,* 18. Retrieved January 31, 2008 from http://www.newsrx.com/newsletters/Womens-Health-Law-Weekly/2006-05-28/052520063331098WH.html

American Social Health Association. (2005). *Learn about STIs/STDs. Syphilis: questions and answers.* Retrieved January 31, 2008, from http://www.ashastd.org/learn/learn_syphilis.cfm

Aslan, D. L., Gulbahce, E. H., Stelow, E. B., Setty, S., Brown, C. A., McGlennen, R. C., et al. (2005). The diagnosis of *Trichomonas vaginalis* in liquid-based Pap tests: correlation with PCR. *Diagnostic Cytopathology, 32,* 341–344.

Baeten, J. M., Wang, C., & Celum, C. (2005). Prevention of HIV. In J. Anderson (Ed.). *A guide to the clinical care of women with AIDS.* Retrieved January 31, 2008 from http://hab.hrsa.gov/publications/womencare05/index.htm

Ballweg, M. L. (2005). What women with endometriosis are looking for from their doctors. In *Endometriosis: the mysteries are unraveling—new clinical and scientific insights.* Endometriosis Association. Retrieved January 31, 2008 from http://www.endometriosisassn.org/cme001_coursemain.html

Breast Expert Workgroup. (2005). *Breast cancer diagnostic algorithms for primary care providers* (3rd ed.). California Department of Health Services. Retrieved January 31, 2008 from http://qap.sdsu.edu/screening/breastcancer/bda/algo_booklet/download.html

Brinton, L. A. (2005). Endometriosis and cancer: what the practitioner needs to know. In *Endometriosis: the mysteries are unraveling—new clinical and scientific insights.* Endometriosis Association. Retrieved January 31, 2008 from http://www.endometriosisassn.org/cme001_coursemain.html

Brinton, L. A., Sakoda, L. C., Sherman, M. E., Frederiksen, K., Kjaer, S. K., Graubard, B. I., et al. (2005). Relationship of benign gynecologic diseases to subsequent risk of ovarian and uterine tumors. *Cancer Epidemiology Biomarkers Prevention, 14,* 2929–2935. Retrieved January 31, 2008 from http://cebp.aacrjournals.org/cgi/reprint/14/12/2929

Centers for Disease Control and Prevention (CDC). (2000). *Tracking the hidden epidemics 2000.* Retrieved February 5, 2008 from http://www.cdc.gov/std/Trends2000/default.htm

Centers for Disease Control and Prevention (CDC). (2004a). Increases in fluoroquinolone-resistant *Neisseria gonorrhoeae* among men who have sex with men: United States, 2003, and revised recommendations for gonorrhea treatment, 2004. *Morbidity and Mortality Weekly Report, 53,* 335–338.

Centers for Disease Control and Prevention (CDC). (2004b). *STD facts: genital herpes.* Retrieved February 5, 2008 from http://www.cdc.gov/std/Herpes/STDFact-Herpes.htm

Centers for Disease Control and Prevention (CDC). (2004c). Protocols for confirmation of rapid reactive HIV tests. *Morbidity and Mortality Weekly Report, 53,* 221–222.

Centers for Disease Control and Prevention (CDC). (2005). *Genital candidiasis.* Retrieved January 31, 2008 from http://www.cdc.gov/ncidod/dbmd/diseaseinfo/candidiasis_gen_g.htm

Centers for Disease Control and Prevention (CDC). (2006a). *Sexually transmitted diseases treatment guidelines 2006.* Retrieved January 31, 2008 from http://www.cdc.gov/std/treatment/

Centers for Disease Control and Prevention (CDC). (2006b). Prevention of hepatitis A through active or passive immunization. *Morbidity and Mortality Weekly Report,* 55(RR07), 1–23. Retrieved January 31, 2008 from http://www.cdc.gov/mmwr/preview/mmwrhtml/rr5507a1.htm

Centers for Disease Control and Prevention (CDC). (2006c). Hepatitis B virus infection: a comprehensive immunization strategy to eliminate transmission in the United States. *Morbidity and Mortality Weekly Report,* 55(RR16), 1–25. Retrieved January 31, 2008 from http://www.cdc.gov/MMWR/preview/mmwrhtml/rr5516a1.htm

Centers for Disease Control and Prevention (CDC). (2006d). Revised recommendations for HIV testing of adults, adolescents, and pregnant women in healthcare settings. *Morbidity and Mortality Weekly Report,* 55, 1–17.

Centers for Disease Control and Prevention (CDC). (2007a). *Updated recommended treatment regimens for gonococcal infections and associated conditions—United States.* Retrieved January 31, 2008 from http://www.cdc.gov/std/treatment/2006/updated-regimens.htm

Centers for Disease Control and Prevention (CDC). (2007b). *HIV/AIDs among women.* Retrieved February 5, 2008 from http://www.cdc.gov/hiv/topics/women/resources/factsheets/women.htm

Davidson, T. (2006). Dysfunctional uterine bleeding. In *Gale encyclopedia of medicine.* Retrieved January 31, 2008 from http://www.healthatoz.com/healthatoz/Atoz/common/standard/transform.jsp?requestURI=/healthatoz/Atoz/ency/dysfunctional_uterine_bleeding.jsp

Davey, D. D., Austin, M., Birdsong, G., Buck, H. W., Cox, J. T., Darragh, T. M., et al. (2002). ASCCP patient management guidelines: Pap test specimen adequacy and quality indicators. *Journal of Lower Genital Tract Disease,* 6, 195–199.

Dharmananda, S. (2005). *HIV drugs and herb interactions.* Institute for Traditional Medicine. Retrieved January 31, 2008 from http://www.itmonline.org/arts/hivdrugint.htm

Dodds, N., & Sinert, R. (2006). *Dysfunctional uterine bleeding.* E-medicine. Retrieved January 31, 2008 from http://www.emedicine.com/emerg/topic155.htm

Emmons, L., Callahan, P., Gorman, P., & Snyder, M. (1997). Primary care management of common dermatologic disorders in women. *Journal of Nurse-Midwifery,* 42, 228–253.

Faerstein, E., Szklo, M., & Rosenshein, N. (2001). Risk factors for uterine leiomyoma: a practice-based case-control study. *American Journal of Epidemiology,* 153, 1–10.

Faucher, M. A. & Schuiling, K. D. (2006). Normal and abnormal uterine bleeding. In K. D. Schuiling & F. E. Likis (Eds.). *Women's gynecologic health.* Sudbury, MA: Jones and Bartlett.

Ferenci, P., Dragosics, B., Dittrich, H., Frank, H., Benda, L., Lochs, H., et al. (1989). Randomized controlled trial of silymarin treatment in patients with cirrhosis of the liver. *Journal of Hepatology,* 9, 105–113.

Fogel, C. I. (2006a). Gynecologic infections. In K. D. Schuiling & F. E. Likis (Eds.). *Women's gynecological health.* Sudbury, MA: Jones and Bartlett.

Fogel, C. I. (2006b). Sexually transmitted infection. In K. D. Schuiling & F. E. Likis (Eds.). *Women's gynecologic health.* Sudbury, MA: Jones and Bartlett.

Food and Drug Administration. (2003). *Public health advisory: safety of topical lindane products for the treatment of scabies and lice.* Retrieved February 5, 2008 from http://www.fda.gov/cder/drug/infopage/lindane/lindanePHA.htm

Forna, F. & Gulmezogly, A. M. (2003). Interventions for treating trichomoniasis in women. *Cochrane Database of Systematic Reviews,* Issue 2, Art. No. CD000218.

Foster, S. (1996). *Herbs for your health.* Loveland, CO: Interweave Press.

Galaal, K. A., Deane, K., Sangal, S., & Lopes, A. D. (2007). Interventions for reducing anxiety in women undergoing colposcopy. *Cochrane Database of Systematic Reviews,* Issue 3, Art. No. CD006013.

Gise, L. H. (1994). The premenstrual syndromes. In J. J. Sciarra (Ed.). *Gynecology and obstetrics* (pp. 1–14). Philadelphia: Lippincott-Raven.

Greenwald, J. L., Burstein, G. R., Pincus, J., & Branson, B. (2006). A rapid review of rapid HIV antibody tests. *Current Infectious Disease Reports,* 8, 125–131. Retrieved January 31, 2008 from http://www.cdc.gov/hiv/topics/testing/rapid/index.htm#overview

Grube, W. & McCool, W. (2004). Endometrial biopsy. In H. Varney, J. M. Kriebs & C. L. Gegor (Eds.). *Varney's midwifery* (4th ed.). Sudbury, MA: Jones and Bartlett.

Guidelines and Protocols Advisory Committee. (2005). *Viral hepatitis testing.* British Columbia Ministry of Health. Retrieved January 31, 2008 from http://www.health.gov.bc.ca/gpac/pdf/vihep.pdf

Hepatitis C Technical Advisory Group. (2005). *Alternative therapies for hepatitis C.* National Hepatitis C Program

Office. Retrieved February 5, 2008 from http://www.hepatitis.va.gov/vahep?page=altmed-00-00

Herbs2000.com. (2002). *Syphilis*. Retrieved January 31, 2008 from http://www.herbs2000.com/disorders/syphilis.htm

Hessol, N. A., Ghandi, M., & Greenblatt, R. M. (2005). Epidemiology and natural history of HIV infection in women. In J. Anderson (Ed.). *A guide to the clinical care with women with AIDS*. Retrieved January 29, 2008 from http://hab.hrsa.gov/publications/womencare05/

Holden, J. (n.d.). Nutrient Data Laboratory, Agricultural Research Service. USDA National Nutrient Database for Standard Reference, Release 20. United States Department of Agriculture. Retrieved on January 31, 2008 from http://www.ars.usda.gov/main/site_main.htm?modecode=12354500

Hynes, N. A. (2007). *Vaginal discharge*. Johns Hopkins POC-IT ABX Guide. Retrieved January 31, 2008 from http://prod.hopkins-abxguide.org/diagnosis/gynecologic/full_pelvic_inflammatory_disease__pid_.htm

Indman, P. D. (2006). *Fibroids*. Retrieved January 31, 2008 from http://www.gynalternatives.com/fibroids.htm

ICD9data.com. (2007). *2008 ICD-9-CM Volume 1. Diagnosis codes*. Retrieved January 31, 2008 from http://www.icd9data.com/2008/Volume1/default.htm

Johnson, M. I. & Fauci, A. S. (2007). An HIV vaccine—evolving concepts. *New England Journal of Medicine,* 356, 2073–2081.

Khalili, M. (2006). *Coinfection with hepatitis viruses and HIV*. HIV InSite. Retrieved January 31, 2008 from http://hivinsite.ucsf.edu/InSite?page=kb-05-03-04

Klein, S. (2005). Evaluation of palpable breast masses. *American Family Physician*, 71, 1731–1738.

Kripke, C. (2007). Opioid analgesia during evaluation of acute abdominal pain. *American Family Physician*, 76, 971. Retrieved January 31, 2008 from http://www.aafp.org/afp/20071001/cochrane.html#c2

Leung, A. K. & Pacaud, D. (2004). Diagnosis and management of galactorrhea. *American Family Physician*. Retrieved January 31, 2008 from http://www.aafp.org/afp/20040801/543.html

Madigan Army Medical Center. (2006). *Breast mass*. Tacoma, WA: Madigan Army Medical Center. Retrieved February 5, 2008 from http://www.mamc.amedd.army.mil/referral/guidelines/gensurg_brestmass.htm

MedlinePlus. (2006). Secondary amenorrhea. In *Medical Encyclopedia*. U.S. National Library of Medicine, National Institutes of Health. Retrieved February 5, 2008 from http://www.nlm.nih.gov/medlineplus/ency/article/001219.htm

Mercksource.com. (2002). *Dorland's medical dictionary*. W.B. Saunders. Retrieved February 5, 2008 from http://www.mercksource.com/pp/us/cns/cns_hl_dorlands.jspzQzpgzEzzSzppdocszSzuszSzcommonzSzdorlandszSzdorlandzSzdmd_a-b_00zPzhtm

Mercksource.com. (2003). *Hepatitis*. Retrieved February 5, 2008 from http://www.mercksource.com/pp/us/cns/cns_hl_adam.jspzQzpgzEz/pp/us/cns/content/adam/ency/article/001154.htm

Metzger, D. A. (2005). Treating the big picture of endometriosis. In *Endometriosis: the mysteries are unraveling—new clinical and scientific insights*. Endometriosis Association. Retrieved January 31, 2008 from http://www.endometriosisassn.org/cme001_coursemain.html

Moses, S. (2007a). Female tanner stage. In *Family practice notebook*. Retrieved January 31, 2008 from http://www.fpnotebook.com/END42.htm

Moses, S. (2007b). Colposcopy. In *Family practice notebook*. Retrieved January 31, 2008 from http://www.fpnotebook.com/GYN153.htm

Moses, S. (2007c). Chronic pelvic pain. In *Family practice notebook*. Retrieved January 31, 2008 from http://www.fpnotebook.com/GYN183.htm

Murphy, J. L. (Ed.). (2004). *Nurse practitioner's prescribing reference*. New York: Prescribing Reference.

National Institute of Allergy and Infectious Diseases (NIAID). (2006). *HIV infection in women*. Research On. Bethesda, MD: Author. Retrieved January 31, 2008 from http://www.niaid.nih.gov/factsheets/womenhiv.htm

National Institutes of Health (NIH). (2004). *Uterine fibroids*. Retrieved January 31, 2008 from http://www.nichd.nih.gov/health/topics/uterine_fibroids.cfm

National Institutes of Health (NIH). (2007). WHI updated analysis: no increased risk of breast cancer with estrogen-alone. *NIH News*. Retrieved February 5, 2008 from http://www.nhlbi.nih.gov/new/press/06-04-11a.htm

Nezhat, C. (2005). Safe and effective surgery for endometriosis. In *Endometriosis: the mysteries are unraveling—new clinical and scientific insights*. Endometriosis Association. Retrieved January 31, 2008 from http://www.endometriosisassn.org/cme001_coursemain.html

Niu, M. T., Stein, D. S., & Schnittman, S. M. (1993). Primary human immunodeficiency virus type 1 infection: review of pathogenesis and early treatment interventions in humans and animal retrovirus infections. *Journal of Infectious Diseases*, 168, 1490–1501.

Okun, N., Gronau, K. A., & Hannah, M. E. (2005). Antibiotics for bacterial vaginosis or *Trichomonas vaginalis* in pregnancy: a systematic review. *Obstetrics and Gynecology,* 105, 857–868.

Parker, W. H. (2007). Uterine myomas: management. *Fertility & Sterility,* 88, 255–271.

Patel, M. (2005). *Endometrial biopsy and uterine evacuation*. Birmingham, AL: University of Alabama. Retrieved January 31, 2008 from http://www.obgyn.uab.edu/medicalstudents/obgyn/uasom/documents/EMBx.pdf

Payne, K. (2003). *Gonorrhea test*. Retrieved January 31, 2008 from http://my.webmd.com/hw/sexual_conditions/hw4905.asp

Ross, J., Judlin, P., & Nilas, L. (2007). *European guideline for the management of pelvic inflammatory disease.* International Union Against Sexually Transmitted Infections. *International Journal of STD & AIDS,* 18 (10) 662-666.

Sahelian, R. (n.d.). *Natural options for HIV AIDS*. Retrieved February 5, 2008 from http://www.raysahelian.com/hiv.html

Saslow, D., Runowicz, C. D., Solomon, D., Moscicki, A. B., Smith, R. A., Eyre, H. J., et al. (2003). American Cancer Society guideline for the early detection of cervical neoplasia and cancer. *Journal of Lower Genital Tract Disease*, 7, 67–86.

Sauerland, S., Agresta, F., Bergamaschi, R., Borzellino, G., Budzynski, A., Champault, G., et al. (2006). Laparoscopy for abdominal emergencies: evidence-based guidelines of the European Association for Endoscopic Surgery. *Surgical Endoscopy*, 20, 14–29.

Simpson, J., Dressler, L., Cobau, C. D., Falkson, C., Gilchrist, K., et al. (2000). Prognostic value of histologic grade and proliferative activity in axillary node-positive breast cancer: results from the Eastern Cooperative Oncology Group Companion Study, EST 4189. *Journal of Clinical Oncology*, 18, 2059–2069.

Sinclair, C. (2004). *A midwife's handbook*. St. Louis, MO: Saunders.

Smith, T. (1984). *A woman's guide to homeopathic medicine*. New York: Thorsons.

Soule, D. (1995). *The roots of healing*. Secaucus, NJ: Citadel Press.

Swanton, A., Iyer, L., Reginald, P. W. (2006). Diagnosis, treatment and follow up of women undergoing conscious pain mapping for chronic pelvic pain: a prospective cohort study. *British Journal of Obstetrics & Gynaecolgy*, 113(7): 792–796.

Taylor, D., Schuiling, K. D., & Sharp, B. A. (2006). Menstrual cycle pain and discomforts. In K. D. Schuiling & F. E. Likis (Eds.). *Women's gynecologic health*. Sudbury, MA: Jones and Bartlett.

Thompson, S. R. (2004). Nipple discharge. In *NIH MedlinePlus medical encyclopedia*. Retrieved February 5, 2008 from http://www.nlm.nih.gov/medlineplus/ency/article/003154.htm

University of Maryland Medical Center. (n.d.). *Complementary therapy program herpes simplex*. Retrieved February 5, 2008 from http://www.umm.edu/altmed/ConsConditions/HerpesSimplexViruscc.html

Varney, H., Kriebs, J. M., & Gegor, C. L. (Eds.). (2004). *Varney's midwifery* (4th ed.). Sudbury, MA: Jones and Bartlett.

Wallach, E. E., & Vlahos, N. F. (2004). Uterine myomas: an overview of development, clinical features, and management. *Obstetrics & Gynecology* 104, 393–406.

WholehealthMD.com. (2000). *Evening primrose oil*. Retrieved February 5, 2008 from http://www.wholehealthmd.com/refshelf/substances_view/0,1525,779,00.html10

Wright, T. C. Jr., Massad, L. S., Dunton, C. J., Spitzer, M., Wilkinson, E. J., & Solomon, D. (2007a). 2006 Consensus guidelines for the management of women with abnormal cervical screening tests. *Journal of Lower Genital Tract Disease*, 11, 201–222.

Wright, T. C. Jr., Massad, L. S., Dunton, C. J., Spitzer, M., Wilkinson, E. J., & Solomon, D. (2007b). 2006 Consensus guidelines for the management of women with cervical intraepithelial neoplasia or adenocarcinoma in situ. *Journal of Lower Genital Tract Disease*, 11, 223–239.

Wright, V. C., & Lickrish, G. M. (Eds.). (1989). *Basic and advanced colposcopy: a practical handbook for diagnosis and treatment*. Houston, TX: Biomedical Communications.

BIBLIOGRAPHY

Barger, M. K. (Ed.). (1988). *Protocols for gynecologic and obstetric health care*. Philadelphia: W. B. Saunders.

Barton, S. (Ed.). (2001). *Clinical evidence*. London: BMJ.

Department of Health and Human Services. (2004). *Guidelines for the use of antiretroviral agents in HIV-1 infected adults and adolescents*. Washington, DC: Author.

Gordon, J. D., Rydfors, J. T., Druzin, M. L., & Tadir, Y. (1995). *Obstetrics, gynecology & infertility* (4th ed.). Glen Cove, NY: Scrub Hill Press.

MacLaren, A. & Imberg, W. (1998). Current issues in the midwifery management of women living with HIV/AIDS. *Journal of Nurse-Midwifery*, 43, 502–521.

Murphy, J. (1999). Preoperative considerations with herbal medicines. *AORN Journal*, 75, 173–181.

National Institutes of Health (NIH). (2007b). Effect of hormone therapy on risk of heart disease may vary by age and years since menopause. *NIH News*. Retrieved February 5, 2008 from http://www.nih.gov/news/pr/apr2007/nhlbi-03.htm

Schuiling, K. D. & Likis, F. E. (2006). *Women's gynecological health*. Sudbury, MA: Jones and Bartlett.

Scott, J. R., DiSaia, P. J., Hammond, C. B., Gordon, J. D., & Spellacy, W. N. (1996). *Danforth's handbook of obstetrics and gynecology*. Philadelphia: Lippincott-Raven.

Speroff, L., Glass, R. H., & Kase, N. G. (1999). *Clinical gynecologic endocrinology and infertility*. Philadelphia: Williams & Wilkins.

Walls, D. (2007). *Natural families—healthy homes*. LaVergne, TN: Ingram.

Primary Care in Women's Health

8

Primary health care for women encompasses health promotion, disease prevention, and management of common health problems.

Many women only see a women's health care provider during their reproductive years and may not have ready access to a primary care practitioner when health concerns develop. Women use health care services more often than do men, and they typically make decisions regarding health care for the family. The inclusion of primary health care services within midwifery practice increases opportunities for midwives to provide care, education, and support for women to make positive health choices beyond the childbearing year.

The nature and scope of women's health care provided by midwives in the United States has expanded in recent years (Farley et al., 2006). Historically, midwives have assumed a role as health care providers offering services to childbearing women and their newborns. However, the services midwives offer have evolved over the years to include women's health care for a wider range of clients. During the health care reforms of the early 1990s, the American College of Nurse-Midwives (1997) developed a formal position statement that defines midwives as primary care providers for women from adolescence to senescence and for newborns. Many midwives include primary care within their scope of practice. Skill in assessment and diagnosis of common primary care health problems enhances midwifery care, even when the midwife refers the client for treatment.

The practice guidelines in this section provide a brief overview of selected primary care health conditions. The midwife is responsible for caring only for those conditions that are within her or his scope of practice but may opt to expand that scope with continuing education and experience. Formal continuing education, self-study, and an experienced colleague with which to consult provides a safe basis for learning and optimal care for the midwifery client. The ability to assess general health problems and make appropriate referrals is valued by clients. Clients who have developed a trusting relationship with the midwife do not expect the midwife to provide comprehensive medical care but rather to provide a problem-oriented referral to the health care provider that is best able to meet the clients' needs.

CARE OF THE WOMAN WITH CARDIOVASCULAR PROBLEMS

Key Clinical Information

Heart disease remains the most common cause of death in women in the United States. Although most research about the prevention and treatment of heart disease has been performed using male subjects, information from the American Heart Association (2004) noted that 38% of women who have a heart attack will die within a year. Midwives, who are often accustomed to caring for essentially healthy women, must keep in mind the risk factors, signs, and symptoms of heart disease, hypertension, and stroke (Madankumar, 2003).

Many women may be unaware of a problem until significant symptoms develop. Women with diabetes may develop peripheral vascular problems, whereas atrial fibrillation increases a woman's risk of stroke. Clients should be encouraged to participate in a personal review of fixed and modifiable risk factors and to identify life-style changes to decrease personal risk of coronary artery disease. Hypertension guidelines can be downloaded to a handheld device from http://hin.nhlbi.nih.gov/jnc7/jnc7pda.htm.

Client History and Chart Review: Components of the History to Consider (Hunt et al., 2005; National Heart, Lung, and Blood Institute [NHLBI], 2003)

- Age
- Gravida, para, last menstrual period (LMP)
  - Menstrual status/life stage
  - Current method of contraception
- Medical/surgical history
  - Allergies
  - Medications
    - Contraceptive hormones
    - Hormone replacement therapy
    - Aspirin

- Health conditions
  - Diabetes
  - Dyslipidemia
  - Hypertension
  - Valvular heart disease
  - Coronary or peripheral vascular disease
  - Rheumatic fever
  - Collagen vascular disease
  - Kidney disease
  - Cushing's syndrome
  - Thyroid or parathyroid disease
  - Sleep disorders
- Family history
  - Coronary artery disease (males, age < 55 years; females, age < 65 years)
    - Myocardial infarction
    - Cerebrovascular accident
    - Conduction disorders
    - Tachyarrhythmias
    - Sudden death
  - Hypertension
  - Diabetes
- Social history
  - Drugs and alcohol
    - Alcohol use, more than one drink a day
    - Ephedra
    - Cocaine
    - Amphetamines
  - Tobacco use (cigarettes, snuff, chewing tobacco)
  - Life stressors
  - Usual coping methods
  - Support systems
  - Physical activity patterns
  - Usual diet and intake of
    - Sodium
    - Caffeine
    - Saturated fat
- ⊛ Elevated coronary vascular disease risk (American Heart Association, 2004)
  - African-American: hypertension/stroke
  - Hispanic: stroke

- Mexican-Americans: labile hypertension
- Native Americans: labile hypertension
- Symptoms related to cardiovascular disorders
  - ⚠ Women maybe asymptomatic with progressive disease
  - Ability to perform daily tasks without resting, such as
    - Bathe
    - Dress
    - Climb stairs
    - Carry groceries or small children
    - Vacuum
  - Type, severity, and duration of symptoms
    - Headache
    - ⚠ Visual or cognitive changes
    - ⚠ Numbness or weakness
    - ⚠ Chest pain
    - Palpitations
    - Shortness of breath with or without exertion
    - ⚠ Syncope
    - Peripheral and/or dependent edema
    - Nocturnal dyspnea
    - Nocturia
- Review of systems

Physical Examination:
Components of the Physical Exam to Consider
(Wyner et al., 2007)

- General inspection
  - Abdominal girth and body habitus
  - Signs of prior stroke/cerebrovascular accident
- Height, weight, and body mass index (BMI)
- Vital signs: blood pressure (BP) goals for hypertensive patients (NHLBI, 2003; Pearson et al., 2002)
  - Measure supine and standing
  - BP 140/90
  - BP 130/85 in renal insufficiency or heart failure
  - BP 130/80 with diabetes

- Diagnosis of hypertension (NHLBI, 2003)
  - Normotensive: <120 mm Hg/<80 mm Hg
  - Prehypertension: 120–139 mm Hg/ 80–89 mm Hg
  - Stage I hypertension: 140–159 mm Hg/ 90–99 mm Hg
  - Stage II hypertension: ≥160 mm Hg/ ≥100 mm Hg
- Skin and soft tissue
  - Color
    - Pallor
    - Cyanosis
    - Blanching
- Pulse
  - Rate and rhythm
  - Atrial fibrillation
  - Bruits
  - Decreased pulsed in carotids or extremities
- Eyes
  - Funduscopic examination
- Chest
  - Contour
  - Respiratory rate and effort
    - Auscultate breath sounds
    - Use of accessory muscles
  - Cardiac evaluation
    - Auscultation of heart
    - Rate and rhythm
    - Presence or absence of
      - Murmur
      - Thrills
  - Percussion of chest
- Abdomen
  - Masses
  - Bruits
- Extremities
  - Temperature
  - Capillary refill
  - Evaluation for nonhealing wounds/ulcers
  - Edema
- Neurologic examination
  - Speech patterns
  - Gait
  - Focal deficits

Clinical Impression:
Differential Diagnoses and Code Groups to Consider
Additional suffix may apply (ICD9data.com, 2007)

- Hypertension (ICD-9 codes 401–405)
- Dyslipidemia (ICD-9 codes 272)
- Coronary artery disease (ICD-9 codes 414)
- Valvular heart disease (ICD-9 codes 394–396)
- Diabetes mellitus (ICD-9 codes 250)
- Metabolic syndrome (ICD-9 codes 277.7)
- Chronic obstructive pulmonary disease (ICD-9 codes 490–496)

Diagnostic Testing:
Diagnostic Tests and Procedures to Consider (Hunt et al., 2005; Wyner et al., 2007)

- Complete blood count
- Urinalysis for protein, glucose
- Fasting serum lipid profile
  - Cholesterol < 200 mg/dl
  - High-density lipoprotein (HDL) > 40 mg/dl
  - Low-density lipoprotein (LDL) < 100 mg/dl
  - Triglycerides < 150 mg/dl
- Chemistry profile
  - Blood urea nitrogen (BUN)
  - Creatinine (>1.3 mg/dl)
  - Fasting blood glucose (<110 mg/dl)
  - Renal and hepatic function profiles
- Serum electrolytes, including
  - Calcium
  - Magnesium
- Serum uric acid
- Thyroid-stimulating hormone (TSH)
- Electrocardiogram, 12 lead
- Chest x-ray
- Cardiac stress test
- Echocardiogram
- Holter monitoring
- Pulmonary function testing
- Sleep evaluation

Providing Treatment:
Therapeutic Measures to Consider (Smith et al., 2006; Wyner et al., 2007)

- Life-style modifications
  - Weight reduction goal of optimal BMI
  - Dietary Approaches to Stop Hypertension (DASH) diet (NHLBI, 2006)
  - Smoking cessation
  - Alcohol moderation, one or fewer drinks per day
- Vaccination against influenza
- Initiation of medical therapies
  - By primary care provider or referral specialist
  - As indicated by client condition
  - Per scope of practice/practice setting
- Hypertension (NHLBI, 2003)
  - Angiotensin-converting enzyme inhibitors
  - Angiotensin receptor blockers
  - Calcium channel blockers
  - Beta-blockers
  - Alpha-1 blockers
  - Central alpha agonists
  - Thiazide-type diuretics
- ⚠ Avoid estrogen with hypertension
- Elevated cholesterol
  - Statins
  - Niacin
  - Bile-acid binding resins
  - Fibrates
- Aspirin
  - Avoid with aspirin intolerance
  - Use low-dose 75–160 mg as preventive therapy

Providing Treatment:
Alternative Measures to Consider

- ⚠ Alternative measures are not a substitute for medical treatment in a client who does not have a favorable response with life-style changes
- Avoid herbs that may increase BP
  - Licorice
  - Ephedra

- Ma huang
- Bitter orange
- Measures to promote healing or well-being
  - Adequate rest
  - Nutritional support
  - Well-balanced diet
- Vegetarian or whole foods diet
  - DASH diet (Dietary Approaches to Stop Hypertension) (NHLBI, 2006)
  - Fish/fish oils
  - Garlic
  - Sea vegetables for minerals
  - Vitamin C
- Herbs (Foster, 1996)
  - Atherosclerosis
    - Billberry promotes microcirculation
  - Hypertension
    - Garlic
    - Hawthorn
    - Reishi
  - High cholesterol
    - Garlic
    - Omega-3 fatty acids
    - Dietary fiber, such as flaxseed meal
- Exercise or physical activity
  - At least 10 minutes daily
  - Increase as tolerated to 30–60 min/day (NHLBI, 2003)
  - Resistance training twice a week
- Stress-reduction activities
  - Biofeedback
  - Relaxation techniques
  - Meditation or yoga
  - Support groups
  - Dedicated personal time
- Review personal life goals

Providing Support:
Education and Support Measures to Consider
(NHLBI, 2003; Smith et al., 2006; Wyner
et al., 2007)
- Review Joint National Commision 7 (JNC-7) recommendations
  - BP control

- Weight management
  - BMI greater than 25, encourage weight loss of 10% from baseline
  - Waist circumference at iliac crest greater than 35 inches
- Physical activity 30 minutes daily
  - Resistance training
  - Flexibility training
  - Aerobic activity
- Tobacco cessation
- Dietary recommendations
- Low-fat heart-healthy diet
  - Grains
  - Fruits, vegetables
  - Legumes, nuts
  - Lean meat
  - Low-fat dairy
  - Reduce
    - Saturated fats
    - Cholesterol
    - Trans-fatty acids
  - Limit alcoholic beverages to one a day or less
  - Limit salt intake
- Provide information as applicable
  - Diabetes management
  - Treatment of chronic atrial fibrillation
  - Personal cardiac risk assessment
  - Potential cardiac risks of hormone use
- Medication information
  - Correct dosing
  - Anticipated benefits
  - Side effects
  - Need for long-term treatment and follow-up
- Criteria for
  - Emergency care
  - Prompt care
  - Referral
  - Return office visit

Follow-up Care:
Follow-up Measures to Consider
- Document
  - Risk factors
  - Diagnosis

- Discussions with client
- Treatment plan
- Return for continued care
  - As indicated by laboratory results
  - Evaluation of life-style changes
  - BP monitoring
  - Evaluation of medication side effects
  - For reproductive health care
  - For support during
    - Smoking cessation (See Smoking Cessation, Chapter 6)
    - Dietary and life-style changes
- Coronary heart disease risk assessment (NHLBI, 2003; Pearson, et al., 2002)
  - Begin assessment at age 20
  - Update coronary heart disease family history annually
  - Each visit assess
    - Tobacco use
    - Physical activity
    - Nutritional status
    - Alcohol intake
  - Every 2 years (minimum) assess
    - BP
    - Pulse
    - BMI
    - Waist circumference
  - Every 2–5 years, based on risk profile assess (NHLBI, 2003)
    - Fasting serum lipids
    - Fasting blood glucose
- Ten-year global coronary heart disease risk estimation
  - Calculates risk based on
    - Age
    - Gender
    - Total cholesterol
    - High-density lipoprotein (HDL) cholesterol
    - Tobacco use
    - Systolic BP
  - Online risk calculator available at http://hin.nhlbi.nih.gov/atpiii/calculator.asp?usertype=prof

Collaborative Practice:
Criteria to Consider for Consultation or Referral

- Emergency service
  - BP: systolic > 200 or diastolic > 120
  - Signs or symptoms suspicious for stroke or myocardial infarction
- Medical service
  - Suspected cardiovascular dysfunction
  - Elevated lipid levels consistent with dyslipidemia
  - Hypertension
  - Metabolic syndrome
  - Diabetes
- Behavior modification programs
  - Smoking cessation
  - Drug and/or alcohol reduction
  - Weight management
  - Stress management
  - Heart healthy cooking
- For diagnosis or treatment outside the midwife's scope of practice

CARE OF THE WOMAN WITH DERMATOLOGIC DISORDERS

Key Clinical Information

The skin is the largest organ of the body, functioning as a protective barrier and thermoregulatory organ. As the body's first line of defense against the environment, the skin is subject to injury, infection, pigment changes, burns, stings, tumors, rashes, and other conditions. Many systemic illnesses and conditions exhibit dermatologic signs. Although skin lesions may represent localized conditions, they may also be a cutaneous manifestation of a systemic condition, such as the rash associated with rubella virus infection or an allergic response. Many disorders can be accurately diagnosed by careful evaluation of lesion appearance. A comprehensive dermatologic text with color plates is a useful tool when evaluating dermatologic conditions. Online color images are also available. To be most effective examination of the skin includes areas inaccessible to self-examination, because this may yield additional information necessary to make an accurate diagnosis.

People of all races and ethnicity have differences in skin pigmentation and hair primarily due to genetic variation. Endogenous and exogenous environmental factors, such as exposure to the elements, hormonal influences, medications, and immune response, also influence skin thickness and color and hair distribution and quality and must be taken into account when assessing skin conditions.

Client History and Chart Review:
Components of the History to Consider
- Age
- Medical/surgical history
  - Allergies and sensitivities
  - Current medications (especially recent onset of use)
  - Chronic and acute conditions
  - Previous surgery
  - Previous skin conditions
- Skin type
  - Tanning ability
  - Sensitivities
  - Durability
- Family history
  - Melanoma
  - Psoriasis
  - Skin sensitivities
- Symptom profile
  - Onset, duration, severity of symptoms
    - Associated event or injury
    - Rapid or gradual onset
    - Effect of symptoms related to severity
  - Location and distribution of lesions/changes
    - Local
    - Diffuse
  - Characteristics of skin lesion(s)
    - Color changes
      - Red
      - Black or brown
      - Blue
    - Texture
      - Raised or flat
      - Scaly or coarse
      - Crusted or oozing
      - Blistered
    - Borders
      - Geographic
      - Clearly demarcated
      - Gradual or diffuse
    - Exudate or discharge
      - Clear or serous
      - Purulent
      - Bloody
    - Presence of inflammation
      - Redness
      - Heat
      - Pain
  - Associated factors/additional symptoms
    - Itching
    - Fever/chills
    - Nausea/vomiting
    - Pain
    - Swelling
    - Hair loss
  - Remedies used and their effects
- Potential exposures
  - Infections
  - Infestations
  - Bites and stings
    - Animals
    - Insects
    - Snakes
    - Spiders
    - Jellyfish
  - Sun exposure
  - Chemicals, toxins
- Review of systems

Physical Examination:
Components of the Physical Exam to Consider
(Rousseau, 2007)
- General physical examination, with focus on presenting concern
- Vital signs, including temperature
- Thyroid
- Lymph nodes
- Signs of systemic disease

- Observation and palpation of the lesion(s) for
  - Location and distribution of lesion(s)
  - Size and number of lesion(s)
  - Symmetry of lesion(s)
  - Surface contour of lesions
    - Flat
    - Raised
    - Macular
    - Papular
    - Bullous
    - Annular
  - Margin characteristics
    - Geographic, irregular
    - Clear, smooth, linear
    - Blended
    - Raised
    - Rolled
    - Varied
  - Coloration of lesion(s)
    - Pigment color(s)
    - Patchy
    - Confluent
  - Appearance of lesion(s)
    - Scaling
    - Crusting
    - Ulceration
    - Erosion
    - Presence of exudate
- Acne (Strauss et al., 2007)
  - Vulgaris and/or nodulocystic
    - Comedones, open or closed
    - Inflammatory papules and pustules
    - Postinflammatory erythema and scarring
    - Lesions primarily facial, back, and shoulders
  - Rosacea: chronic acneform conditions (Emmons et al., 1997; Wilkin et al., 2002)
    - Subtype 1: Erythematotelangiectatic rosacea
      - Flushing
      - Persistent erythema
      - Scattered telangiectases
    - Subtype 2: Papulopustular rosacea
      - Symptoms of subtype 1 with
        - Papules and pustules
        - Prominent facial pores
    - Subtype 3: Phymatous rosacea
      - Thickening skin
      - Irregular surface nodularity
      - Peau d'orange texture and enlargement
    - Subtype 4: Ocular rosacea
      - Photophobia
      - Conjunctivitis, iritis
      - Chronically inflamed eye margins
- Bacterial infections (Emmons et al., 1997)
  - Cellulitis
    - Acute spreading lesion
    - Red, hot, tender skin and subcutaneous tissue
    - Borders are irregular and raised due to edema
  - Impetigo
    - Acute purulent infection
    - Characterized by 1–3 cm denuded weeping areas
    - Surrounded by honey-colored crust
    - Erythematous halo suggests strep infection
    - Large confluent lesions may occur
  - Abscesses
    - Furuncles, folliculitis, or carbuncles
    - Characterized by
      - Local cellulitis
      - Regional lymphadenopathy
      - Formation of a fluctuant mass
  - Lyme disease (Centers for Disease Control and Prevention, 2007)
    - Caused by a spirochete transmitted by minute ticks
    - Stage I
      - "Bull's-eye" lesion of 3–15 cm at site of bite
      - Flulike symptoms
      - Lymphadenopathy may develop

- ◆ Stage II
  - ➤ Severe fatigue and malaise
  - ➤ Dermatologic symptoms
    - ▸ Erythema migrans
  - ➤ Cardiovascular symptoms
    - ▸ Palpitations
    - ▸ Dizziness
  - ➤ Musculoskeletal symptoms
    - ▸ Muscle and joint pain
    - ▸ Arthritis
  - ➤ Neurologic symptoms
    - ▸ Bell's palsy
    - ▸ Headache
    - ▸ Stiff neck
    - ▸ Cognitive decline
- • Dermatitis
  - ▪ Contact dermatitis
    - ◆ Erythema
    - ◆ Scale and plaque formation
    - ◆ Desquamation
    - ◆ Moist epidermis and lacy border
    - ◆ Associated symptoms
      - ➤ Pruritus
      - ➤ Burning
      - ➤ Stinging
  - ▪ Eczema (atopic dermatitis)
    - ◆ Intensely itching skin lesions character-ized by
      - ➤ Erythema
      - ➤ Papules
      - ➤ Scaling
      - ➤ Excoriations
      - ➤ Crusting
    - ◆ Common locations
      - ➤ Crease of elbow and/or knees
      - ➤ Behind the ears
      - ➤ Hands and feet
  - ▪ Lichen simplex
    - ◆ Chronic inflammation of the skin
    - ◆ Characterized by
      - ➤ Severe itching
      - ➤ Dry scaling skin
      - ➤ Lichenified plaques

- • Infestations
  - ▪ Pediculosis
    - ◆ Capitis: Pruritus of scalp is primary complaint
    - ◆ Corporis: Pruritus of shoulders, buttock, and belly is common
    - ◆ Pubis: Pruritus of pubic area is primary complaint
  - ▪ Scabies
    - ◆ Lesions appear as gray or skin colored
    - ◆ Linear or wavy ridges end in minute vesicle or papule
    - ◆ Associated with severe itching
- • Viral infections
  - ▪ Rubella
    - ◆ Reddish-pink rash
    - ◆ Begins on face
    - ◆ Spreads to trunk
  - ▪ Herpes
    - ◆ Herpes simplex
      - ➤ Blisters and ulcerated sores
      - ➤ Oral or genital
      - ➤ May occur anywhere on body
    - ◆ Herpes varicella
      - ➤ Vesicular lesions become ulcerated, then crust
    - ◆ Herpes zoster
      - ➤ Grouped vesicles
        - ▸ Erythematous base
        - ▸ Along nerve path
      - ➤ Lesions become pustular, then crust
  - ▪ Human papillomavirus
    - ◆ Common wart
      - ➤ Flat flesh-colored papule
      - ➤ Elbows, knees, fingers, and palms
    - ◆ Flat wart
      - ➤ Smooth, small, grouped lesions
      - ➤ Hands, legs, face
    - ◆ Plantar wart
      - ➤ Small to large singular or grouped nodules
      - ➤ Plantar surfaces of feet

- ◆ Genital warts
  - ➤ Single or clustered flat or peduncu-lated nodules
  - ➤ Genital region
  - ➤ Some varieties are microscopic
- ■ Molluscum contagiosum
  - ◆ Dome-shaped papules 2–5 mm
  - ◆ Umbilicated centers
  - ◆ Central waxy core
  - ◆ Genital area
- Human immunodeficiency virus (HIV)-related skin disorders
  - ■ Hairy leukoplakia
    - ◆ Painless white plaque
    - ◆ Lateral tongue borders
  - ■ Herpes simplex and herpes zoster, see above
  - ■ Kaposi's sarcoma
    - ◆ Malignant red to purplish macules, papules, and nodules
    - ◆ Lesions may ulcerate and become painful
    - ◆ Legs, feet, or mouth
  - ■ Thrush
    - ◆ White plaques adherent to mucous membranes
    - ◆ May cause tenderness
    - ◆ Mouth, tongue, and throat
- Fungal infections
  - ■ Tinea pedis
    - ◆ Scaling, fissures, and maceration
    - ◆ Feet and between toes
  - ■ Tinea manuum
    - ◆ Scaling, papules, and clustered vesicles
    - ◆ Usually on dominant hand
  - ■ Tinea corporis
    - ◆ Sharply circumscribed annular lesions
    - ◆ Trunk or extremities
  - ■ Tinea unguium
    - ◆ Brown or yellowish discoloration of nail
    - ◆ Spreads under the nail
  - ■ Tinea versicolor
    - ◆ Scaly hypo- or hyperpigmented areas
    - ◆ Trunk, arms, and neck

- Psoriasis
  - ■ Characterized by intense pruritus
  - ■ Plaque type
    - ◆ Deeply erythematous, sharply defined oval plaques
    - ◆ May have overlying silvery scale
  - ■ Guttate
    - ◆ Papules 1–2 cm
    - ◆ Primarily seen on the trunk
  - ■ Erythrodermic
    - ◆ Generalized intense erythema
  - ■ Pustular
    - ◆ Sterile pustules 2–3 mm
    - ◆ Coalesce, then desquamate
- Skin cancer
  - ■ Basal cell
    - ◆ Nodular
      - ➤ Pigmented or translucent nodular growth
      - ➤ May bleed, ulcerate, and appear to heal
    - ◆ Superficial
      - ➤ Pink or red scaly patches
      - ➤ May burn or itch
  - ■ Squamous cell
    - ◆ Flat, red, scaly patches
    - ◆ Often form a crust
  - ■ ⚠ Malignant melanoma
    - ◆ Pigmented lesions
    - ◆ May form from a preexisting mole or freckle
    - ◆ Warning signs of melanoma include
      - ➤ Asymmetry of lesions shape
      - ➤ Border irregularity
      - ➤ Color variation: blue, black, brown
      - ➤ Diameter larger than 6 mm
- Disorders of hair growth
  - ■ Alopecia
    - ◆ Diffuse hair thinning
      - ➤ Genetic variation of normal
    - ◆ Patchy hair loss
      - ➤ Autoimmune disorder
      - ➤ Spontaneous recovery in about 6 months

- Hirsutism
  - New-onset hair growth
  - Androgen-dependent areas
  - Rarely associated with masculinizing
- Benign skin conditions
  - Keloid scarring
    - Scar hypertrophy
    - Extends beyond original scar borders
  - Seborrheic keratosis
    - "Age spots"
    - Flat or raised
    - Smooth, velvety, or papillated
    - Variable in color

Clinical Impression:
Differential Diagnoses and Code Groups
to Consider
Additional suffix may apply (ICD9data.com, 2007)

- Alopecia (ICD-9 codes 704.0)
- Hirsutism (ICD-9 codes 704.1)
- Cellulitis and abscess (ICD-9 codes 681–682)
- Impetigo (ICD-9 codes 684)
- Viral infection with exanthem (ICD-9 codes 050–057)
- Acne (ICD-9 codes 706.1)
- Rosacea (ICD-9 codes 695.3)
- Lupus (ICD-9 codes 695.4)
- Atopic dermatitis (ICD-9 codes 698.1)
- Contact dermatitis and eczema (ICD-9 codes 692)
- Psoriasis (ICD-9 codes 696)
- Pruritus (ICD-9 codes 698)
- Pediculosis (ICD-9 codes 132)
- Seborrheic keratosis (ICD-9 codes 702.1)
- Keloid scar (ICD-9 codes 701.4)
- Dermatitis to substances taken internally (ICD-9 codes 693.0)
- Skin cancers (ICD-9 codes 172–173)

Diagnostic Testing:
Diagnostic Tests and Procedures to Consider

- Wet preparation of exudate
- Culture of lesions
  - Fungal—dermatophyte test medium

- Bacterial—routine culture, consider Gram stain
- Herpes—viral culture medium
- Skin biopsy
  - Punch biopsy
  - Excisional biopsy
  - Skin scraping
- Serology and titers
  - Rubella
  - Rapid plasma reagin (RPR)
  - HIV
- Testing for systemic disorders
  - TSH
  - Antinuclear antibody (lupus)
  - Lyme titer

Providing Treatment:
Therapeutic Measures to Consider

- General relief measures
  - Acetaminophen
  - Ibuprofen
  - Benadryl
  - Topical aloe vera with lidocaine
- Acne
  - Topical agents (Murphy, 2004; Strauss et al., 2007)
    - Tretinoin—0.025% cream or 0.01% gel, increase strength as tolerated and indicated
    - Benzoyl peroxide—gel or wash 2.5–10%
    - Clindamycin phosphate—gel, lotion, and solution
    - Erythromycin—gel, ointment, or solution
    - Tetracycline (Topicycline)
    - Salicylic acid
- Oral agents for moderate to severe acne
  - Minocycline
  - Doxycycline
  - Tetracycline
  - Erythromycin
    - Pregnancy
    - Children under 8 years
  - Sulfa-trimethoprim

- Oral contraceptives
  - Ortho-TriCyclen
  - Estrostep
- Spironolactone
  - Antiandrogen blocks androgen receptors
  - Dosages of 50–200 mg effective in acne
  - May cause hyperkalemia
- Acne rosacea
  - Benzoyl peroxide
  - Erythromycin—ointment or solution, apply BID
  - Metronidazole—gel, apply BID
  - Ketoconazole 2%—apply once or twice daily
  - Clindamycin phosphate
    - ◆ Gel, lotion, or solution
    - ◆ Apply BID
- Bacterial infections
  - Treat any underlying condition (e.g., tinea)
  - Cellulitis: requires prompt antibiotic therapy for 7–10 days
    - ◆ Dicloxacillin 250–500 mg PO every 6 hours, or
    - ◆ 🕿 Intravenous antibiotics
  - Impetigo: topical or systemic antibiotics
    - ◆ Scrub with soap and water or Hibiclens
    - ◆ Apply topical mupirocin (Bactroban)
    - ◆ Oral therapy, 7–10 days
      - ➤ Dicloxacillin 500 mg PO QID
      - ➤ Ciprofloxin 500 mg PO BID
      - ➤ Sulfa-trimethoprim DS 1 PO BID
- Lyme disease, early diagnosis (Beers & Berkow, 1995–2005)
  - Amoxicillin 500 mg PO TID for 10–21 days (full 21 days for pregnancy)
  - Doxycycline 100 mg PO BID for 10–21 days (not for use in pregnancy)
  - Cefuroxime axetil 500 mg BID for 10–21 days
  - 🕿 Refer for evaluation and treatment when symptomatic
- Dermatitis (Emmons et al., 1997; Murphy, 2004)
  - Topical corticosteroid preparations (many other products are available)
  - Use lowest effective potency

- Do not cover with occlusive dressing
  - ◆ Highest potency, such as
    - ➤ Betamethasone dipropionate 0.05 % cream, ointment, or solution (Diprolene AF)
  - ◆ High potency, such as
    - ➤ Fluocinonide 0.05% cream, gel, ointment, or solution (Lidex)
  - ◆ Medium-high potency, such as
    - ➤ Amcinonide 0.1% cream (Cyclocort)
  - ◆ Medium potency, such as
    - ➤ Hydrocortisone valerate 0.2% ointment (Westcort)
  - ◆ Low potency, such as
    - ➤ Triamcinolone acetonide 0.1% cream or lotion (Aristocort, Kenalog)
  - ◆ Mild potency, such as
    - ➤ Desonide 0.05% cream (Tridesilon)
  - ◆ Lowest potency, such as
    - ➤ Dexamethasone 0.1% gel (Decadron)
- Infestations (see Pediculosis, above)
- Viral infections
  - Symptomatic treatment
  - Herpes (see Herpes simplex, above)
    - ◆ Varicella: acyclovir 800 mg five times a day for 7 days
    - ◆ Zoster: oral famciclovir, valacyclovir, or acyclovir
    - ◆ Immunosuppressed client: IV acyclovir 10 mg/kg every 8 hours for 7 days (Moon, 2007)
- Human papillomavirus
  - Nongenital warts
    - ◆ Topical salicylic acid plaster, pad, solution
    - ◆ Cryotherapy
    - ◆ Electrodesiccation
  - Genital warts, see Care of the Woman with Human Papilloma Virus, Chapter 7
- Molluscum contagiosum: topical ablative therapy with tri- or bi-chloroacetic acid (TCA, BCA)

- Fungal infections (Emmons et al., 1997; Murphy, 2004)
  - Topical agents, such as
    - Allylamine
    - Ciclopirox olamine
    - Haloprogin
    - Imidazole
  - Apply to affected areas BID
  - All listed: Pregnancy Category B
  - Oral antifungals (not recommended for pregnancy)
    - Griseofulvin 250–500 mg BID
      - Two weeks to 12 months based on indication
    - Ketoconazole 200–400 mg daily
      - Three to 18 months based on indication
    - Itraconazole 200 mg daily for 3 months, *or*
      - 200 mg BID for 7 days monthly for 2–4 months

Providing Treatment:
Alternative Measures to Consider

- Measures to promote healing and foster immune response
  - Well-balanced diet
  - Avoid alcohol, spicy foods, hot drinks
    - Cause vasodilation
  - Adequate rest
  - Exposure to light and air (unless contraindicated by medication use)
  - Limit occlusive skin coverings
- Symptomatic relief
  - Itching
    - Cool colloidal oatmeal baths
    - Herbal wash
      - Chamomile
      - Calendula
      - Aloe
      - Marshmallow
- Acne
  - Vitamin and mineral supplements
  - Vitamin B_6 50 mg/day

- Vitamin E 200–400 IU/day
- Zinc 30–50 mg/day
- Omega-3 oils: flaxseed, fish oils
- Herbal extract of sarsaparilla, yellow dock, burdock, and cleavers (Wong, n.d.)
- Tea tree oil applied topically (Strauss et al., 2007)
- Homeopathics (Holisticonline.com, n.d.)
  - Itching with acne: kali bromatum 6× TID
  - Pus-filled pimples: antimonium tartaricum 6× TID
  - Rough sweaty skin: sulfur 6× TID
- Dermatitis
  - Nutritional support
    - Elimination diet to identify contributing factors
    - Vitamin E 200–400 IU/day
    - Zinc 30–50 mg/day
    - Omega-3 oils: flaxseed, fish oils
  - Stress management
    - Yoga or other planned physical activity
    - Hypnotherapy (Kantor, 1990)
- Tinea (Ledezma et al., 1996; Tong et al., 1992)
  - Nutritional support
    - Limit simple carbohydrates/sugars
    - Beta-carotene 15,000 IU/day
    - Vitamin C 1000 mg/day
    - Garlic: orally or topically applied to affected area
  - Vinegar solution soaks
  - Tea tree oil applied topically
  - Allow ventilation of affected area(s)
  - Homeopathics
    - Sepia
    - Graphites

Providing Support:
Education and Support Measures
to Consider

- Provide information regarding
  - Working diagnosis
    - Testing recommendations
    - Relief measures

- ◆ Skin care
- ◆ Care of contacts, as applicable
- ■ Treatment plan options
  - ◆ Medication instructions
  - ◆ Prevention methods
  - ◆ Warning signs and symptoms
- ■ Instructions to return for care
  - ◆ As indicated by diagnosis, *or*
  - ◆ If condition worsens or recurs

Follow-up Care:
Follow-up Measures
to Consider

- ● ▽ Dermatologic terms
  - ■ Macule or macular patch
  - ■ Papule or plaque
  - ■ Vesicle or bulla
- ■ Fissure, erosion, or ulceration
- ■ Pustule
- ■ Nodule
- ■ Petechiae
- ● Document
  - ■ Document lesion(s)
    - ◆ Location(s)
    - ◆ Appearance
    - ◆ Size/spread
    - ◆ Margins
  - ■ Discussions with client
  - ■ Criteria for diagnosis
  - ■ Treatment and follow-up plan
- ● Return for continued care
  - ■ Persistent or worsening symptoms
  - ■ Medication reaction(s)
  - ■ Routine follow-up

DEFINITIONS OF COMMON DERMATOLOGIC TERMS

Abscess: a lesion which contains pus and extends into the dermis or subcutis

Atrophy: a thinning of epidermis or dermis

Bulla: a blister

Crust: an accumulation of dried serum, blood, or purulent exudate

Cyst: a sac containing liquid or semisolid material usually in the dermis

Erosion: a loss of epidermis above the basal layer leaving denuded surface

Excoriation: linear crusts and erosions due to scratching

Keloid: tough, irregularly shaped scar tissue that progressively enlarges

Lichenification: thickening of epidermis marked by the presence of fine papules

Macule: a circumscribed change in skin color without elevation or depression

Nodule: a palpable solid lesion, greater than 0.5 cm and less than 2 cm in diameter

Papule: a solid elevated lesion usually 0.5 cm or less in diameter

Plaque: a raised lesion that has greater surface area than elevation

Purpura: a non-blanching red or violet color from extravasation of blood into tissue

Pustule: a circumscribed elevated lesion which contains pus

Scale: a heaping up of stratum corneum or keratin

Scar: fibrous tissue replacing normal skin in areas of healing

Sclerosis: a hardening or induration of skin

Telangiectasia: dilated superficial blood vessels

Ulcer: a loss of epidermis and part or all of dermis leaving depressed moist lesion

Vesicle: an elevated lesion which contains free fluid, 0.5 cm or less in diameter

Wheal (hive): a rounded or flat-topped elevated lesion formed by local dermal edema

Adapted from: Drugge, R. J. (1996). *Electronic Textbook of Dermatology*. Retrieved on February 15, 2008 from http://telemedicine.org/terms.htm

Collaborative Practice:
Criteria to Consider for Consultation or Referral
- Medical service
  - Skin lesions accompanied by fever, malaise, or other constitutional symptoms
  - Initial diagnosis of HIV infection or evidence of progressive disease
  - Documented or suspected systemic illness, such as
    - Lyme disease
    - Lupus
- Dermatology service
  - Care of chronic dermatologic conditions
  - Treatment of resistant acne with isotretinoin
  - Suspected or biopsy-proven skin cancer
- For diagnosis or treatment outside the midwife's scope of practice

CARE OF THE WOMAN WITH ENDOCRINE DISORDERS

Key Clinical Information

The endocrine system regulates and affects nearly all body systems. Disruption within the endocrine system may cause a multitude of symptoms that may initially appear to be unrelated. Women are more likely than men to be affected by endocrine disorders; therefore the endocrine system and its function must be considered during evaluation of women's health problems. The primary endocrine disorders affecting women are diabetes mellitus and thyroid conditions (Avery & Baum, 2007. Menstrual dysfunction is often the primary presenting complaint to alert the clinician of an increased likelihood of an endocrine disorder (American College of Obstetricians and Gynecologists, 2000). Other evidence of endocrine disorders includes such changes as unusual hair loss, weight gain or loss, pronounced thirst, enlarged thyroid, or skin changes. Identification of endocrine disorders typically prompts consultation or referral to an endocrine specialist for definitive diagnosis, formulation of the treatment plan, and, when appropriate, collaborative care (Avery & Baum, 2007).

Client History and Chart Review:
Components of the History to Consider
(American College of Obstetricians and Gynecologists, 2000; Avery & Baum, 2007; Payton et al., 1997)
- Age
- Menstrual and reproductive history
  - LMP, gravida, para
    - Potential for pregnancy
    - Method of birth control
    - History of infertility
  - Usual menstrual pattern
    - Cyclic versus noncyclic
    - Prolonged versus scant
    - Heavy versus light or absent
    - Presence of mittelschmerz
    - Change in menses
      - Duration
      - Type of change
      - Associated symptoms
        - Weight gain
        - Hirsutism
        - Galactorrhea
- Recent symptoms
  - Onset, duration, severity
  - Description
  - Contributing or mitigating factors
  - Self-help measures used and results
  - Effect of symptoms on client
- Medical/surgical history
  - Allergies
  - Current medications
    - Drugs affecting thyroid function or TSH levels include
      - Glucocorticoids
      - Dopamine and dopamine antagonists
      - Phenytoin
      - Octreotide
      - Amiodarone
  - Chronic conditions
  - Surgeries
  - Illness or disorders

- Family history
  - Chronic and acute conditions
  - Endocrine disorders
- Social history
  - Nutrition and activity patterns
    - Use of iodized salt
    - Changes in energy level
    - Sleep patterns
  - Life stresses
    - Living situation
    - Drug or alcohol use
    - Domestic violence
- Signs and symptoms of endocrine disorders
  - Hypothyroid
    - Lethargy, malaise
    - Cold intolerance
    - Weight gain
    - Menorrhagia, amenorrhea
    - Depression, irritability, apathy
  - Hyperthyroid
    - Nervousness
    - Anxiety
    - Heat intolerance
    - Diplopia
    - Shortness of breath
    - Weakness
    - Oligomenorrhea
  - Hyperparathyroid
    - Asymptomatic, or
    - Vague generalized symptoms, such as
      - Fatigue
      - Anorexia
      - Weakness
      - Arthralgia
      - Polyuria
      - Constipation
      - Nausea and vomiting
      - Mental disturbance
  - Hypoparathyroid
    - Paresthesia of hands, feet, and circum-oral area
    - Derangement of mental and emotional status
    - Lethargy
- Hypopituitary
  - Failure to lactate
  - Symptoms associated with
    - Luteinizing hormone (LH) deficiency
    - Follicle-stimulating hormone (FSH) deficiency
    - Thyroid stimulating hormone (TSH) deficiency
    - Adrenocorticotropic hormone (ACTH) deficiency
- Hyperpituitary
  - Amenorrhea
  - Galactorrhea
  - Infertility, decreased libido, vaginal dryness
  - Hirsutism
  - Tumor impingement, resulting in
    - Headache
    - Visual field changes
- Diabetes mellitus
  - Polydipsia
  - Polyuria
  - Polyphagia
  - Weight loss
  - Blurred vision
  - Paresthesias
  - Fatigue
- Hypofunction of adrenal cortex
  - Fatigue and weakness
  - Anorexia, nausea, and vomiting
  - Cutaneous and mucosal hyperpigmentation
  - Weight loss
  - Hypotension
  - Abdominal pain, constipation, and diarrhea
  - Salt craving
  - Syncope
  - Personality changes and irritability
- Hyperfunction of adrenal cortex
  - Thick body, thin extremities, round face
  - Cervicodorsal and supraclavicular fat pads

- ◆ Thin fragile skin, easy bruising, poor wound healing
- ◆ Acne, hirsutism
- ◆ Hypertension
- ◆ Hyperglycemia
- • Review of systems

Physical Examination:
Components of the Physical Exam to Consider
(EndocrineWeb.com, 2005; Payton et al., 1997)
- • Complete physical examination, including vital signs
- • Hypothyroid
  - ▪ Signs may be subtle
  - ▪ Skin changes
    - ◆ Cool, pale, tough, dry skin
  - ▪ Head, eyes, ears, nose and throat (HEENT)
    - ◆ Thinning, brittle hair
    - ◆ Hoarse husky voice
    - ◆ Thyroid enlargement
  - ▪ Circulatory
    - ◆ Bradycardia
    - ◆ Cardiomyopathy
    - ◆ Pericardial effusion
    - ◆ Anemia
  - ▪ Neurologic
    - ◆ Cerebellar ataxia
- • Hyperthyroid
  - ▪ General
    - ◆ Tremors
    - ◆ Weight loss
    - ◆ Brisk reflexes
    - ◆ Increased perspiration
  - ▪ Skin changes
    - ◆ Warm moist skin
  - ▪ HEENT
    - ◆ Exophthalmos
    - ◆ Lid lag
    - ◆ Thyroid
      - ➤ Enlargement
        - ‣ Diffuse, and/or
        - ‣ Nodular
      - ➤ Mass

- ▪ Circulatory
  - ◆ Thyroid bruit
  - ◆ Palpitations
  - ◆ Tachycardia
  - ◆ Atrial fibrillation
- • Hyperparathyroid
  - ▪ General
    - ◆ Weakness
    - ◆ Sleep disturbance
  - ▪ Musculoskeletal
    - ◆ Arthralgia
    - ◆ Osteoporosis
  - ▪ Genitourinary
    - ◆ Polyuria
    - ◆ Renal calculi
- • Hypoparathyroid
  - ▪ Typically results from damage to or excision of parathyroid gland
  - ▪ HEENT
    - ◆ Cataract development
  - ▪ Neurologic
    - ◆ Increased neuromuscular excitability
      - ➤ Muscle cramps
      - ➤ Tetany
  - ▪ Abnormalities of skin, hair, teeth, and nails
- • Diabetes mellitus
  - ▪ General
    - ◆ Obesity or recent weight loss
  - ▪ Skin
    - ◆ Striae
    - ◆ Fungal infections
      - ➤ Intertriginous candida
      - ➤ Vulvovaginitis
  - ▪ Circulatory
    - ◆ Diminished peripheral circulation
    - ◆ Poor wound healing
  - ▪ Elevated blood glucose/ inadequate insulin
    - ◆ Fruity odor to breath (ketoacidosis)
- • Hypofunction of adrenal cortex
  - ▪ General
    - ◆ Weight loss
    - ◆ Personality changes and irritability

- Skin
  - Cutaneous and mucosal hyperpigmentation
- Circulatory
  - Hypotension
  - Syncope
- Hyperfunction of adrenal cortex
  - General
    - Thick body, thin extremities, round face
    - Cervicodorsal and supraclavicular fat pads
  - Skin changes
    - Thin fragile skin, easy bruising, poor wound healing
    - Acne, hirsutism
  - Circulatory
    - Hypertension
  - Endocrine
    - Hyperglycemia

Clinical Impression:
Differential Diagnoses and Code Groups
to Consider
Additional suffix may apply (ICD9data.com, 2007)
- Diabetes mellitus (ICD-9 codes 250)
- Menstrual dysfunction (ICD-9 codes 626)
- Thyroid disorders (ICD-9 codes 240–246)
  - Enlarged thyroid (ICD-9 codes 240)
  - Thyroid nodule or mass (ICD-9 codes 241)
  - Hypothyroid (ICD-9 codes 244)
  - Hyperthyroid (ICD-9 codes 242)
- Polycystic ovary syndrome (ICD-9 codes 256.4)
- Hypothalamic dysfunction (ICD-9 codes 253.9)
- Pituitary dysfunction (ICD-9 codes 253)
- Adrenal dysfunction (ICD-9 codes 255)

Diagnostic Testing:
Diagnostic Tests and Procedures to Consider
(EndocrineWeb.com, 2005)
- General testing
  - Urinalysis
  - Chemistry profile
  - Lipid profile

- Thyroid testing
  - Normal ranges (verify ranges with laboratory)
    - TSH, 0.45–4.5 mIU/l
    - Free T_4 (0.8–2.0 ng/dl)
  - Hypothyroidism
    - TSH high (>4.5 mIU/l)
      - Repeat in 2 weeks, with
      - Free T_4 low (0.8 ng/dl)
  - Subclinical hypothyroidism
    - Elevated TSH
    - Normal Free T_4
  - Hyperthyroid
    - TSH low
    - Free T_4 high to normal
    - T_3 high
  - Additional thyroid tests include
    - Thyroid binding globulin
    - Thyroid antibodies for autoimmune disorder of thyroid
    - Thyroid scans
      - Iodine uptake
      - Radioactive uptake
      - Evaluates for presence of nodule
      - Indicates likelihood of malignancy
    - Ultrasound
    - Fine-needle biopsy
  - Pituitary insufficiency
    - TSH normal or low
    - Free T_4 low
    - Free T_3 low/normal
- Parathyroid disorders
  - Abnormal serum calcium, usually found incidentally on chemistry screening
  - Hyperparathyroid
    - Serum calcium elevated (>10.5 mg/dl)
    - Serum phosphate low (<2.5 mg/dl)
    - Elevated serum parathyroid hormone levels confirm diagnosis
  - Hypoparathyroid
    - Serum calcium low (<8.8 mg/dl)
    - Serum phosphate elevated (>4.5 mg/dl)
    - Low or absent parathyroid hormone levels confirm diagnosis

- Disorders of glucose metabolism
  - Fasting plasma glucose
    - $\geq$ 126 g/dl diagnostic for diabetes mellitus
    - 100 g/dl < 125 g/dl = abnormal glucose metabolism
    - 70–99 g/dl = normal glucose metabolism
  - Oral glucose tolerance test
    - Eight- to 16-hour fast
    - 75 g glucose
    - Glucose levels drawn
      - Pretesting, *and*
      - ½-hour, 1-hour, 2-hour, and 3-hour postglucose
    - Glucose of ($\geq$200 mg/dl at 2 hours = diabetes
  - Hemoglobin A_{1c} normal = <7.0%
- Evaluation of adrenal function
  - Consider referral for testing and evaluation

Providing Treatment:
Therapeutic Measures to Consider
- Initiation of medical therapies by diagnosis
- Maintenance by midwife in consultation
- Hypothyroid
  - Synthroid 25–50 mg PO daily
  - Titrate to euthyroid based on
    - Clinical profile
    - Laboratory testing 4 weeks after dose change
- Type 2 diabetes
  - Diet and life-style therapy
  - Oral drug therapy
    - Sulfonylureas, such as glyburide (Micronase)
    - Biguanides, such as metformin (Glucophage)
    - Alpha-glucosidaseinhibitors, such as acarbose (Precose)
    - Meglitinides, such as nateglinide (Starlix)
    - Thiazolidinediones, such as pioglitazone (Actos)

Providing Treatment:
Alternative Measures to Consider
- ⚠ Alternative measures may help to restore balance but are not a substitute for medical evaluation and treatment
- General measures to promote well-being
  - Emotional support
  - Balanced nutrition
    - Avoid simple carbohydrates
    - Maintain optimal BMI
  - Adequate rest
  - Regular physical activity
    - Balance with nutritional intake
    - Helps regulate blood glucose
  - Stress reduction
- Dietary supplements
  - Bilberry (Foster, 1996; MedlinePlus, 2006)
    - Lowers blood sugar
    - Lowers blood pressure
    - Improves microcirculation
  - Blue-green algae
  - Chromium
  - Cinnamon ¼–½ tsp daily (Hlebowicz et al., 2007)
    - Delays gastric emptying
    - Lower blood glucose
  - Sea vegetables
    - Trace minerals
    - Iodine

Providing Support:
Education and Support Measures
to Consider
- Provide information regarding diagnosis
  - Potential effects on
    - Client and family
    - Reproductive capacity
  - Testing recommendations
  - Signs and symptoms indicating a need to return for care
  - Recommended follow-up
  - Local resources
- Listen to and address client concerns

Follow-up Care:
Follow-up Measures to Consider
- Document
  - Diagnosis
  - ⬚ Criteria for consultation
  - Individualized plan of care
    - Follow-up testing—type and frequency
    - Medications—type, dose, titration parameters
    - Physician notification parameters
- 🕐 Consultation or referral
  - Develop management recommendations
  - Delineate individualized best care parameters
  - Delegate ongoing and follow-up care
- Return for continued care as indicated for
  - Support
  - Reproductive health care
  - Ongoing surveillance of endocrine disorders
  - Care of select problems in medically stable client

Collaborative Practice:
Consider Consultation or Referral
- Medical or endocrinology service
  - Clients with evidence of endocrine dysfunction
    - Relevant workup
    - Initiation of treatment
    - Collaborative care of endocrine disorders
    - Ongoing care of endocrine disorders
  - Clients with confusing presentation
- Reproductive endocrinology
  - Endocrine-related infertility
- Social support services
  - Support groups
    - Diabetes
    - Infertility
- For diagnosis or treatment outside the midwife's scope of practice

CARE OF THE WOMAN WITH GASTROINTESTINAL DISORDERS

Key Clinical Information

Problems of the gastrointestinal (GI) tract may range from simple nausea to the presence of obstructing colon cancer. Inquiry into usual bowel function is an essential component of the client history. GI symptoms may present as a signal of a GI disorder or may be a sign or symptom of an endocrine, reproductive, or nervous system disorder. Many women react to stress with GI symptoms such as nausea, diarrhea, or "butterflies in the stomach." Social history may reveal a psychosocial component to GI disorders. Validation of the women's concerns is a first step in addressing this very real problem. Evaluation of the GI system begins with the oral cavity and ends with the anus. Multiple factors, such as poor dentition, poor dietary habits, and alcohol and drug abuse, may contribute to the primary presenting condition.

Client History and Chart Review:
Components of the History to Consider
(Angelini et al., 2007)
- Age
  - Reproductive history
    - LMP, gravida, para
    - Menstrual status
    - Potential for pregnancy
    - Method of birth control
    - Last examination, Pap smear, and sexually transmitted infection testing, as applicable
- Medical/surgical history
  - Allergies
  - Current medications
    - Aspirin
    - Nonsteroidal antiinflammatory drugs (NSAIDs)
    - Oral contraceptive pills
    - Antibiotics
    - Laxatives, fiber, stool softeners

- ◆ Antidiarrheals
- ◆ Narcotics
- ◆ Cardiac medications
- ■ Chronic and acute conditions
  - ◆ Diverticulitis
  - ◆ Gallbladder disease
  - ◆ Peptic ulcer disease
  - ◆ Diabetes
  - ◆ Migraine
  - ◆ Hyperthyroidism
- • Past surgical history
  - ■ Cholecystectomy
  - ■ Oophorectomy
  - ■ Appendectomy
- • Symptom profile
  - ■ Type of symptoms
    - ◆ Onset, duration, location
    - ◆ Severity and character
    - ◆ Associated symptoms
  - ■ Changes in GI/genitourinary function
  - ■ Effect of symptoms on daily living
  - ■ Exacerbating or alleviating factors
  - ■ Self-help measures used and effectiveness
  - ■ Common GI symptoms include
    - ◆ Abdominal pain or cramping
    - ◆ Bloating
    - ◆ Bloody stool or vomitus
    - ◆ Constipation
    - ◆ Diarrhea
    - ◆ Flatus
    - ◆ Heartburn or dyspepsia
    - ◆ Nausea and vomiting
    - ◆ Weight gain or loss
- • GI history
  - ■ Usual diet
  - ■ Eating patterns
  - ■ Elimination patterns
  - ■ Pica or food cravings
- • Family history
  - ■ Diabetes mellitus
  - ■ Diverticular disease
  - ■ Duodenal ulcers

- ■ Gallbladder disease
  - ◆ Increased risk in Native Americans
- ■ Gastroesophageal reflux disorder
- ■ Colon cancer
- • Social history
  - ■ Living situation
  - ■ Travel to or habitation in areas with intestinal parasites
  - ■ Stressors
  - ■ Drug, alcohol, and tobacco use
  - ■ Support systems
- • Review of systems

Physical Examination:
Components of the Physical Exam to Consider
(Angelini et al., 2007)

- • Vital signs, including weight, BMI
- • General physical examination with focus directed by history
  - ■ Current level of discomfort
  - ■ Observe for evidence of
    - ◆ Dehydration
    - ◆ Light sensitivity
    - ◆ Ketoacidosis
    - ◆ Alcohol or drug abuse
    - ◆ Endocrine dysfunction
- • Head, eyes, ears, nose and throat (HEENT)
  - ■ Examination of mouth and throat
    - ◆ Presence and condition of teeth
    - ◆ Presence and size of tonsils
    - ◆ Ability to swallow
  - ■ Lymph nodes
  - ■ Palpate thyroid
- • Thorax and chest
  - ■ Auscultation of heart and lungs
  - ■ Costro-vertebral angle tenderness (CVAT)
- • Abdominal examination
  - ■ Inspection for shape, symmetry, pulsations
  - ■ Auscultation for bowel sounds, bruits
  - ■ Percussion
    - ◆ Organ margins
    - ◆ Masses
    - ◆ Ascites

- Palpation, light and deep
  - Pain
  - Rigidity
  - Involuntary guarding
  - Rebound tenderness
  - Masses
- Bimanual abdominopelvic examination
  - Pain
  - Masses
- Rectal examination
  - Appendiceal inflammation
  - Hemorrhoids
  - Masses

Clinical Impression:
Differential Diagnoses and Code Groups
to Consider
Additional suffix may apply (ICD9data.com, 2007)
- Gastrointestinal symptoms
  - Abnormal bowel sounds (ICD-9 codes 787.5)
  - Diarrhea (ICD-9 code 787.91)
  - Difficulty swallowing (ICD-9 codes 787.2)
  - Heartburn (ICD-9 codes 787.1)
  - Nausea and vomiting (ICD-9 codes 787.0)
- Upper GI disorders
  - Dyspepsia (ICD-9 codes 536.8)
  - Gallbladder disease (ICD-9 codes 574–576)
  - Gastroesophageal reflux disorder (ICD-9 code 530.81)
  - Gastroenteritis (ICD-9 codes 555–558)
  - Hiatal hernia (ICD-9 codes 553.3)
  - *Helicobacter pylori* infection (ICD-9 code 041.86)
  - Lactose intolerance (ICD-9 codes 271.3)
  - Pancreatitis (ICD-9 codes 577)
  - Peptic ulcer disease (ICD-9 codes 533)
  - Pica (ICD-9 code 307.52)
- Lower GI disorders
  - Bowel obstruction (ICD-9 codes 560)
  - Constipation (ICD-9 codes 564)
  - Colitis (ICD-9 codes 555–558)
  - Diarrhea, functional (ICD-9 codes 564.5)
  - Diverticular disease (ICD-9 codes 562)

- Hemorrhoids (ICD-9 codes 455)
- Hernia (ICD-9 codes 550–553)
- Intestinal parasites (ICD-9 codes 120–129)
- Irritable bowel syndrome (ICD-9 codes 564.1)
- Rectal bleeding (ICD-9 codes 569.3)
- Obstetrics/gynecologic disorders
  - Ectopic pregnancy (ICD-9 codes 633)
  - Endometriosis (ICD-9 codes 617)
  - Ovarian cyst (ICD-9 codes 620.0)
  - Pelvic inflammatory disease (ICD-9 codes 614)
  - Pregnancy, diagnosis (ICD-9 codes V72.4)
  - Pregnancy, nausea and vomiting (ICD-9 codes 643)
- Other disorders with GI symptoms
  - Dehydration (ICD-9 codes 276)
  - Endocrine dysfunction (ICD-9 codes 240–259)
  - Hepatitis (ICD-9 codes 070)
  - GI malfunction from mental factors (ICD-9 codes 306.4)
  - Malignancy (ICD-9 codes 140–239)
  - Pyelonephritis (ICD-9 codes 590)
  - Renal calculi (ICD-9 codes 592)
- Abdominal pain, unknown etiology (ICD-9 codes 789)

Diagnostic Testing:
Diagnostic Tests and Procedures to Consider
- Testing based on history and examination findings
- Human chorionic gonadotropin
- Urinalysis or urine culture
- Wet preparation
- Chlamydia and/or gonorrhea cultures
- Complete blood count with peripheral smear
- Erythrocyte sedimentation rate (ESR)
- *H. pylori* testing
- Stool testing
  - Occult blood
  - Ova and parasites
  - Culture
- Liver function testing
- Hepatitis screen

- Amylase and lipase levels
- CA-125
- Endoscopy
  - Upper endoscopy
  - Sigmoidoscopy
  - Colonoscopy
- Ultrasound
  - Pelvic
  - Gallbladder and pancreas
- Computed tomography or magnetic resonance imaging of abdomen

Providing Treatment:
Therapeutic Measures to Consider (Angelini et al., 2007; Drug Digest, 2007; Murphy, 2004)

- Treatment based on differential diagnosis
- Constipation
  - Bulk-forming agents: Metamucil, Fiberall, Perdiem
  - Emollients: docusate products
  - Saline derivatives: magnesium, sodium, or potassium salts
  - Lubricants: mineral and olive oil products
  - Hyperosmotics: glycerin suppositories
  - Stimulants: aloe, cascara sagrada, danthron, senna
  - Enemas
- Diarrhea
  - Opiates: paregoric, codeine
  - Absorbents: polycarbophil
  - Antiperistaltics: loperamide, diphenoxylate
  - Traveler's diarrhea, after stool culture results
    - Ciprofloxin
    - Metronidazole
- Nausea and vomiting
  - Antihistamines: promethazine, cyclizine, meclizine
  - Phenothiazines: prochlorperazine, promazine, trimethobenzamide hydrochloride
  - Serotonin antagonists: ondansetron, granisetron
  - Fluid and electrolyte replacement
  - Vitamin B_6 or B complex

- Heartburn
  - H_2 receptor antagonists
    - Cimetidine (Tagamet)—400 mg BID or 800 mg at bedtime
    - Ranitidine (Zantac)—150 mg BID or 300 mg at bedtime
    - Famotidine (Pepcid)—20 mg BID or 40 mg at bedtime
    - Nizatidine (Axid)—150 mg BID
  - Proton pump inhibitors (PPIs)
    - Esomeprazole (Nexium)
    - Lansoprazole (Prevacid)
    - Omeprazole (Prilosec)
    - Pantoprazole (Protonix)
    - Rabeprazole (Aciphex)
- Antimicrobial treatment for *H. pylori* infection (Drug Digest, 2007)
  - Most effective treatment regimens contain
    - Proton Pump Inhibitors, *plus*
    - Clarithromycin, *and*
    - Amoxicillin, *or*
    - Metronidazole
  - Duration of treatment ranges from 7 to 14 days
    - Shorter treatment improves compliance
    - Failed short-term therapy requires 14-day retreatment
  - Treatment options include
    - Three-drug regimens
      - Clarithromycin + metronidazole + PPI
      - Amoxicillin + metronidazole + PPI
      - Tetracycline + metronidazole + sucralfate
    - Four-drug regimens
      - Bismuth + metronidazole + clarithromycin + PPI
      - Bismuth + metronidazole + tetracycline + PPI
      - Bismuth + metronidazole + tetracycline + H_2 blocker
        - H_2 blocker needs to be taken for 4–6 weeks

- ◆ Combination product
  - ➤ Helidac + H$_2$ blocker
- ■ Irritable bowel syndrome
  - ◆ Diarrhea: Imodium or Lotronex
  - ◆ Constipation: fiber supplements
  - ◆ GI spasm: tricyclic antidepressants or Zelnorm
  - ◆ Depression/anxiety: antidepressants or anxiolytics

Providing Treatment:
Alternative Measures to Consider

- ⚠ Alternative therapies are not a substitute for medical evaluation of acute symptoms
- Nausea and vomiting
  - ■ Acupuncture or acupressure
  - ■ Ginger: tea, candied, or gingersnaps
- Diarrhea
  - ■ Increase fiber to regulate fluid balance in stool
  - ■ Acidophilus capsules
  - ■ Herbs
    - ◆ Peppermint
    - ◆ Slippery elm
    - ◆ Bilberry
- Constipation
  - ■ Increase fiber and fluids
  - ■ Cascara sagrada—10 gtts fluid extract, stimulates bowel function
  - ■ Flaxseed meal
    - ◆ Increases bulk to stool
    - ◆ Omega-3 fats
  - ■ Senna—use sparingly; very effective but may cause cramping
- Reflux
  - ■ Chamomile tea
  - ■ Slippery elm
  - ■ Papaya enzyme tablets with meals and at bedtime
  - ■ Hazelnuts with meals and at bedtime

Providing Support:
Education and Support Measures
to Consider

- Dietary recommendations
  - ■ Hydration
    - ◆ Drink ample fluid
    - ◆ Limit caffeine and alcohol intake
  - ■ Lactose intolerance
    - ◆ Limit all dairy products
    - ◆ Check labels for dairy in packaged products
  - ■ Fiber intake; high-fiber foods
    - ◆ Peas, beans, and lentils
    - ◆ Fresh and dried fruit
    - ◆ Uncooked vegetables
    - ◆ Whole grain breads and cereals
- Physical activity
  - ■ Twenty to 60 minutes daily
    - ◆ Increases endorphins
    - ◆ Improves blood flow to gut
    - ◆ Improves bowel function
- Provide information related to
  - ■ Working diagnosis
  - ■ Testing recommendations
  - ■ Recommended medications and treatment
    - ◆ Anticipated results
    - ◆ Side effects
  - ■ Warning signs and symptoms
  - ■ Referral criteria and mechanism

Follow-up Care:
Follow-up Measures to Consider

- Document
  - ■ Criteria for diagnosis
  - ■ Treatment and follow-up plan
  - ■ Indications for specialty care or consultation
- Return for continued care
  - ■ As indicated by test results
  - ■ Follow-up of chronic problems
  - ■ Five to 10 days with no improvement, *or*
  - ■ Sooner with worsening signs or symptoms

Collaborative Practice:
Criteria to Consider for Consultation or Referral

- Emergency service
  - Acute abdomen
  - Intestinal obstruction
- Medical/surgical service
  - Confirmed or suspected
    - Gallbladder disease
    - Colorectal malignancy
    - GI bleeding
  - For nonacute GI problem unresponsive to therapy within 7–21 days
- OB/GYN service
  - Ectopic pregnancy
  - Reproductive malignancy
  - Hyperemesis gravidarum
  - Hydatidiform mole
- For diagnosis or treatment outside the midwife's scope of practice

CARE OF THE WOMAN WITH MENTAL HEALTH DISORDERS

Key Clinical Information

Mental health is a state of psychological and emotional well-being that allows individuals to form relationships, resolve conflicts, and adapt their own behavior to changing circumstances. About one in four adults in America will suffer from a diagnosable mental health disorder in a given year (National Institute of Mental Health, 2007). Striking gender differences are found in patterns of mental illness: Women are more likely than men to suffer depression, anxiety, somatic complaints, and posttraumatic stress syndrome (World Health Organization [WHO], 2004). Caregiver stress is an issue that affects women disproportionately and will increase as the U.S. population ages (NIMH, 2007).

Although midwifery assessment of mental health conditions may include diagnosis and treatment of mild self-limiting disorders, all women with ongoing psychiatric problems should be referred to a mental health professional for further evaluation and treatment. Active listening is a crucial part of the midwifery assessment process, and it places the midwife in a prime position to evaluate the mental well-being of each woman who presents for care. As with other health issues, a strong network of referral options is beneficial in directing women to the type of care that best meets their needs.

Client History and Chart Review:
Components of the History to Consider

- Chief complaint, in client's own words
- History of current problem
  - Symptoms
    - Onset, duration
    - Precipitating factors
  - Client's feelings of danger to self or others
  - Suicide attempts or ideation
  - Expectations for care
- Mental health status
  - Description and theme of mood
    - Effect on daily life
      - Appetite
      - Activities
      - Sleep patterns
    - Delusions
    - Paranoia
    - Suicidal ideation; thoughts, plans, intent, means
  - General cognitive status
    - Orientation
    - Memory
    - Attention
    - Abstract thinking and reasoning
    - Speech patterns
    - Thought processes (e.g., emotional organization and content)
      - Persistent unwanted thoughts
      - Worry
      - Pessimistic thinking
      - Rage
      - Panic

- ➤ Guilt
- ➤ Worthlessness
- ➤ Hopelessness
- ➤ Agitation
- ➤ Forgetfulness
- ➤ Fatigue
- ➤ Sadness
- ➤ Indecision
- ➤ Inability to concentrate
- ➤ Irritability
- ➤ Anxiety
- ➤ Libido
  - Previous diagnosis or treatment
- Reproductive history
  - LMP, current menstrual status
  - Gravida, para, children at home
  - Losses and emotional sequelae
  - Current method of contraception
- Medical and surgical history
  - Allergies
  - Current medications
    - ◆ Hormones
    - ◆ Antidepressants
    - ◆ Analgesics
    - ◆ Other medication
  - Medical conditions
    - ◆ Viral infection
    - ◆ Endocrine problems
    - ◆ Chronic pain
    - ◆ Chronic fatigue
    - ◆ Multiple sclerosis
    - ◆ Cancer
  - Previous surgery
  - Repeated visits to health care providers for vague symptoms
- Social history
  - 🌐 Cultural background
    - ◆ Effect on primary complaint
    - ◆ Social stigma related to seeking help
    - ◆ Cultural variations in symptoms presentation
  - Nature of primary affiliate relationships: partner, spouse, children
  - Housing and occupant situation

- Extended family and community support systems
- Alcohol, drug, or tobacco abuse
- Emotional, sexual, or physical abuse
- Employment or financial status
- Life stresses, transitions, and coping techniques
- Related family history
  - Mental illness
  - Alcohol or drug abuse/addiction
  - Chronic illness
  - Loss of a loved one
- Review of systems

Physical Examination:
Components of the Physical Exam to Consider
- Vital signs
- Weight, height, BMI
- Mental status assessment
  - Posture
  - Mood
  - Body language and movements
  - Personal hygiene and dress
  - Cooperation, participation, eye contact
  - Affect
- Physical manifestations of mental health issues
  - Tics, agitation
  - Diminished affect
  - Slow speech
  - Obsessive/compulsive behaviors
  - Auditory or visual hallucinations
  - Low BMI
- Evaluate for physiologic basis of symptoms
  - Thyroid
  - Cardiopulmonary status
  - Neurologic functioning
  - Reproductive (hormonal) systems

Clinical Impression:
Differential Diagnoses and Code Groups
to Consider
Additional suffix may apply (ICD9data.com, 2007)
- ⚠ Consider the possibility of dual diagnosis: for example, a client with both an emotional

or psychiatric problem and a substance abuse problem
- Affective disorders (ICD-9 codes 296)
- Anxiety disorders (ICD-9 codes 300)
- Posttraumatic stress disorder (ICD-9 code 309.81)
- Eating disorders
  - Anorexia nervosa (ICD-9 codes 307.1)
  - Bulimia (ICD-9 code 307.51)
- Personality disorders (ICD-9 codes 301)
- Psychosis or schizophrenia (ICD-9 codes 295–299)
- Alzheimer's disease (ICD-9 codes 331.0)
- Endocrine dysfunction (e.g., thyroid, diabetes, adrenal) (ICD-9 codes 250–259)
- Hormone-related disorders
  - Premenstrual tension syndromes (ICD-9 codes 625.4)
  - Menopausal/postmenopausal mood disorder (ICD-9 codes 627.8)
  - Postpartum depression (ICD-9 codes 648.4) (See Peripartum Mood Disorders, Chapter 5)
- Substance abuse (ICD-9 codes 304–305)
- Seizure disorders (ICD-9 codes 345)
- Caregiver stress (ICD-9 codes 309)

Diagnostic Testing:
Diagnostic Tests and Procedures to Consider
- Evaluate for physical disorder based on
  - History
  - Physical examination
- Laboratory values
  - Electrolytes
  - Toxicology
  - TSH
  - Follicle-stimulating hormone (FSH)
  - Luteinizing hormone (LH)
- Evaluate for symptoms of mental/ emotional disorders
  - 🌐 Use appropriate screening tools
    - Age appropriate
    - Developmentally appropriate
    - Culturally appropriate
  - Clinician resource (WHO, 2004)

- http://www.mentalneurological primarycare.org/index.asp
- Affective (mood) disorders
  - Depression (Sanders, 2006)
    - Depressed mood
    - Diminished interest in all activities
    - Weight loss/gain
    - Insomnia/hypersomnia
    - Psychomotor agitation/retardation
    - Fatigue or loss of energy
    - Feelings of worthlessness or guilt
    - Inability to concentrate
    - Recurrent thoughts of death: suicidal ideation, plan, or intent
  - Mania
    - Decreased need for sleep
    - Rapid or "pressured" speech
    - Distractibility
    - Flight of ideas
    - Increased goal-directed activity
    - Inflated self-esteem or grandiosity
    - Engaging in risk-taking behaviors
  - Bipolar disorders
    - Symptoms of depression and mania
    - Symptoms alternate
- Anxiety disorders
  - Generalized anxiety disorder
    - General anxiety about "everything"
  - Panic disorder
    - Subjective symptoms of panic attack
      - Tightness in the chest or throat
      - Difficulty breathing without evidence of obstruction
      - Dry mouth
      - Trembling
      - Palpitations
    - Physical symptoms of panic attack
      - Elevated BP, tachycardia, tachypnea
      - Restlessness, trembling, exaggerated startle response

- ➤ Pallor, sweating, erythema, cold, and clammy hands
- ➤ Vomiting, loss of bowel or bladder control
- Phobias
  - ◆ Irrational fear out of proportion to stimulus
- Obsessive-compulsive disorder
  - ◆ Persistent recurrence of
    - ➤ Intrusive thoughts (obsessions)
    - ➤ Ritualized behaviors (compulsions)
- Posttraumatic stress disorder
  - ◆ Development of symptoms after a significant traumatic event
  - ◆ Symptoms include
    - ➤ Flashbacks to the event
    - ➤ Emotional numbing to external stimuli
    - ➤ Autonomic, cognitive, and dysphoric symptoms
    - ➤ Eating disorders (Mitchell & Bulik, 2006)
- Bulimia
  - ◆ Preoccupation with weight and food intake
  - ◆ Feelings of being out of control related to food intake
  - ◆ Binge eating
  - ◆ Purging
  - ◆ Fasting
  - ◆ Over-exercising
  - ◆ Laxative or diuretic abuse
- Anorexia nervosa
  - ◆ Preoccupation with weight and food intake
  - ◆ Focus on control of food intake
  - ◆ Loss of more than 15% of body weight
  - ◆ Amenorrhea for at least three consecutive cycles
  - ◆ Denial
  - ◆ Self-repulsion
  - ◆ Distortion of body image
- Personality disorders
  - Person with a set of inflexible and maladaptive character traits

- Ingrained patterns of perceiving and relating to others and environment
- Classifications
  - ◆ Cluster A: paranoid, schizoid, schizo-typical
  - ◆ Cluster B: histrionic, narcissistic, antisocial, and borderline
  - ◆ Cluster C: avoidant, dependent, obsessive-compulsive, and passive aggressive
- Psychoses (thought disorders)
  - Presence of two or more of the following within a 1-month period
    - ◆ Delusions
    - ◆ Auditory hallucinations
    - ◆ Disorganized speech
    - ◆ Grossly disorganized or catatonic behavior
    - ◆ Negative symptoms (e.g., flat affect or psychomotor retardation) (WHO, 2007)
- Caregiver stress (U.S. Department of Health and Human Services, 2006)
  - Providing for the daily needs of other(s)
    - ◆ Typically an older relative or spouse
    - ◆ Has other demands on time, such as children, job, housework
    - ◆ Somatic symptoms, anxiety, depression

Providing Treatment:
Therapeutic Measures to Consider
- Take care of yourself
  - Diet, exercise, sleep
  - Relaxation, yoga, massage, hobbies
  - Talk with a friend, keep a journal of your feelings
  - Seek and accept help with your problems
- Interactive psychotherapy
  - Individual or group counseling
  - Art therapy
  - Music therapy
  - Expressive therapy
  - Cognitive therapy
  - Behavioral therapy

- Electroconvulsive therapy for major depression (Rabheru, 2001)
- Consider trial of hormone replacement therapy for new-onset mild mental health dysfunction in perimenopausal or menopausal women with no precipitating events (See Hormone Replacement Therapy, Chapter 6)
- Commonly prescribed medications by class
    - ⚠️ All have potentially serious side effects—check profile before prescribing and against client symptoms/presentation
    - 📞 When in doubt, consult
- Antidepressants (Sanders, 2006)
    - Selective serotonin reuptake inhibitors (SSRI) (ACOG, 2006)
        - May cause decrease in libido.
        - Avoid in pregnancy or preconception (Louik, et al, 2007)
            - ➤ Associated with increased risk of persistent pulmonary hypertension in the newborn
            - ➤ To avoid withdrawal symptoms, wean down slowly (ACOG, 2007).
        - Prozac 20–80 mg daily (Pregnancy Category C)
        - Paxil 10–60 mg daily
            - ➤ Do not use in pregnancy (ACOG, 2007)
            - ➤ Fetal echocardiography should be considered for women exposed in first trimester
        - Zoloft 50–200 mg daily (Pregnancy Category C)
        - Celexa 20–60 mg daily (Pregnancy Category C)
        - Lexapro 10–20 mg daily (Pregnancy Category C)
    - Serotonin and norepinephrine reuptake inhibitors
        - Consider weaning off serotonin and norepinephrine reuptake inhibitors in the third trimester of pregnancy

- Effexor 37.5 mg BID (Pregnancy Category C)
- Cymbalta 20–60 mg BID (Pregnancy Category C)
    - Tricyclics—long history of use
        - Elavil 50–200 mg daily (Pregnancy Category D)
        - Tofranil 50–150 mg daily (Pregnancy Category D)
        - Pamelor 50–150 mg daily (Pregnancy Category D)
- 📞 Monoamine oxidase inhibitors (Sanders, 2006)
    - ⚠️ Not recommended for CNM prescription
    - Nardil 15 mg TID (pregnancy category—not rated)
    - Marplan 20–60 mg daily (pregnancy category C)
- Other antidepressants (Sanders, 2006)
    - Wellbutrin 150–450 mg daily (Pregnancy Category C)
    - Trazodone 200–300 mg at bedtime (Pregnancy Category C)
    - Remeron 15–45 mg at bedtime (Pregnancy Category C)
- Anxiolytics and hypnotics
    - 📞 Benzodiazepines
        - Xanax 0.5–6 mg daily, half-life 6–20 hours (Pregnancy Category D)
        - Klonopin 0.5–8 mg daily, half-life 18–50 hours (Pregnancy Category D)
        - Valium 2–60 mg daily, half-life 30–100 hours (Pregnancy Category D)
    - Other
        - BuSpar 10–40 mg daily (Pregnancy Category B)
        - Atarax 200–400 mg daily (Pregnancy Category C)
        - Ambien 5–10 mg at bedtime (Pregnancy Category B)
- 📞 Mood stabilizers
    - Lithium carbonate 600–1800 mg daily (Pregnancy Category D)

- Lithium carbonate slow-release 450–1350 mg daily (Pregnancy Category D)
- Lithium citrate 10–30 ml daily (Pregnancy Category D)
- (K) Anticonvulsants (used as mood stabilizers)
  - Tegretol 400–1200 mg daily (Pregnancy Category D)
  - Depakene/Depakote 500–1250 mg daily (Pregnancy Category D)
- (K) Neuroleptics (antipsychotics)
- (▽) Medication use by diagnosis
  - Affective (mood) disorders
    - ◆ Depression
      - ➤ Antidepressants for
        - ▪ Flat or depressed mood
        - ▪ Sleep dysfunction
        - ▪ Obsessive self-flagellation
      - ➤ Anxiolytics if anxiety also present
    - ◆ Bipolar disorders and mania
- Mood stabilizers (lithium and anticonvulsants)
  - Anxiety disorders
    - ◆ Anxiolytics for acute and chronic anxiety or panic
    - ◆ Antidepressants for panic attacks, phobias, or obsessive-compulsive disorders
  - Posttraumatic stress disorder
    - ◆ Antidepressants for depression or obsessive thoughts or behaviors
    - ◆ Anxiolytics for panic, general anxiety, or mild paranoia
    - ◆ Antipsychotics for
      - ➤ Agitation
      - ➤ Anxiety if anxiolytics have poor response or contraindicated
      - ➤ For persistent paranoid thinking
  - Eating disorders
    - ◆ Antidepressants for mood disorder and obsessive thinking
    - ◆ Anxiolytics if anxiety present
    - ◆ Antipsychotics if thinking is delusional
  - Psychoses (thought disorders)
    - ◆ (K) Neuroleptics (antipsychotics) referral for prescription

- Caregiver stress
  - ◆ Antidepressants for mood disorder
  - ◆ Anxiolytics if anxiety present
  - ◆ Sleep induction medication if insomnia present

Providing Treatment: Alternative Measures to Consider
- Warm, loving, safe environment
  - Supportive friends and family
  - Basic needs met for food, shelter, safety
- Herbal or homeopathic support for minor mood disorders
  - Anxiety
    - ◆ Hops
    - ◆ Kava-kava
    - ◆ Passion flower
    - ◆ Reishi
    - ◆ Valarian
  - Depression
    - ◆ Chamomile
    - ◆ Lemon balm
    - ◆ St. John's wort
- Hormonal effects
  - Red clover
  - Dong quai
  - Black cohosh
  - Evening primrose
- Support groups
  - Women's groups
  - Bereavement support
  - Related to other medical diagnosis (e.g., breast cancer support)
  - Religious

Providing Support: Education and Support Measures to Consider
- Engage client in self-care (U. S. Department of Health and Human Services, 2006)
  - Eat well-balanced diet
  - Get regular rest, adequate sleep

- Set attainable goals
  - Set priorities
  - Break large tasks into small ones
  - Assume a tolerable amount of responsibility
- Be with other people when able
- Participate in activities that may improve mood
  - Mild exercise
  - Engage in pleasurable activities such as going to a movie, a ball game
  - Participating in religious, social, or other activities
- Expect mood to improve gradually
- Postpone important decisions until improvement occurs
- Practice positive thinking
- Let family and friends help
  - With child or elder care
  - In specific tangible ways such as meals, laundry
- Provide information related to community resources
  - Health education services
  - Support groups
  - Crisis hotline number(s)
  - Women with abusive partners
    - Safety planning
    - How to access safe-housing
    - Effects of medications on ability to be vigilant
  - Women with medical treatment and/or referral
    - Medication
      - Name
      - Dosing instructions
      - Indication
      - Desired effects
      - Potential side effects
      - Interactions
      - Pregnancy category (as needed)
    - Referral information and goal of referral
    - Midwifery plan for continued care

- Signs and/or symptoms indicating need for
  - Return for care
  - Immediate care
  - Emergency care

Follow-up Care:
Follow-up Measures to Consider
- Document
  - ⚠ If positive suicide ideation, note timely referral/crisis intervention
  - ▽ Verify client compliance with referral(s)
- Provide, as appropriate
  - Support and education related to diagnosis
  - 🕐 Treatment
    - Counseling
    - Continuing medication use
  - Routine women's health care and contraception as needed

Collaborative Practice:
Consider Consultation or Referral
- Mental health service
  - 🕐 Psychiatric emergency
    - Suicidal or homicidal ideation
    - Psychosis
    - Need for hospitalization
  - Symptoms that suggest a complex psychiatric disorder
  - Failure to respond to medication or prescribed treatment
  - Formal psychotherapy indicated or requested
- Emergency service
  - Potential life-threatening drug reaction
- Social services
  - Concomitant substance abuse
  - Persistent psychosocial problems
  - Counseling
  - Nontraditional therapy options
- For diagnosis or treatment outside the midwife's scope of practice

CARE OF THE WOMAN WITH MUSCULOSKELETAL PROBLEMS

Key Clinical Information

The midwife may assess for musculoskeletal conditions during a college, sports, or school physical; before recommending a client begin a vigorous exercise program; or as a result of new-onset symptoms. The two most frequently diagnosed musculoskeletal problems diagnosed in women are osteoarthritis and back strain. Rheumatoid arthritis occurs two to three times more often in women than in men. Lupus and fibromyalgia also occur more frequently in women. Lupus is three times more common in African-American women than in white women. Obesity can result in increased complaints of musculoskeletal problems such as chronic pelvic, knee or back pain. Psychosocial stressors often result in somatic complaints in the musculoskeletal system. It is therefore vital that the midwife pay attention not only to presenting physical symptoms but also the circumstances surrounding the presentation of symptoms in order to make the correct diagnosis or referral.

Client History and Chart Review: Components of the History to Consider

- Primary indication for visit
- Evaluation of symptoms
  - Location
    - Unilateral versus bilateral
    - Symmetric
    - Joint versus muscle
  - Onset
    - Precipitating factors
    - Mechanism of injury
    - Gradual versus sudden
    - Effect of time of day/weather
  - Duration
    - Chronic versus acute
    - Constant versus intermittent
  - Severity of symptoms

- Relief measures used and their effects
  - Over-the-counter or prescription medications
  - Heat/ice
  - Rest
  - Compression
  - Brace or splint
- Symptoms of possible tumor or infection
  - Atypical pain
  - Fever
  - Chills
  - Weight loss
- Medical/surgical history
  - Age (consider client's life stage)
  - Allergies
  - Current medications
  - Last tetanus, diphtheria immunization
  - History of GI upset or bleeding with prior NSAID use
  - Osteoporosis risk (See Screening, Diagnosis, and Treatment of Osteoporosis, Chapter 6)
- Family history
  - Osteoarthritis
  - Osteoporosis
- Social history
  - Ethnic heritage
  - Physical activity patterns
    - Typical activity
    - Recent unusual activity
  - Nutritional status
  - Physical abuse/neglect
  - Physical exertion/strain related to
    - Job, child care
    - Hobby
    - School
    - Sports
    - Housework
  - Drug or alcohol use
- Review of systems
- Common symptoms of rheumatoid arthritis (National Institute of Arthritis and Musculoskeletal and Skin Diseases, 2004)
  - Swelling in one or more joints
  - Joint stiffness that lasts over 1 hour on arising

- Constant or recurring pain or tenderness in a joint
- Difficulty using or moving a joint normally
- Warmth and redness in a joint

Physical Examination:
Components of the Physical Exam
to Consider

- Vital signs, including temperature
- BMI
- Overall muscle to fat ratio
- Evaluate for neurovascular status of tissues distal to site of injury
- Evaluate affected area for
  - Heat, redness, or swelling
  - Range of motion, crepitus, clicks
  - Muscle tension or limitation
- Palpation
  - Tenderness
  - Point tenderness
  - Soft tissue spasm
  - Mass
- Neurologic assessment
  - Strength/weakness
  - Muscle wasting
  - Sensation
- Vascular assessment
  - Color
  - Pulses
  - Capillary refill
- Presence or absence of
  - Ecchymosis
  - Hematoma
  - Limb or joint deformity

Clinical Impression:
Differential Diagnoses and Code Groups
to Consider

Additional suffix may apply (ICD9data.com, 2007)

- Osteoarthritis (ICD-9 codes 715)
- Back strain (ICD-9 codes 846–847)
- Physical abuse (ICD-9 code 995.81)
- Joint strain or sprain (ICD-9 codes 840–848)
- Malignancy or tumor (ICD-9 codes 170–175)

- Systemic disorders
  - Multiple sclerosis (ICD-9 codes 340)
  - Chronic fatigue syndrome (ICD-9 code 780.71)
  - Lupus erythematosus (ICD-9 code 710.0)
  - Fibromyalgia (ICD-9 codes 729.1)
- Peripheral neuropathy and/or radiculopathy (ICD-9 codes 729.2)
- Fracture (ICD-9 codes 800–829)
- Carpal tunnel syndrome (ICD-9 code 354.0)
- Rotator cuff tendonitis (ICD-9 codes 726.1)

Diagnostic Testing:
Diagnostic Tests and Procedures to Consider

- Bone mineral density testing
- Anticipated NSAID administration > 3 months
  - Baseline testing
    - Liver function
    - Platelets
- Inflammatory process versus infection
  - Complete blood count with differential
  - Erythrocyte sedimentation rate
  - C-reactive protein
  - Rheumatoid factor antibody
  - Creatinine
- Evaluation of mass
  - Ultrasound
  - X-ray
  - Computed tomography, magnetic resonance imaging, positron emission tomography
- Bony tenderness, with night pain
  - Referral for diagnostic evaluation

Providing Treatment:
Therapeutic Measures to Consider

- NSAIDs are frequently the first line of therapy
  - Naproxen sodium (Pregnancy Category B, D in third trimester)
  - Ibuprofen (Pregnancy Category B, D in third trimester)
- Muscle relaxants
  - Be alert for drug seekers complaining of chronic pain

- Equagesic—musculoskeletal pain with anxiety (Pregnancy Category D)
  - ◆ Dose: one to two tablets TID or QID
  - ◆ Short-term use only
- Flexeril—muscle spasm (Pregnancy Category B)
  - ◆ Dose: 10 mg TID; maximum 60 mg daily
  - ◆ Limit use to 21 days or less
- Robaxin—painful musculoskeletal conditions (Pregnancy Category C)
  - ◆ Dose: 1.5 mg QID for 2–3 days
  - ◆ Maintenance: 4 g daily in divided doses (Murphy, 2004)
- Sprain or strain
  - Air cast (ankle)
  - Compression bandage
  - Splinting
  - Consider physical therapy
- Fibromyalgia
  - Trial of selective serotonin reuptake inhibitor antidepressants (See Care of the Woman with Mental Health Disorders).

Providing Treatment:
Alternative Measures to Consider
- Rest affected area
- Ice to affected area for first 24 hours followed by heat
- Elevation of affected area when possible
- Weight loss, as indicated
- For soft tissue injury
  - Comfrey leaf compresses
  - Castor oil warm packs
  - Homeopathic arnica montana
  - Massage therapy
  - Hydrotherapy
- Antiinflammatory herbs as tea, tincture, or capsule
  - Ginger
  - Tumeric
  - Feverfew
  - Rosehips
  - Flaxseed meal 2 T daily with water

- Activities to maintain flexibility, balance, and strength
  - Yoga
  - Dance
  - Pilates
  - Resistance training
  - Swimming
- Arthritis
  - Low-fat vegan diet
    - ◆ May decrease pain, swelling, and progression of disease
  - Planned exercise programs
    - ◆ Range of motion: swimming, dance
    - ◆ Strengthening: resistance training, weight lifting
    - ◆ Aerobic and endurance: walking, bicycling
  - Chondroitin and/or glucosamine
  - Heat and cold therapy
  - Use of assistive devices

Providing Support:
Education and Support Measures to Consider
- Provide information related to diagnosis
  - Review mechanism of injury, as applicable
  - Evaluation and treatment recommendations
  - Provide exercise recommendations
    - ◆ Limitations and restrictions
    - ◆ Range of motion
    - ◆ Strengthening
    - ◆ Aerobic and endurance
  - Long-term sequelae
    - ◆ Chronic pain may result in depression
    - ◆ Changes in activities of daily living, range of motion
    - ◆ Warning signs
  - Medication information
- Teach/reinforce proper body mechanics
  - Wide base of support
  - Lift with object close to body
- Teach/reinforce proper weight for height
  - Well balanced diet
  - Portion control
  - Adequate rest/exercise

Follow-up Care: Follow-up Measures to Consider
- Document
- Return for continued care
  - As needed within 7–14 days
  - If problem worsens or persists
  - Depression related to chronic pain syndrome(s)
  - As needed for medication management

Collaborative Practice:
Criteria to Consider for Consultation or Referral
- Orthopedic services
  - After limited results from treatment for
    - Bursitis
    - Tendonitis
    - Carpal tunnel syndrome
    - Sprain or strain
    - Knee effusion
    - Epicondylitis
  - Osteoporotic and other fractures
- Podiatric or orthopedic services
  - Bunion
  - Plantar fasciitis
  - Morton's neuroma
- Rheumatology services
  - Suspected or diagnosed arthritis
  - Suspected fibromyalgia (Kriebs & Burgin, 1997)
- Physical or occupational therapy
  - Evaluation of body mechanics
  - Strength training
  - Ergonomic training
- Mental health services
  - Chronic pain syndromes
  - Depression related to diagnosis
- Neurologic services
  - Herniated disc
  - Suspected multiple sclerosis
- Persistent back pain, without evidence of pathology consider referral to
  - Osteopath
  - Chiropractor
- Acupuncturist
- Neurologist
- Chronic pain center
- Orthotic services for assistive devices
  - Splints
  - Braces
  - Inserts/insoles
  - Arch support
- Surgical services
  - Gastric bypass surgery
  - Carpal tunnel surgery
  - Hip/knee replacement
- For diagnosis or treatment outside the midwife's scope of practice

CARE OF THE WOMAN WITH RESPIRATORY DISORDERS

Key Clinical Information

The most common respiratory disorders seen in primary care include sinusitis, bronchitis, asthma, and chronic cough. However, less common problems such as tuberculosis, pneumonia, and respiratory malignancies should also be kept in mind. Lung disease affects women of all ages and is a common cause of illness and death. The provision of primary care to women who present with respiratory illness during pregnancy is not uncommon. There may be a relationship between acute and chronic respiratory conditions and spontaneous premature rupture of membranes in term or preterm pregnancies, and early treatment may have some preventive benefit (Getahun, 2007). Black women with asthma may warrant particular care in management as they may be at very high risk of PROM at term. Nasal mucosa and lung function may be affected by allergies, air quality, and environmental toxins such as cigarette smoke, chemical fumes, or particulate matter. The primary presenting complaint in the woman with metastatic cancer to the lungs is cough. Women with HIV/AIDS may present with *Pneumocystis carinii* or drug-resistant tuberculosis.

Client History and Chart Review:
Components of the History to Consider
- Primary complaint
  - Symptom review
    - Onset, duration, severity of symptoms
      - Cough
      - Sputum production
      - Color of sputum/nasal discharge
      - Shortness of breath
      - Difficulty with respiration; wheezing
      - Frontal headache
      - Fever and/or chills
    - Other symptoms
      - Weight loss
      - Night sweats
      - Malaise
      - Loss of appetite
      - Weakness
      - Nasal congestion
      - Impaired or loss of sense of smell
      - Snoring/nasal obstruction
      - Bloody sputum
  - Relief measures used and their effects
- Medical and surgical history
  - Allergies
  - Medications
  - Medical conditions
    - Nasal polyposis
    - Heart disease
    - Respiratory disease
      - Asthma
      - Chronic obstructive pulmonary disease
      - Emphysema
      - Sinus infection(s)
      - Pneumonia
      - Cystic fibrosis
      - Cancer
    - Exposure to asthma triggers
      - Allergens
      - Irritants
      - Drugs
      - Exercise or cold air
    - HIV status, if known

- Social history
  - 🌐 Risk of type of lung disease varies with ethnicity (American Lung Association, 2007)
  - Clinician resource: American Lung Association (2007)
  - IV drug, alcohol, or tobacco use
  - Exposure to respiratory irritants
  - Air quality and living conditions (Hackley et al., 2007)
  - Nutritional status
- Review of systems

Physical Examination:
Components of the Physical Exam
to Consider
- Vital signs
- Color
  - Pallor
  - Rubor
  - Cyanosis
- HEENT
  - Nasal septum and turbinates
  - Palpate sinuses
  - Palpate lymph nodes
  - Throat
  - Tonsils
  - Tympanic membranes
- Respiratory evaluation
  - Rate and pattern of breathing
  - Depth and symmetry of lung expansion
  - Auscultation
    - Quality and intensity of breath sounds
    - Adventitious breath sounds
      - Pneumonia
        - Crackles
      - Asthma
        - Diffuse wheezes or rhonchi
        - Prolonged expiratory phase
  - Percussion
    - Resonant—normal, asthma or interstitial lung disease
    - Dull—consolidation or pleural effusion
    - Hyperresonant—emphysema or pneumothorax

- Evidence of respiratory distress
  - Nasal flaring
  - Intercostal or supraclavicular retractions
  - Peripheral cyanosis
  - Elevated pulse and respiratory rate
  - Grunting or wheezing

Clinical Impression:
Differential Diagnoses and Code Groups
to Consider
Additional suffix may apply (ICD9data.com, 2007)

- Asthma (ICD-9 codes 493.0)
- Bronchitis (ICD-9 codes 466.0)
- Chronic cough, due to
  - Smoking (ICD-9 codes 491.0)
  - Postnasal drip (ICD-9 code 784.91)
- Allergic rhinitis (ICD-9 codes 477)
- Sinusitis (ICD-9 codes 461)
- Nasal polyposis (ICD-9 codes 471)
- Deviated nasal septum (ICD-9 codes 470)
- *Pneumocystis carinii* (ICD-9 codes 136.3)
- Tuberculosis (ICD-9 codes 010–018)
- Community-acquired pneumonia (ICD-9 codes 482.9)
- Respiratory malignancies (ICD-9 codes 160–165)

Diagnostic Testing:
Diagnostic Tests and Procedures
to Consider

- Complete blood count (CBC)
- Nasal endoscopy
- Chest x-ray
  - Fever plus abnormal breath sounds
  - Suspicion of tuberculosis
- Gram stain and culture of purulent sputum
  - Suspected pneumonia
- HIV counseling and testing
- Pertussis serology
  - Afebrile client
  - Normal breath sounds
  - Cough > 2 weeks duration
- Pulse oximetry and blood gases

- Peak flow or spirometry to assess
  - Lung function
    - Restrictive
    - Obstructive
  - Progression of disorder
    - Severity
    - Medication effectiveness
- X-ray, MRI or CAT scan of sinuses
  - Chronic cough
- Tuberculosis testing (Centers for Disease Control and Prevention, n.d.)
  - TB Mantoux (purified protein derivative)
    - 0.1 ml injected intradermally
    - Two-step procedure indicated for select groups
    - Purified protein derivative interpretation based on mm of induration, considered positive in following conditions
      - ≥5 mm
        - HIV-infected patients
        - Close contact of newly diagnosed patient with active tuberculosis
        - Scars on x-ray suggest prior healed active tuberculosis
      - ≥10 mm
        - Immigrants from areas with endemic tuberculosis prevalence
        - Low income and/or medically underserved
        - IV drug users
        - Chronic illness or exposure that may increase risk of contracting tuberculosis
        - Infants and young children
      - ≥15 mm
        - No known risk factors for tuberculosis

Providing Treatment:
Therapeutic Measures to Consider

- Community-acquired pneumonia or bronchitis
  - Erythromycin 250–500 mg QID for 10 days (Pregnancy Category B)

- Azithromycin 500 mg on day 1, then 250 mg every day for 4 additional days (Pregnancy Category B)
- Sulfa-trimethoprim 1 DS tablet BID for 10 days (Pregnancy Category C/D in third trimester)
- Amoxicillin—clavulanic acid 250–500 TID for 10 days (Pregnancy Category B)
- Cefuroxime 250–500 mg BID for 10 days (Pregnancy Category B)
- Asthma
  - ⚠ Pregnant women on asthma medications should be maintained on these medications during pregnancy. It is safer for these women and their babies than asthma symptoms and exacerbations (ACOG, 2008; NHLBI, 2004).
  - Bronchodilators/rescue therapy (fast acting for acute attacks)
    - Albuterol (Pregnancy Category C)
      - Inhaled β-agonist
      - Two puffs every 4–6 hours as needed
    - Ipratropium (Pregnancy Category B)
      - Anticholinergic
      - Three to six puffs every 6 hours
    - Metaproterenol (Pregnancy Category C)
      - Inhaled β-agonist
      - Two puffs every 4–6 hours as needed
    - Salmeterol and fluticasone (Advair) (Pregnancy Category C)
      - Inhaled long-acting β-agonist and steroid
      - Two puffs every 12 hours
  - Antiinflammatory medications/ long term control
    - Decrease airway edema and secretions
    - Beclomethasone (Pregnancy Category C)
      - Inhaled steroid
      - Two to five puffs QID
    - Cromolyn sodium (Pregnancy Category B)
      - Mast cell stabilizer
      - Two to four puffs QID

- Flunisolide (Pregnancy Category C)
  - Inhaled steroid
  - Two to four puffs BID
- Leukotriene modifiers/long term control
  - Accolate 20 mg BID (Pregnancy Category B)
  - Singulair 10 mg daily (Pregnancy Category B)
  - Zyflo CR 1200 mg BID (Pregnancy Category C)
- Bronchitis
  - Cough suppressants
  - Tessalon perles (Pregnancy Category C)
    - 100-200 mg po TID as needed
    - Swallow capsules whole
    - Reduces cough reflex by anesthetizing stretch receptors in respiratory passages
  - Promethazine with codeine cough syrup (Pregnancy Category C)
    - One tsp PO every 4 to 6 hours as needed
    - Drowsiness precautions
    - Narcotic precautions
  - Antibiotics generally not indicated, unless bacterial pneumonia is suspected
  - Albuterol inhaler (afebrile but diffuse abnormal breath sounds) (Pregnancy Category C)
    - Two puffs every 4 hours as needed
  - Mometasone nasal (Pregnancy Category C)
    - One to two sprays each nostril daily
- Pertussis—suspected or confirmed
  - Erythromycin 1 g daily in divided doses for 14 days (Pregnancy Category B)
  - Sulfa-trimethoprim DS 1 PO BID for 14 days (Pregnancy Category C/D in third trimester)
- Chronic cough
  - Treatment based on definitive diagnosis
- Tuberculosis
  - 🔎 See Centers for Disease Control and Prevention guidelines for treatment of tuberculosis (http://www.cdc.gov/nchstp/ tbdailyefault.htm)

Providing Treatment:
Alternative Measures to Consider

- General measures to promote healing
  - Rest, adequate nutrition
  - Increase fluid intake, especially hot liquids
  - High-protein high-calorie diet
  - Use positioning to aid drainage of secretions
- Saline nasal irrigation daily (National Jewish Medical and Research Center, 2006)
  - Neti pot
- Eucalyptus steams
- Herbal remedies
  - Marshmallow root
  - Horehound
  - Mullein
- Astragalus (safe for those with immune disorders) (Foster, 1996)

Providing Support:
Education and Support Measures
to Consider

- Provide information and recommendations
  - Diagnosis
  - Medication regimen(s)
    - Dosage, frequency
    - Potential side effects
    - Indications for cough suppressants
  - Signs of improvement
    - Symptoms diminish within 1–3 days
    - Afebrile within 2–5 days (pneumonia)
  - Warning signs and symptoms, such as
    - Persistent cough
    - Fever with chills
    - Bloody sputum
    - Shortness of breath
  - Environmental controls
    - Pets/allergens
    - Air conditioning
    - Mask or respirator
  - Limitations, such as
    - Isolation precautions with family
    - Decreased activity

Follow-up Care:
Follow-up Measures to Consider

- Document
- Return for continued care
  - Contact within 7–10 days (phone or visit)
  - As indicated by test results
  - Symptoms persist or worsen in spite of therapy
  - Persistent symptoms at revisit, reevaluate for asthma

Collaborative Practice:
Criteria to Consider for Consultation
or Referral

- Medical services
  - Respiratory illness requiring hospitalization
  - Symptoms of respiratory distress
    - Respiratory rate ≥ 30
    - Superclavicular or intercostal retractions
    - O_2 saturation of $<95\%$
    - Cyanosis
  - Diagnosis of
    - Tuberculosis
    - Pertussis
    - *Pneumocystis carinii*
    - Pneumonia
    - HIV/AIDS
- For diagnosis or treatment outside the midwife's scope of practice

CARE OF THE WOMAN WITH URINARY TRACT PROBLEMS

Key Clinical Information

Acute urinary symptoms are a frequent presenting problem in primary care outpatient settings. Women are much more likely to develop urinary tract infections (UTIs) in their lifetime than men (O'Dell and Labin, 2006). Urinary tract problems include bladder infections, pyelonephritis, renal lithiasis, incontinence issues, and structural problems such as cystocele. Urinary tract problems may create significant discomfort for the woman, whether it be physical, emotional, or social. Many women restrict their activities due to urinary frequency or fear of incontinence. Often women do not address the issue of incontinence with their midwife or health care provider out of embarrassment or the belief that it is an expected consequence of aging (Koch, 2006). Thoughtfully worded questions during the history may encourage discussion of this problem and exploration of potential solutions.

Client History and Chart Review: Components of the History to Consider (Koch, 2006; O'Dell and Labin, 2006)

- Age
- Urinary history
  - Frequency, volume, and timing of voids
  - Changes in life-style related to urinary tract
  - Urogenital hygiene habits
  - Onset, duration, type, and severity of symptoms
    - Incontinence
    - Urgency or frequency
    - Flank pain and/or dysuria
    - Fever and chills
    - Malaise
    - Relief measures used and results
  - Previous UTI or problem with urination
- Risk factors for UTI
  - New sex partner or multiple partners
  - More frequent or intense intercourse
  - Diabetes
  - Pregnancy
  - Postmenopausal
  - Use of irritating products
    - Skin cleansers
    - Diaphragms and spermicides
  - Blockage in the urinary tract
  - History of UTIs
- Urge incontinence
  - Characterized by involuntary bladder contractions
  - May be neurologic or caused by irritant

- Stress incontinence
  - Occurs when intraabdominal pressure is greater than urethra's closing pressure
  - May be worsened by
    - Childbearing, regardless of mechanism of birth
    - High-impact activities
    - Heredity
    - Atrophy
- Mixed incontinence
  - Stress and urge incontinence
- Overflow incontinence
  - Obstruction
  - Detrusor muscle dysfunction
  - Urethral torsion
- Iatrogenic incontinence
  - Surgical scarring or trauma
  - Medications
- Reproductive history
  - Gravida, para, LMP
  - Vaginal or cesarean births
  - Sexually transmitted infections
  - Sexual activity
    - Anal/vaginal intercourse
    - Lubrication
    - Sex toys
  - Vasomotor symptoms
- Medical/surgical history
  - Allergies
  - Current medications
  - Neurologic disorders
  - Medical conditions, such as
    - Lung disease
    - Elevated BMI
    - Diabetes
  - Genital or pelvic surgery
- Diet history
- Social history
  - Smoking
  - Caffeine and alcohol intake
  - Fluid intake
  - Heavy lifting
- Review of systems

Physical Examination:
Components of the Physical Exam
to Consider
(O'Dell and Labin, 2006)

- Vital signs, including temperature
- Weight, height, BMI
- Thorax
  - Costovertebral angle tenderness (CVAT)
  - Flank pain
- Abdominal palpation
  - Suprapubic pain
- Pelvic examination with focus on
  - Urethra
  - Presence of cystocele or rectocele
  - Signs or symptoms of
    - Reproductive tract infection
    - Genital atrophy
    - Genital trauma
  - Evaluation of pelvic floor strength and function

Clinical Impression:
Differential Diagnoses and Code Groups
to Consider
Additional suffix may apply (ICD9data.com, 2007)

- UTI (ICD-9 codes 599.0)
  - Cystitis (ICD-9 codes 595.0)
  - Urethritis (ICD-9 code 597.89)
  - Pyelonephritis (ICD-9 code 590.10)
- Urinary incontinence (ICD-9 codes 788.30)
  - Urge (ICD-9 code 788.31)
  - Stress (ICD-9 codes 625.6)
  - Mixed (ICD-9 code 788.33)
  - Overflow (ICD-9 code 788.38)
  - Iatrogenic (ICD-9 code 788.30)
- Interstitial cystitis (ICD-9 codes 595.1)
- Sexually transmitted infection affecting the urinary tract
  - Chlamydia (ICD-9 code 079.98)
  - Gonorrhea (ICD-9 code 098.0)
  - Herpes (ICD-9 codes 054.9)
  - Trichomoniasis (ICD-9 code 131.01)

- Vaginitis
  - Candidiasis (ICD-9 code 112.1)
  - Bacterial vaginosis (ICD-9 code 616.10)
- UTI in pregnancy (ICD-9 code 646.63)

Diagnostic Testing:
Diagnostic Tests and Procedures to Consider

- UTIs
  - Urinalysis (dip and/or microscopic) (Rosenfeld, 1997)
    - Leukocyte esterase, frequent false positives
    - Nitrites, first morning urine more accurate
    - Positive leukocytes and positive nitrites more predictive of UTI
  - Culture
    - Most common pathogens *Escherichia coli, Staphylococcus saprophyticus,* proteus, enterococcus
    - Diagnosis considered positive if >100,000 colony count in clean-catch specimen
    - Recurrent or persistent symptoms
    - Pregnancy
    - Urinary calculi
- Human chorionic gonadotropin (HCG), serum or urine
- Ultrasound
  - Renal calculi
- Strain urine
  - Renal calculi
- Incontinence (O'Dell and Labin, 2006)
  - 🔊 Urodynamics
  - Postvoid catheterization to determine residual
  - Simple cystometrogram
  - Cough stress test
- 🔊 Cystoscopy (National Kidney and Urologic Diseases Information Clearinghouse, 2003)
  - Recurrent UTIs
  - Hematuria
  - Incontinence or overactive bladder

- Unusual cells in urine sample
- Painful urination, chronic pelvic pain, or interstitial cystitis
- Urinary stricture
- Stone in the urinary tract

Providing Treatment:
Therapeutic Measures to Consider
- UTI
  - Pyridium for pain relief 200 mg TID for 2 days (Pregnancy Category B)
  - Appropriate antibiotic therapy (Table 8-1)
- Pyelonephritis
  - IV fluids
  - Pain relief
  - Appropriate IV antibiotic therapy
- Urge incontinence (O'Dell and Labin, 2006)
  - Detrol 2 mg BID (Pregnancy Category C)
  - Ditropan XL 10–30 mg PO daily (Pregnancy Category B)
  - Sanctura IR 2 mg BID (Pregnancy Category C)
  - VESICare ER 5-10 mg daily (Pregnancy Category C)
  - Enablex ER 7.5-15 mg daily (Pregnancy Category C)

- Stress Incontinence
  - Hormonal treatment for urogenital atrophy
    - Estring
    - Vaginal estrogen cream
  - Medications
    - Pseudoephedrine HCl (Pregnancy Category C)
  - Pessary fitting
    - Ring
    - Ring with support
    - Gellhorn
    - Use vaginal cream with pessary
      - Trimo-san
      - Acigel
      - Estrogen cream

Providing Treatment:
Alternative Measures to Consider
- Incontinence
  - Scheduled toileting
  - Bladder retraining (biofeedback)
  - Pelvic muscle rehabilitation
  - Weight loss of 5-15% if high BMI (O'Dell and Labin, 2006)

Table 8-1   Medications for Urinary Tract Infections

MEDICATION	DOSE	SIDE EFFECTS
Amoxicillin/clavulanate	250/125 mg q 8 hr	Rash, GI upset
Cefaclor	250–500 mg q 8 hr	Caution if penicillin allergic
Cephalexin	250 mg q 6 hr or 500 mg q 8 hr	Caution if penicillin allergic
Ciprofloxacin	250–500 mg BID	Dizziness, headache, GI upset
Fosfomycin	Single-dose packet	Diarrhea, headache
Lomefloxacin	400 mg once daily	Dizziness, headache, GI upset
Nitrofurantoin	50–100 mg q 6 hr	Nausea, pulmonitis, neuropathy
Ofloxacin	400 mg BID	Dizziness, headache, GI upset
Sulfa/trimethoprim	800/160 mg BID	Rash, Stevens-Johnson syndrome
Trimethoprim	100 mg q 12 hr	GI upset, delayed rash

Source: Physicians' desk reference (61st ed.). (2007). Montvale, NJ: Thomson Healthcare.

- UTI
  - Cranberry tablets, capsules, or juice (Avorn et al., 1994)
  - Flush urinary system
    - Drink water or herbal tea
    - Avoid caffeine, sugar, and alcohol
  - Vitamin C 250–500 mg BID
  - Beta-carotene 25,000–50,000 IU daily
  - Zinc 30–50 mg daily
  - Homeopathic remedies (Jonas & Jacobs, 1996)
    - Aconitum—for early recent infection, with or without flank pain
    - Cantharis—searing lancing pain accompanied by urgency and frequency
  - Herbal teas (Soule & Szwed, 2000; University of Maryland Medical Center, 2006)
    - Echinacea
    - Urinary antiseptics
      - Pipsissewa
      - Bearberry (uva-ursi) (not for use in pregnancy)
      - Thyme
    - Soothing inflammation
      - Corn silk
      - Marshmallow root
      - Cleavers
        - Drink ½ cup every hour until symptoms subside
        - Continue three to five times daily for 10 days

Providing Support:
Education and Support Measures
to Consider

- Provide information regarding
  - Diagnosis
  - Treatment options
  - Medication instructions
- UTI recommendations
  - Avoid caffeine, alcohol, and sugar
  - Drink plenty of water

  - Void frequently
  - Void after intercourse
  - Blot from front to back after voiding
- Urge incontinence
  - Void
    - Frequently
    - With initial urge
    - Do not limit fluids
  - Kegel exercises daily
  - Medication instructions
- Stress incontinence
  - Kegel exercises daily
  - Biofeedback plan
  - Pessary use and fitting instructions as indicated
  - Limit increased intra-abdominal pressure, such as with
    - Heavy lifting
    - Straining at stool
    - Coughing
- Signs and symptoms requiring return for continued care
  - Signs of infection/stones
  - Worsening symptoms
- Option for referral for surgical evaluation and treatment

Follow-up Care:
Follow-up Measures to Consider

- Document
- Plan for continued care
  - UTI
    - Reculture after treatment for
      - Acute pyelonephritis
      - Recurrent symptoms
      - Pregnancy
  - Urge/stress incontinence
    - Keep 2- to 5-day urinary diary
    - Follow-up for
      - Biofeedback
      - Reevaluation of
        - Pelvic floor strength
        - Response to medications

> ▶ Need for pessary
> ▶ Need for surgical consult
- Pessary use
  - ◆ Check every 3 months
  - ◆ Clean
  - ◆ Evaluate for tissue breakdown

Collaborative Practice:
Criteria to Consider for Consultation or Referral
- OB/GYN services
  - Acute pyelonephritis
  - Persistent UTI during pregnancy
  - Evaluation of persistent urinary incontinence
  - Pelvic prolapse
  - Pessary fitting
  - Surgical treatment
- Urology services
  - Unresolved, recurrent, or persistent infection
  - Persistent renal calculi
  - Suspected
    - ◆ Obstruction
    - ◆ Interstitial cystitis
  - Surgical treatment
- For diagnosis or treatment outside the midwife's scope of practice

REFERENCES

American College of Nurse-Midwives. (1997). *Certified nurse-midwives certified midwives as primary care providers/case managers.* Silver Spring, MD: American College of Nurse-Midwives.

American College of Obstetricians and Gynecologists. (2000). Practice Bulletin No. 14. Management of anovulatory bleeding. In *2006 Compendium of selected publications.* Washington, DC: Author.

ACOG Committee on Obstetric Practice. (2006). Treatment with selective serotonin reuptake inhibitors during pregnancy. *Obstet Gynecol,* 108, 1601-3

American College of Obstetrics and Gynecology. (2007). Practice Bulletin No. 87. Use of psychiatric medications during pregnancy and lactation. *Obstetrics and Gynecology,* 110, 1179-1198.

American College of Obstetrics and Gynecology. (2008). Practice Bulletin No. 90. Asthma in pregnancy. *Obstetrics and Gynecology,* 111, 457-464.

American Heart Association. (2004). *Women and coronary heart disease.* Retrieved February 17, 2008 from http://www.americanheart.org/presenter.jhtml?identifier=2859

American Lung Association. (2007). *State of lung disease in diverse communities.* Retrieved February 17, 2008 from http://www.lungusa.org/site/pp.asp?c=dvLUK9O0E&b=308853

Angelini, D., Hodgman, D. & McConaughey, E. (2007). Gastrointestinal. In B. Hackley, J. M. Kriebs, and M. E. Rousseau (Eds.). *Primary care of women: a guide for midwives and women's health providers.* Sudbury, MA: Jones and Bartlett.

Avery, M.D. & Baum, K. D. (2007). Endocrine. In B. Hackley, J. M. Kriebs, and M. E. Rousseau (Eds.). *Primary care of women: a guide for midwives and women's health providers.* Sudbury, MA: Jones and Bartlett.

Avorn, J., Monane, M., Gurwitz, J. H., Glynn, R, J., Choodnovskiy, I., & Lipsitz, L. A. (1994). Reduction of bacteriuria and pyuria after ingestion of cranberry juice. *Journal of the American Medical Association,* 271, 751–754.

Beers, M., & Berkow, R. (Eds.). (1995–2005). Recommendations for antibiotic treatment of adult Lyme disease. In *Merck manual of diagnosis and therapy* [online edition]. Retrieved February 17, 2008 from http://www.merck.com/mrkshared/mmanual/tables/157tb5.jsp

Centers for Disease Control and Prevention. (n.d.). *Tuberculosis guidelines and recommendations.* Retrieved February 17, 2008 from http://www.cdcnpin.org/scripts/tb/cdc.asp

Centers for Disease Control and Prevention. (2007). *Lyme disease.* Retrieved February 17, 2008 from http://www.cdc.gov/ncidod/dvbid/lyme/index.htm

Clark, T. & Fitzgerald, L. (2007). Malaria, tuberculosis and HIV/AIDS. *Journal of Midwifery and Women's Health,* 52, e33–e35.

Drug Digest. (2007). *Helicobacter pylori treatment regimens.* Retrieved February 17, 2008 from http://www.drugdigest.org/DD/Comparison/NewComparison/0,10621,550540-21,00.html

Drugge, R. J. (1996). *Electronic Textbook of Dermatology.* Retrieved on February 15, 2008 from http://telemedicine.org/terms.htm

Emmons, L., Callahan, P., Gorman, P. & Snyder, M. (1997). Primary care management of common dermatologic disorders in women. *Journal of Nurse-Midwifery,* 42, 228–253.

EndocrineWeb.com. (2005). *Endocrine disorders and endocrine surgery.* Retrieved February 17, 2008 from http://www.endocrineweb.com/index.html

Farley, C. L., Tharpe, N., Miller, L. & Ruxer, D. (2006). Women's health care minimum data set: pilot testing and validation for use in clinical practice. *Journal of Midwifery and Women's Health,* 51, 493–501.

Foster, S. (1996). *Herbs for your health.* Loveland, CO: Interweave Press.

Getahun, C., Ananth, C., Oyelese, Y., Peltier, M., Smulian, J. & Vintzileos, A. (2007). Acute and chronic respiratory diseases in pregnancy: associations with spontaneous premature rupture of membranes. *The Journal of Maternal-Fetal and Neonatal Medicine, 20,* 669-675.

Haas, A. (2004). Prematurity is preventable. *Midwifery Today,* 72, 14–16, 64.

Hackley, B., Feinstein, A. & Dixon, J. (2007). Air pollution: impact on maternal and perinatal health. *Journal of Midwifery and Women's Health,* 52, 435–443.

Hlebowicz, J., Darwiche, G., Björgell, O. & Almér, L. O. (2007). Effect of cinnamon on postprandial blood glucose, gastric emptying, and satiety in healthy subjects. *American Journal of Clinical Nutrition,* 85, 1552–1556.

Holisticonline.com. (n.d.). *Conventional, holistic, and integrative treatments for acne.* Retrieved February 17, 2008 from http://holisticonline.com/Remedies/acne.htm

Hunt, S. A., Abraham, W. T., Chin, M. H., Feldman, A. M., Francis, G. S., Ganiats, T. G., et al. (2005). ACC/AHA 2005 guideline update for the diagnosis and management of chronic heart failure in the adult: a report of the American College of Cardiology/American Heart Association Task Force on Practice Guidelines. *Circulation,* 112, e154–e235. Retrieved February 17, 2008 from http://circ.ahajournals.org/cgi/reprint/112/12/e154

ICD9data.com. (2007). *2008 ICD-9-CM. Volume 1. Diagnosis codes.* Retrieved multiple dates from http://www.icd9data.com/2008/Volume1/default.htm

Jonas, W. B. & Jacobs, J. (1996). *Healing with homeopathy: the doctors' guide.* New York: Warner Books.

Kantor, S. D. (1990). Stress and psoriasis. *Cutis,* 46, 321–322.

Koch, L. H. (2006). Help-seeking behaviors of women with urinary incontinence: an integrative review. *Journal of Midwifery and Women's Health,* 51, e39–e44.

Kriebs, J. & Burgin, K. (1997). Pharmacological management of common musculoskeletal disorders in women. *Journal of Nurse-Midwifery,* 42, 207–227.

Ledezma, E., DeSousa, L., Jorquera, A., Sanchez, J., Lander, A., Rodriquez, E., et al. (1996). Efficacy of ajoene, an organosulphur derived from garlic, in the short-term therapy of tinea pedis. *Mycoses,* 39, 393–395.

Louik, C., Lin., A., Werler, M., Hernandez-Diaz, S., & Mitchell, A. (2007). First trimester use of selective serotonin—reuptake inhibitors and the risks of birth defects. *New England Journal of Medicine,* 356, 2675-2683.

Madankumar, R. (2003). An overview of hypertensive disorders in women. *Primary Care Update for OB/GYNs,* 10, 14–18.

MedlinePlus. (2006). *Drugs and supplements.* Retrieved February 17, 2008 from http://www.nlm.nih.gov/medlineplus/druginformation.html

Mitchell, A. M. & Bulik, C. M. (2006). Eating disorders and women's health: an update. *Journal of Midwifery and Women's Health,* 51, 193–201.

Moon, J. (2007). Herpes zoster. *E-Medicine.* Retrieved February 17, 2008 from http://www.emedicine.com/med/topic1007.htm

Murphy, J. L. (Ed.). (2004). *Nurse practitioner's prescribing reference.* New York: Prescribing Reference.

National Heart, Lung, and Blood Institute (NHLBI). (2003). *The seventh report of the joint national committee on prevention, detection, evaluation, and treatment of high blood pressure.* Retrieved February 17, 2008 from http://www.nhlbi.nih.gov/guidelines/hypertension/express.pdf

National Heart, Lung, and Blood Institute (NHLBI). (2004). National Asthma Education and Prevention Program. *Working group report on managing asthma during pregnancy: recommendations for pharmacologic treatment—update 2004.* Retrieved February 17, 2008 from http://www.nhlbi.nih.gov/health/prof/lung/asthma/astpreg/astpreg_full.pdf

National Heart, Lung, and Blood Institute (NHLBI). (2006). *Your guide to lowering your blood pressure with DASH.* Retrieved February 15, 2008 from http://www.nhlbi.nih.gov/health/public/heart/hbp/dash/new_dash.pdf

National Institute of Arthritis and Musculoskeletal and Skin Diseases. (2004). *Rheumatoid arthritis.* Retrieved February 17, 2008 from http://www.niams.nih.gov/Health_Info/Rheumatic_Disease/default.asp

National Institute of Mental Health. (2007). *The numbers count: mental disorders in America.* Retrieved February 17, 2008 from http://www.nimh.nih.gov/health/publications/the-numbers-count-mental-disorders-in-america.shtml

National Jewish Medical and Research Center. (2006). *Nasal wash.* Retrieved February 17, 2008 from http://www.nationaljewish.org/disease-info/treatments/alt-ther/nasal-wash.aspx

National Kidney and Urologic Diseases Information Clearinghouse. (2005). *Cystoscopy and ureteroscopy.* Retrieved February 17, 2008 from http://kidney.niddk.nih.gov/kudiseases/pubs/cystoscopy/index.htm

O'Dell, K. K. & Labin, L. C. (2006). Common problems of urination in non pregnant women: causes, current management and prevention strategies. *Journal of Midwifery and Women's Health,* 51, 159–173.

Payton, R. G., Gardner, R. & Reynolds, D. (1997). Pharmacologic considerations and management of common endocrine disorders in women. *Journal of Nurse-Midwifery,* 42, 186–206.

Pearson, T. A., Blair, S. N., Daniels, S. R., Eckel, R. H., Fair, J. M., Fortmann, S. P., et al. (2002). AHA guidelines for primary prevention of cardiovascular disease and stroke: 2002 update. Consensus panel guide to comprehensive risk reduction for adult patients without coronary or other atherosclerotic vascular diseases. *Circulation,* 106, 388–391.

Rabheru, K. (2001).The use of electroconvulsive therapy during pregnancy. *Hospital Community Psychiatry,* 46, 710-719.

Rosenfeld, J. A. (1997). *Women's health in primary care.* Baltimore, MD: William & Wilkins.

Rousseau, M. E. (2007). Dermatology. In B. Hackley, J. M. Kriebs and M. E. Rousseau (Eds.). *Primary care of women: a guide for midwives and women's health providers.* Sudbury, MA: Jones and Bartlett.

Sanders, L. B. (2006). Assessing and managing women with depression: a midwifery perspective. *Journal of Midwifery and Women's Health,* 51, 185–192.

Smith, S. C. Jr., Allen, J., Blair, S. N., Bonow, R. O., Brass, L. M., Fonarow, G. C., et al. (2006). AHA/ACC guidelines for secondary prevention for patients with coronary and other atherosclerotic vascular disease: 2006 update. *Circulation,* 113, 2363–2372.

Soule, D. & Szwed, S. (2000). *The roots of healing: a woman's book of herbs.* Secaucus, NJ: Citadel Press.

Strauss, J. S., Krowchuk, D. P., Leyden, J. J., Lucky, A. W., Shalita, A. R., Siegfried, E. C., et al. (2007). Guidelines of care for acne vulgaris management. *Journal of the American Academy of Dermatology,* 56, 651–663. Retrieved February 17, 2008 from http://www.guideline.gov/summary/summary.aspx?doc_id=10797

Tong, M. M., Altman, P. M. & Barnetson, R. S. (1992). Tea tree oil in the treatment of tinea pedis. *Australian Journal of Dermatology,* 33, 145–149.

U.S. Department of Health and Human Services. (2006). *Caregiver stress.* Retrieved February 17, 2008 from http://www.4women.gov/faq/caregiver.htm

University of Maryland Medical Center. (2006). *Urinary tract infections in women.* Retrieved February 17, 2008 from http://www.umm.edu/altmed/articles/urinary-tract-000169.htm

Wilkin, J., Dahl, M., Detmar, M., Drake, L., Feinstein, A., Odom, R., et al. (2002). Standard classification of rosacea: report of the National Rosacea Society Expert Committee on the classification and staging of rosacea. *Journal of the American Academy of Dermatology,* 50, 584–587.

World Health Organization (WHO). (2004). *WHO guide to mental and neurological health in primary care: diagnostic checklists.* Retrieved February 17, 2008 from http://www.mentalneurologicalprimarycare.org/index.asp

Wong, C. (n.d.). *Natural treatments for acne.* Retrieved February 17, 2008 from http://altmedicine.about.com/cs/conditionsatod/a/acne.htm

Wyner, E., Marfell, J., Karsnitz, D. & Rousseau, M. E. (2007). Cardiovascular disease in women. In B. Hackley, J. M. Kriebs, and M. E. Rouseau (Eds.). *Primary care of women: A guide for midwives and women's health providers.* Sudbury, MA: Jones and Bartlett.

BIBLIOGRAPHY

Alliance for Aging Research. (1997). *Controlling high blood pressure in older women: clinical reference manual.* Washington, DC: National Heart, Lung, and Blood Institute.

American Heart Association. (1998). Cardiovascular disease in women: a scientific statement from the AHA. *Clinician Reviews,* 8, 145–160.

Benetti, M. C. & Marchese, T. (1996). Primary care for women: management of common musculoskeletal disorders. *Journal of Nurse-Midwifery,* 41, 173–187.

Blumenthal, D. (2003). *The ABC clinical guide to herbs.* Austin, TX: American Botanical Council.

Brucker, M. C. & Faucher, M. A. (1997). Pharmacologic management of common gastrointestinal health problems in women. *Journal of Nurse-Midwifery,* 43, 145–162.

Clark, C. & Paine, L. L. (1996). Psychopharmacologic management of women with common mental health problems. *Journal of Nurse-Midwifery,* I, 254–274.

Davis, L. & Stecy, P. (1997). Pharmacologic management of cardiovascular problems in women. *Journal of Nurse-Midwifery,* 42, 176–185.

Drazen, J. M. & Weinberger, S. E. (1998). Disorders of the respiratory system. In A. S. Fauci, E. Braunwald, et al. (Eds.). *Harrison's principles of internal medicine* (14th ed., pp. 1407–1410). New York: McGraw-Hill.

Fauci, A. S., Braunwald, E., et al. (Eds.). (1998). *Harrison's principles of internal medicine* (14th ed.). New York: McGraw-Hill.

Gladstar, R. (1993). *Herbal healing for women.* New York: Simon and Schuster.

Hackley, B., Kriebs, J. M. & Rousseau, M. E. (2007). *Primary care of women: a guide for midwives and women's health providers.* Sudbury, MA: Jones and Bartlett.

Harris, G. D. (1999). Managing hypertension in female patients. *Women's Health in Primary Care,* 2, 395–417.

MacLaren, A. & Imberg, W. (1998). Current issues in the midwifery management of women living with HIV/AIDS. *Journal of Nurse-Midwifery,* 43, 502–521.

Maldondo, A. & Barger, M. (1995). Primary care for women: comprehensive assessment of common musculoskeletal disorders. *Journal of Midwifery and Women's Health,* 40, 202–215.

Mays, M. & Leiner, S. (1996). Primary care for women: management of common respiratory problems. *Journal of Nurse-Midwifery,* 41, 139–154.

Mays, M. & Leiner, S. (1997). Pharmacologic management of common lower respiratory tract disorders in women. *Journal of Nurse-Midwifery,* 42, 163–175.

McIntyre, A. (1994). *The complete woman's herbal.* New York: Henry Holt.

Moser, M. (1996). *Clinical management of hypertension.* Caddo, OK: Professional Communications.

National Cholesterol Education Program. (1993). *Second report on the detection, evaluation and treatment of high blood cholesterol in adults.* Washington, DC: National Institutes of Health.

Payton, R. G., Gardner, R. & Reynolds, D. (1997). Pharmacologic considerations and management of common endocrine disorders in women. *Journal of Nurse-Midwifery,* 42, 186–206.

Rovner, E. S. & Weine, A. J. (2000). Overactive bladder and urge incontinence: establishing the diagnosis. *Women's Health in Primary Care,* 3, 117–126.

Schmitt, M. (March 1999). Skills workshop: evaluating the shoulder. *Patient Care for the Nurse-Practitioner,* 42–50.

Shaw, B. (1996). Primary care for women: management and treatment of gastrointestinal disorders. *Journal of Nurse-Midwifery,* 41, 155–172.

Siris, E. S. & Schussheim, D. H. (1998). Osteoporosis: assessing your patient's risk. *Women's Health in Primary Care,* 1, 99–106.

Smith, T. (1984). *A woman's guide to homeopathic medicine.* New York: Thorsons.

Speroff, L., Glass, R. H. & Kase, N. G. (1994). *Clinical gynecologic endocrinology and infertility* (5th ed.). Philadelphia: Williams & Wilkins.

Swartz, M. H. (1994). *Textbook of physical diagnosis: history and examination* (2nd ed.). Philadelphia: W. B. Saunders.

Walls, D. (2007). *Natural families—healthy homes.* LaVergne, TN: Ingram.

Weintraub, T. A., Paine, L. L. & Weintraub, D. H. (1996). Primary care for women: comprehensive assessment and management of common mental health problems. *Journal of Nurse-Midwifery,* 41, 125–138.

Appendix A: An Herbal Primer

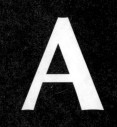

Plants and herbs provide not only medicines but also vitamins, minerals, and macronutrients for optimum benefits.

Plants and botanical medicines have been used for women's health and healing for centuries, as preventive and therapeutic treatments during pregnancy, birth, and breast-feeding. Natural medicines have been shown, through traditional wisdom and modern science, to relieve symptoms, promote health, and provide support for the childbearing year.

Natural medicines are often less toxic and safer than many pharmaceuticals, but that does not mean that all natural medicines are safe. Like nature, there is both good and bad; many botanicals have side effects or may be toxic if not used wisely. The most common side effects that occur with herbal use are headaches, rash, indigestion and nausea, vomiting, or allergic reaction to the plant. Education on safe herbal use is imperative for practitioners and patients alike.

HERBAL PREPARATIONS

There are many sources of herbal medicines: plants, including the aerial parts and roots; trees; shrubs; seeds; berries; fruits; and vegetables. Most herbs can be used in several forms; the most common are teas, tinctures, syrups, decoctions, capsules, compresses, infused oils, and herbal baths.

Teas (infusions)—This is the traditional way of taking herbal medicines. One to two teaspoons of fresh or dried plant material is steeped in 6–8 oz hot water for 5–10 minutes. For children a lower "dose" can be accomplished by steeping only 2–3 minutes. Plant material is strained, and the tea can be sweetened with honey or other sweetener. Organic plants are preferred, and many medicinal teas include a blend of several herbs. For a medicinal dose, usually two to three cups a day should be consumed. Teas or infusions may also be applied topically.

Decoction—A decoction is a tea (or infusion) made from the bark or woody parts of plants. The plant part is broken or crushed and simmered in water for 20–30 minutes to extract the medicinal qualities and then strained and used as a tea or topical application.

Tincture—Another way of preparing and storing botanical medicines is to take fresh or dried plant material (for fresh, use one half the amount) and soak it in an alcohol base for 2 weeks. A clean clear glass jar should be used and sealed tightly during the soaking process. The formula for preparation is creating a ratio of 1:4 plant-to-liquid:

> One part plant material
> One part *distilled* water
> Three parts 80-proof vodka

A "part" can be 1 tablespoon, ½ cup, or any desired amount.

Label the jar with the herb name and date. Seal tightly and set out of sunlight. Gently shake jar twice daily for 2 weeks. Strain plant material and store tincture in amber glass jar, out of direct sunlight. Tinctures maintain their potency for 2–3 years. The medicinal dose of a tincture is 20–30 drops in water or juice two to three times daily.

Nonalcoholic forms of tinctures are available for children or others preferring not to have the alcohol base. These tinctures are prepared with glycerin or vinegar.

Syrup—A syrup is produced when a prepared infusion or decoction is heated and honey is added to the desired thickness and taste to make it more palatable.

Capsules—Plant material is dried or flash frozen, ground into a fine powder, and placed in gelatin or vegetable-based capsules. In commercial products doses vary; label directions should be followed.

Compress (poultice)—Dry or moistened herb is placed in a gauze pad, cheese cloth, or soft porous fabric; folded into a "packet" and placed directly onto the affected area for 10–20 minutes three to four times daily. Gauze or fabric compresses may also be soaked in an infusion and placed directly on the affected area.

Infused oil—To extract the plant's medicinal quality in an oil-based form, tightly pack plant material in a clean clear jar. Completely cover the herbs with a base or carrier oil (such as olive, sweet almond, apricot kernel, jojoba, or wheat germ). Seal well and place in a sun-exposed window for 2 weeks. Strain plant material and store infused oil in an amber jar out of direct sunlight. Apply infused oil to affected area two to three times daily.

Salve (ointment)—Warm (do not boil) two to three cups of infused oil (above). Add 1 oz of beeswax and slowly warm until beeswax is melted. Pour into clean jars and allow to cool before sealing. Apply a small amount to affected area two to four times daily. For a softer ointment use three cups oil to 1 oz beeswax. For a firmer ointment use two cups oil to 1 oz beeswax.

PREGNANCY SAFETY GUIDELINES

1. Use smaller doses
2. Use milder herbs
3. Use only herbs and essential oils deemed safe for pregnancy
4. Use a 2% or low range of 4% dilution (6-12 drops) of essential oils
5. Avoid in first trimester
6. Avoid uterine stimulant herbs (emmenagogues) before 37 weeks
7. Tea/infusion forms may cause less indigestion
8. Discontinue essential oils if headache or nausea presents
9. Discontinue herbs if nausea/vomiting, rash, or headache presents

Herbs Not Recommended in Pregnancy

Barberry	Licorice
Bladderwack	Lobelia
Cascara	Mandrake
Chaparral	Pennyroyal
Damiana	Pleurisy root
Ephedra	Rue

Fenugreek

Gentian

Ginseng (caution)

Goldenseal

Juniper

Saw palmetto

Sage

Tansy

Uva ursi

Yarrow

Herbs Generally Regarded as Safe in Pregnancy

Alfalfa

Arnica (external only
  or homeopathic)

Astragalus

Bilberry

Black haw

Burdock

Calendula

Catnip

Chamomile

Corn silk

Dandelion

Echinacea

Elderberry

Evening primrose oil

Fennel

Feverfew (after
  first trimester)

Flax

Garlic

Ginger Marshmallow

Hawthorn

Horehound

Horse chestnut

Lemon balm

Meadowsweet

Milk thistle

Mullein

Nettle

Oatstraw

Parsley

Passionflower

Peppermint

Red raspberry

Slippery elm

St. John's wort

Skullcap

Wild yam

Valerian

Yellow dock

Vitex

Emmenagogues (Uterine Stimulants)

Use only after 37 weeks:

Blue cohosh

Black cohosh

Birthwort

Cottonroot

Dong quai

Motherwort

Shepherd's purse

Squaw vine (partridgeberry)

AROMATHERAPY

How To Use Essential Oils

Inhalation—The essential oil can be infused with electric, battery, reed, or candle diffusers or by placing a small amount on fabric or cotton ball. This is good for relaxation and calming essential oils.

Topical—Pure essential oils should not be used undiluted on the skin. Dilute the essential oil with a base oil (olive, sweet almond, jojoba, apricot kernel, or any cold pressed oil) or distilled water for direct application or misting of the skin

Hydrotherapy—Essential oils are added as drops to baths, including foot or sitz baths.

Most healthy adults should use the 4% dilution for most topical applications. Children, the elderly, or health-compromised people should use the 1% dilution. Pregnant women should use the 2% or lower range of 4% dilutions.

Essential Oils Considered Toxic and Harmful

Bitter melon

Buchu

Camphor

Cassia

Mugwort

Pennyroyal

Rue

Sassafras

Tansy

Thuja

Wintergreen

Wormwood

Essential Oils to Avoid in Pregnancy

Ginger (do not use in
  first trimester)

Juniper

Mugwort

Nutmeg

Pennyroyal

Tansy

Thuja

Thyme

Wormwood

DILUTIONS FOR TOPICAL USE			
Carrier Oil	**Essential Oil and Dilution Percent**		
½ oz or 1 T	3–5 drops = 1%	6–8 drops = 2%	12–15 drops= 4%
1 oz or 2 T	6–10 drops = 1%	12–16 drops = 2%	24–30 drops = 4%

Essential Oils Generally Regarded as Safe in Pregnancy

Bergamot	Marjoram
Cedarwood	Neroli
Chamomile	Patchouli
Citrus (in small amounts)	Rose
Clary sage	Rose geranium
Cypress	Rosemary
Eucalyptus	Sandalwood
Jasmine	Tea tree
Lavender	Ylang ylang

BIBLIOGRAPHY

Low Dog, T. & Micozzi, M. (2005). *Women's health in complementary and integrative medicine: a clinical guide.* St. Louis, MO: Elsevier.

Walls, D. (2007). *Natural families—healthy homes.* LaVergne, TN: Ingram.

Food Sources of
Selected Nutrients

B

APPENDIX B TABLE OF CONTENTS

APPENDIX B-1. FOOD SOURCES OF POTASSIUM

Food sources of potassium ranked by milligrams of potassium per standard amount; also showing calories in the standard amount. (The adequate intake (AI) for adults is 4700 mg/day potassium.)

FOOD, STANDARD AMOUNT	POTASSIUM (MG)	CALORIES
Sweet potato, baked, 1 potato (146 g)	694	131
Tomato paste, ¼ cup	664	54
Beet greens, cooked, ½ cup	655	19
Potato, baked, flesh, 1 potato (156 g)	610	145
White beans, canned, ½ cup	595	153
Yogurt, plain, nonfat, 8-oz container	579	127
Tomato puree, ½ cup	549	48
Clams, canned, 3 oz	534	126
Yogurt, plain, low fat, 8-oz container	531	143
Prune juice, ¾ cup	530	136
Carrot juice, ¾ cup	517	71
Blackstrap molasses, 1 Tbsp	498	47
Halibut, cooked, 3 oz	490	119
Soybeans, green, cooked, ½ cup	485	127
Tuna, yellowfin, cooked, 3 oz	484	118
Lima beans, cooked, ½ cup	484	104
Winter squash, cooked, ½ cup	448	40
Soybeans, mature, cooked, ½ cup	443	149
Rockfish, Pacific, cooked, 3 oz	442	103
Cod, Pacific, cooked, 3 oz	439	89
Bananas, 1 medium	422	105
Spinach, cooked, ½ cup	419	21
Tomato juice, ¾ cup	417	31
Tomato sauce, ½ cup	405	39
Peaches, dried, uncooked, ¼ cup	398	96
Prunes, stewed, ½ cup	398	133
Milk, nonfat, 1 cup	382	83
Pork chop, center loin, cooked, 3 oz	382	197
Apricots, dried, uncooked, ¼ cup	378	78
Rainbow trout, farmed, cooked, 3 oz	375	144
Pork loin, center rib (roasts), lean, roasted, 3 oz	371	190
Buttermilk, cultured, low fat, 1 cup	370	98

(continues)

FOOD, STANDARD AMOUNT	POTASSIUM (MG)	CALORIES
Cantaloupe, ¼ medium	368	47
1% to 2% milk, 1 cup	366	102–122
Honeydew melon, ⅛ medium	365	58
Lentils, cooked, ½ cup	365	115
Plantains, cooked, ½ cup slices	358	90
Kidney beans, cooked, ½ cup	358	112
Orange juice, ¾ cup	355	85
Split peas, cooked, ½ cup	355	116
Yogurt, plain, whole milk, 8-oz container	352	138

Source: U.S. Department of Health and Human Services and U.S. Department of Agriculture. (2005). *Dietary guidelines for Americans* (6th ed.). Washington, DC: U.S. Government Printing Office.

APPENDIX B-2. FOOD SOURCES OF VITAMIN E

Food sources of vitamin E ranked by milligrams of vitamin E per standard amount; also calories in the standard amount. (All provide ≥10% of the Recommended Daily Allowance (RDA) for vitamin E for adults, which is 15 mg α-tocopherol [AT]/day.)

FOOD, STANDARD AMOUNT	AT (MG)	CALORIES
Fortified ready-to-eat cereals, ~1 oz	1.6–12.8	90–107
Sunflower seeds, dry roasted, 1 oz	7.4	165
Almonds, 1 oz	7.3	164
Sunflower oil, high linoleic, 1 Tbsp	5.6	120
Cottonseed oil, 1 Tbsp	4.8	120
Safflower oil, high oleic, 1 Tbsp	4.6	120
Hazelnuts (filberts), 1 oz	4.3	178
Mixed nuts, dry roasted, 1 oz	3.1	168
Turnip greens, frozen, cooked, ½ cup	2.9	24
Tomato paste, ¼ cup	2.8	54
Pine nuts, 1 oz	2.6	191
Peanut butter, 2 Tbsp	2.5	192
Tomato puree, ½ cup	2.5	48
Tomato sauce, ½ cup	2.5	39
Canola oil, 1 Tbsp	2.4	124
Wheat germ, toasted, plain, 2 Tbsp	2.3	54
Peanuts, 1 oz	2.2	166
Avocado, raw, ½ avocado	2.1	161
Carrot juice, canned, ¾ cup	2.1	71
Peanut oil, 1 Tbsp	2.1	119
Corn oil, 1 Tbsp	1.9	120
Olive oil, 1 Tbsp	1.9	119
Spinach, cooked, ½ cup	1.9	21
Dandelion greens, cooked, ½ cup	1.8	18
Sardine, Atlantic, in oil, drained, 3 oz	1.7	177
Blue crab, cooked/canned, 3 oz	1.6	84
Brazil nuts, 1 oz	1.6	186
Herring, Atlantic, pickled, 3 oz	1.5	222

Source: U.S. Department of Health and Human Services and U.S. Department of Agriculture. (2005). *Dietary guidelines for Americans* (6th ed.). Washington, DC: U.S. Government Printing Office.

APPENDIX B-3. FOOD SOURCES OF IRON

Food sources of iron ranked by milligrams of iron per standard amount; also calories in the standard amount. (All are ≥10% of RDA for teen and adult females, which is 18 mg/day.)

FOOD, STANDARD AMOUNT	IRON (MG)	CALORIES
Clams, canned, drained, 3 oz	23.8	126
Fortified ready-to-eat cereals (various), ~ 1 oz	1.8–21.1	54–127
Oysters, eastern, wild, cooked, moist heat, 3 oz	10.2	116
Organ meats (liver, giblets), various, cooked, 3 oz[a]	5.2–9.9	134–235
Fortified instant cooked cereals (various), 1 packet	4.9–8.1	Varies
Soybeans, mature, cooked, ½ cup	4.4	149
Pumpkin and squash seed kernels, roasted, 1 oz	4.2	148
White beans, canned, ½ cup	3.9	153
Blackstrap molasses, 1 Tbsp	3.5	47
Lentils, cooked, ½ cup	3.3	115
Spinach, cooked from fresh, ½ cup	3.2	21
Beef, chuck, blade roast, lean, cooked, 3 oz	3.1	215
Beef, bottom round, lean, 0″ fat, all grades, cooked, 3 oz	2.8	182
Kidney beans, cooked, ½ cup	2.6	112
Sardines, canned in oil, drained, 3 oz	2.5	177
Beef, rib, lean, ¼″ fat, all grades, 3 oz	2.4	195
Chickpeas, cooked, ½ cup	2.4	134
Duck, meat only, roasted, 3 oz	2.3	171
Lamb, shoulder, arm, lean, ¼ ″ fat, choice, cooked, 3 oz	2.3	237
Prune juice, ¾ cup	2.3	136
Shrimp, canned, 3 oz	2.3	102
Cowpeas, cooked, ½ cup	2.2	100
Ground beef, 15% fat, cooked, 3 oz	2.2	212
Tomato puree, ½ cup	2.2	48
Lima beans, cooked, ½ cup	2.2	108
Soybeans, green, cooked, ½ cup	2.2	127
Navy beans, cooked, ½ cup	2.1	127
Refried beans, ½ cup	2.1	118
Beef, top sirloin, lean, 0″ fat, all grades, cooked, 3 oz	2.0	156
Tomato paste, ¼ cup	2.0	54

[a] High in cholesterol.

Source: U.S. Department of Health and Human Services and U.S. Department of Agriculture. (2005). *Dietary guidelines for Americans* (6th ed.). Washington, DC: U.S. Government Printing Office.

APPENDIX B-4. NONDAIRY FOOD SOURCES OF CALCIUM

Nondairy food sources of calcium ranked by milligrams of calcium per standard amount; also calories in the standard amount. The bioavailability may vary. (The AI for adults is 1000 mg/day.)[a]

FOOD, STANDARD AMOUNT	CALCIUM (MG)	CALORIES
Fortified ready-to-eat cereals (various), 1 oz	236–1043	88–106
Soy beverage, calcium fortified, 1 cup	368	98
Sardines, Atlantic, in oil, drained, 3 oz	325	177
Tofu, firm, prepared with nigari,[b] ½ cup	253	88
Pink salmon, canned, with bone, 3 oz	181	118
Collards, cooked from frozen, ½ cup	178	31
Molasses, blackstrap, 1 Tbsp	172	47
Spinach, cooked from frozen, ½ cup	146	30
Soybeans, green, cooked, ½ cup	130	127
Turnip greens, cooked from frozen, ½ cup	124	24
Ocean perch, Atlantic, cooked, 3 oz	116	103
Oatmeal, plain and flavored, instant, fortified, 1 packet prepared	99–110	97–157
Cowpeas, cooked, ½ cup	106	80
White beans, canned, ½ cup	96	153
Kale, cooked from frozen, ½ cup	90	20
Okra, cooked from frozen, ½ cup	88	26
Soybeans, mature, cooked, ½ cup	88	149
Blue crab, canned, 3 oz	86	84
Beet greens, cooked from fresh, ½ cup	82	19
Pak-choi, Chinese cabbage, cooked from fresh, ½ cup	79	10
Clams, canned, 3 oz	78	126
Dandelion greens, cooked from fresh, ½ cup	74	17
Rainbow trout, farmed, cooked, 3 oz	73	144

[a]Both calcium content and bioavailability should be considered when selecting dietary sources of calcium. Some plant foods have calcium that is well absorbed, but the large quantity of plant foods that would be needed to provide as much calcium as in a glass of milk may be unachievable for many. Many other calcium-fortified foods are available, but the percentage of calcium that can be absorbed is unavailable for many of them.

[b]Calcium sulfate and magnesium chloride.

Source: U.S. Department of Health and Human Services and U.S. Department of Agriculture. (2005). *Dietary guidelines for Americans* (6th ed.). Washington, DC: U.S. Government Printing Office.

APPENDIX B-5. DAIRY FOOD SOURCES OF CALCIUM

Dairy food sources of calcium ranked by milligrams of calcium per standard amount; also calories in the standard amount. (All are ≥20% of AI for adults aged 19–50, which is 1000 mg/day.)

FOOD, STANDARD AMOUNT	CALCIUM (MG)	CALORIES
Plain yogurt, nonfat (13 g protein/8 oz), 8-oz containe	452	127
Romano cheese, 1.5 oz	452	165
Pasteurized process Swiss cheese, 2 oz	438	190
Plain yogurt, low fat (12 g protein/8 oz), 8-oz container	415	143
Fruit yogurt, low fat (10 g protein/8 oz), 8-oz container	345	232
Swiss cheese, 1.5 oz	336	162
Ricotta cheese, part skim, ½ cup	335	170
Pasteurized process American cheese food, 2 oz	323	188
Provolone cheese, 1.5 oz	321	150
Mozzarella cheese, part skim, 1.5 oz	311	129
Cheddar cheese, 1.5 oz	307	171
Fat-free (skim) milk, 1 cup	306	83
Muenster cheese, 1.5 oz	305	156
1% low-fat milk, 1 cup	290	102
Low-fat chocolate milk (1%), 1 cup	288	158
2% reduced fat milk, 1 cup	285	122
Reduced fat chocolate milk (2%), 1 cup	285	180
Buttermilk, low fat, 1 cup	284	98
Chocolate milk, 1 cup	280	208
Whole milk, 1 cup	276	146
Yogurt, plain, whole milk (8 g protein/8 oz), 8-oz container	275	138
Ricotta cheese, whole milk, ½ cup	255	214
Blue cheese, 1.5 oz	225	150
Mozzarella cheese, whole milk, 1.5 oz	215	128
Feta cheese, 1.5 oz	210	113

Source: U.S. Department of Health and Human Services and U.S. Department of Agriculture. (2005). *Dietary guidelines for Americans* (6th ed.). Washington, DC: U.S. Government Printing Office.

APPENDIX B-6. FOOD SOURCES OF VITAMIN A

Food sources of vitamin A ranked by micrograms Retinol Activity Equivalents (RAE) of vitamin A per standard amount; also calories in the standard amount. (All are ≥20% of RDA for adult men, which is 900 mg/day RAE.)

FOOD, STANDARD AMOUNT	VITAMIN A (μG RAE)	CALORIES
Organ meats (liver, giblets), various, cooked, 3 oz[a]	1490–9126	134–235
Carrot juice, ¾ cup	1692	71
Sweet potato with peel, baked, 1 medium	1096	103
Pumpkin, canned, ½ cup	953	42
Carrots, cooked from fresh, ½ cup	671	27
Spinach, cooked from frozen, ½ cup	573	30
Collards, cooked from frozen, ½ cup	489	31
Kale, cooked from frozen, ½ cup	478	20
Mixed vegetables, canned, ½ cup	474	40
Turnip greens, cooked from frozen, ½ cup	441	24
Instant cooked cereals, fortified, prepared, 1 packet	285–376	75–97
Various ready-to-eat cereals, with added vitamin A, ~1 oz	180–376	100–117
Carrot, raw, 1 small	301	20
Beet greens, cooked, ½ cup	276	19
Winter squash, cooked, ½ cup	268	38
Dandelion greens, cooked, ½ cup	260	18
Cantaloupe, raw, ¼ medium melon	233	46
Mustard greens, cooked, ½ cup	221	11
Pickled herring, 3 oz	219	222
Red sweet pepper, cooked, ½ cup	186	19
Chinese cabbage, cooked, ½ cup	180	10

[a]High in cholesterol.

Source: U.S. Department of Health and Human Services and U.S. Department of Agriculture. (2005). *Dietary guidelines for Americans* (6th ed.). Washington, DC: U.S. Government Printing Office.

APPENDIX B-7. FOOD SOURCES OF MAGNESIUM

Food sources of magnesium ranked by milligrams of magnesium per standard amount; also calories in the standard amount. (All are ≥10% of RDA for adult men, which is 420 mg/day.)

FOOD, STANDARD AMOUNT	MAGNESIUM (MG)	CALORIES
Pumpkin and squash seed kernels, roasted, 1 oz	151	148
Brazil nuts, 1 oz	107	186
Bran ready-to-eat cereal (100%), ~1 oz	103	74
Halibut, cooked, 3 oz	91	119
Quinoa, dry, ¼ cup	89	159
Spinach, canned, ½ cup	81	25
Almonds, 1 oz	78	164
Spinach, cooked from fresh, ½ cup	78	20
Buckwheat flour, ¼ cup	75	101
Cashews, dry roasted, 1 oz	74	163
Soybeans, mature, cooked, ½ cup	74	149
Pine nuts, dried, 1 oz	71	191
Mixed nuts, oil roasted, with peanuts, 1 oz	67	175
White beans, canned, ½ cup	67	154
Pollock, walleye, cooked, 3 oz	62	96
Black beans, cooked, ½ cup	60	114
Bulgur, dry, ¼ cup	57	120
Oat bran, raw, ¼ cup	55	58
Soybeans, green, cooked, ½ cup	54	127
Tuna, yellowfin, cooked, 3 oz	54	118
Artichokes (hearts), cooked, ½ cup	50	42
Peanuts, dry roasted, 1 oz	50	166
Lima beans, baby, cooked from frozen, ½ cup	50	95
Beet greens, cooked, ½ cup	49	19
Navy beans, cooked, ½ cup	48	127
Tofu, firm, prepared with nigari,[a] ½ cup	47	88
Okra, cooked from frozen, ½ cup	47	26
Soy beverage, 1 cup	47	127
Cowpeas, cooked, ½ cup	46	100
Hazelnuts, 1 oz	46	178
Oat bran muffin, 1 oz	45	77

(continues)

FOOD, STANDARD AMOUNT	MAGNESIUM (MG)	CALORIES
Great northern beans, cooked, ½ cup	44	104
Oat bran, cooked, ½ cup	44	44
Buckwheat groats roasted, cooked, ½ cup	43	78
Brown rice, cooked, ½ cup	42	108
Haddock, cooked, 3 oz	42	95

[a]Calcium sulfate and magnesium chloride.

Source: U.S. Department of Health and Human Services and U.S. Department of Agriculture. (2005). *Dietary guidelines for Americans* (6th ed.). Washington, DC: U.S. Government Printing Office.

APPENDIX B-8. FOOD SOURCES OF DIETARY FIBER

Food sources of dietary fiber ranked by grams of dietary fiber per standard amount; also calories in the standard amount. (All are ≥10% of AI for adult women, which is 25 g/day.)

FOOD, STANDARD AMOUNT	DIETARY FIBER (G)	CALORIES
Navy beans, cooked, ½ cup	9.5	128
Bran ready-to-eat cereal (100%), ½ cup	8.8	78
Kidney beans, canned, ½ cup	8.2	109
Split peas, cooked, ½ cup	8.1	116
Lentils, cooked, ½ cup	7.8	115
Black beans, cooked, ½ cup	7.5	114
Pinto beans, cooked, ½ cup	7.7	122
Lima beans, cooked, ½ cup	6.6	108
Artichoke, globe, cooked, 1 each	6.5	60
White beans, canned, ½ cup	6.3	154
Chickpeas, cooked, ½ cup	6.2	135
Great northern beans, cooked, ½ cup	6.2	105
Cowpeas, cooked, ½ cup	5.6	100
Soybeans, mature, cooked, ½ cup	5.2	149
Bran ready-to-eat cereals, various, ~1 oz	2.6–5.0	90–108
Crackers, rye wafers, plain, 2 wafers	5.0	74
Sweet potato, baked, with peel, 1 medium (146 g)	4.8	131
Asian pear, raw, 1 small	4.4	51
Green peas, cooked, ½ cup	4.4	67
Whole-wheat English muffin, 1 each	4.4	134
Pear, raw, 1 small	4.3	81
Bulgur, cooked, ½ cup	4.1	76
Mixed vegetables, cooked, ½ cup	4.0	59
Raspberries, raw, ½ cup	4.0	32
Sweet potato, boiled, no peel, 1 medium (156 g)	3.9	119
Blackberries, raw, ½ cup	3.8	31
Potato, baked, with skin, 1 medium	3.8	161
Soybeans, green, cooked, ½ cup	3.8	127
Stewed prunes, ½ cup	3.8	133
Figs, dried, ¼ cup	3.7	93
Dates, ¼ cup	3.6	126

(continues)

FOOD, STANDARD AMOUNT	DIETARY FIBER (G)	CALORIES
Oat bran, raw, ¼ cup	3.6	58
Pumpkin, canned, ½ cup	3.6	42
Spinach, frozen, cooked, ½ cup	3.5	30
Shredded wheat ready-to-eat cereals, various, ~1 oz	2.8–3.4	96
Almonds, 1 oz	3.3	164
Apple with skin, raw, 1 medium	3.3	72
Brussels sprouts, frozen, cooked, ½ cup	3.2	33
Whole-wheat spaghetti, cooked, ½ cup	3.1	87
Banana, 1 medium	3.1	105
Orange, raw, 1 medium	3.1	62
Oat bran muffin, 1 small	3.0	178
Guava, 1 medium	3.0	37
Pearled barley, cooked, ½ cup	3.0	97
Sauerkraut, canned, solids, and liquids, ½ cup	3.0	23
Tomato paste, ¼ cup	2.9	54
Winter squash, cooked, ½ cup	2.9	38
Broccoli, cooked, ½ cup	2.8	26
Parsnips, cooked, chopped, ½ cup	2.8	55
Turnip greens, cooked, ½ cup	2.5	15
Collards, cooked, ½ cup	2.7	25
Okra, frozen, cooked, ½ cup	2.6	26
Peas, edible-podded, cooked, ½ cup	2.5	42

Source: U.S. Department of Health and Human Services and U.S. Department of Agriculture. (2005). *Dietary guidelines for Americans* (6th ed.). Washington, DC: U.S. Government Printing Office.

APPENDIX B-9. FOOD SOURCES OF VITAMIN C

Food sources of vitamin C ranked by milligrams of vitamin C per standard amount; also calories in the standard amount. (All provide ≥20% of RDA for adult men, which is 90 mg/day.)

FOOD, STANDARD AMOUNT	VITAMIN C (MG)	CALORIES
Guava, raw, ½ cup	188	56
Red sweet pepper, raw, ½ cup	142	20
Red sweet pepper, cooked, ½ cup	116	0.19
Kiwi fruit, 1 medium	70	46
Orange, raw, 1 medium	70	62
Orange juice, ¾ cup	61–93	79–84
Green pepper, sweet, raw, ½ cup	60	15
Green pepper, sweet, cooked, ½ cup	51	19
Grapefruit juice, ¾ cup	50–70	71–86
Vegetable juice cocktail, ¾ cup	50	34
Strawberries, raw, ½ cup	49	27
Brussels sprouts, cooked, ½ cup	48	28
Cantaloupe, ¼ medium	47	51
Papaya, raw, ¼ medium	47	30
Kohlrabi, cooked, ½ cup	45	24
Broccoli, raw, ½ cup	39	15
Edible pod peas, cooked, ½ cup	38	34
Broccoli, cooked, ½ cup	37	26
Sweet potato, canned, ½ cup	34	116
Tomato juice, ¾ cup	33	31
Cauliflower, cooked, ½ cup	28	17
Pineapple, raw, ½ cup	28	37
Kale, cooked, ½ cup	27	18
Mango, ½ cup	23	54

Source: U.S. Department of Health and Human Services and U.S. Department of Agriculture. (2005). *Dietary guidelines for Americans* (6th ed.). Washington, DC: U.S. Government Printing Office.

Index

hysterectomy
    and cytologic screening, 291
    for uterine fibroids, 332

I

ibandronate sodium (Boniva), for osteoporosis, 274
ICD-9 codes, 7–8. *See also* code groups
Icon Key, 4
identification, client, in documentation of care, 11
identity, cultural, 20
IFN. *See* fibronectin
imiquimod cream 5%, for HPV, 351
immigrant women, individualized care for, 21
immunizations, 46
    for adult women, 233
    in documentation of care, 15
    in preconception evaluation, 242
    in well-baby care, 208
impetigo, 356
    evaluation of, 388
    treatment for, 392
implanon contraceptives, 251–252, 253
incontinence, urinary, 420
    treatment for, 422–423
    types of, 420
Incorporation of New Procedures into Nurse-Midwifery
    Practice, ACNM Guidelines for, 259
induction of labor
    contraindications to, 146–147
    follow-up care for, 149
    indications for, 146
    physical examination in, 147
    therapeutic measures in, 148
infant care
    anticipated, 46
    assessment for deviations from normal, 196–199
    breastfeeding, 199–204
    initial evaluation of, 193–196
    neonatal circumcision, 204–206
    newborn resuscitation, 190–193
    well-baby care, 206–209
infant feeding
    at breast, 201
    problems in, 202
infestations. *See also* parasitic infestation
    evaluation of, 389
    treatment for, 392
influenza vaccine, in prenatal care, 45
information. *See also* education
    about breast cancer, 290
    for cardiovascular problems, 385
    about GBS disease, 145
    about hepatitis, 345
    in neonatal circumcision, 205
informed choice, advocacy for, 73

informed consent
    in Cesarean delivery, 137
    documentation of, 14
    elements of, 21–22
    in neonatal circumcision, 205
    in VBAC, 183
infused oil, 430
insomnia, in prenatal care, 59–61
International Classification of Diseases, Ninth Revision,
    Clinical Modification (ICD-9-CM), 7
International Confederation of Midwives
    ethical principles of, 29
    practice standards of, 35
    professional standards defined by, 27
International Normalized Ratio (INR), 344
interpreter services, 19–20
intrauterine device and/or system (IUD/IUS), 243, 244,
    245, 246
    and client history, 255–256
    code groups for, 256
    follow-up care for, 258
    hormonal, 251
    insertion of, 257
    physical examination in, 256
    removal of, 257
    types of, 255
intrauterine growth restriction (IUGR), 78
intravenous (IV) therapy
    during labor, 123–124
    for nausea and vomiting, 64, 65
    in postpartum hemorrhage, 161
Ipratropium, in asthma, 418
iron, food sources of, 437
iron deficiency anemia, 74–76
iron replacement therapy, 75
iron salts, 75
iron supplementation, in prenatal care, 45
irritable bowel syndrome, 404
itching, treatment for, 393. *See also* urticarial papulres
    and plaques
Itraconazole, for fungal infections, 393
IUD/IUS. *See* intrauterine device and/or system
Ivermectin, in parasitic infestation, 356

J

jaundice, in hepatitis, 344
justice, in midwifery practice, 29

K

Kaposi's sarcoma, 390
keloid scarring, 391
ketoconazole, for fungal infections, 393
Kleihauer-Betke quantitative testing, in Rh
    alloimmunization, 101